• • • • • •

The Cognitive Neuroscience of Memory

THE
COGNITIVE
NEUROSCIENCE
OF MEMORY

an introduction

• • • • • • • • • • • • •

Howard Eichenbaum

Laboratory of Cognitive Neurobiology
Boston University
Boston, Massachusetts

OXFORD
UNIVERSITY PRESS
2002

OXFORD

UNIVERSITY PRESS

Oxford   New York
Athens   Auckland   Bangkok   Bogotá   Buenos Aires   Cape Town
Chennai   Dar es Salaam   Delhi   Florence   Hong Kong   Istanbul   Karachi
Kolkata   Kuala Lumpur   Madrid   Melbourne   Mexico City   Mumbai   Nairobi
Paris   São Paulo   Shanghai   Singapore   Taipei   Tokyo   Toronto   Warsaw

and associated companies in
Berlin   Ibadan

Published by Oxford University Press, Inc.
198 Madison Avenue, New York, New York 10016
http://www.oup-usa.org
1-800-334-4249

Oxford is a registered trademark of Oxford University Press.

Library of Congress Cataloging-in-Publication Data
Eichenbaum, Howard.
The cognitive neuroscience of memory : an introduction/
Howard Eichenbaum.
p.;cm   Includes bibliographical references and index.
ISBN 0-19-514174-1 (cloth)—ISBN 0-19-514175-X (pbk.)
1. Memory. I. Title
[DNLM: 1. Memory—physiology. 2. Brain—physiology.
3. Cognition—physiology.
WL   102 E338c 2002]   QP406 .E334 2002   612.89—dc21   2001036607

3 5 7 9 8 6 4
Printed in the United States of America
on acid-free paper.

• • • • • •
Preface

This book is written for undergraduate students and others who seek an overview of progress in understanding how the brain accomplishes one of its most marvelous acts, memory. At the outset I review the history of thinking and research on the biological bases of memory, and highlight discoveries made in a "Golden Era" that spanned from the late nineteenth century into the twentieth century. During this period major breakthroughs were made, revealing secrets about the fundamental elements of the brain and how they work. Although these discoveries were about brain function in general, many of the researchers were interested in the applicability of their findings to the phenomenon of memory. Also, during the Golden Era four main themes in memory research were initiated. In my introduction, I attempt to give the reader an appreciation for how those themes emerged from the discoveries made in that period.

Those four themes provide the framework for the remainder of the book. The first theme is "connection," and it considers how memory is fundamentally based on alterations in the connectivity of neurons. This section of the book covers the most well-studied models of cellular mechanisms of neural plasticity that may underlie memory. The second theme is "cognition," which involves fundamental issues in the psychological structure of memory. This section of the book considers the competition among views on the nature of cognitive processes that underlie memory, and tells how the controversy was eventually resolved. The third theme is "compartmentalization," which is akin to the classic problem of memory localization. However, unlike localization, the notion of "compartments" is intended to avoid the notion that particular memories are pigeonholed into specific loci, and instead emphasize that different forms of memory are accomplished by distinct modules or brain systems. This section of the book surveys the evidence for multiple memory systems, and outlines how they are mediated by different brain structures and systems. The fourth and final theme is "consolidation," the process by which memories are transformed from a labile trace into a permanent store. In this section of the book, I summarize our current understanding of two distinct stages in memory consolidation. One stage involves molecular and cellular mechanisms that underlie a fixation of changes in the connection strengths introduced earlier. The other stage of consolidation occurs at the level of brain systems and involves a reorganization and restructuring of the circuits that store and retrieve memories. For heuristic purposes I attempt to deal with these two stages separately, although they are highly interrelated by the brain mechanisms involved.

I hope the book will be of use to cognitive scientists, biologists, and psychologists who seek an introduction to biological investigations of memory, and to undergraduate students seeking an expanded coverage of the neurobiology of memory for courses in learning and memory or behavioral and cognitive neuroscience. Readers will benefit from a solid background in basic molecular biology and neurobiology. However, a brief overview of the necessary biological background is included.

It bears mentioning that substantial portions of the material presented in this book are derived from another recent book, *From Conditioning to Conscious Recollection: Multiple Memory Systems of the Brain* (Oxford University Press), coauthored by myself and Neal Cohen. Although there is overlap in the materials of the two books, they differ substantially in two ways. First, the earlier book has a much more limited scope. It is a comprehensive presentation and synthesis, as well as an attempt at reconciliation of current controversies, on the specific topic of multiple memory systems. Its aim is focused on a thorough analysis of one of the central themes of the present book, the theme of "compartmentalization." By contrast, the scope of the present book is much broader. It provides a general introduction to the history of brain and memory research, and is constructed as a comprehensive survey of topics in memory research, including the molecular and cellular bases of memory in cells, invertebrate model systems, and vertebrate systems, the psychological foundations of learning theory, and the phenomena of memory consolidation, as well as the topic of multiple memory systems. Second, the earlier book is constructed for an advanced readership, primarily scientific colleagues and graduate students with considerable previous background in relevant areas of neuroscience and the neurobiology of memory. By contrast, the treatment of topics in the present book is introductory. This book intentionally makes no effort at being detailed or thorough in the described experiments in any research area. Rather, it is aimed to show how we address central questions in brain mechanisms of memory, and seeks to provide a basic understanding of each of several central issues through a presentation of a selected set of classic and recent exemplary experiments.

In addition, for students and instructors who plan to use this book as a text, I have included a set of heuristic aids. First, I emphasize a historical perspective at the outset, with a review of memory research from its very beginnings. Second, the book is divided into four sections, each of which distinguishes a fundamental theme in memory research. Each section is introduced with a theoretical and historical overview. Third, each chapter begins with a set of "Study Questions" aimed to guide the student toward the central issues in that chapter. I encourage students to think about these questions as they read the text, and then write out detailed answers in preparation for exams. Fourth, each chapter ends with a "Summing Up" section that recaps the major take home points in that chapter and attempts to synthesize the several issues that arose. Fifth, I have included a Glossary that contains definitions of frequently used and important terms. In addition, it may be useful to have a basic neuroscience text available as an adjunct reference for the course. Such a text will help orient students to anatomical terms and provide supplementary information about the anatomy and physiology of brain structures described here. It is hoped that these aids will help students in formulating their "schemas" for the topics in this book and permit them to take more away from the information in it.

Considerable appreciation goes to Michelle Barbera who created the illustrations for this book, and to Fiona Stevens of Oxford University Press for her counsel on its organization and content. Thanks also to Neal Cohen, my long time collaborator in thinking and writing about memory, including the related co-authored book described above. More generally, I am indebted to the many students whom I have had the pleasure of teaching over the last couple of decades; they have contributed by asking the hard questions and demanding clear explanations, some of which I hope are conveyed in this text. Finally, I owe a fundamental debt to Edith Eichenbaum, a professional teacher like me, who has provided generous encouragement and guidance throughout my scholarly life.

Contents

1. Introduction: Four Themes in Research on the Neurobiology of Memory, 1

Part I   Connection:
The Cellular and Molecular Bases of Memory, 27

2. Neurons and Simple Memory Circuits, 29

3. Cellular Mechanisms of Memory: Complex Circuits, 53

Part II   Cognition:
Is There a "Cognitive" Basis for Memory? 79

4. Amnesia—Learning about Memory from Memory Loss, 85

5. Exploring Declarative Memory Using Animal Models, 105

6. Windows into the Workings of Memory, 139

Part III   Compartmentalization:
Cortical Modules and Multiple Memory Systems, 171

7. The Cerebral Cortex and Memory, 175

8. Multiple Memory Systems in the Brain, 195

9. A Brain System for Declarative Memory, 213

10. A Brain System for Procedural Memory, 237

11. A Brain System for Emotional Memory, 261

Part IV Consolidation:
The Fixation and Reorganization of Memories, 283

12. Two Distinct Stages of Memory Consolidation, 285

13. Working with Memory, 311

Final Thoughts, 339

Glossary, 341

References in Figure Captions, 353

Index, 357

● ● ● ● ● ●
The Cognitive Neuroscience of Memory

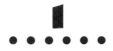

Introduction:
Four Themes in Research on
the Neurobiology of Memory

STUDY QUESTIONS

What is the neurobiology of memory?

What major questions about memory are pursued with a neurobiological approach, and how are these questions addressed in experimental analyses?

What are meant by "connection," "cognition," "compartmentalization," and "consolidation"?

Our memories reflect the accumulation of a lifetime of experience and, in this sense, our memories are who we are. Surely the background of our makeup is determined largely by our genes; genetics sets the range of what we can aspire to be. However, by contrast to generality of genetic limitations, the specifics are a matter of *memory*. We learn to walk, to dance, to drive a car, to throw a ball, and to play a video game—a myriad of acquired skills we come to take for granted. We learn to fear dangerous situations, to appreciate particular types of music and styles of art— a broad range of aversions and enjoyments we have assumed as elements of our preferences and personality. We learn to speak, and to speak and understand our particular language. We learn world history, and we learn our own family tree and personal autobiography—all of these, and much, much more, compose the vast contents and intricate, complex organization of memories that make each of us a unique human being. So, the analysis of memory is a search for self-understanding, an adventure that promises to reveal the inner secrets of how we came to be who we are.

The nature of memory—its basic biological structure, its psychological character and organization, and its longevity—has been the subject of investigations by philosophers, writers, and scientists for hundreds of years, and each approach offers its own distinct avenue for understanding memory. Recently, with the rise of modern methods of cognitive science and neuroscience, and their combination, many new and deep insights about the mechanisms of memory have emerged. These observations have also led us to a greater general understanding about the mind and about brain functions that mediate cognition, emotion, behavior, and consciousness. The aim of this book is to explore memory from the perspective of cognitive neuroscience, offering a historical and a current overview of how brain functions in memory have been studied and what we have learned about memory as an encompassing aspect of the mind.

The present chapter introduces some of the philosophical and historical underpinnings of research on the biological bases of memory. I begin by presenting four central themes that have guided memory research for over a hundred years. Substantial preliminary evidence regarding each of these themes emerged during a "Golden Era" for neuroscience in the latter half of the nineteenth century and the beginning of the twentieth century. A brief introduction to some of these accomplishments provides the background for a subsequent, more detailed summary of progress on each of the four central themes in the remainder of the book.

The four "C's"

At the outset of systematic investigations of the nervous system four major themes dominated considerations of brain function of relevance to memory. In part to facilitate your memory for them, I refer to these themes as the four "C's": *connection, cognition, compartmentalization*, and *consolidation*.

The first theme—*connection*—concerns the most basic level of analysis of memory function, the basic nature of the circuitry of the brain including the elements of information processing and how they communicate with one another in the service of memory. The emphasis on "connection" here reflects the major conclusion that has emerged in this research—that memory is encoded within the dynamics, that is, the changeability or plasticity, of connections between nerve cells. More specifically, the consensual view from the perspective of memory as a phenomenon of brain cells is that memories are instantiated by alterations of the strength ern research has shown that there are two general kinds of consolidation. One of these—which I call "fixation"—involves a cascade of molecular and cellular events during which the changes in connections between cells become permanent in several minutes to hours after a memory is formed. This process can be influenced by many factors, including among them a specific brain system for modulation of memory fixation. The other kind of consolidation process is called "reorganization" because this process involves a prolonged period during which distinct brain structures interact with one another, and the outcome is that newly acquired information is integrated into one's previously existing body of knowledge. This reorganizational process therefore involves an entire brain system, and discovering how it works involves a consideration of both the individual contributions of particular parts of the brain system and the nature of interactions among the parts.

The Golden Era

The aim of this chapter is to set the stage for the succeeding sections that will review our understanding of each of the four major themes in memory research, and in doing so provide a framework for understanding the neurobiological bases of memory. I pursue an historical approach, elaborating on each of the four "Cs," beginning with a summary of discoveries made at the threshold of modern neuroscience research on memory in the latter half of the 1800s.

Before that period, some of the critical background had already long been established. In 1664 the early anatomist Willis published the first description of the anatomy of the brain and had suggested that different brain areas controlled distinct functions. Simplified views of the brain and its main components are provided in Figures 1–1 and 1–2. Also, in 1791 Galvani introduced the notion that electricity is the mechanism of nervous conduction. But around the turn of the twentieth century several additional major discoveries formed the full beginning of a scientific analysis of the brain, a Golden Era in which several key findings led toward real progress in understanding brain function and memory. Some of these contributions represented major advances to the field of neuroscience in general, and others pertained to memory research in particular. Here I highlight a few of the major insights of that period that have had lasting impact. Put together, these observations should give the reader a sense of the field of neuroscience, and especially about the neurobiology of memory, upon which all subsequent progress is based.

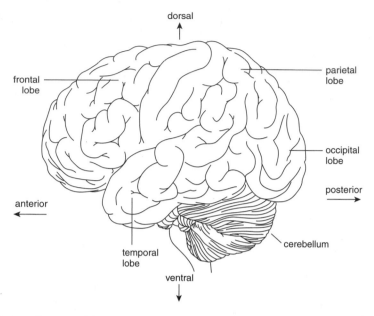

Figure 1–1. Side view of the human brain, showing the major subdivisions of the cerebral cortex, the cerebellum, and terminology used to describe relative locations in the brain.

Connection: Cellular substrates of brain communication and memory

One main set of advances that laid the foundation for memory research involved discoveries about the basic building blocks of brain circuits. These discoveries identified the fundamental elements of the brain, characterized

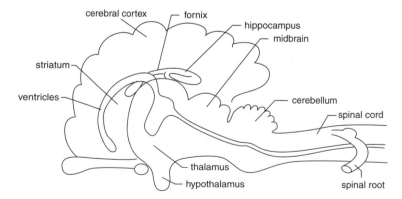

Figure 1–2. Cut-away side view schematic of a generic mammalian brain and spinal cord, showing locations of major subcortical brain structures and the system of ventricles (a hollow circulatory system running throughout).

how they are assembled into simple functional circuits, and demonstrated that they can be modified during learning.

The neuron doctrine

One major area of discovery about the brain that contributed directly to our understanding of the cellular and molecular substrates of memory was the development of the "neuron doctrine" by the Spanish anatomist Santiago Ramon y Cajal. The neuron doctrine is the notion that the brain is composed of discrete nerve cells, and that these cells are the essential units of information processing, connected to one another so as to transfer and integrate information in large-scale networks. At the time of Cajal, this view was not entirely new, but it was also not widely accepted. Rather, Cajal's work addressed a major controversy about the nature of connections between neurons. In the debate, one camp, called the "reticularists," argued that the brain is a single unified interconnected network of fibers in which all the cells were fused to one another. By contrast, the other camp, called the "antireticularists," suspected that the brain was composed of independent nerve cells as units, but they had no definitive evidence. Before Cajal, the strongest argument for independent cells came from the observation that small lesions in one area resulted in sharply defined areas of degeneration, not what one would expect of a fused network.

Cajal's success was based on his adoption of a new staining method that was developed by another anatomist named Camillo Golgi in 1873. The method involved a "black reaction," a new silver stain that had the remarkable quality of darkening the entire cell membrane of a neuron. At the same time, the staining was selective to only a small fraction of the neuron population in an area of brain tissue. Thick sections of the brain stained this way provided a full view of individual cells standing out clearly against the background of many other surrounding pale cells. Using this method Cajal was able to provide the most striking confirmation of the already existing identification of the major elements of nerve cells. As shown in Figure 1–3, these include the cell body, the multiple fine processes that extended from one end of the cell body called dendrites, and the single larger process extending from the other end of the cell body called the axon. Also, he noted the specialization of the axon as it contacted the dendrites of other cells; this specialization would later be called the synapse (see next section).

Cajal attempted many variations of the procedure. He found that tissue with less myelin, the insulation layer of axons, produced the clearest images of neuronal processes, and the best cases were found in young brains and in birds. He also found that thicker sections allowed one to examine all of the extensions of the cell membrane that connect with other

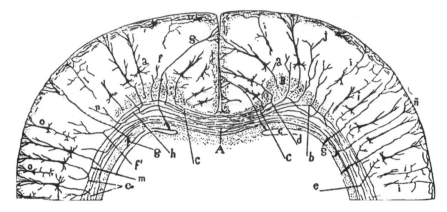

Figure 1–3. Drawing by Cajal based on a section through the cortex of a 20-day-old mouse. Note the different types of cells, all oriented vertically from the superficial layer at the top to the corpus callosum (indicated by the letter A) at the bottom, where the axons of the cortex bundle (from DeFelipe and Jones, 1988).

cells. In each of several different preparations he found elaborate endings of axons in nests or baskets of axonal "arborization"—a treelike branching—of the axon connecting it to multiple parts of another cell or multiple cells. In no case did he observe the stain continuing into the next cell, as would be expected if there was a fusion of the axonal ending with dendrites of another cell. Cajal concluded that there must be some method of communication between cells that did not involve a joining of their membranes. Cajal's preparations and the evidence they provided were elegant, and convinced other anatomists and physiologists that each cell was contained within a membrane and was separate although in contact with other cells. These observations won him the Nobel Prize in 1906.

Cajal was also able to make key conclusions about the function of neurons from his observations on their anatomy. As said previously, he confirmed the existence of all of the major components of the nerve cell. Moreover, in his studies on visual and olfactory sensory structures, Cajal noted that the dendrites pointed toward the outside world and that the axon pointed toward the brain. From these observations he deduced that nerve cells were functionally polarized, such that information flows from the dendrites to the axon and is subsequently conveyed by the specialized connection to the dendrites of another nerve cell.

These conclusions established the essential view that the integration of information occurred by the summation of signals converging from the axons of several neurons onto the dendrites of cells receiving those inputs. In addition, Cajal developed some important and prescient ideas directly relevant to the basic memory mechanism. He studied the brains of several species and observed that the vertebrates higher in the phylogenetic scale had a greater number of connections between nerve cells. He concluded that the increase in connectivity could be the basis of greater intellectual power of the higher species. He suggested that mental exercise could facilitate increased connectivity through a greater number and intensity of the connections, and that these changes in connectivity could coincide with the acquisition of skills such as playing a musical instrument. Cajal's insights have become key axioms for the study of neuronal function and communication. Moreover, his suggestion that "plasticity" in number and strength of neuronal connections underlies learning guides the search for molecular and cellular substrates of memory.

The reflex arc

In the same period other major advances were made from studies on the physiology of the nervous system. Perhaps most important among these were Charles Sherrington's observations on the nature of reflexes in the spinal cord. Before Sherrington the existence of involuntary muscle actions was already well recognized, including the basic observation that specific sensory stimulation could be "reflected," as if by a mirror, to generate muscle movements—hence the "reflex arc" (Fig. 1–4). In addition it was known that complex reflexes, such as those mediating jumping in frogs or coordinated flying movements in birds, could be elicited even following decapitation, suggesting control of complex coordination could happen at a level below the brain—at the level of the spinal cord. And it was clear that reflex arcs accomplished within the spinal cord could be inhibited by higher level control. However, there was very little understanding of the underlying circuitry that accomplished either simple or complex reflexes.

Sherrington made many contributions that provided the foundations for our understanding of neural circuitry that are as relevant today as they were when he made his discoveries. Even before Cajal's convincing anatomical evidence was provided, Sherrington had reached the conclusion that neurons must be independent elements. Part of the evidence came from his studies on neural degeneration, showing that cortical lesions, damage induced by heat or cutting, resulted in restricted, not diffuse patterns of degeneration. He also realized that the neuron doctrine, and the detailed evidence showing the connection was from axons to dendrites, could explain why neural transmission was one-way. And the discontiguity between cells provided a mechanism for why there was a time lag in reflexes such that they were much slower than predicted from the speed of conduction of the neural impulse—the loss of time in long-range conduction had to involve the extra time re-

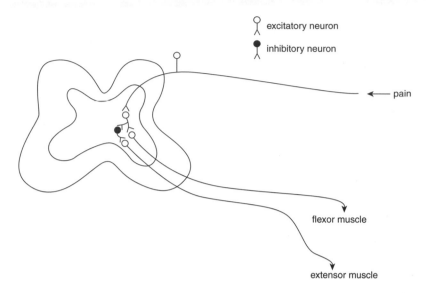

Figure 1–4. A schematic diagram of some components of the pain withdrawal reflex arc. Pain to the skin activates a sensory neuron whose cell body is just outside the spinal cord. The axon synapses with an interneuron within the spinal cord, which excites a motor neuron that causes contraction of the relevant flexor muscle, and excites an inhibitory interneuron that decreases activity in motor neurons that activate the extensor muscles in the same limb.

quired for an impulse to jump a "gap" between the neural elements. Sherrington is credited for inventing the term *synapse* to describe the hypothetical junction between neurons where transmission occurs.

In his classic studies on the "knee jerk" reflex, Sherrington demonstrated the details of his model reflex arc, wherein specific sensory information is gathered at the input end of the arc and then relayed to turn specific muscles on and off at the output end. He provided critical evidence for the existence of the "sixth sense"—specialized sensory receptors in the muscle that monitor muscle length and tension, and showed that these sensory elements send nerves into the spinal cord. He also contributed to the characterization of the maps of sensory inputs from the skin surface into the spinal cord, the so-called dermatomes. By isolating and stimulating sensory roots he could determine which regions of the skin evoked reflexive movements. Conversely, to map the output pattern, he stimulated individual spinal cord motor roots and characterized which muscles were activated.

Important as these discoveries were, perhaps Sherrington's most outstanding contribution was elucidating some of the complexities of the circuitry that underlie reflexes. He concluded that, even at the level of the spinal cord, reflex arcs are not entirely separate or independent. In these circuits the initial sensory neurons in the spinal cord receive dedicated inputs, but the output neurons of even the simplest reflexes received information from many of those input cells (Fig. 1–4). Thus, consistent with Cajal's observations on the anatomy of nerve cells, there was a summation or integration of both inputs into a common path that could guide complex behavioral actions. And there were two major kinds of inputs that combined in this integration. There were excitatory inputs by which an impulse from the input cell increased the likelihood of impulse generation in the next cell. And there were inhibitory inputs by which an impulse in the input cell decreased the likelihood of impulse generation in the next cell. He also made major discoveries about the phenomenon of reciprocal innervation, the basic mechanism by which excitatory and inhibitory influences are coordinated to mediate movement. Within this scheme every action by one muscle is coordinated with an opposing action of complementary muscles. For example, the simple act of walking involves the coordinated actions of flexing one group of muscles during the extension of others, followed by the opposite complementary actions in executing the next step in walking.

In addition, Sherrington employed the technique of decerebration, cutting the spinal cord just behind the brain, to show that complex coordinated actions existed even without higher level cerebral control. He showed, for example, in a decerebrate cat, when a forelimb was excited to move forward, the hindlimb on the same side moved back and the two legs on the other side of the body exhibited the opposing movements, producing the pattern seen in normal walking, but without conscious cerebral control. In studies on the "scratch reflex" he showed the specificity of arm movements for scratching evoked in response to small areas of skin stimulation. Furthermore, in extensions of these studies he revealed that coordinated and directed scratching movement patterns could be played out over time, with alternating extension and flexion of muscles at different levels of the limb to produce repeated scratching movements, plus postural adjustments in the other limbs to support standing without the use of the scratching limb.

Sherrington envisioned all of this as accomplished within the spinal cord, by a "chaining" of reflexes wherein successive coordinated movements are elicited by their predecessors. These elements provided the outline for his formulation on the integrative action of the nervous system. In this prototype for modern views, Sherrington proposed a hierarchy of coordinated control wherein the cerebral cortex is acknowledged as the newest and most complicated switchboard of reflexes, and successively lower centers in the brain stem and spinal cord to mediate more and more specific, yet still complex and coordinated actions.

The conditioned reflex

Initially unrelated to this course of research, the Russian physiologist Ivan Pavlov was making landmark discoveries about the nervous control of digestion. He discovered that the release of digestive fluids was controlled by the nervous system, contrary to the prevailing view that digestive fluids were released as a consequence of mechanical stimulation by food directly onto the stomach wall. To test his hypothesis that the nervous system was involved, Pavlov developed a surgical procedure in which he severed the gullet and attached both open ends to the skin of the neck. This allowed him to either introduce food into the mouth and upper gullet and then retrieve it without going to the stomach, or introduce food directly into the stomach. He found that food stimulation associated with ingestion caused the release of gastric fluids in the stomach, even when the food never reached its normal target. He concluded that food excites the gustatory sensory apparatus in the mouth and gullet, transmitting signals into the brain stem, which, via the vagus nerve, controls the release of gastric fluids. From a neurophysiological perspective, one can say that Pavlov identified a reflex arc for digestion, and for this he received the Nobel Prize in 1904.

But by the time he received the prize, Pavlov had already turned his interest to an intriguing report that gastric juices of a horse could begin to flow not only with a direct application of gustatory stimuli but also even when the animal only caught sight of hay. Pavlov replicated the phenomenon of "psychic secretion" using dogs and measured the generation of fluids from the salivary glands. He found that the sight of a piece of beef indeed caused salivation, but he also found that the phenomenon was unreliable. The salivation tended to decrease following repeated presentations of the sight of beef. Conversely, sometimes salivation was initiated by events that preceded the sight of beef, for example, when the person who regularly provided the food merely appeared in the testing room.

Pavlov set out to meticulously control the stimuli available to the animal, and he tried out many arbitrary stimuli—including the famous bell rung prior to the presentation of food. Based on the results from a broad range of experimental manipulations, Pavlov concluded there were two kinds of reflexes. One kind of reflex is "unconditioned," identical with the innate and stable reflexes of Sherrington. The unconditioned reflex is composed of a particular unconditioned stimulus (US) that inevitably elicits its characteristic unconditioned response (UR). The other kind of reflex is "conditioned," that is, acquired through experience. This kind of reflex is the unstable one, and is composed of an arbitrary conditioned stimulus (CS) that when paired with a US comes to elicit a conditioned response (CR) similar in form to the UR. Pavlov identified the critical importance of two parameters in establishing and maintaining the conditioned reflex: the close temporal contiguity of the CR and US—the CS must lead the US by a particular time interval, and the CS must consistently predict the US.

Combined, the contributions of Cajal, Sherrington, and Pavlov, as well as many others, laid the basic framework for succeeding views of brain circuitry and function, as well as its role in memory. They showed that the basic elements of the circuits are independent neurons that communicate across synapses, that these elements are integrated within complex patterns of circuitry for coordinated action built up from simple reflex arcs, and that these circuits can be modified to support learned reflexes. These insights set the stage for future investigations on the mechanisms of how connections between neurons are modified during learning, and guided the development of views on the organization of memory for both simple and complex behaviors.

Cognition and memory

During the same period, distinct developments were made toward characterizing the nature of memory from a purely psychological perspective. Two main and competing lines of theorizing developed. One school, called "behaviorism," developed out of a desire to provide a rigorous science of memory consistent with the findings on the neurophysiology of conditioned reflexes, and attempted to explain all of learned behavior on the basis of elements of association and conditioned responses. The other school, called "cognitivism," emphasized the complexity of learned behavior, and its promoters could not be persuaded that all aspects of cognition, insight, and planning could be captured in an elaborate account of associations or reflex chains and instead required a more elaborate conception and, correspondingly, a more complex neural instantiation.

Behaviorism

The tradition of rigorous methodology in memory research began with Herman Ebbinghaus, who admired the mathematical analyses that had been brought to the psychophysics of perception, and he sought to develop similarly precise and quantitative methods for the study of memory. Basing his work on a large number of pioneering studies, in 1885 Ebbinghaus published a monograph that set a new standard for the systematic study of memory. Ebbinghaus rejected the use of introspection as a methodology that was prominent in previous conceptual schemes about memory. In its place he developed several key new techniques that would control the nature of the material to be learned and provide quantitative objective assessments of memory performance. To create learning materials that were both simple and homogeneous in content Ebbinghaus invented the "nonsense syllable," a meaningless letter string composed of two consonants with a vowel between (e.g., "ket," "poc." "baf"). With this invention he avoided the confounding influences of what he called "interest," "beauty," and other features that he felt might affect the memorability of real words. In addition, the nonsense syllable simultaneously equalized the length and meaningfulness of the items, albeit by minimizing the former and eliminating the latter. Furthermore, to measure memory Ebbinghaus invented the use of "savings" scores that measured retention in terms of the reduction in trials required to relearn material. In addition, he was the first to employ mathematical–statistical analyses to test the reliability of his findings.

It was also in this period that systematic studies on animal learning and memory had their beginnings. In 1901 Small introduced the maze to studies of animal learning, inspired by the famous garden maze at Hampton Court in London (Fig. 1–5). He began what would become an industry of systematic and quantitative studies to identify the minute details of how rats acquired specific responses in repetitions of turns taken in the maze. But he observed that within a trial or two rats prefer a shortcut over the response route that had been reinforced on many previous trials, leading Small to conclude that future experiments should investigate the natural biological character of the animal if one is to be able to interpret the findings. These initial observations set forth a major controversy in the field of animal learning. Can learning be reduced to a set of arbitrary associations between external stimuli and behavioral responses, or must one consider issues such as cognition, insight, and motive?

At the turn of the century, Edward Thorndike had invented a "puzzle box" in which he observed cats learning to manipulate a door latch to allow escape from a holding chamber. Based on his observations he proposed the "law of effect," which stated that rewards reinforced repetitions of the specific behaviors that preceded them. (This simple law would be reinvented and extensively elaborated by B.F. Skinner in the 1950s to explain all of learned behavior.) In the same period John Watson published his accounts on maze learning by rats. In one of his most famous experi-

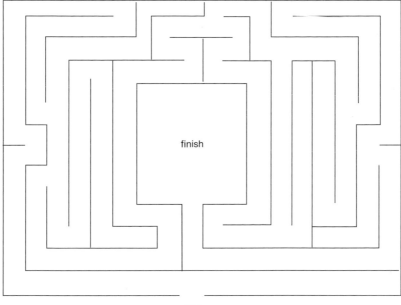

finish

start

Figure 1–5. Small's maze, based on the maze at Hampton Court. The animal entered at the bottom of the maze and had to find its way to the central open area.

ments, Watson trained rats to run a maze and then searched for the underlying stimulus control by eliminating one sense after another. He found the rats could still run the maze with only the kinesthetic (muscle) sense remaining, leading him to conclude that the learning must be mediated by a chain of reflexes, consistent with the evidence from physiology. By 1913 he had accumulated sufficiently compelling evidence for the reductionist strategy that he wrote a "behaviorist manifesto," formalizing the view that learning could be understood in terms of simple stimulus and response associations without resorting to considerations of vague concepts such as consciousness.

Cognitivism

William James captured prevalent views of the time on the origins of both the behaviorist and cognitivist perspectives in his classic *The Principles of Psychology*. Within this treatise, James considered reflex mechanisms and pathways as the essential building blocks of memory, and he called these the mechanisms for the formation of a "habit." James viewed habits as built upon a very primitive mechanism that is common among biological systems and due to an inherent plasticity of organic materials. Within the nervous system he viewed the mechanism of habit in terms of its known electrical activity, and suggested that electrical currents should more readily traverse paths previously taken. Thus, James felt that a simple habit was nothing more than the discharge of a well-worn reflex path, entirely consistent with the views of emerging behaviorism. Furthermore, James expanded on this notion, attributing great importance to habits as the building blocks of more complicated behavioral repertoires. He suggested that well-practiced behaviors and skills, including walking, writing, fencing, and singing, are mediated by concatenated discharges in connected reflex paths, organized to awaken each other in succession to mediate the serial production of learned movement sequences.

However, while acknowledging the importance of habits as the fundamental mechanism that underlies memory, James recognized real "memory" as something altogether different from habit. James argued that there were two forms of memory, differentiated by their timing and by their role. He suggested that initially there is a *primary memory,* what we today call short-term or working memory, a short-lived state where new information has achieved consciousness and belongs to our stream of thought. Primary memory also serves as the gateway by which material would enter *secondary memory,* what we now call long-term memory. James emphasized that secondary memory involves both the intellectual content of information we have learned and the additional consciousness of the experience during learning.

In addition to the feature of personal consciousness, the full characterization of memory was framed in terms of its structure as an elaborate network of associations. James argued that, while memory is based on the habit mechanism, it is vastly elaborated such that the formation of associations among habits supports the richness of our experience of a memory. Thus, the underlying foundation of recall involves a complex, yet systematic set of associations between any particular item and many other co-occurring items during one's experiences.

It is of interest that James also offered speculations that touched on the biological basis of memory. He suggested that memory depends on two aspects of the habit mechanism. First, how good a memory is depends on the strength or persistence of the pathway—this aspect James suggested was innate. Second, he suggested that memory depends on the number of pathways through which an item is associated. He emphasized the latter as more malleable, and argued that the key to a good memory is to build diverse and multiple associations with one's experiences, weaving information and experiences into systematic relations with each other. The capacity to search through one's network associations was held to be the basis of conscious recollection, and could lead to creative use of memory to address new problems. Conversely, James admonished his students not to simply rehearse learned materials. This, he argued, could lead only to the concatenation of habit pathways that could only be expressed by repetition.

James never contrasted "habit" and "memory" as distinct forms of memory. A more direct recognition of two forms of memory can be attributed to the philosopher Henri Bergson, who in 1911 explicitly proposed that representations of the past survive under two distinct forms, one in the ability to facilitate repetition of specific actions, and the other in independent recollections. The suggestion that habits and memories might both have a common cellular basis, and at the same time exist as distinct forms of memory, would ultimately resolve the controversy between the behaviorist and cognitivist schools. In addition, the notion of different forms of memory would reappear in the solution to the controversy about the compartmentalization of memory discussed next.

Compartmentalization of cortical function and memory

In this same period as advances were made in characterizing reflex circuitry, and the controversy about the nature of memory was brewing, a separate battle was engaged over another critical puzzle about the brain and memory. This controversy focused on the organization of the cerebral cortex. There was already scattered evidence from studies of patients with circumscribed brain damage that the anterior (front) and posterior (back) regions of the cerebral cortex played different functional roles. But no clear functional specifications arose from the early observations. Two dramatically different views emerged during the nineteenth century.

"Organology"

The earliest specific and systematic formulation on cortical localization came in the early 1800s from the German physician Franz Joseph Gall. Following a trend early in the eighteenth century in which scientists were attempting to associate body features with aspects of personality, Gall sought to determine whether there existed variation in structure and function of the brain. He developed a theory of cortical localization, which he called organology, in which each of many independent psychological faculties is mediated by a specialized organ in the brain. The central axiom of this theory was that individual differences in specific faculties were reflected in greater development of the mediating brain organ and, correspondingly, the size of the overlying skull area. The theory was developed using a combination of observations on individual variation in specific psychological faculties and skull areas in humans and on comparisons between the abilities and skulls of animals versus humans. Gall's detailed investigations on humans included a variety of individuals that represented extreme variations in behavioral capacities. He sought out people with a special talent, such as writers, statesmen, and musical and mathematical prodigies, or with a behavioral abnormality, such as lunatics, the feeble-minded, and criminals. For each he would interview the person extensively to characterize their unusual behavioral qualities and carefully examine the head for irregularities. Based on his insights about the functional aspects of their abilities and on discovery of unusual skull features, he envisioned a tight correlation between the skull and brain anatomy and a direct link to the unusual aspect of behavior. For example, among his earliest findings on humans was the observation that some people who were outstanding in memorizing verbal material had bulging eyes, suggesting to Gall an enhanced development of an organ in the frontal lobes specialized for verbal memory.

In addition, Gall collected hundreds of skulls from animals and made detailed comparisons between the anatomical features of those skulls and those of humans. The same sort of loose correlation was applied, in this case comparing the psychological abilities of animals both between different species and with humans. From a combination of all this material he devised a system of faculties, some shared by humans and animals and some exclusively human (Fig. 1–6). An example of his reasoning comes

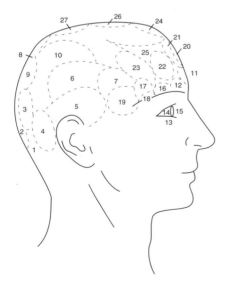

Figure 1–6. Gall's organology scheme. The assignments were: 1. Instinct for reproduction. 2. Love of offspring. 3. Affection. 4. Instinct of self-defense. 5. Carnivorous instinct, tendency to murder. 6. Guile. 7. The feeling of property, theft, hoarding. 8. Pride. 9. Vanity, ambition. 10. Forethought. 11. Educability. 12. Places. 13. Memory of people. 14. Words. 15. Language and speech. 16. Colors. 17. Sounds, music. 18. Sense of connections between numbers. 19. Mechanics of construction. 20. Wisdom. 21. Metaphysics. 22. Satire. 23. Poetry. 24. Kindness. 25. Ability to imitate. 26. Religion. 27. Perseverance.

from his deductions about the faculty of "destructiveness, carnivorous instinct, or tendency to murder," localized to an area above the ears. This designation was strongly based on a combination of observations on animals and humans. That area was larger in carnivores than in grass-eating animals. And the area was overly large in a successful businessman who gave up his profession to become a butcher, in a student who was fond of torturing animals and became a surgeon, and in a pharmacist who became an executioner.

Gall's early attempts to make functional assignments of cortical areas were considerably off-base, due to two major flaws in his methodology. First, Gall's methods were based on individual cases, each of which was subject to considerable interpretation about the nature of the basis of their unusual abilities. Second, Gall simply assumed a close correlation between skull and brain anatomy, and had little interest in examining brain directly. Gall's assumptions led him in the wrong direction in almost every case. Later clinical and experimental studies consistently failed to confirm Gall's specific functional assignments. However, these later studies would demonstrate localization of cortical functions, albeit with different functional designations. Thus, quite rightfully Gall is given considerable credit for the basic insight that the cortex is composed of multiple, functionally distinct areas.

Case studies of human patients with localized cortical damage

More compelling evidence for specific functional designations within the cerebral cortex came from observations of neurological case studies of patients with selective brain damage, and from parallel physiological studies. Among the most important of the case studies on brain pathology was one made by the French physician Paul Broca in 1861. The study involved a 51-year-old man named Lebourgne who had suffered from epilepsy since birth and had later lost the power to speak and developed a right side paralysis and loss of sensitivity. This patient came to Broca's attention when he was admitted to Broca's surgical ward at the hospital for an unrelated disorder, and died within a week. The autopsy revealed a circumscribed area of damage in the third convolution of the frontal lobe on the left side of the cerebral cortex. The patient's disorder was also well circumscribed. He was virtually unable to speak—indeed, he acquired the nickname "Tan" from the only sound he made—but his mouth was not paralyzed and he retained the capacity to hear and understand speech. This case provided a compelling demonstration of a highly severe and selective behavioral disorder related to a specific cortical zone. The argument for localization of higher functions was made all the more compelling with the description of a complementary case by Carl Wernike in 1894. In this case the patient was severely impaired in speech comprehension, without hearing loss or a disorder of speech production, and the damage was circumscribed to a zone within the left temporal cortex.

Experimental neurology and neurophysiology

The evidence from neurological cases was strongly supported by concurrent findings from experimental work on animals. The earliest studies on animals, specifically aimed to test Gall's theory, were reported in 1824 by Flourens. He failed to find localization of sensory and motor functions following cortical damage in birds. These findings and other studies that could not demonstrate selective losses in mammals became the strongest evidence against localization of cortical function. However, the use of birds and other animals with relatively less differentiated cortical areas turned out to be a poor choice for an experimental model in analyses of cortical function. The case for localization was eventually made, from studies using brain stimulation in dogs, by Gustav Fritsch and Eduard Hitzig published in 1870, and with the careful work of David Ferrier using brain lesions in monkeys, presented in 1874.

Based on earlier work showing that stimulation of the head or cortex could produce twitching movements of the musculature, Fritsch and Hitzig employed minimal levels of electrical stimulation to map the cortex of dogs. They found that stimulation of a zone within the frontal cortex resulted in specific muscle movements. Moreover, they discovered that minimal stimulation of one cortical area more anterior and dorsal produced selective movements of the forepaw on the contralateral side of the body, whereas nearby regions of stimulation resulted in muscle movements in adjacent body areas. Low-level stimulation of other cortical areas did not produce movements in any part of the body, indicating that they had isolated a specialized motor area of the cortex and that area was organized as a kind of mapping of the musculature of the body.

Based on the physiological findings of Fritsch and Hitzig, Ferrier was convinced there had to be separate cortical areas that mediated specific sensory functions, such as vision, hearing, smell, and touch, and other areas that controlled movement. He suspected that previous studies had failed to find selective behavioral–anatomical correlations because the lesions were too small or the animals selected did not have sufficiently differentiated cortical areas. He prepared two monkeys, and in each showed a selective disorder associated with a specific area of cortical damage. One monkey had a severe paralysis on the right side of the body associated with a circumscribed lesion within the left frontal area. The other monkey was completely deaf following a bilateral removal of the temporal lobe. Ferrier's evidence held up to close scrutiny by his colleagues and provided the most compelling initial evidence of distinct sensory and motor functional areas in the cerebral cortex.

This combination of studies settled the debate on localization, making it clear that the cerebral cortex does not operate as a unitary organ, but rather is composed of many functionally distinct compartments. Subsequently, the localization controversy would arise again, this time about the locus of memory traces *per se*, as distinct from the more general issue of functional localization. This time, the strong localizationist view would not hold, at least with regard to the cortex. However, a new perspective, based on anatomical considerations beyond the cortex, would show that memory is subdivided according to larger pathways or compartments that involve connections between the cortex and other brain regions.

Consolidation

A major topic in research of the Golden Era directly associated with the phenomenon of memory involved studies on memory performance in neurological patients with memory disorders, as well as in normal human subjects. Two phenomena of amnesia following brain damage were prominent. First, patients with memory deficits could acquire new information and remember it briefly, but showed an abnormally rapid amount and rate of forgetfulness. This phenomenon in amnesia, called anterograde amnesia, was intimately tied to the diagnosis of memory impairment, in that the disorder of memory could be contrasted with intact perception and comprehension, as well as a spared ability to hold information long enough to demonstrate the latter capacities. Second, and even more impressive, was the observation of retrograde amnesia, the loss of memories acquired before the brain trauma. Both phenomena of memory loss were systematically studied first in the Golden Era.

The neuropathology of memory

In 1882, the French philosopher and psychologist Theodore Ribot reviewed a large number of cases of retrograde amnesia associated with brain damage and head trauma. He observed that in those cases where memory impairment is the major consequence, memories acquired remotely before the insult were relatively preserved compared to those acquired recently just before. His formulation, which came to be known as Ribot's law, was stated as a "law of regression" by which the loss of memory is inversely related to the time elapsed between the event to be remembered and the injury. Ribot thus concluded that memories required a certain amount of time to be organized and fixed.

Further early systematic characterizations of memory disorders, and the incumbent insights they provide about normal memory, began with the descriptions of two forms of dementia in which memory loss plays a prominent role. In 1906, Alois Alzheimer reported on an institutionalized female patient with progressive dementia. Her first symptoms involved personality changes, but soon after she exhibited a profound memory impairment. After being shown objects and recognizing them, she immediately forgot them and the circumstances in which she had learned about them. Patients with Alzheimer's disease exhibited a set of prototypical symptoms including the cardinal signs of anterograde and retrograde amnesia. Initially, the patients would show mild memory lapses. As the disease progressed, the patients would become profoundly forgetful, remembering things said for only a few minutes and then completely losing them. Consistent with the law of regression Ribot had described for retrograde amnesia following head injury, the impairment in Alzheimer's disease was more severe for memories recently acquired than for those acquired earlier in life.

Another disease with prominent loss of memory was first described by Sergei Korsakoff in 1887. His initial report involved a group of patients with an odd combination of peripheral neuromuscular symptoms (polyneuritis) and memory disorder. Many of these patients were chronic alcoholics, who came to the clinic in a global confusional state that gradually resolved, leaving an outstanding selective impairment in memory as the outstanding prominent symptom. The characterization of the memory loss in Korsakoff syndrome was similar to that for the early stage of Alzheimer's disease. These patients could follow a train of conversation, but, when distracted even for a brief period, they lost both the contents of the conversation and the memory that it had taken place. The patients also showed the signs of retrograde amnesia, including the temporal gradient in which remote memories were more preserved than recent ones.

Consolidation and normal human memory

In a monograph published in 1900 Georg Muller and Alfons Pilzecker reported a large number of experiments performed on normal human subjects. They had adapted Ebbinghaus's method for learning "nonsense syllables," short and pronounceable but meaningless character strings, presenting a list of them in pairs and then asking subjects to recall the second item in each pair upon subsequent probing with the first item. A major finding involved the observations of a strong tendency for subjects to spontaneously become aware of the training pairs during the retention phase, even when they tried to suppress rehearsal. They called this phenomenon "perseveration" and linked it to the additional observation that errors made during recall involved items in the same list much more often than those from separate lists. Also, both phenomena of perseveration followed a regular time gradient—they were much more prominent for a few minutes after original learning than later. Muller and Pilzecker speculated that the perseveration reflected a transient brain activity that might play an important role in establishing and strengthening the word associations. They postulated that if this were the case, then the disruption of perseveration should have a deleterious effect on recall.

To test their hypothesis Muller and Pilzecker evaluated the effects on recall performance of interpolated material given in between the initial presentations and the recall test. They tested the effects of presenting an additional list in between training and recall on an initial list, finding that indeed recall was poorer if an additional list was presented, as compared to the results with no intervening material. They called this phenomenon "retroactive interference." They varied the nature of the interpolated material by assessing the effects of presenting pictures instead of another verbal list, and found that this distraction was also effective in producing retroactive interference. Furthermore, they varied the timing of presentation of the interpolated material, and found that delaying the distraction by more than a few minutes diminished its interfering effects considerably. These studies led them to the conclusion that there is a brain activity that normally perseverates following new learning and that this activity serves to consolidate the memory.

These findings were shortly after linked to the reports of retrograde amnesia in patients with brain insult or damage. Thus, temporally graded amnesia was explained as a disruption of the perseveration process caused by a direct functional interruption of the underlying brain activity. In 1903 William Burham described the effect of brain trauma as disrupting a natural physical process of organization associated with a psychological process of repetition and association, processes that required time to mature.

Succeeding decades of progress

In the following chapters we explore in greater detail all of the issues raised in this chapter. The plan for the remainder of the book is to follow up on each of the four central themes, one at a time. This might seem to suggest that these issues are entirely independent, but this is very much *not* the case. The discovered characteristics of conditioned reflexes guided much of the succeeding work that unsuccessfully addressed the issue of compartmentalization of memory in the cortex. Conversely, the results of succeeding studies on the nature of cognition in memory also strongly influenced the ultimately successful advances in the compartmentalization of memory functions. And succeeding studies on both the basis of cellular connections and cognitive mechanisms have led to a more sophisticated understanding of processes underlying memory consolidation. So, while I will proceed to separate these themes as a heuristic, the research that guides them, the issues themselves, and the findings on each of them are strongly interrelated.

Part I of the book updates you on our understanding of the cellular and molecular bases of memory. Chapter 2 reviews the basic anatomy of physiology of neurons, and shows how these basic principles can be put to use in explaining how memory works in relatively simple nervous systems. Chapter 3 describes parallel successes in understanding the cellular bases of a form of plasticity characteristic of mammalian brain areas, and summarizes research indicating that this form of neural plasticity may be the fundamental mechanism of learning in many more complex brain systems.

The Part II of the book builds on the discussion of the nature of cognition in memory. I will update you on how the controversy between behaviorists and cognitivists played out in the middle of the twentieth century, and then how it was resolved by discoveries in neuroscience. In particular I consider a major discovery in the neurology of memory, a case study of amnesia that ultimately showed that memory could be isolated as a cognitive function and that laid the groundwork for resolving the controversy between cognitivist and behaviorist views of memory. Then I elaborate on our understanding of a memory system that mediates "cognitive" or, as it is called today, "declarative" memory. Chapter 4 reviews the evidence from studies of amnesia in humans, and chapter 5 covers the additional evidence from animal models of amnesia. Chapter 6 summarizes complementary evidence from observations on brain activity during declarative memory in humans and animals.

In Part III, I summarize progress on the issue of compartmentalization. In Chapter 7, I begin by describing how the controversy over cortical localization became a central issue in research on memory *per se*, and I show how this controversy was resolved by our modern understanding of cortical modules in information processing and memory. Then I summarize the current psychological, anatomical, and physiological evidence about multiple memory systems in the brain. Chapter 8 introduces substantial direct evidence for the existence and initial localization of multiple memory systems in the brain. Chapter 9 elaborates the anatomy and workings of the full system that mediates declarative memory. Chapters 10 and 11 elaborate on two major systems, one for procedural (habit and skill) learning and the other for emotional memory.

In Part IV, I consider progress on the issue of memory consolidation. In Chapter 12, I describe how modern research has distinguished between two different kinds of consolidation, a short-term cellular fixation process and a long-lasting reorganization process. This chapter reviews the evidence for modulation of memory fixation and considers brain mechanisms that mediate memory reorganization.

Finally, Chapter 13 returns to an emphasis on a particular part of the cerebral cortex, the prefrontal area, and how this area along with other cortical areas works to orchestrate memory. Throughout the text you will see that the issues laid out a century ago are as relevant today as when they were introduced. But now we are truly beginning to resolve the anatomy and mechanisms of memory at a level of sophistication that could not have been envisioned so long ago.

Summing up

There are four main themes in studies on the neurobiology of memory: *connection, cognition, compartmentalization,* and *consolidation.*

Connection concerns the most basic level of analysis of memory function, the fundamental nature of the circuitry of the brain including the elements of information processing and how they communicate with one another in the service of memory. Neurons are independent elements of information processing that are connected via synapses. In the simplest circuits, neurons connect sensory inputs to motor outputs to mediate reflex arcs. However, most reflex circuitries involve more complex arrangements that offer considerable coordination and control over behavior. There are also conditioned reflexes that involve the association of an arbitrary stimulus and an unconditioned stimulus, such that the conditioned stimulus comes to produce a conditioned response that is similar in form to the unconditioned or reflexive response. Conditioning is thought to be mediated by an enhancement or elaboration of the connections between neurons involved in reflex arcs.

Cognition refers to the nature of memories at the highest level of analysis, the psychological level. The central issue in the understanding of the psychological nature of memory involves the debate between behaviorism, which espouses that all learning can be reduced to conditioned responses, and cognitivism, which argues that more complex phenomena such as insight and inference are required to explain complex learned behavior. Over most of the twentieth century evidence for both views has been accumulated.

Compartmentalization refers to the notion that memory as a whole is distributed widely in the brain, and at the same time, there are different kinds of memory that are accomplished by specific brain modules, circuits, pathways, or systems. Gall first proposed the first detailed function mapping of the cerebral cortex, which he called "organology." However, his flawed methods led to incorrect assignments of function–structure relations. Later neurologists discovered case studies of humans with specific cortical damage and consequent specific deficits in language. Also, physiologists demonstrated that specific cortical areas in monkeys had identifiable delimited functional roles in sensory or motor processing.

Consolidation is a hypothetical phenomenon derived from the observation that memories are initially labile and later become resistant to loss, suggesting an extended process during which memories take on a permanent form. The existence of consolidation has been shown in studies on patients with damage to the brain showing a temporally graded retrograde loss of memories, that is, intact memories for material acquired remotely prior to the damage and lost memories for materials learned recently prior to the damage. The existence of consolidation can also be observed in normal humans by interposing interfering materials briefly, but not delayed, following initial learning.

READINGS

Eichenbaum, H., and Cohen, N.J. 2000. *From Conditioning to Conscious Recollection: Multiple Memory Systems in the Brain.* New York: Oxford University Press.

Finger, S. 1994. *Origins of Neuroscience: A History of Explorations into Brain Function.* New York: Oxford University Press.

Finger, S. 2000. *Minds Behind the Brain.* New York: Oxford University Press.

Lechner, H.A., Squire, L.R., and Byrne, J.H. 1999. 100 years of consolidation— Remembering Muller & Pilzecker. *Learn. Mem.* 6:77–87.

McGaugh, J.L. 2000. Memory—a century of consolidation. *Science* 287: 248–251.

Milner, B., Squire, L.R., and Kandel, E.R. 1998. Cognitive neuroscience and the study of memory. *Neuron* 20:445–468.

Polster, M.R., Nadel, L., and Schacter, D.L. 1991. Cognitive neuroscience analyses of memory. A historical perspective. *J. Cog. Neurosci.* 3:95–116.

Tolman, E.C. 1948. Cognitive maps in rats and men. *Psychol. Rev.* 55:189–208.

Zola-Morgan, S. 1995. Localization of brain function: The legacy of Franz Joseph Gall (1758–1828). *Annu. Rev. Neurosci.* 18:359–383.

CONNECTION:
THE CELLULAR AND MOLECULAR
BASES OF MEMORY

The parallel anatomical, physiological, and behavioral studies of Cajal, Sherrington, and Pavlov provided an immensely strong foundation for the conditioned reflex as a central model of the basic memory circuit. And this model became the centerpiece of the biological instantiation of the learning mechanism for behaviorists. In succeeding decades further major advances in our understanding of the basic elements of neural connections would be made. In particular, one major discovery was that the nature of transmission of information between neurons is chemical.

The key experiment was performed by Otto Loewi in 1921. He was familiar with current work that had shown that chemical agents could stimulate and modulate the actions of the autonomic nervous system. The general view was that communication across neurons was by an electrical impulse, but the notion that there might be chemical transmission was being considered seriously. Loewi devised an experiment that would provide proof of a chemical mechanism. He removed the heart of a frog and bathed it in a neutral solution, where he stimulated the still attached vagus nerve, producing a well-known inhibition of contractions in the heart. Loewi then removed some of the bathing solution and placed it into a chamber holding another frog heart for which the vagus nerve had been removed. The second heart also slowed, demonstrating that a chemical agent that had been produced in the stimulated heart caused the inhibition. Loewi also performed the complementary experiment, showing that other stimulation that produced an acceleration of the first heart resulted in the release of a chemical agent that also accelerated the second (nonstimulated) heart.

It turns out that the inhibitory agent is the neurotransmitter acetylcholine, the major neurotransmitter of the parasympathetic system, and the accelerating agent is noradrenaline, the major neurotransmitter of the sympathetic system. Since the discovery of neurotransmitters, two major lines of research have refined our understanding of the mechanisms of chemical communication between neurons. First, the pioneering work of Bernard Katz in the 1950s showed that neurotransmitters are released at the synaptic ending of the axon in small packets of molecules called synaptic vesicles. Second, a long list of other neurotransmitters and neuromodulators has now been described, allowing for a range of effects that can be accomplished via neurotransmission.

In addition, interest in the molecular and cellular basis of synaptic modification has intersected with the issue of memory consolidation. In the 1960s and 1970s considerable effort was placed on showing that protein synthesis was required for permanent modifications of cells for lasting memory. Many studies showed that interfering with the synthesis of proteins, using drugs that prevent specific stages of gene expression, blocked the establishment of long-term memory without affecting short-term memory. Moreover, these drugs were effective in blocking later expression of memory even if they were given a few minutes after training, but not if treatment was delayed by an hour or more. The results of these experiments paralleled the time course of effects of other types of interference or brain insult that characterized the earlier studies demonstrating memory consolidation. In addition, the studies on protein synthesis inhibition provided a much more specific mechanism, suggesting that gene expression leading to proteins is a critical part of the consolidation process. As you will see in Chapters 2 and 3, this search has now narrowed substantially toward investigations on particular types of neurotransmitters that are activated during learning and on the identification of specific molecular pathways of subsequent gene expression.

The following two chapters review the state of our understanding about the cellular mechanisms of memory. In Chapter 2, I summarize our knowledge about the basic anatomy and physiology of neurons. Then I show how these basic anatomical and physiological elements are modified to mediate memory within model systems in invertebrate species. Chapter 3 builds on these observations, introducing a mammalian model system for cellular plasticity that shares many of the features of the invertebrate models and expands on them and other mechanisms within more complex circuitries. Then I consider how well this model works in accounting for cellular mechanisms of real memory in mammals.

2

• • • • • •

Neurons and Simple Memory Circuits

STUDY QUESTIONS

What are the elements of neuronal structure?

How do the electrical properties of neurons arise?

What distinguishes different forms of neural conduction and transmission?

Why are simple invertebrate systems useful for understanding the cellular mechanisms of memory?

What are the molecular and cellular bases of simple forms of learning, including habituation, sensitization, and classical conditioning?

Neurons encode memories by modifications in the strength of the functional connections. In this chapter I summarize some of the key fundamental concepts about the anatomy and physiology of neurons, including the molecular basis of the unusual electrical properties of neurons, different forms of electrical conduction, and transmission of information between neurons. Then I show how these concepts can be put to work toward understanding the cellular bases of basic forms of learning. Three elemental forms of learning that are accomplished within the circuitry of relatively simple animals have served as model systems for the study of memory. These studies have provided a clear understanding of the mechanisms of neuronal plasticity that mediate habituation, sensitization, and classical conditioning mediated within well-identified circuits of a marine invertebrate.

Neuron structure

As recognized at the time of Cajal, neurons are composed of four main elements, the dendrites, the soma or cell body, the axon, and the synapse (Fig. 2–1). There are typically many dendrites and they are often highly branched, such that most neurons receive inputs at the synaptic connections with axons of many other neurons. Each neuron has only one cell body, although the axons of many other cells can contact the cell body directly and these contacts are particularly effective. Each neuron also has only one axon, although in many situations the axon can branch extensively to make a large number of contacts onto one or more other neurons. These basic anatomical facts dictate that neurons receive and integrate information from a substantial number and variety of inputs, and then sum them up to a single main output that can affect one or many cells that are next in the circuit.

The synapse is a complicated structure, composed of two main parts, the presynaptic and the postsynaptic elements. The presynaptic element is an enlargement of axonal ending that contains specialized machinery for the process of neuronal transmission. This machinery includes cellular organelles that produce energy and elements that are involved in the recycling and packaging of neurotransmitters into synaptic vesicles. In addition, there are specialized docking stations for the vesicles from which the neurotransmitter is released. There is a narrow separation between the presynaptic element and postsynaptic cell membrane of the neuron to which it is connected; this separation is known as the synaptic cleft. When released from the presynaptic element, neurotransmitters must diffuse

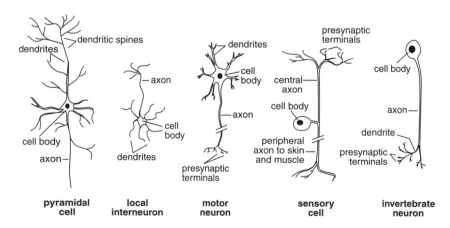

Figure 2–1. Examples of different types of neurons and their major components.

across the synaptic cleft to reach specialized receptors in the postsynaptic element. There are many different kinds of receptors, including distinct types of receptors for the same neurotransmitter, providing for a variety of effects of transmission on the target cell's activity. The structure of these receptor molecules and mechanisms of their activation are only now becoming known.

Within the overall design described above, the elements of neurons can take many configurations suited to specific applications in different parts of the nervous system (Fig. 2–1). A prototypical *principal neuron* is the pyramidal cell of the cortex and hippocampus. These neurons have a long branching dendrite that extends upward from the cell body and receives inputs from other regions, as well as multiple dendrites that branch laterally from the cell to receive inputs from local neurons. The axon extends downward and branches. It may connect with other local cells or extend many millimeters to another brain region. *Interneurons* are neurons that receive inputs and send their outputs within a local brain region. *Motor neurons* of the spinal cord have many branching dendrites that extend in all directions, and a single long axon that extends very long distances to innervate skeletal muscles. Its axon branches extensively and has specialized presynaptic terminals to make contact with muscle cells. *Sensory cells*, conversely, have specialized endings of their dendrites to receive information from specific sensory organs. Some of them may have the cell body displaced such that it is connected to a single main dendritic and axonal element. There are many other variations on these patterns.

The physiology of neurons

As I describe the physiology of neurons, it should be kept foremost in mind that communication in the nervous system involves three main stages that are mediated by different physiological mechanisms (Fig. 2–2). Two of these stages involve electrical mechanisms for *conduction* of neuronal signal over substantial distances through the dendrites and axon, and the third involves chemical mediation of *transmission* of the signal between neurons. The initial phase of conduction, known as *electrotonic conduction,* typically begins at the postsynaptic site, and proceeds to the cell body. This type of electrical conduction is remarkably fast, but dissipates over relatively short distances. The second type of electrical conduction, called the *action potential*, is initiated by a special mechanism at the cell body and conducted down the axon to the presynaptic elements. This type of electrical conduction is relatively slow compared to passive conduction, but involves a mechanism that maintains the signal over very long distances. When the action potential

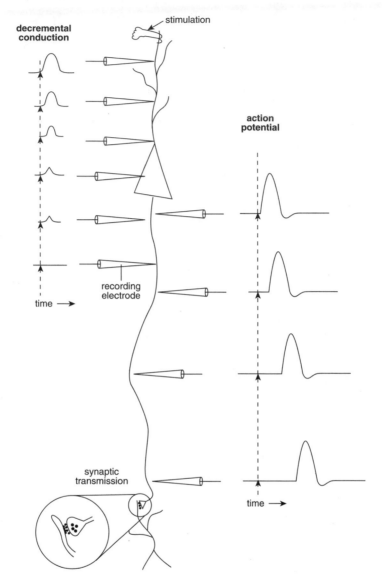

Figure 2–2. Comparison of decremental conduction and action potentials. On the left are idealized waveforms of synaptic potentials recorded at successive loci indicated by the site of the recording electrode. Note that the latency after stimulation until onset of the potential is very short for all recordings. On the right are idealized waveforms of action potentials recorded at successive loci indicated by the sites of recording electrodes. Note that the latency increases substantially between recordings, showing the slow conduction of action potentials as compared with electrotonic conduction.

reaches the presynaptic element, the molecular processes of synaptic transmission are initiated and carry a chemical signal across the synaptic cleft to the presynaptic elements of the next cell. In the following sections, I summarize and compare the different forms of electrical conduction and then describe the mechanisms of synaptic transmission.

The resting potential

To understand the mechanisms of electrical conduction it is important to appreciate that nerve cells, as well as other types of cells throughout the body, have a natural electrical potential known as the *resting potential*. This potential arises from two features common to most living cells (Fig. 2–3). First, there is a natural concentration of molecules inside the cell

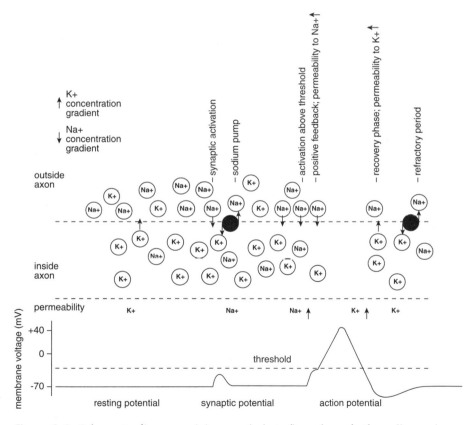

Figure 2–3. Schematic diagram of ions and their flow through the cell membrane (dashed lines) associated with the resting potential, synaptic potential, and action potential.

membrane relative to the fluid outside the cell (called the extracellular fluid), and many of these molecules are polarized in that they have a positive or negative charge. Major contributors to the high intracellular (i.e., inside) concentration are large protein molecules that have a negative charge that is balanced out by small positively charged molecules such as sodium (Na^+) and potassium (K^+) in the intracellular fluid. Second, the membrane that surrounds the cell and contains its contents is typically somewhat permeable in that it contains pores or channels that allow the diffusion of molecules between the inside and outside of the membrane. These two situations conspire to create a situation in which a potential difference between the inside and outside of the cell membrane is established.

The potential difference across the membrane arises because of two natural and competing forces that are consequences of these properties of neurons. One of these forces comes about because of the difference in concentration of molecules inside and outside the membrane. The accumulation of large molecules inside the cell creates a substantial *concentration gradient,* such that the interior fluid of the cell is much more concentrated than the fluid of the exterior of the cell. If the membrane pores or channels were indifferently permeable to all molecules, the difference in concentration would disappear as molecules from the inside diffused out until the concentration on both sides of the membrane was equal. However, the membrane channels are actually quite selective, typically allowing small molecules such as Na^+ and K^+ to flow, and even the passage of those molecules is tightly regulated. Indeed, in the natural resting state, the cell membrane is mostly permeable only to K^+. Because of this selective permeability and because there is typically much more K^+ inside the cell than out, some K^+ flows from inside to outside following the concentration gradient, and this creates a situation where the inside of the cell has a net negative charge due to the loss of some positively charged potassium molecules. If the concentration gradient was the only force involved, K^+ would continue to flow outside the cell until its concentration was equal on both sides.

This overall potential difference, with the inside negatively charged and the outside positively charged, invokes the second force that affects the resting potential. The interior-to-exterior charge difference constitutes an overall *electrostatic gradient* across the cell membrane that tends to repel positively charged molecules from the positively charged exterior. At the same time, because the interior of the cell has become negatively charged, there is an overall attraction of positive charges to the inside of the cell. Because the cell membrane is selectively permeable to K^+, and so it is the only molecule that can pass, the combination of repellant force from the outside and attractive force from the inside draws some K^+ molecules back into the cell. If the electrostatic gradient was the only force involved, K^+ would flow back into the cell until there was no charge difference.

Thus, there are two competing forces on the K^+ molecules. The concentration gradient pushes K^+ outside, whereas the electrostatic gradient pulls K^+ inside. These two forces eventually reach an equilibrium in which K^+ molecules leave the cell to decrease the concentration gradient only somewhat, resulting in an overall net electrostatic gradient in one direction and a concentration gradient of equal force in the opposite direction. This final electrostatic gradient is called the resting potential, and its magnitude is typically about -70 millivolts (inside relative to outside the membrane). The exact magnitude of this potential depends on many factors, including the concentrations of K^+ and other molecules for which the cell membrane is typically less permeable.

Electrotonic conduction

In the natural situation the resting potential is disturbed when chemical processes at the synapse result in a change in the permeability to a molecule, typically Na^+ (Fig. 2–3). Unlike K^+, Na^+ is more concentrated outside the cell membrane. This is because there is an active mechanism, embedded in the cell membrane, that pumps Na^+ molecules from the inside to the outside of the cell. This pump is metabolically expensive, consuming as much as 40% of the energy needs of a neuron. But it is a very valuable mechanism for the conduction of signals.

When synaptic transmission results in a transient increase in permeability to Na^+ at the receptor site, Na^+ follows its concentration gradient and flows into the cell. Because Na^+ is positively charged, this results in movement of the membrane potential in the positive direction, from -70 millivolts to something closer to zero, with the magnitude depending on the strength of the synaptic transmission. This relative positive charge gradient spreads passively and almost instantaneously, like electricity, decreasing the polarization of the membrane for some distance along the dendrite toward the cell body. However, as this *depolarization* spreads, it also diffuses across the membrane surface and so diminishes in size. Thus, electrotonic conduction is fast but it is also *decremental*, in that it decreases in magnitude so that a smaller depolarization reaches the cell body (see Fig. 2–2). The size of the potential depends critically on the distance it must travel, such that synapses on very distant dendrite branches are usually much less effective than those near the cell body.

The action potential

Something truly magical happens at one end of the cell body, and it involves a mechanism that defines the special physiology of the neuron. This special property, which involves a dramatic alteration in the membrane permeabilities, typically occurs only in axons. At the postsynaptic site in dendrites and in most of the cell body, the membrane does not generally change its permeabilities substantially. So, potentials created at the synapse are propagated only by electrotonic conduction of the transient perturbation of the resting potential at the synapse when transmission occurs. As described previously, this perturbation is conducted rapidly, at the speed of electricity, but it also decrements rapidly along the length of the dendrite. So electrotonic conduction is not a mechanism that would support long-range communication of signals down the axon for distances of up to a meter or more, as required in some pathways of the brain.

At the end of the cell body where the axon originates, the membrane takes on a profound new quality, one that allows it to change its permeabilities in a large and very useful way. At this locus, called the initiation zone, the channels in the membrane change their permeability when they are depolarized to a specific threshold, and hence they are called *voltage-gated channels*. The mechanisms of these channels in mediating the action potential were first discovered by Alan Hodgkin and Andrew Huxley in the 1940s. They showed that depolarization of the axon membrane above the threshold, typically about a 15–20 millivolt depolarization, results initially in an increase in permeability selectively to Na^+ molecules. As was the case at the synapse, Na^+ is in greater concentration outside the axon, and therefore an increase in Na^+ permeability results in an influx of positively charged sodium molecules, and consequently a further depolarization of the cell membrane. This sets up an unusual "regenerative" situation, a positive feedback mechanism by which the initial depolarization above threshold causes an influx of Na^+, which further depolarizes the cell, which causes more Na^+ channels to open, which allows more Na^+ in, which additionally depolarizes the cell, and so on. When does this regenerative loop end? Sooner or later, the membrane becomes fully permeable to Na^+ and it will reach its equilibrium potential, that is, its balance between concentration and electrostatic gradients. Thus, the maximum potential is a fixed number for a given cell (whose value depends on factors such as the initial inside and outside Na^+ concentrations, and the temperature). Because the pump makes the Na^+ concentration greater outside the cell, its equilibrium is reached when the inside of the membrane reaches an overall positive value, typically about 40 millivolts.

Importantly, once the threshold of depolarization is achieved, this regenerative process runs itself inevitably and precisely to the equilibrium potential for Na^+. The magnitude of the action potential is much larger than the potentials associated with decremental conduction, and its appearance is "all-or-none." Either the threshold for activation of the voltage-gated channels is not reached, and very little potential is obtained and dissipates rapidly, or threshold is reached, and the mechanism regenerates itself up to the full value of the equilibrium potential for Na^+. Furthermore, when an action potential is generated in the initiation zone, the potential spreads electrotonically. This spread would decrement, but over a short distance would be more than sufficient to take the adjacent voltage-gated channels of axon membrane to threshold. This would regenerate the full magnitude of the action potential at that neighboring locus, and that potential would itself spread, reinitiating a full-blown action potential at its neighboring loci, and so on, continuing to reduplicate the action potential through the length of the axon. This simple regenerative mechanism, therefore, not only insures that the action potential achieves its full size at each locus but also insures its propagation for the full length of the axon regardless of the distance involved.

The action potential also includes a mechanism for recovery. Shortly after the Na^+ channels are activated, voltage-gated channels for K^+ also open. During the resting phase, K^+ channels were open to some extent, allowing the establishment of the resting potential. In addition, just after the initiation of the Na^+ current, other K^+ channels are activated, allowing even greater permeability to this molecule. Because K^+ is more concentrated on the inside of the cell, it flows out, and does so especially strongly because the Na^+ onrush has made the inside of the cell move to a positive potential. The result of this series of events is that the rise in the membrane potential to a positive state is short-lived. The membrane potential rapidly returns to its initial level (indeed to even below that level—an overshoot—because of the especially high K^+ permeability). At that point the membrane has more or less reachieved its normal potential but the molecular balance is not the same as its initial status. There is a lingering high concentration of Na^+ inside the cell, and extra K^+ has left the cell. The pumping mechanism sets this imbalance right, but during this recovery period a new action potential cannot be initiated, and so the cell is said to be in a *refractory period*.

Synaptic transmission

When the action potential reaches the end of the axon, at the presynaptic site, another mechanism takes over to mediate synaptic transmission (Fig. 2–4). The spreading of the action potential to the membrane of the presynaptic element activates voltage-gated channels in that area for a different molecule, calcium (Ca^{2+}). Calcium is more highly concentrated on the outside of the cell, in the synaptic cleft, and so the depolarization of the presynaptic element results in a substantial influx of Ca^{2+} into the presynaptic element. It takes time for these channels to open, in part accounting for the delay in synaptic transmission of signals, but Ca^{2+} is the critical catalyst to initiate synaptic transmission. It appears that Ca^{2+} plays a central role in facilitating the docking of synaptic vesicles at specific sites in the end of the presynaptic membrane. When this docking has been accomplished, the vesicle fuses with the end of the cell membrane and re-

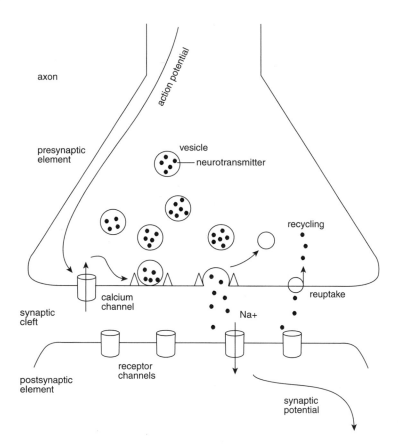

Figure 2–4. Schematic diagram of events in synaptic transmission.

leases its contents, the neurotransmitter, into the synaptic cleft. Quickly the vesicular material is recaptured and recycled, to be filled again with neurotransmitter.

Meanwhile, the neurotransmitter diffuses across the synaptic cleft and finds its way onto and binds with specific receptors. The receptors briefly bind the neurotransmitter, and in doing so, activate channels that control the permeability of the postsynaptic membrane to local molecules. The binding is typically transient, interrupted by an unbinding and diffusion of the neurotransmitter, or by other molecules that destroy the neurotransmitter. The neurotransmitter or its breakdown products are not allowed to remain in the synaptic cleft for long, however. They are reabsorbed by the presynaptic membrane and recycled.

One main action of these receptors is to initiate changes in the postsynaptic membrane already described, the opening of Na^+ channels to initiate an *excitatory* postsynaptic potential that can be propagated electronically along the dendrite. However, there are many types of neurotransmitters and many types of receptors, even for the same neurotransmitter molecule. This provides considerable capacity for regulation of the duration and type of potential produced at the postsynaptic element. One major variant is the capacity to generate *hyperpolarization,* rather than depolarization, of the postsynaptic element. This is accomplished, at least in some of these *inhibitory* synapses, by transmitter-gated chloride channels in the postsynaptic element. Chloride is a negatively charged molecule that is more concentrated outside the cell membrane. When its channels are activated, the negatively charged chloride molecules flow inside, making the postsynaptic element become even more polarized than normal. This hyperpolarization also flows via electrotonic conduction across the dendrite and can serve to inhibit the generation of an action potential in the activation zone.

Integration of synaptic potentials

In most cases the synaptic potentials that are initiated by synaptic transmission are relatively small, about 5–20 millivolts. As described earlier, these subthreshold potentials decrement in magnitude as they travel to the initiation zone in the axon. Therefore, in most cases, an action potential does not occur as a result from a single activation of one synapse. Instead, the initiation of an action potential typically requires summation of many synaptic potentials. This summation can occur across time if the same synapse is activated repeatedly quickly enough so that the synaptic potentials can build up. Also, summation can occur by the concurrent activation of many spatial distant synapses on the same dendrite or different dendrites. The combination of excitatory (depolarizing) and inhibitory (hyperpolarizing) synaptic potentials offers considerable fine tuning of the likelihood of an action potential. In addition to these forms of temporal and spatial summation, the degree to which individual synapses control the action potential depends to a great extent where on the dendrite it is initiated—synapses close to or on the cell body are most effective, because they will suffer less from the effects of decremental conduction, as described earlier.

These aspects of integration are complemented by a variety of mechanisms that regulate the efficacy of synapses and their consequent contribution to initiation of action potentials. The efficacy of a synapse is determined by the supply of neurotransmitter, and by the amount and duration of Ca^{2+} influx that determines how much neurotransmitter is released. The sensitivity and duration of receptor activation can be regulated by substances in the synaptic cleft, and, indeed, many drugs operate by interfering with or enhancing the operation of receptors. The number and sensitivity of receptors also determine the efficacy of the synapse. As you will see, alterations in each of these parameters provides a mechanism for changes in synaptic efficacy that underlie memory storage.

Cellular biology of simple memory circuits

To provide examples of how the cellular and molecular mechanisms of neural conduction and transmission become important in memory, the remainder of this chapter summarizes a program of study on the behavior and physiology of a relatively simple invertebrate species. Invertebrates are superb animals in which to study the cell biology of nervous function because their nervous systems involve many fewer neurons than those of most vertebrates, and many of their neurons are quite large and unique. These qualities allow researchers to individually identify exactly the same set of cells in each animal, and to study virtually all of the major cells involved in a functional circuit.

In pioneering studies, Eric Kandel and his colleagues have examined the behavioral, anatomical, and physiological properties of simple forms of memory in *Aplysia*, a large sea snail. Most of their studies have focused on one particular reflex circuit, called the gill withdrawal reflex. When the snail is quiescent, it extends its gills from the abdominal region, as well as a fleshy continuation of the gill called the siphon. Ordinarily the siphon serves to assist the flow of aerated water over the gills as they function in respiration. However, the gills are a delicate organ, one that is easily damaged. Therefore, when there are signs of danger, the snail can withdraw the gill and siphon. In the laboratory, a mantle shelf that ordinarily completely covers the gill and siphon can be retracted, and then when the animal is relaxed, the gill and siphon are extended. The defensive reflex is initiated by a gentle stroke of the siphon with a paint brush. This results in the rapid withdrawal of the gill under the mantle shelf.

This reflex has been studied extensively, using behavioral paradigms that examine three simple forms of learning, *habituation, sensitization*, and *classical conditioning*. For each form of learning the anatomical circuit of the relevant neurons has been characterized, and the cellular and molecular mechanisms that underlie learning have been explored. A review of the findings of these studies provides a solid introduction to central principles of the cellular mechanisms that mediate learning.

Habituation

Perhaps the simplest form of learning is habituation. All of us use habituation every day to help us learn *not* to attend or respond to irrelevant stimuli. For example, if you ever moved from a small to a big city, your attention to the noise of traffic may have initially made it difficult for you to sleep through the night. Each time a car blew its horn or a siren went off, you woke up. However, after several days, you probably came to ignore the noises, that is you habituated to them, and your sleep was undisturbed by them.

Rapid and lasting habituation can also be observed in the gill withdrawal reflex of *Aplysia*. Following elicitation of the reflex and subsequent relaxation, if the siphon is stimulated again the reflex is smaller, and following several repetitions it becomes quite reduced in magnitude. Furthermore, following only 10 stimulations, the reflex may remain habituated for only 15 minutes. But, after 4 days of such training, the habituation can last weeks. The longer-lasting habituation is a very simple form of learning, to be sure, but it has the lasting property that indicates it is indeed a form of long-term memory.

Now the researchers sought to characterize the circuit of nerve cells involved in the reflex and to determine the mechanism of lasting habituation. A highly schematic sketch of this circuit that shows just one of each type of cell is provided in Fig. 2–5. It turns out that all the relevant cells of the circuit are in a single ganglion, or cluster of cells in the abdomen. There are about 40 sensory cells that innervate the siphon skin, and these connect with six motor neurons that innervate the gill musculature. The neurotransmitter for this synapse is glutamate, and this will become important later. There are also clusters of both excitatory and inhibitory in-

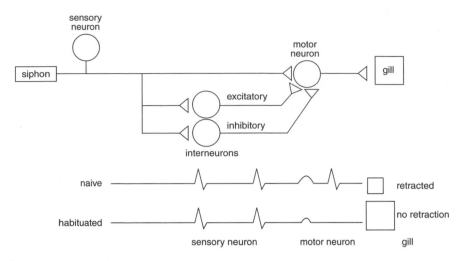

Figure 2–5. Schematic diagram of an idealized circuit for habituation in *Aplysia*, and recordings of action potentials at successive stages in the circuit.

terneurons, cells that receive input from the sensory cells and innervate the motor neurons. When the stimulus is initially applied to the siphon, the sensory neurons are excited, and these excite the interneurons and gill motor neurons. These inputs converge and cause the motor neuron to discharge action potentials repeatedly, producing a vigorous withdrawal response.

Following repetitions of the siphon stimulation, the sensory neurons still produce action potentials, indicating that the habituation is not mediated by a sensory adaptation or any other change in the responsiveness of the sensory elements (Fig. 2–5). However, the magnitude of the synaptic potential in the interneurons and motor neurons is reduced, such that the likelihood of generating an action potential in the motor neuron, and the number of them generated, is smaller. Eventually, even though the sensory neuron is still responding vigorously, no action potentials are produced in the motor neurons. This means that the locus of the memory is to be found in the physiology of the connections between the sensory neurons (as well as the excitatory interneurons) onto motor neurons. This was confirmed by closely examining the synaptic potentials in the motor neurons and confirming that the magnitude and longevity of their depression closely mirror that of the behavioral response.

Now, Kandel and colleagues asked what stage in the process of conduction or transmission was affected by habituation. They found that the receptors in the postsynaptic site were equally sensitive, so the locus of the depression had to be presynaptic. Indeed, they found that the depression was due to a decrease in the number of synaptic vesicles released for each action potential. They then used an electron microscope to examine the number and locations of synaptic vesicles in the presynaptic element before and after habituation, and found that the number of available vesicles did not decrease but fewer of them became docked onto release sites in habituated animals. Furthermore, following extended training, physiological assessments indicated that many fewer sensory neurons had effective connections with motor neurons, and anatomical examination showed that the number of synaptic contacts between sensory neurons and interneurons and motor neurons was substantially reduced. These findings showed that memory can be mediated by changes in synaptic efficacy, both through intracellular mechanisms that control transmitter release and through changes in anatomical connectivity.

Sensitization

A second simple form of nonassociative learning observed in *Aplysia* is sensitization. This kind of learning is, in a way, the opposite of habituation in that it involves an *increase* in reflex magnitude as a result of stimulation. In this case though, the circuit involves a combination of two inputs such that strong stimulation of one input sensitizes, or makes more vigorous, responses to the other input. An everyday example is when we encounter a fearful stimulus, such as a loud noise, we become for some time more likely to startle, or startle more vigorously, to many other sounds as well.

In *Aplysia*, sensitization has been studied using a protocol in which initially the tail of the animal is stimulated with an electric shock, which results in an increase in the robustness of the gill withdrawal to siphon stimulation. A single tail shock produces sensitization that lasts for minutes, whereas a series of 4–5 tail shocks produces sensitization that lasts for a few days. The circuit that mediates this form of learning involves the same set of cells involved in habituation, plus sensory neurons that innervate the tail and additional interneurons (Fig. 2–6). Thus, one way or another, the same set of cells can mediate both habituation and sensitization, two different forms of learning. In the case of habituation, the synaptic depression that occurs is said to be *homosynaptic,* because the mediating events occur within the same pathway that constitutes the reflex itself. However, in the case of sensitization, there must be a facilitation that is mediated by a *heterosynaptic* mechanism because it involves modulation of the reflex pathway by another set of cells, in this situation in the tail sensory pathway.

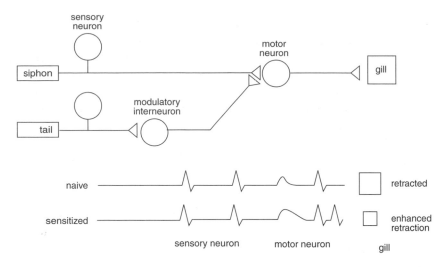

Figure 2–6. Schematic diagram of an idealized circuit for sensitization in *Aplysia*, and recordings of action potentials at successive stages in the circuit.

The central events that underlie sensitization do not involve direct modifications of the siphon sensory neuron, as was the case in habituation. Rather, the tail shocks activate sensory neurons for the tail, which in turn activate modulatory interneurons that synapse onto the cells bodies and presynaptic elements of the siphon sensory neurons. These modulatory neurons affect the strength of synaptic signal produced by the siphon sensory neurons, and so use an indirect mechanism to support the facilitation of reflexes. Specifically, the facilitation is due to forms of modulation that act to increase the number of synaptic vesicles released by the siphon sensory neuron onto its targets, resulting in a substantial increase in the response of the gill motor neurons.

The key to the modulation of sensory neuron synaptic potentials lies in a distinction between two types of receptors (Fig. 2–7). As described before, the conventional receptors, called ionotropic receptors, are found in postsynaptic elements, are transmitter-gated, and allow charged molecules to flow briefly inducing the postsynaptic excitatory and inhibitory potentials. There is also a second class of receptors, called metabotropic receptors. These are activated by transmitters or other molecules, but do not open channels and directly cause changes in the membrane potential. Rather, they produce other changes in the cell that can have lasting effects on its responsiveness.

The changes resulting from metabotropic receptor activation typically involve a cascade of molecular events. Thus, when a neurotransmitter binds

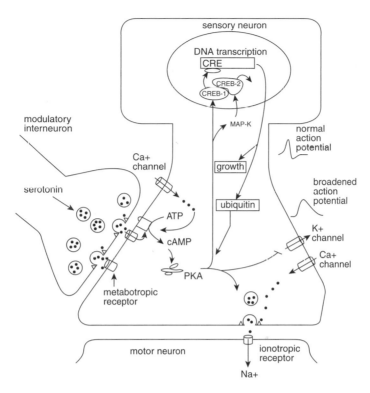

Figure 2–7. Schematic diagram of cellular events that mediate long-term changes in synaptic efficacy of the presynaptic site in *Aplysia*.

onto a metabotropic receptor, an enzyme is activated which in turn alters the concentration of an intracellular signaling molecule called a *second messenger* (distinguishing it from the neurotransmitter as the "first" messenger). In this and many other situations the second messenger is cyclic adenosine monophosphate (cAMP), which is synthesized by the enzyme from the common metabolic molecule adenosine triphosphate (ATP). The action of cAMP is to turn on a number of cellular processes through activation of a special protein called cAMP protein kinase, also known as PKA. In turn, PKA mediates its effects by adding a phosphate group to a variety of proteins, activating them to play any of a variety of roles in cell regulation. Thus, the second messenger signaling system is different from the primary synaptic mechanism in having a variety of long-lasting effects.

In the case of sensitization in *Aplysia*, the specific neurotransmitter of the modulatory interneurons is serotonin, which acts on the metabotropic receptors of the sensory neurons to increase their intracellular cAMP, which in turn activates PKA. This was found by showing that direct application of serotonin is sufficient to activate cAMP, and direct intracellular injection of cAMP is sufficient to enhance transmitter release by the sensory neuron, and to induce the facilitation of the reflex. Furthermore, intracellular infusion of the main subunit of PKA also produces the facilitation, and inhibiting the action of PKA blocks the facilitation. Thus, the full cascade of events associated with the second messenger is both sufficient and necessary for mediation of sensitization. Furthermore, a key specific effect on the physiology of the synapse has been identified. Both cAMP and PKA (or some of its subunits) act to close one of the K^+ channels in the presynaptic membrane of the sensory neuron, reducing the action of this channel in terminating the action potential. This results in a broadening of the action potential, opening the Ca^{2+} channels of the presynaptic element for a longer period, and allowing a greater amount of Ca^{2+} to enter the presynaptic element. The increased Ca^{2+} concentration in the presynaptic element increases the number of vesicles docked per action potential, increasing the release of neurotransmitter, which, of course, leads to a greater response of the motor neurons.

Classical conditioning

Habituation and sensitization are considered very elementary forms of learning, because they do not involve the acquisition of an association between stimuli, but rather a change in responsiveness to repeated stimulation of one kind. The simplest form of associative learning is classical conditioning, the kind of learning that was the focus of the pioneering studies of Pavlov described in Chapter 1. In this form of learning two different stimuli are presented in close temporal proximity, such that typically a form of stimulation that does not ordinarily produce a response is presented before another stimulus that does produce the response. After multiple pairings the first stimulus acquires the ability to produce the response. In that sense, classical conditioning involves the acquisition of an association between the first, or conditioned stimulus, and the second, unconditioned stimulus. In Pavlov's dogs the conditioned stimulus was a tone, that did not initially elicit salivation. It was presented repeatedly prior to injection of food into the mouth (the unconditioned stimulus), which did directly elicit salivation. After several pairings, the tone came to elicit the conditioned response of salivation.

In the *Aplysia* model, a protocol for classical conditioning was established using an elaboration of the habituation and sensitization paradigms and their neural circuits (Fig. 2–8). Added to the already described ele-

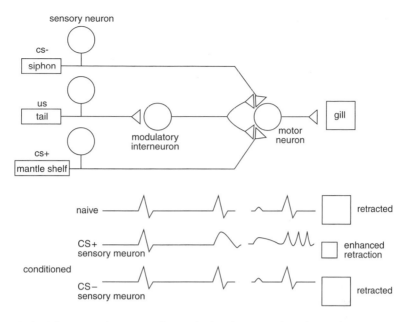

Figure 2–8. Schematic diagram of an idealized circuit for classical conditioning in *Aplysia*, and recordings of action potentials at successive stages in the circuit.

ments is an additional reflex pathway from the sensory neurons of the skin on the mantle shelf that connect to the same set of motor neurons that withdraw the gill. This pathway is essentially the same as the pathway from the siphon to the gill, and offers the ability to differentially condition one of those paths, and not the other, consistent with the selectivity of associations in classical conditioning in mammals. In this differential classical conditioning protocol, then, on some trials the mantle shelf is lightly stimulated and then the tail is shocked. The mantle shelf stimulation is referred to as the positive conditioning stimulus (CS+) and the tail stimulation is the unconditioned stimulus (US). On other trials, the siphon is stimulated and no tail shock is given, and this stimulation is referred to as the CS−. The animals come to have vigorously enhanced withdrawal responses to the mantle stimulation, the conditioned response (CR), but not to the siphon stimulation, that is, they become differentially conditioned to the mantle conditioned stimulus.

As is the case in mammalian examples of classical conditioning, timing is everything. In this case strong tail stimulation simply produces a generalized sensitization. But in the case of classical conditioning, the protocol produces differential conditioning for the paired stimulus. How is this accomplished within the cells of this circuit? The critical steps occur both in the presynaptic and postsynaptic elements of the reflex circuit. At the presynaptic element, it turns out that when an action potential reaches the site, the influx of Ca^{2+} not only induces transmitter docking and release, but Ca^{2+} also binds to the protein calmodulin. The calcium–calmodulin complex binds to the enzyme (adenyl cyclase) that generates cAMP. Additionally, bound to calmodulin, the adenyl cyclase becomes more sensitive to activation by serotonin, consequently releasing a greater amount of cAMP and subsequently enhancing the influx of Ca^{2+}. Thus, the critical timing involves first a priming step in which the CS+ (mantle shelf stimulation) generates calcium–calmodulin bound to adenyl cylase, and then the closely following US (tail stimulation) acts via the modulatory interneurons to induce cAMP and PKA responses—the closely timed combination produces especially large cAMP responses only in the conditioned stimulus sensory neurons.

In addition, there is a change in the postsynaptic element that also mediates the conditioned response. As you should recall, the neurotransmitter for the reflex pathway is glutamate. This neurotransmitter activates two types of ionotropic receptors on the postsynaptic elements. One is a conventional receptor that regulates Na^+ influx. The other is a special receptor, called the N-methyl-D-aspartate (NMDA) receptor, that regulates Ca^{2+} flow. Under normal operation of the reflex, and under habituation and sensitization, the NMDA receptor is blocked by another charged molecule, magnesium (Mg^{2+}). However, NMDA receptors have the unusual property of being modulated by the voltage of the cell membrane such that when the membrane is depolarized the magnesium block is eliminated and Ca^{2+} can flow into the cell. During the protocol for classical conditioning this is accomplished when the CS+ activates the conventional ionotropic receptors, allowing Na^+ influx and producing the typical synaptic depolarization. This transiently unblocks the NMDA channels, so that if a US occurs briefly afterward, facilitating the synapse so that the motor neuron generates a long train of action potentials, the NMDA receptor opens allowing in Ca^{2+}. This results in a cascade of molecular events that results in lasting modifications of the postsynaptic element. The NMDA receptor and its role in memory in mammalian systems is considered again in greater detail in the next chapter.

Substrates of permanent memory traces in cellular mechanisms

The sensitization and classical conditioning studies so far described have focused on the local mechanisms within synaptic elements that mediate short-term memory. To create long-lasting memories, it has long been recognized that additional mechanisms are likely required—mechanisms that rely on structural changes involving the growth of existing synapses or the addition of new synapses. These changes surely involve protein synthesis. Early experiments showed repeatedly that inhibition of protein synthesis, at any stage in the activation of the genes to the production of protein molecules, blocks the formation of memories. Furthermore, the role of protein synthesis in memory formation is a somewhat prolonged one, as demonstrated in studies showing that inhibition of protein synthesis for several minutes after learning also blocks later expression of memory. Following that period, however, inhibition of protein synthesis does not block memory, showing that the process is completed in due course.

What are the mechanisms that connect the activation of intracellular mechanisms at the synapse to the production of proteins and the fixation of memory? There is evidence that the first steps begin with the molecular cascade already described (see Fig. 2–7). For example, in the sensitization protocol described earlier, single stimulations with serotonin result in the release of a small amount of cAMP, sufficient to generate small amounts of PKA that have local effects. But the amount of PKA is not sufficient to diffuse in quantity to the nucleus of the cell where the genetic machinery lies. However, repeated stimulations raise the concentration of cAMP to a level where it interacts with the PKA to break up its form into separate functional units. One type of unit, called the catalytic subunit, then diffuses in sufficient quantity to the nucleus to activate the genetic decoding machinery.

When the active unit of PKA translocates to the nucleus it phosphorylates (adds a phosphorous-containing molecule) to several factors that activate the transcription of RNA from the DNA code (see Fig. 2–7). The most relevant of these for our purposes is a protein called cAMP-response element binding protein (CREB). One form of CREB, called CREB-1, binds to a special element on DNA called CRE and switches on the genes that code for molecules critical to the fixation of memory. This was confirmed in experiments showing that inhibiting the binding of CREB-1 prevents sensitization whereas infusing phosphorylated CREB-1 into the sensory neuron produces lasting facilitation. This combination of findings indicates that CREB-1 is both necessary and sufficient for the fixation of this simple form of memory.

In addition, there are mechanisms for fine tuning the process of fixation. In particular, within the same sensitization paradigm, another form of CREB, called CREB-2, has been identified. CREB-2 appears to suppress CREB-1 and therefore acts as an inhibitory transcription regulator, that is, a repressor. Evidence indicates that CREB-2 is regulated by a different protein kinase called mitogen-activated protein kinase, or MAP kinase. MAP kinase acts by preventing CREB-2's blockade of CREB-1, and thus activation of MAP kinase facilitates CREB-1 and memory. This was shown in an impressive demonstration of enhanced learning in *Aplysia*. Whereas a single stimulation of the sensory neuron ordinarily produces only a short-lasting sensitization, following a treatment that blocked CREB-2, the facilitation was lasting.

The precise set of genes activated by the CREB mechanism, and their specific actions in mediating memory fixation, are not well understood. Because of the rapidity of the gene expression following stimulation, it has been suggested that the critical steps may involve a special class of genes called immediate-early genes that are activated quickly and transiently. Within the *Aplysia* sensitization model, there is evidence that one of these genes may control the production of an enzyme called ubiquitin hydrolase, which appears to diffuse back toward the synapse where it helps release the active subunits of PKA and consequently produce a lasting alteration in synaptic physiology.

In addition, there must be a production of as yet unknown molecules that regulate growth of synapses. It has been shown, for example, that long-term sensitization results in a major increase in the number of synaptic terminals of the sensory neurons. Dendritic processes also grow to accommodate the increase in synaptic contacts. Thus, there has to be a coordination of presynaptic and postsynaptic growth that would mediate long-lasting changes in efficacy of the reflex.

Other "simple" systems

Parallel observations on other model systems indicate that the cellular events and molecular cascade described for *Aplysia* are conserved in evolution. In particular, one prominent model based on another invertebrate often used in genetic studies provides substantial converging evidence of the scheme outlined above. These studies involve a kind of olfactory learning in fruit flies. In this behavioral paradigm, groups of animals are placed in chambers that contain a particular odor and then shocked briefly. On other trials, the same animals are placed in a different chamber that contains another odor and no shock is given. Finally, the animals are placed in an apparatus that allows the animal to migrate between the two familiar chambers and they typically express memory as a preference for the safe chamber. Several different mutant flies have been tested in this protocol, and a number of them turn out to have specific amnesic deficits.

One of these flies, called *dunce*, had a defect in the gene that regulates cAMP and had a severe learning deficit. Another with a defect in adenyl cyclase, the enzyme that synthesizes cAMP from ATP, is called *rutabaga* (one of several named after vegetables, as a reflection on their intelligence), and other flies with defects in genetic regulation of PKA also show deficient memory capacity.

Recently, in this model, the role of CREB has also been examined. These studies found that a genetic manipulation that led to overexpression of a CREB repressor blocked the fixation of memory. More strikingly, and similar to the studies on *Aplysia*, overexpression of a CREB activator reduced the training required to have lasting memory. Usually a single training trial with each odor is sufficient to produce only a short-lived memory. However, when the CREB activator was overexpressed, a single training trial was sufficient to fixate the memory.

Summing up

Neurons are composed of three main elements: dendrites that are specialized for receiving signals from other cells, the cell body, and the axon that is specialized for conduction of the neural impulse. In addition, there are specialized areas of these cellular components that mediate communication between cells, called synapses, each composed of a presynaptic element where neurotransmitters are stored and released and a postsynaptic element where there are receptors that recognize the neurotransmitter and generate signals in the postsynaptic cell.

There are two electrical mechanisms for conduction of the neuronal signal over substantial distances through the dendrites and axon. The initial phase, called *electrotonic conduction*, typically begins at the postsynaptic site and proceeds to the cell body, and involves passive and fast, but decremental conduction of an electrical signal. The later phase is called the *action potential*, which typically begins at the origin of the axon, and involves active and relatively slow, but faithful conduction of a signal over long distances. Neural transmission occurs at the synapse and involves the action potential causing the fusion of synaptic vesicles and release of neurotransmitter from the presynaptic element. The neurotransmitter activates voltage-gated channels in the postsynaptic receptor site, which depolarizes the postsynaptic cell in excitatory synapses and hyperpolarizes the postsynaptic cell at inhibitory synapses.

These basic mechanisms of neuronal physiology are important to understanding the nature of neural plasticity that underlies memory. These and other aspects of the molecular physiology of neurons have been put to use in simple invertebrate systems to understand three fundamental types of learning: habituation, the decrementing of responsiveness to repeated sensory stimulation without reinforcement, sensitization, the incrementing of responsiveness to sensory stimulation following strong stimulation, and classical conditioning, the association of an arbitrary external stimulus with a stimulus that produces a reflexive response.

The findings from the studies of relatively simple invertebrate learning models have provided fundamental insights about the representation of memories in the brain of all animals. These basic insights can be summed up as follows: First, Cajal was right in his conjecture that alterations in synaptic efficacy provide the basic cellular mechanism for memory. Second, the nature of the chemical mechanisms involved in memory are not unique "memory molecules," but rather involve a set of adaptations of natural molecular mechanisms by which synaptic activity is regulated. Indeed, the most common mechanisms involve clever uses of ubiquitous molecules, such as cAMP and the genetic code regulators. Third, the changes that mediate memory do not involve special "memory cells," but rather the same cells that perform sensory, modulatory, and motor functions in the reflex pathway. Fourth, and closely related to the last point, the cells of the nervous system seem to be highly adaptable. It takes very few activations of the right type to induce an adaptation of the cellular mechanisms to support memory, and not many more to incite the permanent fixation process. Fifth, and finally, several mechanisms are employed in memory formation at the cellular level, allowing for different forms of memory to be encoded within the same cells, and allowing for a variety of ways to fine tune the memory and its time course at the various stages in a cascade of cellular events.

READINGS

Bear, M.F., Connors, B.W., and Paradiso, M.A. 2000. *Neuroscience: Exploring the Brain*. New York: Williams & Wilkins.

Carew, T.J. 1996. Molecular enhancement of memory formation. *Neuron* 16:5–8.

Squire, L.R., and Kandel, E.R. 1999. *Memory: From Mind to Molecules*. New York: Scientific American Library.

Tully, T., Bowling, G., Chistensen, J., Connoly, J., Delvechhio, M., DeZazzo, J., Dubnau, J., Jones, G., Pinto, S., and Regulski, M., et al. 1996. A return to the genetic dissection of memory in Drosophila. *Cold Spring Harbor Symposium in Quantitative Biology* 61:207–218.

3

• • • • • •

Cellular Mechanisms of Memory: Complex Circuits

STUDY QUESTIONS

What is LTP?

Why is LTP a good model for the plasticity that underlies memory?

What are the cellular mechanisms for the induction of LTP?

What are the molecular mechanisms for the preservation and expression of LTP?

What is the evidence that something like LTP occurs during learning?

What is the evidence that the mechanisms of LTP are required for learning?

The previous chapter showed how understanding cellular and molecular mechanisms can provide clear insights into the bases for memory in relatively simple nervous systems. Indeed, to the extent that the most important aspects of the relevant circuitry have been included in those model systems, it might not be too vain to conclude that we truly *understand* how memory works in those circuits.

In the present chapter, we aim higher: Can we also understand the nature of learning and memory in more complex systems, such as those of mammals, through a characterization of cellular and molecular properties in the key brain areas involved in memory functions? There is certainly a long history of the expectation that a simple reflex modification mechanism will be conserved across species and in complex as well as simple systems. Pavlov and Sherrington, from distinct behavioral and physiological perspectives, recognized that modification of synaptic function—synaptic plasticity—is the basic substrate of the conditioned reflex mechanism in mammals. In 1949 Donald Hebb broadened this notion beyond that of stimulus and response associations, outlining a cascade of events that begins with synaptic plasticity as the fundamental associative mechanism and extends to the development of "cell assemblies" that represent specific percepts, thoughts, and actions, in all species including humans.

Modern neuroscience since Hebb's time has made tremendous advances in understanding synaptic plasticity mechanisms and their possible role in memory using mammalian model systems. This chapter reviews some of the recent progress toward a full characterization of one particular form of synaptic plasticity observed in the mammalian brain called long-term potentiation (LTP). LTP is a laboratory phenomenon, but its mechanisms are now quite well understood. It can be induced in many brain structures that are involved in memory, and there is substantial evidence that the same cellular mechanisms that mediate LTP are required for lasting memory. Therefore, this chapter reviews the state of our understanding of this important phenomenon as a likely candidate for memory coding in mammalian systems.

Hippocampal long-term potentiation as a model memory mechanism

Long-term potentiation is most commonly studied in the hippocampus, a brain structure that you will come to know quite well in this book. The hippocampus is a complex structure, but it is easy to find in the brain, and its inputs, outputs, and intermediate pathways are largely segregated, making it an excellent model system for studying its circuitry. We now know a lot about the initial steps in the molecular and synaptic basis of LTP, particularly as seen in the hippocampus. The elucidation of these mechanisms has been facilitated greatly by the development of the *in vitro* hippocampal "slice" preparation in which thick transverse sections of the hippocampus are taken from the brain and kept alive in a Petri dish (Fig. 3–1). This preparation lacks the complex influences of the normal inputs and outputs of the hippocampus, but provides an especially clear access to cells and intrinsic connections of the hippocampal circuit. Most of these studies have focused on area CA1 of the hippocampus, where the in vitro preparation allows multiple input and output pathways to be preserved intact and to be manipulated independently for recording and stimulation (Fig. 3–2A).

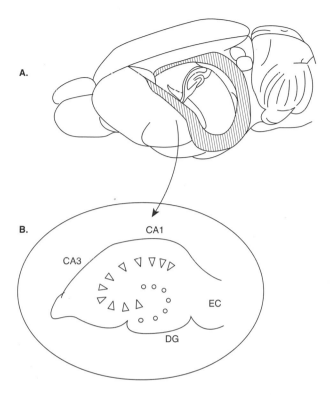

Figure 3–1. The hippocampal slice preparation. *A:* A view of the rodent brain. The hippocampus is a large structure inside the cerebral hemispheres. A slice is taken in a plane transverse to the long axis of the hippocampus. *B:* The hippocampal slice in vitro, with indications of its major subdivisions, CA1, CA3, DG = dentate gyrus, EC = entorhinal cortex.

The phenomenon of LTP was first discovered by Terje Lomo, a PhD student working in Oslo. Lomo was exploring the physiology of the circuitry of the hippocampus, and in particular he was examining the phenomenon of frequency potentiation, an increase in the magnitude of responsiveness of cells following a series of rapidly applied activations. Lomo observed that repetitive high-frequency electrical stimulation (called tetanus) of one pathway resulted in a steeper rise time (slope) of the excitatory synaptic potential to a subsequent single pulse. He also observed that following a tetanus there was recruitment of a greater number of cells reaching the threshold for an action potential, reflected in a greater "population spike," the spike observed when many cells fire together (see examples in Fig. 3–2B). Lomo found that the tetanus-induced changes in the synaptic and cellular responses to single pulses lasted for several hours,

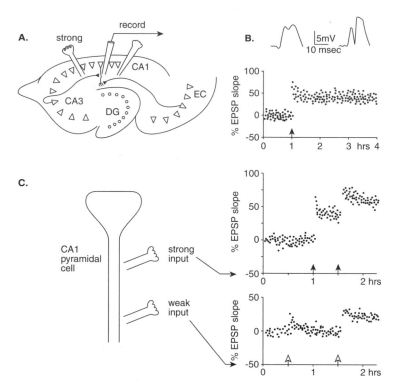

Figure 3–2. Hippocampal long-term potentiation (LTP). *A:* Illustration of a horizontal section through the hippocampus showing the pathways by which pyramidal cells in CA1 are stimulated by either a strong input from CA3 or a weak input from the entorhinal cortex (EC). *B:* Excitatory postsynaptic potentials (EPSPs) recorded after single pulse stimulations of the strong path before (left) and after (right) tetanus. Below is the standard method for tracking the changes in the EPSP slope over a period of hours. *C:* Associative LTP. A schematic diagram of a CA1 pyramidical cell and loci of strong and weak stimulation, and measurements of the EPSP slopes following single pulses of each type of input. The weak input stimulation alone (open arrow at 0.5 hr on lower graph) produces only a transient change, but strong stimulation alone (filled arrow at 1 hr) produces LTP. Combined strong and weak stimulation (both arrows at 1.5 hr) result in LTP at both synaptic sites (data from Bliss and Collingridge, 1993).

leading him to distinguish this phenomenon from short-lasting facilitations. And so, he called it *"long-term potentiation."* In subsequent years several investigators have characterized the basic properties of the synaptic and cellular components of LTP, creating considerable excitement about this phenomenon as a model for lasting history-dependent synaptic change. The findings have spawned a veritable cottage industry within the field of neuroscience.

What fascinated researchers at the outset were the remarkable parallels between properties of LTP and memory. In 1989 Richard Morris identified five fundamental properties that make LTP such an attractive model of memory. First, LTP is a prominent feature of the physiology of the hippocampus, a brain structure universally identified with memory. Subsequent work has made clear that the hippocampus is not the only site of LTP, but its functional role as a component of one of the brain's major memory systems would seem to demand that it possess a memory mechanism.

The second and third properties have to do with temporal characteristics. LTP develops very rapidly, as one would require of a plausible memory mechanism, typically within 1 minute after a single stimulus train delivered with the proper parameters. Moreover, like a good memory, LTP can be long-lasting. In in vivo preparations it can be observed for hours after a single stimulation train, or for weeks or more after repetitive stimulations that might act as "reminders."

Fourth, LTP has the sort of *specificity* one would require of a memory mechanism: Only those synapses activated during the stimulation train are potentiated. Other neighboring synapses, even on the same neurons, are not altered. This phenomenon parallels the natural specificity of our memories, in which we are able to remember many different specific episodes with the same person (e.g., one particular date you had, out of many, with a given individual) or object (e.g., where you parked your car today rather than last week), and thus would be a key requirement of any useful cellular memory mechanism. In addition, the property of specificity may be key to the magnitude of the storage capacity of brain structures. Each cell can participate in the representation of multiple memories, each composed of distinct subsets of its many synaptic inputs.

Fifth, and perhaps most definitively important for memory, LTP is *associative* in that potentiation occurs best when multiple inputs are stimulated simultaneously during the tetanus (Fig. 3–2C). This phenomenon has been demonstrated most elegantly in studies that employ activation of separate pathways that synapse on the same hippocampal neurons. In these studies the two pathways involve the combination of a "weak" input, designated as one that does not produce potentiation at any stimulation level, plus a "strong" input for which a threshold level of stimulation suffices to produce LTP. Associativity is observed when the weak input is activated at the same time as the strong input, resulting in LTP of the weak as well as the strong pathway. The time window for this sort of association was initially thought to be quite brief, on the order of a few milliseconds, and thus quite limited in the extent to which it could support Pavlovian conditioning, which usually involves hundreds of milliseconds separation between conditioned stimulus (CS) and unconditioned stimulus (US). However, there is new evidence that a form of associativity may be possible within a broader, and more behaviorally meaningful, time window. An intriguing 1997 study by Frey and Morris indicated that activity at hippocampal synapses that produces only a short-lived potentiation can nonetheless create a synaptic "tag" that lasts a few hours. Subsequent strong activation of a neighboring pathway within that period leads to lasting potentiation of both the "strong" pathway and the previously "tagged" synapses. Thus, LTP could serve to associate or integrate patterns of activity over a time window that has obvious behavioral significance.

The property of associativity is especially appealing because it offers a cellular model of the mechanism for structural change in neural connections, a change that would increase synaptic "efficacy," the strength of the postsynaptic response resulting from a presynaptic activation. When Hebb proposed his theory of cell assemblies (see Part III), he recognized the need for alterations in the cells so that a whole assembly could be reactivated to recall a memory. He suggested that the essential trigger for changing synaptic efficacy involved the repeated activation of a presynaptic element AND its participation in the success in firing the postsynaptic cell. The simultaneous activation of many inputs of the hippocampus during a tetanus provides a perfect situation to accomplish the co-occurrence of presynaptic and postsynaptic activity. Furthermore, the property of associativity, by permitting the ability to integrate patterns of activity, simultaneously satisfies the induction requirement of LTP—that there be a combination of presynaptic and postsynaptic activation—and offers a fundamental mechanism for encoding associations between functionally meaningful activation patterns.

Cellular basis for the induction of hippocampal LTP

Many studies have shown that the induction of LTP in area CA1 requires two fundamental synaptic events—activation of presynaptic inputs and depolarization of the postsynaptic cell. Both are ordinarily accomplished within a single high-frequency stimulus train—the initial stimulation depolarizes the cell for a relatively prolonged period during which the following stimulations provide simultaneous postsynaptic activations. However, high-frequency stimulation is not required *per se*. Instead, for example, direct depolarization of the postsynaptic cell by injection of current through an intracellular electrode, combined with low-frequency presynaptic input, will suffice. Conversely LTP induction can be blocked by preventing depolarization, or by hyperpolarization of the postsynaptic cell. These findings show that the conditions of Hebb's postulate about the critical conditions for cellular events are both necessary and sufficient to provide a synaptic mechanism for memory.

Molecular bases for the induction and maintenance of hippocampal LTP

The molecular mechanism that underlies the major type of LTP induction in CA1 involves special properties of a combination of synaptic receptors, some of which should be familiar from your reading of Chapter 2 (see Fig. 3–2). Considerable evidence points to the amino acid glutamate as the primary excitatory transmitter in the hippocampus and elsewhere where LTP is found. There are several types of glutamate receptors, most prominently divided into those that are excited by N-methyl-D-aspartate (NMDA receptors, already introduced in Chapter 2) and those that are activated by a-amino-3-hydroxy-5-methyl-4-isoxazolepropionate (AMPA receptors). These two types of receptors can be dissociated functionally by pharmacological manipulations. In particular, the NMDA receptors are selectively and competitively blocked by the antagonist D-2-amino-5-phosphono-valerate (AP5). A major discovery in revealing the mechanism of LTP was that AP5 has little effect on excitatory postsynaptic potentials (EPSPs) elicited by low-frequency stimulation, indicating that AMPA receptors, and not NMDA receptors, mediate normal synaptic transmission in the hippocampus. In contrast, AP5 completely blocks LTP following high-frequency stimulation trains, indicating that glutamate activation of NMDA receptors is critical to this form of synaptic plasticity.

Discoveries about two major differences between NMDA and AMPA receptors in their regulation of postsynaptic ion permeability in CA1 offer an explanation of the role of these receptors in LTP (Fig. 3–3). First, activation of AMPA receptors increases the permeability of the postsynaptic membrane to both sodium (Na^+) and potassium (K^+) ions, but does not alter cell permeability to calcium (Ca^{2+}). By contrast, activation of NMDA receptors increases permeability to Ca^{2+} as well as to Na^+ and K^+ ions. Second, unlike for AMPA receptors, ion flow through NMDA receptors is highly dependent on the voltage state of the postsynaptic cell at the time of NMDA receptor activation. In the resting state, NMDA receptor channels are blocked by another doubly charged ion, magnesium (Mg^{2+}), which prevents the flow of the other ions even in the presence of glutamate at the receptor. However, when the membrane of the postsynaptic cell is depolarized, Mg^{2+} is expelled from the receptor channel, al-

A. Normal synaptic transmission

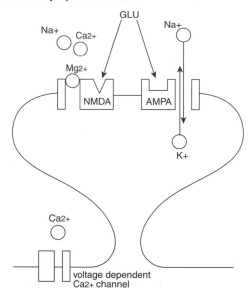

B. During depolarization

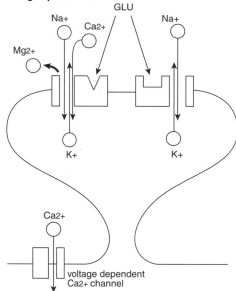

Figure 3–3. Molecular mechanism of the induction of long-term potentiation (LTP). GLU = glutamate; See text for explanation (adapted from Nicoll et al., 1988).

lowing glutamate to bind and the ions including Ca^{2+} to flow. Thus, the effect of the initial activations in the high-frequency stimulus train is to activate the AMPA receptors, depolarizing the postsynaptic cell membrane. This unblocks the NMDA receptor channels so that succeeding stimuli activate the NMDA receptor, allowing Ca^{2+} to enter the postsynaptic cell.

The entry of Ca^{2+} to the intracellular space is a key step in the induction of LTP. This is shown in at least three lines of evidence. First, LTP is prevented when Ca^{2+} is bound by intracellular injection of a calcium chelator (a molecule that binds up calcium). Second, LTP is triggered by intracellular injection of a caged Ca^{2+} compound that releases calcium molecules. Third, the entry of Ca^{2+} into the postsynaptic cell following stimulation trains has been directly imaged using a sophisticated technique called confocal fluorescence microscopy. There is evidence, however, that Ca^{2+} entry does not, by itself, lead to lasting synaptic potentiation; rather, some sort of NMDA receptor activation seems to be required. One possibility under scrutiny is that glutamate also activates metabotropic receptors that mediate release of intracellular stores of Ca^{2+} as an amplification mechanism.

The succeeding steps in the permanent maintenance of LTP are less well understood, and can only be provided in outline form at this time (Fig. 3–4). The leading view is that the role of Ca^{2+} is to activate kinases, enzymes that phosphorylate proteins, transforming them into their active

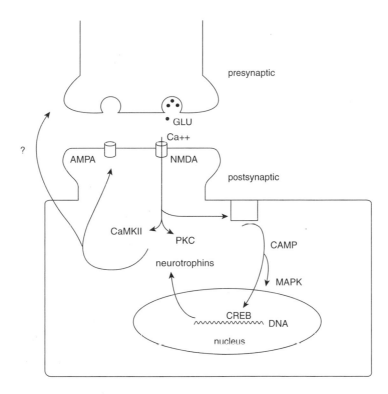

Figure 3–4. Model of the molecular mechanisms of short-term and long-term processes following long-term potentiation induction.

configuration, and some of these will be familiar from your reading about invertebrate systems in Chapter 2. Specific candidates of the critical kinases in the hippocampus include type II Ca^{2+}/calmodulin-dependent kinase (CaMKII), Ca^{2+}/phospholipid-dependent protein kinase C (PKC), and mitogen-activated protein kinase (MAPK).

CaMKII is a very attractive candidate because it is present in large quantities in the postsynaptic area and its initial activation depends on Ca^{2+}. Tetanus stimulates its production, and pharmacological inhibition and genetic elimination of CaMKII block LTP. Furthermore, following activation, CaMKII undergoes an autophosphorylation by which it becomes independent of the transient Ca^{2+} influx to remain phosphorylated. This prolonged activation could mediate long-lasting consequences, one of which might be the conversion of inactive (so-called silent) AMPA receptors into active ones. PKC is also strongly implicated by experiments showing that its activation results in marked potentiation of the EPSP that occludes further potentiation by stimulation trains. Furthermore, intracellular injection of PKC enhances synaptic transmission, and application of PKC antagonists block LTP. MAPK is activated by phosphorylation following LTP or stimulation that results in intracellular Ca^{2+}, and inhibition of MAPK prevents later steps in gene expression.

In addition to modifying existing proteins, there is evidence that the maintenance of LTP also depends on new protein synthesis in the hippocampus. Experiments using protein synthesis inhibitors indicate that proteins synthesized from preexisting mRNA are required for lasting LTP. In addition, there is also evidence that the maintenance of LTP depends upon the cAMP-responsive transcription factor CREB. One possible mechanism for CREB involves the Ca^{2+} influx activating adenylyl cyclase, which in turn activates cAMP. This could in turn activate PKC, leading to the phosphorylation of many proteins, including CREB. The phosphorylated form of CREB is known to modulate the transcription of genes so as to increase the expression of several proteins. There is some evidence indicating that genetically altered mice who lack a form of CREB have deficient LTP maintenance.

One possible target of new protein synthesis in the hippocampus is the production of neurotrophins, molecules long known as regulated by neural activity and having the capacity to promote morphological change and increased connectivity. Stimulation trains capable of inducing LTP increase the gene expression for some neurotrophins in the hippocampus. In turn, some neurotrophins potentiate glutaminergic transmission in CA1, and these effects occur within minutes and last for several hours or longer.

Where is the synaptic alteration?

A major unresolved question is whether the locus of lasting synaptic alteration following LTP is presynaptic or postsynaptic. Of course, changes at both sites are entirely possible. The evidence on both sides of this issue is considerable, and it may not be possible to fully resolve the issue with current methods available to study the hippocampal preparation. Recent attempts to resolve the question have focused on *quantal analysis*, a protocol that involves reducing presynaptic release to a statistical phenomenon. This method allows estimation of the magnitude of the postsynaptic response to a single quantum of transmitter, presumably corresponding to release of a single synaptic vesicle. During LTP there is a decrease in the percentage of failures of postsynaptic response and a decreased variability of responses to presynaptic stimulation, both consistent with an increase in the probability of presynaptic release. However, there is also observed an increase in the amplitude of the response to a single quantum of transmitter, which is consistent with an increase in postsynaptic receptor efficacy. Thus, the current evidence from quantal analyses are consistent with both loci as being involved in plastic change.

Conceptual considerations have also weighed in on this controversy. Possible cellular mechanisms for postsynaptic modification are straightforward to envision, as just discussed. By contrast, because the initial effects of combined pre- and postsynaptic activity evoke cellular mechanisms localized in the postsynaptic cell, an ultimate change in presynaptic physiology would require production and transport of some sort of retrograde messenger, a signal that travels from the activated postsynaptic site to the presynaptic site. Several candidates for the retrograde messenger have been proposed [e.g., arachidonic acid, nitrous oxide (NO), carbon dioxide (CO)], but so far, none has received more than fragmentary support.

Hippocampal long-term depression

If there was only a form of plasticity that *increased* synaptic efficacy, eventually all synapses would become "saturated," that is, raised to a ceiling level of efficacy, and no further learning could occur. So most investigators think that, in addition to the potentiation of synapses, there must be a mechanism of depotentiation or *long-term depression* (LTD) of synaptic efficacy. LTD also can enhance the relative effect of LTP at neighboring synapses, improving the signal-to-noise contrasts, as well as also increasing the range of synaptic coding patterns by a population of synapses providing input to a single postsynaptic cell.

In general, the learning rule for LTD involves activity-dependent plasticity with a direct violation of the Hebb rule for LTP. Thus, LTD has been described under conditions where there is either presynaptic activity or postsynaptic activity, but not both. One can activate presynaptic elements with single pulses at a very low rate that produces no activation, or only weak activation, of the postsynaptic cell. Or one can induce presynaptic activity in the absence of postsynaptic firing, by activating presynaptic elements weakly and out-of-phase with strong stimulation to converging synapses of the same postsynaptic cell. Alternatively, LTD also results from activation of the postsynaptic neuron, without activation of the presynaptic element. This form of LTD can be induced either by stimulation of separate converging synapses on the same postsynaptic cell or by inducing an action potential in the axon that is conducted backward to the cell body (called antidromic activation). All of these forms of LTD have been observed at one pathway or another in the hippocampus, but it remains to be seen if they obey the same induction and maintenance rules and are available at all sites in the hippocampus.

Anatomical modifications consequent to LTP

Most researchers believe that lasting changes in neural connectivity ultimately require altered morphology of synapses. Although this research area has been plagued by technical issues of the proper means of preserving tissue for examination with the electron microscope, there is now substantial evidence that LTP does result in structural alterations in synaptic connections consistent with increases in synaptic efficacy. Most of these data focus on the protruding heads of dendritic spines that are the excitatory synapses of the dentate granule or CA1 pyramidal cells, the same sites that involve NMDA receptor dependent LTP. In the dentate gyrus, the reported structural changes suggest an increase in spine surface area and in the area of the opposing pre- and postsynaptic membranes. In some reports the changes in spines occurred without any appreciable increase in the number of synapses, suggesting an interconversion of spine shapes in which LTP results in increases in synaptic contact area by expansions of the pre- and postsynaptic cell membranes surrounding one another. Studies on CA1 have provided strikingly parallel results, changes in spine dimensions consistent with the overall rounding of spines, although these changes may be transient. Recent studies using newly available high resolution optical methods have detected growth of new spines on postsynaptic dendrites in CA1 shortly after induction of LTP. In addition, lasting changes in spine number have been reported in CA1, and these changes have been characterized as reflecting the transformation of synapses into types with protracted necks as well as sessile types. The coordination of increased presynaptic and postsynaptic active contact, as observed in studies on both the dentate granule and CA1 pyramidal cells, seems to obviate the question of whether the fundamental basis of LTP is pre- or postsynaptic in origin.

LTP beyond the hippocampus

LTP was first discovered in the hippocampus, and it is easily studied there because of the laminar separation of synaptic inputs and outputs. However, there are now reports of potentiation of synaptic efficacy in widespread areas of the brain and LTP is rapidly becoming viewed as a universal plasticity mechanism. Among the areas where LTP, and/or LTD, have been demonstrated are several areas of the neocortex, piriform cortex, amygdala, striatum, cerebellum, and even the spinal cord.

Perhaps best characterized of the nonhippocampal areas is the visual cortex, which has been studied extensively by Mark Bear and his colleagues. In the rat visual cortex, Bear's research group developed an in vitro visual cortex slice preparation in which they would stimulate layer IV input cells and record from layer III principal cells that receive inputs from the layer IV cells (Fig. 3–5). They recorded EPSPs before and after

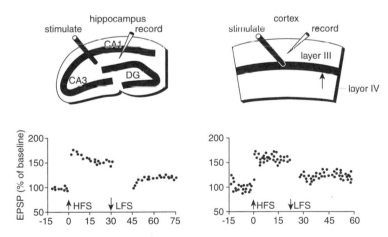

Figure 3–5. Induction of long-term potentiation (LTP) and long-term depression (LTD) in hippocampal and cortical slices. The plots show that in both preparations an increase in the excitatory postsynaptic potentials (EPSP) (LTP) is produced by short bursts of high-frequency stimulation (HFS), and in both preparations a decrease in the field EPSP (LTD) is produced by low-frequency stimulation (LFS) (data from Bear, 1996).

tetanization of the input cells, and found that stimulation of the input layer results in LTP and LTD in principal cells with the same protocols effective for producing these phenomena in the hippocampus. Thus, they demonstrated bidirectional activity-dependent modification of visual cortex synapses such that low-frequency stimulation results in synaptic depression, whereas high-frequency stimulation produces potentiation, just as in the hippocampus. Both forms of synaptic modification are synapse specific and depend on NMDA receptors. Intracellular injections of current that produce postsynaptic depolarization or hyperpolarization paired with low-frequency synaptic activation produce synaptic enhancements or decrements, respectively.

LTP and memory

LTP captures an exciting physiological phenomenon, one that is seen, deservedly, as the most prominent model of synaptic plasticity that might underlie memory. As Charles Stevens once put it, this mechanism is so attractive that it would be a shame if the mechanism underlying LTP turned out not to be a memory mechanism. But there should be no doubt about the fact that LTP is not memory—it is a laboratory phenomenon that involves massive coactivations never observed in nature. The best we can hope is that LTP and memory share a common mechanism. In recent years disappointing evidence has emerged, amidst the more positive findings, regarding all main lines of evidence that have been offered to connect LTP and memory.

Here I attempt just to summarize the history of the research on the possible linkage between LTP and memory. Several relatively direct approaches have been pursued in attempting to demonstrate that LTP and memory share common physiological and molecular bases. Most prominent are demonstrations of changes in synaptic efficacy consequent to a learning experience ("behavioral LTP"), and, conversely, attempts to prevent learning by pharmacological or genetic manipulation of the molecular mechanisms of LTP induction. Examples of each approach are presented here, and discussed in light of the inherent limitations they have in convincingly connecting LTP and memory.

"Behavioral LTP"

Do conventional learning experiences produce changes in synaptic physiology similar to the increases in EPSP and cellular responses that occur after LTP? Seeking changes in synaptic physiology consequent to learning is an ambitious and optimistic approach because one might well expect the magnitude of synaptic change observed in gross field potentials to be vanishingly small following any normal learning experience—a virtual "needle in a haystack." In addition, it is most likely that learning involves changes in synaptic efficacy in both the positive and negative directions, that is, both LTP and LTD. Thus, learning would likely result in changes in the distribution of potentiated and depressed synapses with little or no overall shift, and consequently no change, or even an overall negative change, in the averaged evoked potentials commonly used to measure LTP.

Addressing the first of these concerns by using powerful and extended experience as the learning event, the initial reports showed enhancement of excitatory synaptic potentials and population spikes after different types of learning experience. The early studies include ones in which several aspects of synaptic physiology were observed to change in the perforant pathway response in rats who had been exposed for prolonged periods to an "enriched" as compared to "impoverished" environment. The "enriched" rats lived in a large housing area with littermates, with continuous social stimulation and various forms of environmental stimulation through their opportunity to investigate and interact with many objects placed in their shared cages, whereas the "impoverished" rats had solitary housing, the absence of stimulating objects, and a small living space. In one particularly illustrative study of this type, hippocampal slices were taken from these rats and were tested for various aspects of synaptic and cellular responsiveness. It was found that rats who had lived in the enriched environment, compared to those restricted to the impoverished environment, had an increased slope of the synaptic potential and larger population action potentials, implying more cells recruited, but no change in other physiological parameters. These changes are entirely consistent with the pattern of increased synaptic efficacy observed following LTP. These changes were not permanent, however. They disappeared if the enriched-condition animals were subsequently isolated for 3–4 weeks prior to the analyses.

Recent observations by Joseph LeDoux and his colleagues offer confirming evidence for a connection between the phenomena of LTP and enhanced transmission of relevant sensory inputs in a different neural circuit that supports a specific kind of learning. In this case the learning involved a form of classical (Pavlovian) conditioning in which rats become fearful of tones that have been paired with foot shocks (see Chapter 11). The relevant anatomical pathway involves auditory inputs to a subcortical structure in the thalamus called the medial geniculate nucleus, projections from there to another subcortical area called the lateral amygdala nucleus, and then projections from there to other parts of the amygdala which control the expression of fear responses (Fig. 3–6A; this pathway is described in

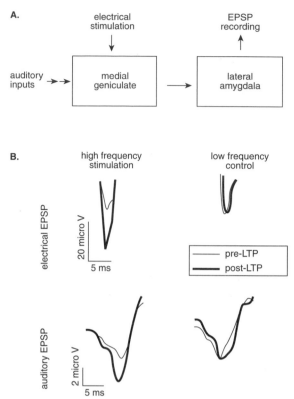

A.

electrical stimulation

EPSP recording

auditory inputs

medial geniculate

lateral amygdala

B.

high frequency stimulation

low frequency control

electrical EPSP

20 micro V

5 ms

pre-LTP
post-LTP

auditory EPSP

2 micro V

5 ms

Figure 3–6. Common mechanisms for long-term potentiation (LTP) and sensory processing. *A:* Anatomical pathway for natural auditory stimulation or electrical stimulation of the medial geniculate nucleus and recording in the lateral amygdala. *B:* Examples of excitatory postsynaptic potentials (EPSPs) evoked by auditory stimulation or electrical stimulation of the medial geniculate before and following high- or low-frequency medial geniculate electrical stimulation that produces LTP in the lateral amygdala recording; note that the same stimulation at low frequency does not produce any potentiation of the EPSP. The induction of LTP in that pathway also results in a large increase in the EPSP response to auditory stimulation in the same pathway (data from Rogan and LeDoux, 1995).

more detail in Chapter 11). In one study they used high-frequency electrical stimulation of the medial geniculate nucleus to induce LTP within the lateral nucleus of the amygdala. Consequently they found an enhancement of synaptic responses within the same area of the amygdala to natural auditory stimulation (Fig. 3–6B). In a complementary study they found the converse evidence that fear conditioning enhances early sensory-evoked responses of neurons in the lateral amygdala.

These findings are illuminating in two ways. First, they support the view that there is nothing special about the hippocampus when it comes to LTP. Second, the approach taken by LeDoux and colleagues points toward a potentially more decisive and therefore possibly more fruitful way to link LTP and memory. The pattern of changes in auditory-evoked synaptic potentials, including the magnitude, direction, and longevity of increased responses, paralleled those parameters for electrically induced synaptic potential, showing us that natural information processing can make use of the very cellular and molecular mechanisms set in place by conventional, artificially induced LTP. Conversely, the observation of increased neuronal sensory responses following conditioning shows us that, like LTP, real learning can enhance information processing relevant to the task.

In subsequent studies the same group has also now shown that repeated pairings of auditory stimuli and foot shocks that train rats to fear the tones also alter evoked sensory responses to the tones in the same way as LTP in that pathway (Fig. 3–7). Thus, in rats with properly timed pairings, tones produce evoked potentials of greater slope and amplitude, just as electrical stimulus trains do when applied to this pathway. No enhancement of field potentials is observed with unpaired tone and foot shock presentations, even though this conditioning control leads to as much of a behavioral response (freezing) as paired presentations (even the unpaired control rats learn to freeze to the environmental context where shocks are received—see Chapter 11). Furthermore, this behavioral LTP is enduring, lasting at least a few days, as long as the behavioral response during extinction trials. Thus, LeDoux and colleagues' approach takes us beyond mere similarities between LTP and memory, bringing into contiguity the identical neural pathways and experimental procedures that define LTP and sensory processing in memory.

A different set of studies on the rat motor cortex by John Donoghue and his colleagues demonstrates the generality of this approach to other brain areas and other forms of learning. In these experiments, rats were trained to reach with one particular paw through a small hole in a food

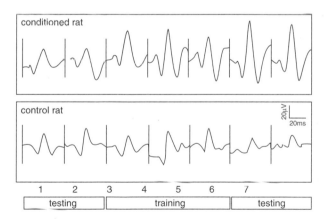

Figure 3–7. Changes in auditory field potentials in the amygdala following fear conditioning. Note the sustained increase in the size of the auditory-stimulation-induced excitatory postsynaptic potentials (EPSP) following paired tone–shock combinations versus no change in the EPSP size under control conditions where tones and shocks were not consistently paired (data from Rogan et al., 1997).

box in order to retrieve food pellets. Initially, the rat's reaching movements are labored and often the food pellets are dropped. However, over the course of one or two hour-long practice sessions, the rats refine their motor coordination and ultimately obtain pellets at a rapid asymptotic rate. Following this kind of motor coordination training, Donoghue and colleagues removed the brain and measured the strength of connections among cells within the area of the motor cortex that controls hand movements. They accomplished this using an *in vitro* preparation of the appropriate brain section and evoking EPSPs in a principal cell layer of the motor cortex by stimulating horizontal fibers that connect neighboring cells to one another (Fig. 3–8). They found that for the same or lower input stimulation intensity, the magnitude of the EPSPs on the side of the brain that controlled the trained paw (i.e., in the contralateral or opposite hemisphere) were consistently larger than those on the side of the brain that controlled the untrained paw. Furthermore, they also found it difficult to induce LTP by electrical stimulation in the trained hemisphere, but not in the untrained hemisphere. Thus, training produced an anatomically localized increase in synaptic efficacy that occluded the capacity for LTP. These observations show in a compelling way that synaptic potentiation results from motor learning, and the real plasticity phenomenon shares common resources with the artificial one, providing strong evidence for common cellular mechanisms of LTP and learning.

Blocking LTP and memory

The major limitation of the preceding approach is that the experiments only provide correlations between aspects of LTP and memory. The con-

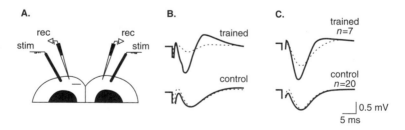

Figure 3–8. Effects of motor skill learning on evoked excitatory postsynaptic potentials (EPSPs) in the motor cortex. *A:* Placement of stimulating and recording electrodes in the two sides of the motor cortex slices. *B:* (example) and *C:* (group average) EPSPs recorded from trained animals and untrained controls. The dark lines represent recordings from the trained hemisphere and dotted lines recordings from the untrained hemisphere (from Rioult-Pedotti et al., 1998).

verse approach is to draw cause-and-effect links between the phenome-nology of LTP and of memory by blocking LTP and determining if mem-ory is prevented. Perhaps the most compelling and straightforward data on a potential connection between the molecular basis of LTP and mem-ory have come from experiments where a drug or genetic manipulation is used to block LTP and, correspondingly, prevent learning. Here again there was the need for optimistic assumptions. It had to be assumed that the drugs were selective to plasticity and not normal information processing in the brain, and that they would knock out a critical kind of plasticity. These assumptions were accepted based on the observation that drugs such as AP5, which selectively blocks the NMDA receptor, prevent hippocam-pal LTP while sparing normal synaptic transmission. Thus, to the extent that the role of the NMDA receptor is fully selective to plasticity, one might predict these drugs would indeed block new learning without af-fecting nonlearning performance or retention of learning normally ac-complished prior to drug treatment.

Consistent with these predictions some of the earliest and strongest ev-idence supporting a connection between LTP and memory came from stud-ies on spatial learning by Richard Morris and his colleagues. Morris de-veloped a maze learning task in which hippocampal function is required. In this task, the maze involves a swimming pool in which the water is made opaque by the addition of a milky powder, and an escape platform is submerged just under the water at a predetermined location. Rats are good swimmers, but prefer to find and climb onto the platform. Typically, they are trained to find the platform from any of four starting positions around the periphery of the maze, and they show learning by shortening the time required to escape from all starting points. At the end of train-ing, their memory is assessed using a probe test where the platform is re-moved, and rats exhibit good memory by swimming in the vicinity of the former escape locus.

Initially Morris and his colleagues showed that AP5-induced blockade of NMDA receptors prevents new spatial learning in the water maze. Drug-treated rats swim normally, but do not reach the same level of rapid es-cape as normal rats. Indeed, the drug-treated rats often adopt a strategy of swimming at a particular distance from the walls of the maze, which reduces their escape latency to some extent without knowing the exact lo-cation of the platform. In the probe tests, normal rats show a distinct pref-erence for swimming in the vicinity of the former escape locus, but drug-treated rats show little or no such bias, indicating the absence of memory for the escape location (see Chapter 5 for further discussion of this task). Additional experiments showed no effect of AP5 on retention when training was accomplished prior to drug treatment. This could be fully predicted because NMDA receptors are viewed as required only for the induction of LTP and not for its maintenance (see Molecular bases for induction and maintenance of hippocampal LTP). Furthermore, the deficit was limited to spatial learning, known from other work to be dependent on the hippocampus, and not to a simple visual discrimination, known to be NOT dependent on hippocampal function.

Additional research by Morris and his colleagues has also shown how NMDA receptor dependent LTP might play a continuing role in updating one's memories. To accomplish this they developed a new version of the water maze task in which the location of the escape platform is moved every day, and animals are given four trials to learn the new location. Across a series of training days the rats became skilled at the task such that they consistently found the platform very rapidly on the second trial it was presented. Subsequent to initial drug-free training, animals were tested with different memory delays inserted between the first and second trial on each day (Fig. 3–9A). On some days, AP5 was infused into the hippocampus, and on other days a placebo was given. AP5 treatment resulted in a deficit on trial 2 performance (Fig. 3–9B). Moreover, this deficit was dependent on the time interval between trial 1 and trial 2, such that no impairment was observed with a 15 second intertrial interval, but significant deficits ensued if the intertrial interval was extended to 20 minutes or longer. These data suggest that memory for specific episodes of spatial learning remains dependent on NMDA receptors and LTP, even after the animals have learned the environment and the general rules of the spatial task.

Genetic manipulations of LTP and memory

Other research has used targeted genetic manipulations to show that blocking the cascade of molecular triggers for LTP also results in severe memory impairments. In one of the early studies of this type, mice with a mutation of one form of CaMKII had deficient LTP and were selectively impaired in learning the Morris water maze. Despite the fact that the genetic manipulation was effective throughout development, the hippocampus appeared normal in architecture and was normal in its basic physiological responsiveness. Since that time, selective memory impairments have been reported in several different types of knockout mice with deficiencies in LTP, with a special emphasis on knockouts of CREB.

The manipulation of biochemical mechanisms by interference with specific genes allows investigators to identify critical molecular events at a very high level of specificity. For example, one study by Alcino Silva and

A.

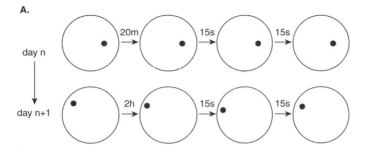

B.

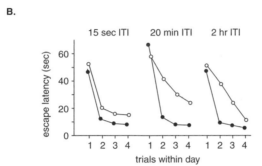

Figure 3–9. Matching-to-place version of the Morris water maze task A: Example test sessions. On each session the animal is given four trials with the escape platform in a novel location. Note that the first intertrial interval is variable, and the others are constant at 15 sec. B: Effects of infusion of AP5. After initial training on the task, rats treated with AP5 or placebo were tested on a series of four-trial sessions with the escape platform in a novel location each day. On some test sessions the interval between trials 1 and 2 was 15 sec. On these sessions rats given AP5 performed as well as normal subjects in showing a substantial reduction in the latency that indicated intact memory On other sessions the interval between trials 1 and 2 was 20 min or 2 hr. On these sessions normal animals also showed good retention, but AP5 rats showed substantially less reduction in their escape latencies, indicating memory impairment. The later intertrial intervals were all 15 sec, and all animals show substantial latency decreases over these brief intervals. Filled circles = controls; open circles = AP5 (data from Morris and Frey, 1997).

his colleagues showed that substitution of a single amino acid in CaMKII that prevents its autophosphorylation results in severe learning and memory deficits. In addition, other new genetic approaches are providing greater temporal- as well as region-specific blockade of gene activation. In another recent study by Susumu Tonegawa and his colleagues, the genetic block was limited to postdevelopment activation of the genes for the NMDA receptor specifically in the CA1 subfield of the hippocampus, which selectively blocked LTP in that region. Despite these highly selective temporal and anatomical restrictions, the mice with this mutation were severely deficient in spatial learning as well as in other types of memory dependent on hippocampal function. A complementary recent study showed that a mutation that results in overexpression of NMDA receptors can enhance several kinds of memory dependent on the hippocampus. There is also growing evidence that interference with other events involved in the LTP molecular cascade, specifically PKC and MAPK, also have deleterious effects on memory. Thus, it is likely that the full set of cellular events that mediate LTP will also be shown to play critical roles in memory.

Blocking LTP and plasticity of hippocampal firing patterns

The studies described previously provide strong evidence in favor of the view that pharmacological and genetic manipulations that prevent hippocampal plasticity selectively block a critical stage in memory formation. However, skeptical neuroscientists are always concerned that a particular drug or genetic manipulation could have its deleterious effects not on memory directly, but rather on the normal information processing in brain structures that play a role in task performance. In general the best evidence offered in pharmacological and genetic studies involves the observation that the drugs or genetic manipulations do not affect synaptic transmission as revealed in evoked potential protocols. However, it is important to realize that large-scale evoked EPSPs never actually occur during normal information processing. So the data available from these studies do not allow us to conclude that other more complex, and more relevant, patterns of hippocampal information processing are fully normal under the influence of drugs such as AP5.

A newer generation of combined electrophysiological and pharmacological-genetic studies is providing evidence critical to this question. Several studies have how examined the nature and persistence of spatial representations of single hippocampal neurons and neuronal populations in animals with compromised capacity for LTP. These studies involve genetically altered mice or rats with pharmacologically blocked LTP and recordings of so-called place cells, hippocampal neurons that fire when the animal is in a particular location in its environment (see Chapter 6 for a detailed explanation of place cells). One of these studies found that mutant mice expressing an active form of CaMKII that impairs one form of LTP and spatial learning have impoverished and unstable hippocampal spatial representations. Hippocampal cells of these mice initially develop

spatially specific firing patterns, albeit in fewer cells, and the spatial specificity of these patterns is reduced. Perhaps most important, unlike normal
mice who have very stable hippocampal spatial representations, the spatial firing patterns in mutant mice are lost or changed if the animal is removed from the environment and later replaced even within a few minutes. Acute pharmacological blockade of NMDA receptors in rats also
resulted in instability of the spatial firing patterns of hippocampal neurons, without affecting the incidence or spatial specificity of previously acquired spatial firing patterns. The drug did not prevent the initial establishment of hippocampal spatial firing patterns or their short-term
retention between repeated recording sessions separated by brief intervals.
By contrast the maintenance of a newly developed spatial representation
across days was severely compromised.

The consequence of LTP blockade for the network processing of hippocampal spatial representations has also been examined. One study examined the spatial firing patterns of groups of neighboring hippocampal
neurons in mice with the CA1-specific knockout of NMDA receptors. They
also reported that these cells had diminished spatial specificity, and characterized a reduction in the coordinated activity of neurons tuned to overlapping spatial locations. Furthermore, they tied these findings to the spatial memory impairment by showing how the loss of coordinated activity
in mutant hippocampal place cells leads to a poorer prediction of sequential
locations during navigation behavior. Another study characterized hippocampal spatial representations in mice with knockouts of CaMKII or
CREB. Similar to the other studies, they observed diminished spatial selectivity in both mutants, as well as diminished stability of the spatial representations when some of the environmental cues were altered. CaMKII
mutant mice could not recover their spatial representations when the environmental cues were returned to their original configuration. However,
the CREB-knockout mice, in whom spatial learning and LTP are partially
preserved, showed they could recover their spatial representations in the
original environment. These results suggest that the network processes that
bind together single neuron representations of spatial cues are particularly
dependent on LTP. Further investigations on the coding of space by hippocampal networks offer a particularly promising direction for relating
synaptic plasticity processes to memory functions.

Blocking LTP and memory outside the hippocampus

Other studies suggest that the cascade of molecular events that is invoked
by LTP may also mediate cortical plasticity that underlies memory. A par-

ticularly good example of this work involves a set of studies by Yadin Dudai and his colleagues focused on taste learning mediated by the gustatory cortex of rats. When rats are exposed to a novel taste and subsequently become ill, they develop a conditioned aversion specifically to that taste, and this learning is known to depend on the gustatory cortex. Blockade of NMDA receptors by infusion of the antagonist AP5 produces an impairment in taste aversion learning, whereas the same injections given prior to retention testing, or into an adjacent cortical area, had no effect. Thus, it is likely that modifications in cortical taste representations depend on LTP. Furthermore, blockade of protein synthesis in the gustatory cortex by infusion of an inhibitor prior to learning also prevents development of the conditioned taste aversion. By contrast, the same injection given into a neighboring cortical area or given to the gustatory cortex hours after learning has no effect. Consistent with this finding, MAP kinase as well as a downstream protein kinase were activated selectively in gustatory cortex within 10 minutes of exposure to a novel taste and activation peaked at 30 minutes, whereas exposure to a familiar taste had no effect. Conversely, a MAP kinase inhibitor retarded conditioned taste aversion. This combination of findings provides complementary lines of evidence that strongly implicate the NMDA mediated plasticity and subsequent specific protein synthesis as playing a critical role in cortical modifications that mediate this type of learning.

Summing up

In mammalian systems, the most popular model for the cellular and molecular mechanisms that underlie memory is long-term potentiation (LTP) and its sister phenomenon long-term depression (LTD). Both phenomena follow Hebb's rule in that increases in synaptic efficacy (facilitation of synaptic transmission) marking LTP occur as a consequence of repeated activation of a presynaptic element and its participation in the success in firing the postsynaptic cell, whereas decreases in synaptic efficacy (decrements in synaptic transmission) marking LTD occur as a consequence of the absence of correspondence between activation of a presynaptic element and postsynaptic cell activation.

An understanding of the molecular and cellular mechanisms of some forms of LTP is emerging. The induction of one prominent form of LTP involves the activation of NMDA receptors, which occurs when a non-NMDA receptor is initially activated to depolarize the postsynaptic cell, causing the release of a magnesium block of the NMDA receptor allowing the transmitter glutamate to activate that receptor. This results in an influx of calcium which begins a molecular cascade of events that both stabilizes the changes in the postsynaptic cell and induces gene expression and permanent cellular modifications.

Does LTP equal memory, and do we now understand memory in mammalian systems? There is certainly no consensus among researchers that LTP and memory are the same thing, or even that the case for common mechanisms is strong and closed. As described here, there are compelling lines of evidence favoring this view. There is evidence that LTP enhances learning-related information processing, and conversely that learning results in enhancement of synaptic potentials in circuits relevant to particular forms of memory. Correspondingly, there is evidence that blocking LTP with drugs or genetic manipulations can result in a pattern of amnesia reflected both in memory impairments and instability of relevant neural representations. So, while there is also some contradictory evidence, not outlined here, at least a provisional case for shared mechanisms has emerged.

In the simpler invertebrate systems discussed in Chapter 2, the circuits that mediated forms of habituation, sensitization, and classical conditioning were mostly identified. So, the additional evidence about cellular changes and their molecular mechanisms seems to offer fairly comprehensive framework for an understanding of memory in those systems. In reading this chapter, though, you were introduced to fragments of a few of the brain circuits involved in learning in mammalian systems, and to a few of the different kinds of learning in which they participate. You have not yet seen the full circuitry involved in any of these systems. Nor have you yet heard about why they mediate different forms of learning, or about how many systems and forms of learning exist. Even for the hippocampus itself, you have only been provided with a glimpse of its role in memory and the nature of the information represented within its circuitry. Completing these stories is a major aim of the remainder of this book.

At this point, you should be impressed with the conservation of fundamental cellular and molecular mechanisms of memory across species and brain systems. In all the examples discussed, changes in synaptic efficacy are central. And these changes seem to be subserved by a relatively small set of pervasive molecular mechanisms that reveal a cascade of events that leads from short-term modulation to permanent structural alteration of synapses. Within simpler, well-understood circuitries, this cascade provides a more or less comprehensive picture of memory accomplished. Within more complex circuitries, a higher level of analysis will be required to reach a full understanding of the systems, circuits, and codes for memory.

READINGS

Bear, M.F. 1996. A synaptic basis for memory storage in the cerebral cortex. *Proc. Nat. Acad. Sci. U.S.A.* 93:13453–13459.

Bliss, T.V.P., and Collinridge, G.L. 1993. A synaptic model of memory: Long-term potentiation in the hippocampus. *Nature* 361: 31–39.

Malenka, R.C. 1994. Synaptic plasticity in the hippocampus: LTP and LTD. *Cell* 78: 535–538.

Morris, R.G.M. 1989. Does synaptic plasticity play a role in information storage in the vertebrate brain. In *Parallel Distributed Processing: Implications for Psychology and Neurobiology*, Morris, R.G.M. (Ed.). Oxford: Clarendon Press, pp. 248–285.

Morris, R.G.M., and Frey, U. 1997. Hippocampal synaptic plasticity: Role in spatial learning or the automatic recording of attended experience? *Phil. Trans. R. Soc. Lond.* 352: 1489–1503.

Rioult-Pedotti, M.-S., Friedman, D., Hess, G., and Donoghue, J.P. 1998. Strengthening of horizontal cortical connections following skill learning. Nat. Neurosci. 1:230–234.

Rogan, M.T., Staubli, U.V., and LeDoux, J.E.. 1997. Fear conditioning induces associative long-term potentiation in the amygdala. *Nature* 390:604-607.

Silva, A.J., Smith, A.M., and Giese, K.P. 1997. Gene targeting and the biology of learning and memory. *Annu. Rev. Gene.* 31:527–547.

Steele, R.J. and Morris, R.G.M. (1999) Delay dependent impairment in matching-to-place task with chronic and intrahippocampal infusion of the NMDA-antagonist D-AP5. *Hippocampus* 9:118–136.

Stevens, C.F. 1998. A million dollar question: Does LTP = memory. *Neuron* 20: 1–2.

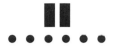

COGNITION:
IS THERE A "COGNITIVE" BASIS
FOR MEMORY?

William James may have best captured the essence of the distinction between the behaviorist and cognitivist views of memory in his turn of the twentieth century text, *The Principles of Psychology*. While acknowledging that habits (learned reflexes) could be chained to mediate even rather complicated and coordinated, sequences, such a form of representation lacked the flexibility and consciousness that characterized real memory. He qualified true memory as "the knowledge of an event, or fact, of which in the meantime we have not been thinking, with the additional consciousness that we have thought or experienced it before" (p. 648). Even in acknowledging that conditioning could revive an image or copy of a prior event, such a revival would not really be a true memory—to be a true memory, the image must not only be conceived of as in the past, but as in one's *own* past, and the memory must contain one's own experience with the item. This, James argued, would come about only by retrieving memories within a network of associated information, and bringing this network-memory up to the realm of consciousness. But, other than suggesting this would require a vastly complicated brain process, James was at a loss to offer details on the mechanisms of conscious recollection.

By contrast, the behaviorist school that emerged in the Golden Era promised tight experimental control and a detailed understanding of the elements of learning within the context of findings emerging from Pavlov's physiological studies. So ignoring James's admonitions, the behaviorists held sway in the thinking of most learning theorists for several decades. Nevertheless, battles between the "behaviorists" and "cognitivists" would continue for that entire period. A major early challenge came from Yerkes, who, based on his extensive observations of problem solving in great apes, concluded that higher animals did not learn by random trial and error with reinforcement guiding behavior, but rather exhibited ideation and insight. A greater degree of success in challenging the reductionist approach was achieved by two later experimentalists, Edward Tolman and Fredric Bartlett, working with rats and humans, respectively.

Tolman and the "cognitive map"

In the 1930s and 1940s Edward Tolman was more successful in challenging behaviorism precisely because he developed operational definitions for mentalistic processes including "purposive behavior" and "expectancy." Moreover, he rigorously tested these ideas using the same species (rats) and maze learning paradigms that were a major focus of prominent behaviorists. Tolman and his students performed several experiments pitting these views against one another in analyses of maze learning by rats. Their studies focused on whether rats could demonstrate "insight" by taking a roundabout route or shortcut in a maze when such strategies were warranted, and were inconsistent with a previous reward history that favored a different route. For example, in an experiment that demonstrated detour taking in rats, Tolman used an elevated maze that involved three diverging and then converging routes from a starting place to a goal box (Fig. II-1). During preliminary training the rat could take any route, and came to prefer the shortest. When this route was blocked (at block A) most rats would prefer to switch to the next shortest route. Only when this route was also blocked would they take the longest path. In the critical test phase, a new block was introduced at the point where the two shorter paths converged (block B). Rats began by running down the shortest path (path 1) as usual. But instead of immediately selecting the next shortest path (path 2), as they had done during the preliminary phase when the shortest route (path 1) was blocked, most rats immediately selected path 3.

In addition to this "detour" ability, Tolman also provided evidence that rats could take shortcuts. In this experiment rats were trained to approach a goal via a single circuitous route, then the maze was substituted with many direct paths, some leading toward and others away from the goal locus. Most rats ran to the path that took them directly to where the entrance of the food box had originally been located. These studies provided compelling operational evidence of Tolman's assertions that rats had inferential capacities revealed in the flexibility of the behavioral repertoire that could be brought to bear in solving problems for which behavioral theory had no explanation.

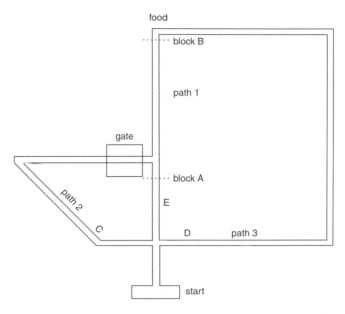

Figure. II-1. Schematic diagram of the maze Tolman used to test the ability of rats to infer a detour.

Thus, Tolman's basic premise was that learning generally involved the acquisition of *knowledge* about the world, and in particular about relationships among stimuli and between stimuli and their consequences, and that this knowledge led to expectancies when the animal was put in testing situations. His views contrasted sharply with those of the behaviorists on three key features of learning. First, the behaviorists argued that the contents of memory involve habits that can be characterized as acquired stimulus–response reflex sequences. But for Tolman learning involved the creation of a "cognitive map" that organized the relations among stimuli and consequences that would guide behavioral solutions to obtain desired consequences.

Second, for the behaviorists reinforcement was the central driving force of learning. Thorndike's "law of effect" attributes all learning to the principle that behaviors that lead to a positive reinforcement strengthen stimulus–response connections and are thus more likely to be repeated. Alternatively, Pavlov had proposed that learning involved the association of conditioned and unconditioned stimulus through temporal contiguity. In Pavlov's paradigm, that key association was between the bell, as conditioned stimulus, and the taste of food as unconditioned stimulus; through the learned association the bell comes to substitute for the food taste in evoking salivation. For Tolman, however, reinforcers served simply as more information on which to confirm one's expectancies about when, where, and how rewards were to be obtained—learning itself was driven not by reinforcement but by curiosity about the environment and seeking of knowledge for expectancies about its predictive structure. Reinforcers would certainly determine what behavior might eventually be emitted, but were not necessary for establishment of the representation.

Third, for the behaviorists the responses emitted are precisely the motor commands that are the end point of stimulus–response reflexes. The range of behavioral responses then is fully determined as the motor patterns that were elicited and reinforced during learning itself. But to Tolman, learning and performance were fundamentally independent events. That is, what an animal knew about the world and what it was going to do about it were surely related (through its expectancies), but were not the same thing, as the behaviorists held. Thus, Tolman argued, animals could use their cognitive maps and expectancies to guide the expression of learned behavior in a variety of ways not limited to repetition of the behavioral patterns exhibited and reinforced during learning. These aspects of expectancy, insight, and flexibility will prove to be important aspects of modern views of memory.

It would be too strong to say that Tolman's arguments were sufficiently compelling to cause learning theorists to abandon the reductionist views. Indeed, as shown by the success of B.F. Skinner's successes in the 1950s and 1960s, the behaviorist school still played out a long run in research laboratories, in the development of some clinical approaches to abnormal behavioral patterns in people, and in the popular press.

Frederic Barlett and the "schema"

Around the same time as Tolman was carrying out his classic studies on maze learning in rats, the British psychologist Frederic Bartlett published a treatise on human memory. And just as Tolman's theory challenged stimulus–response behaviorism, Barlett's work stood in stark contrast to the then established and better known rigorous methods introduced by Ebbinghaus, which guided the pursuits of most of his contemporary psychologists. However, Bartlett's insights about the structure and richness of memory have proven to be critical for modern views of memory. His work was central in bringing the field of memory research back to issues about the nature of the more complex forms of memory that support conscious recollection. Bartlett differed diametrically from Ebbinghaus in two major ways. First, his interest was in the mental processes used to remember. He was not so interested in the probability of recall, as dominated Ebbing-haus's approach, but in what he called "effort after meaning," the mental processing taken to search out and ultimately reconstruct memories. Second, Bartlett shuddered at the notion of using nonsense syllables as learning materials. By avoiding meaningful items, he argued, the resulting memories would necessarily lack the rich background of knowledge into which new information is stored. Barlett's main strategy to study recollection was called the method of repeated reproduction. His best known work examined recollections of a South American Indian folk tale written in a syntax and prose style that were quite different from the culture of his British experimental subjects. In particular the story contents lacked explicit connections between some of the events described, and the tale contained dramatic and supernatural events that would evoke vivid visual imagery on the part of his subjects. These qualities were, of course, exactly the sort of thing Ebbinghaus worked so hard to avoid with his nonsense syllables. But Bartlett focused on these features because he was primarily interested in the content and structure of the memory obtained.

Bartlett did not use rigorous operational definitions or statistical measures, but his analyses were compelling nonetheless. Bartlett concluded that remembering was not simply a process of recovering or forgetting items, but rather that memory seemed to evolve over time. Items were not lost or recovered at random, as Ebbinghaus might predict. Rather, material that was more foreign to the subject, or lacked sequence, or was stated in unfamiliar terms, was more likely to be lost or changed substantially in both syntax and meaning, becoming more consistent with the subject's common experiences. These and many other examples led Bartlett to develop an account of remembering known as "schema" theory, in which a schema is an active organization of past experiences in which, during remembering, one constructs or infers the probable constituents of a memory and the order in which they occurred. He proposed that remembering is therefore a *reconstructive* process and not one of mere *reproduction*, as Ebbinghaus preferred. In Bartlett's terms, remembering required the ability to "turn round" on one's own schemata, using consciousness to search within the simpler learned sequences for rational and consistent order and to reconstruct them anew consistent with one's whole life of experience. In this way Bartlett gave consciousness a function beyond merely being aware. It played a central role in the reconstructive act of remembering, making it consciously mediated, running contrary to current psychological views that would banish references to consciousness.

Ultimately, behaviorist-versus-cognitivist controversy on the nature of memory would be resolved by observations from neuroscience. This work involved examinations of amnesic patients, people who were suffering severe memory loss as a result of specific brain damage. While debilitating, it turns out that the memory capacity lost was selective to aspects of conscious recollection described by James and Bartlett, and had properties shared with Tolman's characterizations of the cognitive map. Other capacities that the behaviorists might recognize as intact stimulus–response learning were spared, even in severe cases of amnesia in humans. Parallel studies on animals with experimental brain damage in the same brain areas implicated in human amnesia provided additional insights into the anatomical psychological bases and fundamental psychological mechanisms of cognitive memory. In addition, related physiological observations provide an understanding of the coding elements that underlie the cognitive mechanisms in conscious memory. These findings are the focus of this section.

READINGS

Bartlett, F.C. 1932. *Remembering*. London: Cambridge University Press.

James, W. 1890. *The Principles of Psychology*. New York: Dover Publications (1950 edition).

Tolman, E.C. 1932. *Purposive Behavior in Animals and Men*. Berkeley: University of California Press (1951 edition).

4
• • • • • •

Amnesia—
Learning about
Memory from Memory Loss

STUDY QUESTIONS

Who is H.M. and why is he so valuable to memory research?

What nonmemory abilities are spared in amnesia?

What memory capacities are spared in amnesia?

How is the kind of memory lost in amnesia best characterized?

Over 50 years of experimentation on the course of normal learning did not resolve the debate between behaviorists and cognitivists. But studies on the loss of memory in humans, the phenomenon of amnesia, provided a pair of breakthroughs that has led to an understanding and validation of both the behaviorist and the cognitivist views.

The first major breakthrough came with the 1957 report by Scoville and Milner on the most famous neurological patient ever, a man known by his initials H.M. This patient had been severely epileptic for several years. In an effort to alleviate his disorder, the medial temporal lobe area was removed, and indeed the surgery did reduce the frequency of his seizures considerably. However, following the surgery this patient became severely amnesic, and yet showed hardly any other neurological deficits. Because of both the severity and the selectivity of his memory deficit, the findings on H.M. changed everything about how we think about the brain and memory. Before H.M. the search for memories was focused on the cerebral cortex—in H.M. the critical damage was in areas underneath the cortex. Before H.M. the generally held view was that memory and other perceptual and cognitive functions were not anatomically separable—H.M. showed a clear dissociation between fully intact perception and cognition versus severely impaired memory. The observations on the pattern of his impairment directly addressed the nature of cognitive processes in memory; these findings are discussed in this chapter in detail. The discovery of a "pure" memory deficit following selective brain damage also addressed how memory is compartmentalized in the brain, and that topic is discussed in the next section of this book. In addition, a prominent component of H.M.'s amnesia is a temporally graded retrograde memory impairment, like that of Ribot's patients introduced in Chapter 1, and the implications of these findings for the phenomenon of consolidation are discussed in greater detail in Chapter 12.

The initial observations did not at first provide clarification about the nature of cognitive processes in memory. H.M.'s loss of everyday memory was "global," that is, it appeared to encompass all kinds of memories, and in this broad scope did not directly reveal anything about the memory processes that underlie the deficit. Yet, even from the outset, exceptions to H.M.'s global amnesia were noted—he was able to learn new motor skills. In addition, another hint of an exception to the otherwise pervasive scope of amnesia came from the observation that prior exposure to picture or words could facilitate later identification of those items from fragmentary information. But these spared capacities at first seemed meager compared to the devastation of his overall memory capacity.

A deeper understanding about the exceptions came in 1980 when Neal Cohen and Larry Squire made a second major breakthrough in understanding the nature of the memory processing deficit behind amnesia. They described a complete preservation of the acquisition, retention over several months, and expression of a perceptual skill in amnesic patients. The behavioral paradigm they explored involved an improvement in fluency during reading of mirror-reversed words. Ordinarily one is slow in deciphering a word that is presented "backward," that is, with each of the letters reversed as if seen in a mirror. However, with practice one improves considerably at this general skill, even when none of the particular words are repeated. Cohen and Squire found that this kind of learning was fully normal in a set of amnesic patients.

In addition, when normal subjects were presented the same mirror-reversed words a second time, they showed an extra level of facilitation in reading them beyond that explained by the general skill acquisition—that is, they showed memory for the particular mirror-reversed words they had seen before. However, the amnesic patients were markedly impaired both in recognizing the familiar words and in recollecting their training experiences. Cohen and Squire were struck by the dissociation between the ability to acquire the general mental procedure of reading reversed text, an ability that appeared fully normal in the amnesic patients, and the capacity to explicitly remember or consciously recollect those training experiences or their contents, which was markedly impaired in the amnesics. They attributed the observed dissociation of these two kinds of memory performance, together with the earlier reported exceptions to amnesia, to the operation of distinct forms of memory. Cohen and Squire suggested that the medial temporal region was specialized for *declarative memory,* the capacity to consciously recollect everyday facts and events, and that other brain regions were sufficient to mediate a collection of learning capacities that they called *procedural memory,* the ability to tune and modify the brain's networks that support skilled performance. Two decades of research have supported this dissociation, and further characterized and distinguished the properties of declarative and procedural memory.

The following sections provide a more detailed overview of the patient H.M., in order to provide a closer perspective on the nature of his amnesia. Then the distinction between declarative and procedural memory is explored further, using several examples from the experimental literature on amnesia.

The amnesic patient H.M.

In 1933, when H.M. was 7 years old, he was knocked down by a bicycle, hit his head, and was unconscious for 5 minutes. Three years after that accident he began to have minor epileptic seizures, followed by his first major seizure while riding in his parents car on his 16th birthday. Because of the epileptic attacks his high school education was erratic, but eventually he graduated in 1947 at age 21 with a "practical" course focus. Subsequently, he worked on an assembly line as a motor winder. However, the seizures became more frequent, on average 10 minor attacks each day and a major one each week, and he eventually could not perform his job. Attempts to control the seizures with large doses of anticonvulsant drugs were unsuccessful, leading to consideration of a brain operation. There was no evidence of localization from electroencephalographic (EEG) studies. Nevertheless, because of the known epileptogenic qualities of the medial temporal lobe areas, an experimental operation was considered justified as an effort to ameliorate his devastating seizure disorder. In 1953, when H.M. was 27, Dr. William Scoville performed the bilateral medial temporal lobe resection.

The surgical approach to this area is difficult, because the relevant tissue lies inside the part of the temporal lobe near the midline, almost in the center of the brain. The surgical procedure involved making a hole above the orbits of the eyes and lifting the frontal lobes. From this approach the anterior tip of the temporal lobe could be visualized, and the medial part resected. Suction was used to remove all of the tissue bordering the lateral ventricle, including the anterior two-thirds of the hippocampus, as well as the amygdala and surrounding cortex very selectively (Fig. 4–1).

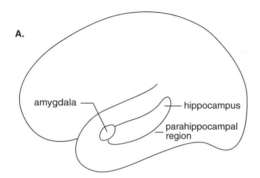

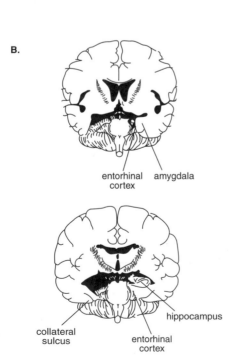

Figure 4–1. A: Position of the hippocampus, amygdala, and surrounding cortex in the human brain. B: Sections through the human brain showing reconstructions of the area of medial temporal lobe removal in the patient H.M., based on MRI scans. Top: A more anterior section showing the area of removal that involved the amygdala (left side) compared to the intact area (right side). Bottom: A more posterior section showing the area of removal that involved the hippocampus (left side) as compared to the intact area on the right. In H.M. the lesions were bilateral (from Corkin et al., 1997).

The operation reduced the frequency of seizures to a point that they are now largely prevented by medication, although minor attacks persist. However, one striking and totally unexpected consequence of the surgery was a major loss of memory capacity. Because of the combination of the unusual purity of the ensuing memory disorder, the static nature of his condition, his cooperative nature, and the skill of the researchers who have protected and worked with him, H.M., is probably the most examined and best known neurological patient ever studied.

After recovery from his operation, H.M. returned home and lived with his parents. There he did household chores, watched TV, and solved crossword puzzles. Following his father's death he attended a rehabilitation workshop and became somewhat of a handyman, doing simple and repetitive jobs. Eventually his mother and then another relative could no longer care for him, so he was moved to a nursing home where he still resides, participating in daily social activities of the home, as well as watching TV and solving difficult crossword puzzles. He is characterized as a highly amiable and cooperative individual. He rarely complains about anything, and has to be quizzed to identify minor problems such as headaches. He never spontaneously asks for food or beverage, or to go to bed, but he readily follows directions for all of his daily activities. His temper is generally very placid, although this author recalls one day when H.M. was depressed about "having not done anything with his life." However, when assured that he was indeed a very important person, his mood returned to its normal rather upbeat state, and he told one of his famous stories about once considering a career in neurosurgery. He is aware of his memory disorder, but is not consistently concerned about it. Sometimes when given a rather difficult memory question he reminds the tester, "You know I have a memory problem." The severe magnitude of his memory disorder has continued unabated since the time of the surgery.

Some of the most compelling examples of the severity of H.M.'s amnesia come from anecdotes of those who have worked with him. I recall my first encounter with H.M., while transporting him from the nursing home to M.I.T. for a testing period in 1980. On the way to the nursing home, I had stopped at a nearby McDonald's for lunch, and had left a coffee cup on the dashboard of the car. When I retrieved H.M., I sat him comfortably in the back seat and we began the trip to Boston. After just a few minutes H.M. noticed the cup and said, "Hey, I knew a fellow named John McDonald when I was a boy!" He proceeded to tell some of his adventures with the friend, and so I asked a few questions and was impressed with the elaborate memories he had of that childhood period. Eventually the story ended and H.M. turned to watch the scenery passing by. After just a few more minutes, he looked up at the dashboard and remarked,

"Hey, I knew a fellow named John McDonald when I was a boy!" and proceeded to relate virtually the identical story. I asked probing questions in an effort to continue the interaction and to determine if the facts of the story would be the same. H.M. never noticed he had just told this elaborate tale, and repeated the story more or less exactly as before. A few minutes later the conversation ended, and he turned to view the scenery again. However, just minutes later, once more H.M. looked up to the dashboard and exclaimed, "Hey, I knew a fellow named John McDonald when I was a boy!" I helped him reproduce, as well as he could, the same conversation yet again, then quickly disposed of the cup under the seat. . . .

The selective nature of H.M.'s memory disorder

H.M.'s disorder is highly selective in two important ways. First, his impairment is almost entirely selective to memory, as distinguished from other higher-order perceptual, motor, and cognitive functions. Second, even within his memory functions, the disorder is selective to particular domains of learning and memory capacity. Some of the details concerning these two aspects of his preserved and impaired capacities are discussed next.

H.M.'s perceptual, motor, and cognitive functions are intact

The results of extensive testing of sensory functions showed that H.M.'s perceptual capacities are entirely normal. He performs well within the normal range on tests of visual acuity, adaptation, and other commonly tested visual-perceptual functions. He can recognize and name common objects. He has some loss of touch and fine motor coordination revealed in sophisticated tests, but these are not noticed in his generally good performance on tasks that require coordination in his daily environment. H.M.'s intelligence was above average in standard IQ tests just before the operation. After the surgery his IQ actually rose somewhat, perhaps because of the alleviation of his seizures. H.M.'s language capacities are largely intact, although he exhibits slight deficits in the fluency of his speech, and his spelling is poor. He appreciates puns and linguistic ambiguities, and communicates well and freely. His spatial perceptual capacities that do not depend on memory are mixed. For example, he has some difficulty copying a complex line drawing, and cannot use a floor plan to walk a route from one room to another in the M.I.T. testing facility. On the other hand, he does well on other complex spatial perceptual tasks, and can draw and recognize an accurate floor plan of his former house.

By contrast, H.M. has almost no capacity for new learning, as measured by a large variety of conventional tests. He was not given standard memory tests prior to the operation. After the surgery his scores on standardized scales indicated a severe memory disorder. In particular, he scores zero on components of the test that assess the persistence of his memory for short stories, lists of words or numbers, pictures, or any of a large range of other materials.

H.M's memories acquired in childhood are intact, and his immediate memory capacity is normal

H.M. can remember material learned remotely prior to his operation. His memory for the English language seems fully intact. He also retains many childhood memories. By contrast, all memory for events for some period preceding the operation was lost. In addition, H.M.'s immediate or short-term memory is intact. He can immediately reproduce a list of numbers as long as that of control subjects—thus the "span" of his short-term memory is normal. However, the memory deficit becomes evident as soon as his immediate memory span is exceeded or after a delay with some distraction. These aspects of H.M.'s spared memory abilities are discussed further in later chapters.

"Exceptions" to H.M.'s impairment in new learning

The early studies on H.M. also revealed a few "exceptions" to his otherwise profound defect in lasting memory. One of these, called mirror drawing, involved the acquisition of sensorimotor skill. In this task the subject sits at a table viewing a line drawing and one's hand only through a mirror (Fig. 4–2). The line drawing contains two concentric outlines of a star, and the task is to draw a pencil line within the outlines. Errors are scored each time an outline border is contacted. This test may seem simple, but in fact normal subjects require several trials before they can successfully draw the line without committing crossover errors. H.M. showed strikingly good improvement over several attempts within the initial session, and considerable retention of this skill across sessions, to the extent that he consistently made very few errors on the third test day. This success in learning this sensorimotor skill contrasted with his inability to recall ever having taken the test.

In addition, H.M. also showed strikingly good performance in perceptual learning in a task called the Gollins partial pictures task, which involves the recognition of fragmented line drawings of common objects. For each of 20 items, subjects are presented with a series of five cards containing fragments of a realistic line drawing of the same object. The first card of each series contains the fewest fragments of the drawing and the last card contains the complete drawing (Fig. 4–3). Subjects are initially

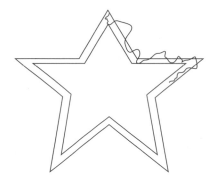

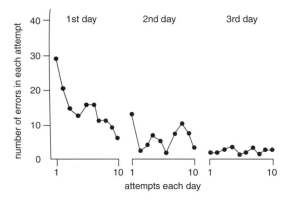

Figure 4–2. The mirror drawing test. *Top:* Sketch of the double-star pattern and the beginning of a typical early attempt at drawing a line between the boundaries. *Bottom:* H.M.'s performance across 10 attempts on 3 successive days (data from Milner et al., 1968).

shown all 20 of the most difficult items and asked to identify the object drawn on each one. Then the second, slightly more complete version of each item is presented with the ordering of the 20 cards randomized, so it is impossible to anticipate an item based on its predecessor. The procedure is continued using successively more complete versions of each item until all are identified. Then, after an hour of intervening activity, the entire test is repeated, and the number of errors (unidentified drawings) is scored. Normal subjects show retention of this perceptual memory reflected in the ability to identify less complete versions of the drawings. H.M.'s scores on the retest were not as good as age-matched controls, but he showed a surprising degree of retention, especially considering he did not remember having taken the initial test.

A broad range of spared learning abilities in amnesia

The observations of Cohen and Squire showing fully intact perceptual skill learning were properly heralded as a revelation about memory processing

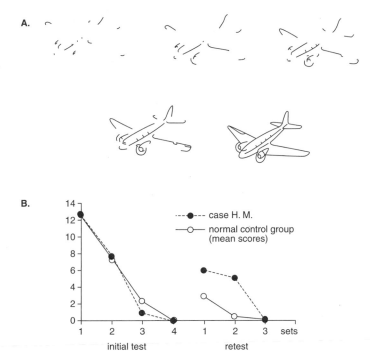

Figure 4–3. The Gollins partial pictures test. *A:* An example of the series of partial figures that compose one item on the test. *B:* Performance of H.M. and normal control subjects measured by the number of errors on the entire series on the initial test and on a delayed retest with the same items (data from Warrington and Weiskrantz, 1968).

functions accomplished by the medial temporal lobe. Subsequently, several laboratories uncovered a variety of examples of spared learning ability in amnesia. Examples from a broad range of those findings are presented next, to provide a view of the scope of preserved learning and memory capacities observed in amnesia. These include a form of perceptual learning called "priming," skill learning, Pavlovian conditioning, and sequence learning.

Priming

Perhaps the most intensively studied form of memory that can be accomplished fully normally in amnesic patients is the phenomenon known as repetition priming, or just "priming." Priming involves initial presentation of a list of words, pictures of objects, or nonverbal materials, and then subsequent reexposure to fragments or very brief presentation of the whole item. In the reexposure phase, learning is measured by increased ability to reproduce the whole item from a fragment (as in the Gollins partial pictures task described earlier) or by increased speed in making a decision about the item.

One example study particularly nicely illustrates a striking dissociation between intact priming and impaired declarative memory performance by amnesic subjects. This experiment used the word stem completion task, a test of verbal repetition priming in which subjects initially study a list of words, then are presented with the first three letters of each word (the word "stem") and asked to complete it. The stimulus words are selected as ones for which the stem can be completed more than one way to compose a high frequency word. For example, the word "MOTEL" is used because its stem "MOT——" can be completed to form either the stimulus word or "MOTHER" (see other examples in Fig. 4–4 top). Priming is measured by the increased likelihood that the subject will complete the stimulus word presented during the study phase. In this experiment, subjects initially studied a list of such words and, to make sure they attended to them, had to identify shared vowels among sets of words or rate the words according to how much they liked them. Then, in the test phase, they were presented with the three-letter word stems and tested for their memory in one of three ways. In the *free recall* condition, subjects were not presented with stems but just asked to recall the studied words. In the *cued recall* condition, subjects were presented with the word stems and told to use them as cues to remember words that were on the list. In the *completion* condition, they were presented with word stems and asked sim-

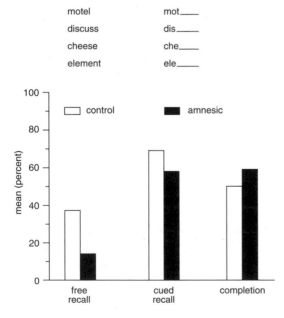

Figure 4–4. Word stem completion test of verbal priming. *Top:* On the left are examples of study words, and on the right, examples of the word stems used for cueing. *Bottom:* Performance of normal control subjects and amnesics on three versions of the test (data from Squire, 1987).

ply to "write the first word that comes to mind." The amnesics were impaired in recall as tested either with cueing or without (Fig. 4–4 bottom). By contrast, they were not impaired on the completion test. A particularly revealing comparison can be made between the performance of amnesics across the different test conditions. They did much better on the cued recall than the free recall condition, but no better on cued recall than on completion. One interpretation of these findings is that performance in cued recall might be entirely supported by priming. By contrast, the normal subjects did much better on cued recall than on priming, suggesting they used the stems to aid an active search in recalling the words.

Intact priming in amnesia is not restricted to nameable objects and verbal material. For example, H.M. also shows normal priming in a task explicitly designed to be refractory to verbalization. In this test H.M. and normal subjects were presented with a set of stimuli each of which consisted of five dots arranged in a unique pattern (Fig. 4–5 top). To establish baseline performance, subjects were asked to draw on the dots any line pattern they wished. Substantially later they were presented with a set of predetermined target patterns and asked to replicate them onto a corresponding dot pattern. After exposure to the entire list plus a distracter task, they were provided with the dot pattern again and asked to complete it any way they wished. Priming scores were calculated based on the incidence of baseline patterns. As shown in Fig. 4–5 (bottom), H.M. showed significant above chance priming for dot patterns, indicating as much memory as the normal subjects. This intact performance stood in contrast to his inability to recognize the same dot patterns when explicitly asked if he had seen them before.

Skill learning

Mirror drawing, described before, is an example of spared capacity for the acquisition of sensorimotor skills. In addition, the intact capacity to learn skills extends to the acquisition of cognitive rules. For example, in one study subjects were presented with strings of letters that were generated by an artificial "grammar" that determined general rules for sequencing and length of the letter strings (Fig. 4–6). They studied these strings by reproducing each item immediately after its presentation. Then subjects were informed that the letter strings were formed by complex rules. Subsequently they were shown novel letter strings one at a time and asked to classify them as "grammatical" or "nongrammatical" according to whether they conformed with the rules. Finally, subjects were tested to determine if they could recognize grammatic letter strings after a brief study phase. Both amnesic and normal subjects were able to correctly classify the letter strings

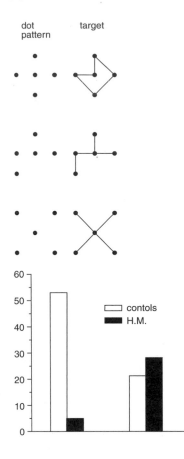

Figure 4–5. Priming for dot patterns test. *Top:* Examples of dot patterns and target completion pattern. *Bottom:* Performance (percentage correct) as measured by recognition of the target and by correct completion in normal control subjects and case H.M. (data from Gabrieli et al., 1990).

on about two-thirds of the trials. By contrast, the amnesic patients were impaired on recognition of studied grammatical items.

Classical (Pavlovian) conditioning

Modern formal studies of classical conditioning in both humans and animals have focused on conditioning of eyeblink reflexes, because these are easy paradigms to control and allow straightforward measures of learning. These studies typically involve repeated pairings of a tone or light as the conditioning stimulus (CS) and an airpuff to the eye as the unconditioned stimulus (US) that produces a reflexive blink. The measure of classical conditioning is the occurrence of eyeblinks during the CS period prior to presentation of the US, that is, conditioned eyeblink responses. Systematic studies comparing amnesic and normal subjects have demonstrated intact classical eyelid conditioning in amnesics, as well as normal extinction of conditioned responses when the CS was presented repeatedly with-

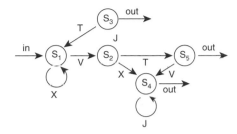

Figure 4–6. Artificial grammar test. A rule system used to string letters into "grammatical" and "nongrammatical" series, and several example items (data from Knowlton et al., 1992).

grammatical	nongrammatical
XXVT	TVT
XXVXJJ	TXXXVT
VXJJ	VXXXVJ
VTV	VJVTX

out the US. The examples of intact eyelid conditioning all involve a procedure known as "delay-conditioning," in which the presentation of the CS is prolonged and overlaps the US. Another procedure, known as "trace-conditioning," involves a brief CS followed by a trace interval during which no stimulus is presented, followed by the US alone. The distinction between these two types of classical conditioning is important because it has been shown that rabbits with hippocampal damage normally acquire the eyelid response with the delay-conditioning procedure but cannot learn under the trace-conditioning procedure. Just like rabbits with hippocampal damage, human amnesics are impaired in trace eyelid conditioning. Moreover, this deficit has been related to the conscious awareness of the stimulus contingencies.

Sequence learning

Another domain of intact learning in amnesia involves the gradual improvement in speed of performance following specific regularities in stimulus–response sequences. A compelling example of intact learning of a specific perceptual–motor habit involves manual sequence learning in a task called the serial reaction time test. On each trial subjects were shown a light at one of four locations on a computer monitor, and had to press one of four keys that corresponded to that light location. On each trial the lights were presented in a consistent pattern, and the entire pattern was presented repetitively in each training session such that subjects could anticipate the position of the next light. As a control, in separate testing blocks the sequence of light positions was randomized. Normal subjects and amnesics decreased their reaction times to press the keys, and did so at an equal rate. Both groups showed minimal improvement when the light position sequence was random, indicating that the improvement on regular sequences involved acquisition of a specific habit and not a general ability to coordinate the pressing of keys for appropriate lights.

Another example of spared learning of a specific habit in human amnesic patients comes from studies of speed reading. Several experiments have shown that amnesics improved their reading times over the course of repeating a story aloud. In these studies there was no general facilitation between stories, indicating that the habit was text-specific. Moreover, this intact capacity does not seem to rely on memory for the content of the story, as demonstrated in an experiment showing that the phenomenon extends to nonwords (pronounceable but meaningless letter strings) as well as text. However, even with nonwords, the facilitation is specific to the sequence of repeated nonwords and is not a reflection of a general learning to read new nonwords.

Characterizing the properties of declarative and procedural memory

There have been numerous attempts to identify the common properties among the types of learning and memory spared in amnesia, and to distinguish them from the common aspects of learning and memory on which amnesics fail. These comparisons have provided insights into the nature and cognitive mechanisms that underlie declarative memory, as well as properties of the domains of procedural memory.

One way to characterize declarative memory is to consider whether there is a set of common or fundamental properties of memory that is spared in amnesia. Some of the earliest findings on H.M. indicated that intact learning in amnesia is limited to motor skills or simple perceptual learning. Other studies have suggested that spared learning always involves the slow incremental acquisition of habitual routines or to specific categories of information.

However, intact learning in amnesia is not limited to general motor skills. Rather, the scope of spared memory in amnesia includes a variety of forms of highly specific new learning. Also, intact learning in amnesia is not limited to simple forms of perceptual learning or other easy tasks, as clearly shown by the improvements in very difficult tasks such as grammar learning and sequence production. In addition, spared learning in amnesia is not limited to types of learning that involve slow incremental improvement, but includes a variety of forms of one-trial learning, such as observed in numerous repetition priming tests. Indeed, priming for single exposures to pictures can be both robust and last at least a week in amnesic subjects. Finally, preserved learning in amnesia is not limited to any particular category of learning materials, as one can see in our broad range of examples, including intact learning for words, nonwords, common objects, tones, nonverbalizable pictures, motor patterns, and spatial patterns. In sum, the domain of intact learning ability is global, and it can be either fast or slow, and include both general skills and highly specific information content. Thus, the common properties among examples of intact memory in amnesia are not to be found in relatively objective parameters such as the modality of information, or the speed or specificity of memory.

Formal characterizations of nondeclarative memory

Several hypotheses have emerged from efforts to characterize the critical features that are common to intact learning in amnesia. Instead of simpler objective parameters such as those listed just previously, these proposals focus on more complex and higher-order properties, and in particular, the form of memory expression, the extent of conscious access to memories, and the structure of the memory representation.

One of the most objective attempts to formalize the general learning abilities of amnesics was provided by Morris Moscovitch in his 1984 list of sufficient conditions for demonstrating preserved memory. He focused on task demands, and argued that amnesics show savings on tests that satisfy three conditions: *(1)* the task has to be so highly structured that the goal of the task and the means to achieve it are apparent, *(2)* the means to achieve the goal are available to the subject (i.e., the response strategies are already in the subject's repertoire), and *(3)* success can be achieved without reference to any particular event or episode. Combining these, he suggested that amnesics will succeed whenever they simply have to perform a task guided by the conditions and strategies at hand. The new memory is revealed in changes of task performance itself, typically either a change in the speed of responding or in a bias of choices that are readily available.

Daniel Schacter made a similar distinction between "explicit" and "implicit" memory. Explicit memory involves conscious recollection generated by direct efforts to access memories. Explicit tests of memory involve direct inquiries that ask the subjects to refer to a specific event of learning or a specific fact in their knowledge. Examples of explicit tests of memory include, "What were the words on the list you studied?" and "Which of these two items did you see before?" The full range of explicit memory tests includes a large variety of direct measures of recall or recognition of word or picture lists, paired associates, story recall, and most of the common tests of memory that are performed so poorly by amnesic patients. Explicit memory expression also includes most everyday instances of memory, such as recalling what one had for breakfast this morning or what the capital of France is. Both examples involve conscious efforts to search for a specific event or fact.

By contrast, implicit memory involves unconscious changes in performance of a task as influenced by some previous experience. Implicit tests of memory involve indirect measures such as changes in the speed of performance or in biases in choices made during performance of a task that can be solved with the information at hand. Examples of implicit memory tests include the full variety of assessments of motor, perceptual, and cognitive skills, habits, conditioning, and repetition priming described earlier at which amnesic patients usually succeed. Notably none of these tests requires the subjects to be aware of their memory, or to "remember," a specific event or fact.

A related proposal is Endel Tulving's distinction between "episodic memory" and "semantic memory." Episodic memory contains representations of specific personal experiences that occur in a unique spatial and temporal context. Episodic memory involves the capacity to reexperience particular events in one's life, what Tulving calls "time traveling." By contrast, according to Tulving, semantic memory is the body of one's world knowledge, a vast organization of memories not bound to any specific experience in which they were acquired. Some investigators have suggested that the pattern of impaired and spared memory capacities in amnesia can be explained as an impaired episodic memory capacity and intact semantic memory. This view readily accounts for the impairment in day-to-day episodic memory ("What did you have for breakfast?"). In addition, episodic memory can strongly facilitate one's performance on many standard tests, such as one's ability to recall or recognize a recently studied list of words. Memory in these situations is stronger in normal subjects because they can refer to their episodic memory for the specific learning experience, in addition to any memory for the materials independent of that specific experience. But, according to this view, amnesics have only the episode-free record and so usually perform less well.

Furthermore, according to this view, amnesic subjects perform well on implicit memory tasks, because the memory demands avoid reference to the temporal or spatial context in which the information was acquired, and do not require the subject to refer to the learning experience directly. In these tests there is typically no advantage conferred on normal subjects in remembering the items. The episodic–semantic distinction shares much with Moscovitch's characterization of successful memory performance whenever amnesics do not have to "conjure up, that is, 'remember,' any previous experience or a newly learned fact." Indeed, the episodic–semantic and implicit–explicit views are fully compatible, to the extent that implicit memory tests always and only require semantic memory.

In support of this view, Tulving et al. described a patient, K.C., with normal intelligence, preserved general knowledge, and fragmentary general knowledge of his past. He also had expert knowledge from work done 3 years before a closed head injury. By contrast, K.C. did not remember a single personal event from his previous life and did not remember new events. He had some capacity to gradually acquire new knowledge, as demonstrated in studies aimed at very gradual accumulation of semantic knowledge by teaching methods that reduce interference associated with making errors. In addition, there are now several cases of childhood brain injury that result in amnesia for everyday life events, but near normal general world knowledge. Some of the latter cases appear to have relatively circumscribed damage to the hippocampus, suggesting specific involvement of this structure in episodic memory.

Disentangling episodic and semantic memory is a difficult problem. Surely these patients forget "facts," such as a list of words, just as rapidly as they forget daily events, such as what they had for breakfast. One study directly addressed the issue of semantic learning in amnesia by attempting to train H.M. on new vocabulary words. H.M. and normal subjects were given implicit test instructions and were directed away from conscious recollection of the events surrounding the learning experiences. Training proceeded in several phases. They first studied word definitions for eight novel vocabulary words created by the experimenters. The subjects were given a recognition test asking them to choose a definition for each word. Then they studied synonyms for the words, and were tested on a sentence completion task where they had to fill in a blank at the end of a sentence with one of the new words. Normal subjects learned the new words readily, completing each phase within a few trials. Despite an exhaustive regimen of testing, H.M. showed virtually no ability to learn new semantic knowledge.

This is not to say that amnesics cannot acquire any semantic knowledge, and indeed there are many examples of highly specific learning even for complex materials. For example, there have been demonstrations of successful learning where subjects were trained to use computer commands and terminology. The training methods used painstaking and very gradual procedures by which the commands were introduced in situations where responses were "error-free" at each stage. These subjects did subsequently show aptitude for learning new computer terms. But the range with which they could use this new learning was highly limited, such that their learning could be expressed only in replications of the precise training conditions. Schacter referred to this characteristic of their successful learning as a "hyperspecificity" of the preserved memory. Such limited applicability is not characteristic of our common use of semantic memory in solving everyday problems across a broad range of one's daily challenges.

Summing up

H.M. was important as much for the selectivity of his deficit as for its severity. Subsequent to the discovery of H.M.'s amnesia, Scoville publicized the findings, and supported Milner, Corkin, and others in their research on H.M., in great part to insure that the operation would not be performed again. H.M. was among a group of patients who underwent the experimental operation for bilateral medial temporal lobe resection. However, all the other patients were severely psychotic, muddling the interpretation of the memory tests. The resection in some of the patients involved only some of the cortex and the amygdala, and these patients' memory was intact. Also, the severity of the amnesic deficit in other patients was related to the amount of hippocampal damage, so it was concluded that the hippocampus and immediately adjacent cortex were the likely critical area for memory.

Combining the data across an enormous range of memory and non-memory assessments, H.M.'s amnesia is characterized by several cardinal features: *(1)* intact perceptual, motor, and cognitive functions, *(2)* intact immediate memory, *(3)* severe and global anterograde amnesia, *(4)* temporally graded retrograde amnesia, *(5)* spared remote memory. At that time, views about memory were most influenced by the notion that different cortical areas contained specific perceptual and memory functions together, such that perception, cognition, and memory were considered inseparable and, by Lashley's proposal, widely distributed in the brain. The case study of H.M. was a breakthrough because it showed that a general memory function could be dissociated from other functions. In addition, the findings of exceptions to severe global amnesia, in successful sensorimotor and perceptual learning, foreshadowed a second major breakthrough that promises to further clarify the nature of hippocampal processing in memory.

Other studies on many amnesic patients have shown that the domain of spared learning in amnesia includes intact repetition priming, skill learning, Pavlovian conditioning, sequence learning, and more. The common features that distinguish the impaired and preserved memory capacities in amnesia have been characterized in several ways, including the distinctions between explicit and implicit memory expression, and between episodic and semantic memory.

Based on considerations from a wealth of data from studies on amnesic patients, the most consistent characterization of the domain of memory impaired in amnesia is captured by the notion of "declarative memory," the memory for facts and events that can be brought to conscious recollection and can be expressed explicitly. Conversely, the most consistent characterization of learning ability spared in amnesia is the notion of "procedural memory," the acquisition of skills and preferences that can be expressed unconsciously by implicit changes in the speed or biasing of performance during a repetition of processing of the learning materials. These characterizations capture all of the features of the distinctions outlined previously. However, they leave unresolved the nature of memory traces that underlie either category of memory. An understanding memory representation at that more fundamental level requires the establishment and exploitation of animal models of different types of memory, because only in such models can the required biological recordings and manipulations be pursued. A consideration of the challenges and successes of animal models of declarative and procedural memory begins in the next chapter.

READINGS

Cohen, N.J. 1984. Preserved learning capacity in amnesia: Evidence for multiple memory systems. In *The Neuropsychology of Memory*, N. Butters, and L.R. Squire, (Eds.) New York: Guilford Press, pp. 83–103.

Cohen, N.J., and Squire, L.R. 1980. Preserved learning and retention of a pattern- analyzing skill in amnesia: Dissociation of knowing how and knowing that. *Science* 210:207–210.

Corkin, S. 1984. Lasting consequences of bilateral medial temporal lobectomy: Clinical course and experimental findings in H.M. *Semin. Neurol.* 4:249–259.

Moscovitch, M. 1984. The sufficient conditions for demonstrating preserved memory in amnesia: A task analysis. In *The Neuropsychology of Memory*, N. Butters, and L.R. Squire (Eds.). New York: Guilford Press, pp. 104–114.

Ogden, J.A., and Corkin, S. 1991. Memories of H.M. In *Memory Mechanisms: A Tribute to G.V. Goddard*, W.C. Abraham, M. Corballis, and K.G. White (Eds.) pp. 195–215.

Schacter, D.L. 1987. Implicit memory: History and current status. *J. Exp. Psychol. Learn. Mem. Cogn.* 13:501–518.

Scoville, W.B., and Milner, B. 1957. Loss of recent memory after bilateral hippocampal lesions. *J. Neurol. Neurosurg. Psychiatry* 20:11–12.

Squire, L.R., Knowlton, B., and Musen, G. 1993. The structure and organization of memory. *Annu. Rev. Psychol.* 44:453–495.

Tulving, E. Schacter, D.L., McLachlin, D.R., and Moscovitch, M. 1988. Priming of semantic autobiographcal knowledge: A case study of retrograde amnesia. *Brain and Cogn.* 8:3–20.

5

• • • • • •

Exploring Declarative Memory
Using Animal Models

STUDY QUESTIONS

What is an animal model of amnesia? Why are such models valuable?

What characteristics of amnesia are well modeled using nonhuman primates?

What characteristics of amnesia are well modeled using rodents?

How good were the initial attempts at each of these models?

What advances led to breakthroughs in each model?

Almost immediately after the early reports on H.M. and other patients suffering the consequences of medial temporal lobe excision, efforts began to reproduce elements of the amnesic syndrome in monkeys, rats, and other animals. The major aim of these early efforts was twofold. First, specific experimental brain damage offered an increase in anatomical specificity over that which occurs in cases of surgeries, accidents, and disease. Increased anatomical specificity of the damage improved the ability of investigators to designate which structures of the temporal lobe are critical to memory. Second, in animals, to a much greater extent than in humans, investigators can control the nature and extent of experience gained prior to the brain damage. Human patients arrive in the clinic with a unique background of learning that differs along many dimensions and to a very great extent among individuals. In addition, the specifics of the history of individual people can only be known to the extent that there is a record of one's history, which is typically rather vague. By contrast, in animals, investigators can dictate all the details of experience the animal brings to the experimental setting where learning will be studied. From many of our considerations so far, it should be obvious that new learning occurs in the context of previously acquired knowledge (one's schema or prior semantic knowledge), and so it is greatly advantageous to know and control the nature and extent of that knowledge.

As in any other situation where an experimental model is desired, it is important at the outset to classify the precise aspects of the human condition that one wishes to model. Fortunately, the properties of a valid animal model of the human amnesic syndrome were clearly outlined in the clinical studies presented earlier: (1) sensory, motor, motivational, and cognitive processes should be intact; (2) short-term memory should be intact. (3) following preserved short-term performance, memory should decline with abnormal rapidity, that is, exceeding the rate of natural forgetting in intact control subjects. (4) the deficit should be global in scope for the to-be-learned materials, that is, the impairment should span sensory and conceptual modalities of new learning. (5) there should be a graded retrograde impairment, such that learning accomplished recently prior to brain damage would be lost, whereas learning accomplished remotely long before the damage should be spared.

Two lines of research in the development of animal models

The efforts to model amnesia associated with damage to the medial temporal lobe followed two parallel approaches, one using monkeys as the experimental subjects and the other using primarily rats. The studies on monkeys began appropriately by reproducing the same pervasive medial temporal damage that was done to H.M. Therefore, this line of research has been most useful in characterizing the nature of the memory mediated by the entire set of structures in the medial temporal lobe. The early studies on rats focused on the hippocampus, leaving out of the experimental ablation other structures that were damaged in H.M. and in experiments on monkeys. Therefore, this line of research has been most useful in characterizing the role of the hippocampus itself. The conclusions derived from these two lines do not entirely overlap, because of differences both in the size and locus of experimental brain damage and in the behavioral tests typically employed in monkeys and rats. The following sections summarize some of the findings from both lines of research.

The development of a model of amnesia in monkeys

The behavioral assays initially used to study the role of the medial temporal lobe in monkeys focused on two type of tasks that were already being used in comparative studies on the cognitive functions of nonhuman primates: visual discrimination and matching to sample. In visual discrimination training, typically there are two stimuli for each problem, usually flat plaques painted with different colors or patterns, or easily discriminated three-dimensional objects (Fig. 5–1A), each placed to cover food wells on a choice platform. One stimulus is arbitrarily assigned as "positive," and displacing the plaque would reveal a hidden reward on each trial. The other stimulus is assigned a "negative" value and never rewarded. The positions of the stimuli are varied randomly across trials, so their spatial position does not correlate with the reward locus. In delayed matching to sample, each trial is composed of three distinct phases (Fig. 5–1B). In the first phase, called the sample phase, a single stimulus is presented. This is followed by a variable delay phase during which the monkey has to remember the stimulus for different periods of time. In the third phase,

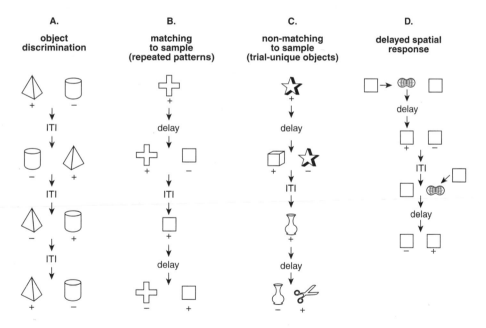

Figure 5–1. Illustration of trials in four memory tests used on monkeys: *A:* Visual discrimination. *B:* Delayed match to sample with trial-repeated stimuli. *C:* Delayed non-match to sample test with trial-unique objects as memory cues. *D:* Delayed spatial response. ITI = intertrial interval.

called the choice phase, two stimuli are presented, one identical to the sample and baited and the other different and not baited. So the requirement of the task is to "match" a choice stimulus to the sample in order to receive the reward. Typically in these early studies, the same two stimuli were two-dimensional patterns reused on every trial, with the sample selected randomly across trials. As described later, there are several important variations on this task, employing different kinds of stimuli, a different "nonmatching" rule by which the subject must select the alternative to the sample item in the choice phase (Fig. 5–1C). Among the variations in stimuli was the use of two identical plain stimuli, and the requirement was for the subject to select the same location it had seen food covered by the plain stimulus on the sample trial. This is called the classic "delayed spatial response" task (Fig. 5–1D).

The early efforts to model amnesia in monkeys using these tests were not impressively successful. The general pattern of results was not inconsistent with the properties of amnesia listed earlier. Also, some of those key properties, including no effect on aspects of the task that did not require memory and normal short-term memory, were very well duplicated in monkeys with medial temporal lobe damage. But the *magnitude* of both the anterograde and retrograde components of the memory deficit were quite modest compared to the apparent almost total loss of memory observed in H.M. Monkeys with substantial removals of all of the medial temporal lobe structures were only mildly impaired on learning new visual pattern, color, object, or auditory discrimination problems. In relearning visual pattern or object discriminations that the monkeys had acquired a few weeks prior to the surgery, deficits were reliably observed. However, the *magnitude* of this retrograde impairment was also disappointing—monkeys with medial temporal lobe damage merely showed less savings from the previous learning and not a complete loss of recently acquired information.

Furthermore, monkeys with medial temporal lobe lesions performed surprisingly well on matching to sample and other delayed response tests. The task was trained preoperatively, and there was a retrograde impairment in reacquisition of the task with short delays. This loss of recent memory was consistent with the characteristics of human amnesia. However, having reacquired the task after the surgery, the monkeys performed well even at memory delay intervals of several seconds. It was a state of affairs that led many to suggest that there might be a true species difference in the role of the medial temporal lobe in memory, such that memory relied much more on hippocampal function in humans than in animals.

Success with a new test of recognition memory

A major breakthrough came with a combination of a novel twist in the procedures used for the delayed matching to sample task combined with a modification in the approach for removing medial temporal lobe structures. The key aspects of the task variant involved the use of new sets of stimulus objects on each trial (the "trial-unique stimulus" procedure) plus a nonmatching reward contingency (Fig. 5–1C). Thus, on each trial, the sample was a novel three-dimensional "junk" object. Then, to obtain a reward during the choice phase, the subject was required to select a different novel junk object over the now-familiar sample object. Because an entirely novel sample is used on each trial, it is appropriate to think of this task as a test of recognition for the newly familiar object. Notably this characterization of the task is quite different from that for the task where the same stimuli are used repeatedly—in such a situation both stimuli are highly familiar, so their potential for recognition would hardly differentiate them.

The distinction between the trial-unique or repetitive stimulus procedures had a profound effect on monkeys' performance in the delayed matching (or nonmatching) task and on the effects of medial temporal lobe damage. Normal monkeys learned the task with the trial-unique procedure exceedingly rapidly. Monkeys with damage to the hippocampal region were impaired in learning the task when the memory delay was short, but they did eventually reach a high performance criterion and continued to perform well when the memory load was low. However, when the delay was extended, a deficit was observed and the severity of the impairment increased as the delay was elongated (Fig. 5–2A). In addition, if a list of items was presented and then memory for each was tested in a sequence of choice trials, a severe deficit was observed.

Monkeys with damage to the medial temporal lobe have a selective memory impairment

The introduction of a new benchmark assessment of amnesia monkeys using the delayed nonmatch to sample (DNMS) task opened up the opportunity to readdress whether this approach would indeed provide a valid model of the fundamental characteristics of human amnesia. Recall that these characteristics include: spared nonmemory functions and short-term memory in the face of rapid forgetting, global scope of amnesia across learning materials, and graded retrograde amnesia.

A central issue is the selectivity of the deficit to memory and the sparing of perceptual, motor, motivational, and attention or other cognitive functions. The DNMS task provides an automatic and ideal control in that

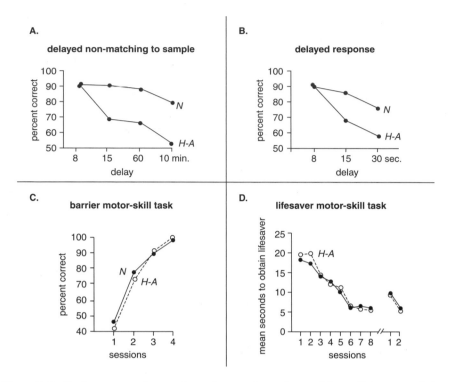

Figure 5–2. Performance of normal monkeys and monkeys with medial temporal damage on different memory tasks. N = normal animals; H-A = animals with hippocampus plus amygdala and cortical damage (data from Squire, 1987).

all of those nonmemory functions are fully required even in the absence of a memory delay. Thus, if monkeys with medial temporal lobe damage perform normally at the shortest delay, it must be that they can attend to, perceive, and encode the object cues, that they can execute the choice responses, that they are motivated to participate in the task, and that they can acquire and retain the nonmatching rule.

Producing a DNMS task with no memory delay at all is problematic because, quite simply, the manually operated apparatus typically used requires 8–10 seconds to exchange sample and choice objects, and deficits in memory can be apparent in human amnesics within 10 seconds. This issue was addressed directly by the development of a computerized version of the DNMS task that employed complex visual patterns presented on a "touch screen" of a video display. Intact subjects required trials to learn the computerized version of the task at the brief delay. Nevertheless, following a medial temporal lobe ablation the rate of learning was fully normal. In subsequent testing with delays up to 10 minutes, normal monkeys showed a gradual forgetting. Monkeys with medial temporal damage performed as well as normal subjects at delays up to 1 second, but at longer delays a deficit became ever more apparent.

Another characteristic of human amnesia is that the deficit can be seen across a variety of learning materials. That is, the impairment is global with regard to the stimulus modality of items to be remembered. Early evidence that addressed this question came from studies of the delayed spatial response task, which is based on memory for a spatial location and not the visual qualities of a particular stimulus. Monkeys with medial temporal damage show the same spared memory at brief delays and increasing impairment at long delays as seen in standard DNMS (Fig. 5–2B).

In addition, this issue was addressed by the development of a tactual variant of the DNMS task. Monkeys were initially trained on the conventional version of the task, and then retrained with the room lights gradually dimmed to complete darkness except for small dim cue-lights signaling the positions of the objects. In this situation the animals had to perceive and encode the objects entirely by tactual cues. Normal monkeys required about twice as many trials to relearn the task in the dark, but performance was excellent in the final preoperative stage of tactual DNMS testing even over long delays. After removal of the medial temporal lobe, relearning at a short delay was substantially impaired, but the animals did eventually succeed and continued to perform well with short delays, as observed with the visual version of the task. More important, the deficit grew as the delay was elongated. Thus, the pattern of sparing of ultimate performance at a short delay and increasing impairment at longer delays was identical to that observed for the visually guided version of the same task, demonstrating that the amnesic deficit extended across specific sensory modalities.

Another central characteristic of the amnesic syndrome is the phenomenon of graded retrograde memory loss. As described in Chapter 4, H.M. and other amnesic patients display a loss of memories backward in time from the moment of brain damage, with the most severe loss in the period just prior to the damage and total sparing of remotely acquired memories, including childhood recollections and general knowledge acquired early in life. However, a major problem in the interpretation of retrograde memory loss in human patients is that the amount and timing of prior learning experiences can only be approximated. Conversely, one of the major advantages of an animal model of amnesia is that one can examine the retrograde loss of memories with a "prospective" design. That is, one can provide measured amounts of learning at specific times prior to brain damage that occurs suddenly. In so doing, one can directly compare the strength of memories acquired at different times in intact animals and one can more accurately measure the period and magnitude of retrograde loss.

Unfortunately, the DNMS task is unsuitable for this kind of study because single exposures to objects do not provide sufficiently strong memories to endure testing weeks or months after learning. To address this issue and develop a task that would be suitable for a study of retrograde memory, experimenters created an object discrimination task where subjects were presented with pairs of novel objects like those used in DNMS testing, and repeatedly reinforced the choice of one object over the other. Normal monkeys learned sets of these pairings rapidly, accumulating 100 successfully acquired problems over 4 months of training. Following completion of the learning series, in half of the animals the hippocampus and nearby cortex were removed and the animals were allowed 2 weeks to recover. Then all the animals were each tested with just one trial on each problem. Normal animals scored well on the most recently acquired problems, and their performance declined a bit, showing some forgetting for problems learned more than 2 months before. By contrast, monkeys with hippocampal damage were substantially impaired, performing at just above that expected by chance, on problems presented within 2 weeks of the surgery. They performed significantly better on remotely learned discriminations, exhibiting normal performance on those acquired 4 months prior to the surgery. This pattern of recent retrograde memory loss and spared remote memory, emphasized most strikingly by worse performance on recent memory than remote memory within the medial temporal group, provides compelling evidence that damage to the medial temporal region results in a graded retrograde amnesia (see Chapter 12 for an extended discussion of this topic).

A domain of spared learning ability in monkeys with medial temporal damage

In addition to the previously described aspects of *impaired* learning and memory following hippocampal damage, there is the critical characterization of a *spared* domain of new learning capacity in H.M. and other amnesic patients. Toward the goal of modeling this phenomenon, there are specific examples that represent a domain of spared learning in monkeys following ablation of the entire medial temporal lobe.

One spared domain that closely parallels intact motor skill learning in human amnesics is the acquisition of manual skills in monkeys. In a study of this kind of learning, experimenters devised two manual skill tests on which monkeys could be trained. One of these involved training the monkeys to reach around a clear barrier to obtain a reward. Another involved challenging the monkeys to obtain a doughnut-shaped candy (a "lifesaver") reward that was presented in the middle of an irregularly bent stiff wire (a coat hanger). To rapidly retrieve the reward the monkey had to improve its manual manipulation of the lifesaver around the turns of the coat hanger. In both tasks monkeys with medial temporal damage improved in performance at the same rate as normal subjects, demonstrating preserved motor skill learning in amnesia (Fig. 5–2C, D).

In addition, monkeys with medial temporal lobe damage perform normally well in the acquisition and retention of single visual discrimination problems that are acquired gradually. This spared learning capacity was described in some of the early studies on medial temporal lobe ablations in monkeys, and was confirmed in studies using the same junk object stimuli employed in DNMS. Notably, the deficit is observed only under conditions where normal learning was slow and gradual (by presenting each pair of object only once per day). In conditions where normal animals learn object discriminations most rapidly (acquisition in a single session with multiple presentations), a deficit is observed. Thus, these findings revealed a common, albeit not universal, aspect of learning by the medial temporal system, that this system acquires information rapidly. Under the conditions where normal acquisition was rapid, animals without that system were disadvantaged. Conversely, under conditions where the rapid learning system conferred no advantage, no learning deficit was observed.

This combination of observations, and several other findings, showed that many of the central features of the phenomenology of human amnesia can be modeled in animals, and specifically in monkeys. This work set the stage for a more detailed examination of which medial temporal lobe structures are critical for memory in monkeys; this work is discussed in Chapter 9. A parallel effort was also ongoing to model amnesia in other animals, particularly rats. The results of this effort are summarized next.

Can declarative memory be modeled using rats?

Scoville and Milner's 1957 report on H.M. had suggested that, among the structures damaged within the temporal lobe, damage to the hippocampus in particular was responsible for the memory deficit. Therefore, following the initial reports on human amnesia, several laboratories developed procedures for ablation of the hippocampus in rats, as well as cats and rabbits. As was the case with monkeys, the first tests to be employed in examining the effects of hippocampal damage were a variety of simple conditioning, discrimination learning, and maze learning tests that were the focus of current research by learning theorists. However, the results using each of these formal tests seemed inconsistent by any simple analysis. The findings were puzzling at best, and certainly did not support a conclusion that hippocampal damage results in severe and global amnesia in rats or other nonprimates. A few of these findings are summarized next to illustrate the confusing state of affairs that ensued from this research.

The earliest assessments of learning and hippocampal function in rodents included two different tests of conditioning animals to avoid noxious stimuli (usually irritating electrical shocks). One of these, called "shuttle-box avoidance," involved training rats to alternate (shuttle) between two adjacent compartments of an alleyway. In one version of this task, each trial began with a buzzer that signaled the rat to shuttle to the alternate chamber before the floor in the currently occupied side was electrified by a mild current. The surprising result was that rats with large ablations of the hippocampus and overlying cortex learned the task in *fewer* trials than normal rats or rats with cortical damage only, and they retained this learning solidly across testing days. Shortly after, and contrasting with the first results, another study reported that rats with hippocampal ablations were *unable* to learn a different sort of avoidance task called "passive avoidance." Initially, hungry rats were trained to approach a chamber that had food. They began each trial in a large compartment, and were then signaled by a door opening to leave that compartment and to approach and enter the small food-containing chamber. After learning to execute the approach behavior immediately upon opening of the door, one day they were shocked while eating and driven out of the reward chamber. Normal rats and rats with hippocampal ablations rapidly learned the initial approach response and, consistent with the earlier experiment, rats with hippocampal ablations had shorter approach latencies and less variability in learning. However, the two groups responded quite differently in the avoidance component of training. After having been shocked just once in the reward chamber, none of the normal rats reentered again. By contrast, each of the rats with hippocampal damage did return to the chamber in which they were shocked. Although there was a learning impairment here following hippocampal damage, the overall pattern of findings did not offer compelling support for a simple amnesic disorder: After outperforming normal rats on the initial learning phase, rats with hippocampal damage showed a deficit in passive avoidance that seemed to reflect an inability to give up the previously acquired response, rather than a failure to learn *per se*. What a confusing state of affairs!

Rats with hippocampal damage also performed perfectly normally, or better than normal rats, in the acquisition of standard Skinnerian conditioning tests in which rats learned to press a bar for food rewards. In addition, the pattern of early findings on the acquisition of simple sensory or spatial discriminations was no easier to reconcile with the deficit in human amnesia than were the findings on approach and avoidance learning. For example, in one of the first of these studies, rats with hippocampal ablations acquired at the same rate as normal animals a visual discrimination in which the stimuli were presented simultaneously. This task employed a Y-shaped maze composed of a start arm and two choice arms: one choice arm was black and the other white, and their left–right positions were randomly changed across trials (Fig. 5–3, left). The rat began each trial at one end of the start arm and then was rewarded for consistently selecting one color choice arm by food placed at the end of that arm.

The opposite result was obtained in another version of the same visual discrimination task where the critical stimuli were presented successively on separate trials (Fig. 5–3, right). On each trial of this test, the rats were

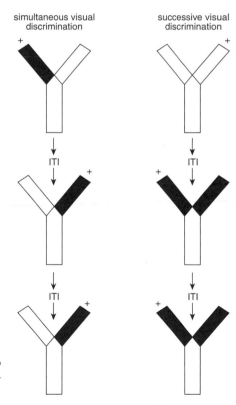

Figure 5–3. A sequence of trials on two different versions of a visual discrimination task using a Y-maze.

presented with one of two mazes, either a maze with two black goal arms or a maze with two white goal arms. The right arm contained food when the goal arms were white, whereas the left arm contained the food when the goal arms were black. In this variant of visual discrimination, rats with hippocampal damage required over twice as many trials as normal rats to reach a learning criterion. However, after a 2-week period, rats with hippocampal ablations showed as good retention as normal rats. As was the case with passive avoidance, although a discrimination learning impairment was observed following hippocampal damage, the overall pattern of results could not be interpreted as supporting a rodent model of global amnesia. Rats with hippocampal damage were not consistently impaired in learning a set of seemingly similar visual discriminations, and there was no impairment in long-term retention in either version of the task.

Many subsequent efforts continued to provide mixed results on the effects of hippocampal damage on simple discrimination learning in rats and other species. There were some kinds of tasks where a disproportionate number of studies showed either impairment or spared learning: Discrimination learning was intact in three times as many experiments as not, although there were also many examples of deficient learning in each situation. This was the case across a broad variety of critical stimuli: nonspatial stimuli including specific visual, auditory, tactile, or olfactory cues, and spatial stimuli including left and right arms of a T- or Y-shaped maze. By contrast, a different result was obtained when animals were required to "reverse" the reward assignments, that is, when they were required to relearn the discrimination for same stimuli but each stimulus had the opposite reward assignment. In these situations animals with hippocampal damage more often showed impairments, although again there were many exceptions. Some researchers suggested that the deficit following hippocampal damage was an impairment in withholding previously learned responses. There was a constituency for this idea, but surely this was not the sort of conclusion that supported a straightforward model of amnesia in animals.

Several new ideas suggested the hippocampus is involved in only one type of memory

In the mid-1970s, several breakthroughs were made in the establishment of a rodent model of amnesia. Parallel to the successful approach in understanding human amnesia, a number of proposals emphasized the critical participation of hippocampus in some aspect of memory and lack of critical involvement in some other aspect of memory processing. Despite major differences in the fundamental processing function assigned to the hippocampus, all the proposals shared two general aspects of their formulations that are very important. First, each proposal espoused the view that the hippocampus plays a selective role in a distinct, higher-order form of memory, whereas hippocampal-independent mechanisms are sufficient to mediate simpler forms of learning and memory. The recognition of multiple forms of memory, only one of which depends on the hippocampus, constituted a major breakthrough of research on rodent memory in that period.

Second, there was substantial agreement on the characteristics of the kind of learning that was successful *in*dependent of hippocampal function. All the proposals that emerged in this period described the capacities of animals with hippocampal damage in a manner consistent with characterizations of "habit" learning. Some characterized learning without the hippocampus as involving dispositions of specific stimuli into approach and avoidance categories, and as involving slow and incremental behavioral adaptation to the stimuli. Others characterized the behavior of animals with hippocampal damage as prone to rigidly adopt permanent assignments of cues and behaviors associated with reinforcement very early. The combination of these qualities remains undisputed in accounting for the success of rats with hippocampal damage in simple approach and avoidance conditioning and in discrimination learning.

Beyond general agreement on what the hippocampus does *not* do, however, the theories differed substantially. In the following section two prominent views are discussed. Both of these proposals received substantial support from a particular key line of experimentation. At the same time each line of experiments challenged the conclusions from the other theory.

A cognitive map in the hippocampus?

In 1978 John O'Keefe and Lynn Nadel proposed that the hippocampus implements the cognitive maps described by Tolman. In a monumental achievement, O'Keefe and Nadel surveyed the extensive research findings on the anatomy and physiology of the hippocampus and on the studies of the effects of hippocampal damage in animals and humans. Each of these areas of knowledge was interpreted as supporting their overall hypothesis that the hippocampus is specifically dedicated to the construction and use of spatial maps of the environment. In their survey of the studies on animals with damage to the hippocampus or its connections, O'Keefe and Nadel emphasized that hippocampal damage typically results in severe impairment in most forms of spatial exploration and learning. Conversely, they noted that impairment of nonspatial learning (such as simple discrimination learning) is less commonly reported. These conclusions were combined with evidence of hippocampal "place cells," hippocampal neurons that signaled the location of the animal in space while it explored its environment (see Chapter 6 for details), leading them to suggest that hippocampal spatial information processing is a critical element of creating maps of space.

It is important to emphasize that O'Keefe and Nadel's analysis went well beyond making a simple distinction between "spatial" and "nonspatial" learning. They proposed that the acquisition of cognitive maps involves a wholly distinct form of cognition from that of habit formation. Cognitive maps involve the representation of places in terms of distances and directions among items in the environment, and are composed as a rough topological map of the physical environment that the animal uses to navigate among salient locations and other important cues. They envisioned cognitive maps as enabling animals to act at a distance, that is, to *navigate* to locations beyond their immediate perception. In addition, cognitive mapping was characterized by a rapid, all-or-none assignment of cues to places within the spatial map. This kind of learning was envisioned as driven by curiosity, rather than reinforcement of specific behavioral responses, and as involving relatively little interference between items because they would be represented separately in a map or in different maps for distinct situations. In short, spatial mapping had most of the qualities of Tolman's cognitive maps, and therefore represented the form of cognitive memory as distinguished from habit learning.

To get a feel for the striking and selective impairment in spatial learning following hippocampal damage in animals, consider the evidence from the water maze test, a spatial memory task that has received widespread use in studies of learning and memory. Originally developed by Richard Morris in 1981, this apparatus involves a large swimming pool filled with tepid water made murky by the addition of milk powder (Fig. 5–4A). An escape platform is hidden just beneath the surface of the water at an arbitrary location. Rats are very good swimmers and rapidly learn to locomote around the pool, but they prefer not to swim and will seek the platform so they can climb onto it. Animals cannot see the platform directly, but instead must use distant spatial cues that are visible above the walls of the pool around the room. On each training trial, the rat begins swimming from one of multiple locations at the periphery of the maze, so that it cannot consistently use a specific swimming course to reach the escape platform. Rats learn to use a spatial navigation strategy to find the platform even after training from a consistent starting

Figure 5–4. The Morris water maze task. *A:* A sketch of the apparatus and two trials of a typical training sequence. In the place navigation version of the task, the rat begins each trial at one of four randomly selected locations and must find a submerged platform (dashed circle) positioned at a constant location. In the cued navigation version, the rat also starts at one of four locations, and the platform is visible (solid circle) and moved randomly across trials. *B:* Performance of rats with hippocampal lesions, cortical lesions, and normal controls in acquiring the water maze task. Place navigation = hidden platform; cue navigation = visible platform. *C:* Performance on the transfer test. Left: Swim path of a control subject; dashed lines indicate quadrant of the maze in which the platform had been located. Right: Swim times of rats in different maze quadrants; black bar corresponds to the training quadrant (data from Morris et al., 1982).

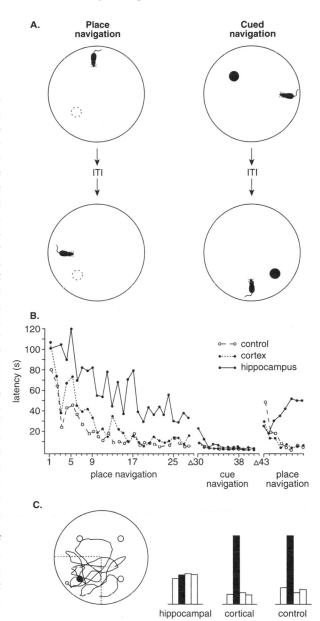

point, as evidenced in their ability after training to locate it efficiently from novel starting points.

Morris and his colleagues showed that hippocampal ablation results in severe impairments in the water maze task (Fig. 5–4B). In the initial trials, all animals typically required 1–2 minutes to find the platform. During the course of repeated trials, normal animals rapidly reduced their escape latency, such that they eventually reached it in less than 10 seconds from every starting point. Rats with hippocampal ablations also reduced their escape latencies, showing some extent of learning. However, they reached asymptotic performance at approximately 35 second latencies, largely due to a reduction of completely ineffective strategies such as trying to climb the walls; however, they never learned to swim directly to the platform location in the manner that normal rats do.

In a subsequent "transfer test" the escape platform was removed and rats were allowed to swim for 1 minute with no opportunity for escape. In this transfer condition, normal rats circled in the close vicinity of the former location of the platform, as measured by a strong tendency to swim within the quadrant of the pool in which it had been located (Fig. 5–4C). Rats with hippocampal ablations showed no preference for the quadrant of the platform, highlighting the severity of their spatial memory deficit. In a different version of the water maze task, when the escape platform could be seen above the surface of the water (cue navigation), both normal rats and rats with hippocampal ablations rapidly learned to swim directly to it. This protocol emphasized the distinction between intact learning to approach the platform guided by a specific local cue, versus no capacity for learning guided by the relation among distant spatial cues. Since Morris and colleagues' original experiment, several studies have confirmed the selective impairment on the spatial version of the Morris water maze task following hippocampal damage, and this task has become a benchmark test of hippocampal function in rodents.

An alternative theory: The hippocampus and remembering recent experiences

In 1979, David Olton and his colleagues proposed an alternative view of the role the hippocampus plays in learning and memory. He argued that the hippocampus is critical when the solution of a problem requires memory for a particular recent experience. He called this "working memory," but note that we will not use this term because it has a different meaning in the current cognitive and neuroscience literatures. In current usage, working memory refers to the ability to temporarily hold information *online* while the subject is working on that information. As described in detail in Chapter 13, this memory capacity has been tied to the function of prefrontal cortex rather than hippocampus. The kind of memory Olton described involved the capacity to remember information that was obtained in a single experience, and to retain and then use it after any delay and over substantial interpolated material, exceeding the properties of working memory. Olton and his colleagues distinguished this kind of memory from "reference memory," which he characterized as memory for information that is constant across trials. Such reference information includes that there is a food reward at the end of each arm, that the rewards are not replaced during a trial but are replaced between trials, etc. On a conceptual level Olton viewed his theory as capturing the distinction raised by Tulving (1972) between "episodic memory" events tied to specific time and place, as contrasted with "semantic memory" for knowledge that is time- and event-independent (see Chapter 4). Accordingly, it is more appropriate to describe Olton's characterization of hippocampal memory as memory for unique episodes.

Olton and colleagues' evidence was generated in great part from experiments using a novel test apparatus called the radial-arm maze. This maze is composed of several (typically eight) runway arms radiating outward like spokes of a wheel from a central platform (Fig. 5–5A), and there are many variants on the number of arms and reward contingencies involved in this task. In the standard version of the task, at the outset of each trial a food reward is placed at the end of each of the arms of the maze. During the course of a trial, the rat is free to enter each arm to retrieve the food rewards. Once retrieved, the food rewards are not replaced during that trial. Rats rapidly learn to approach each arm just once on a given trial. On subsequent trials, all of the arms are baited again just once. The number of arms entered during a trial provides a measure of the ability of the rat to remember which arms it has visited on that particular trial. Notably, this is not a test for memory of spatial locations—typically the spatial cues themselves are never hidden and do not need to be remembered. Instead, the central memory demand is to remember the animal's most recent visits to particular arms of the maze, that is, the recent behavioral episodes as opposed to the many other times each arm has been visited.

In a classic experiment demonstrating the specificity of the impairment following hippocampal damage, Olton and his colleagues compared performance for different maze arms that had distinct reward contingencies (Fig. 5–5B). Some arms of the maze were baited once each trial, following the typical contingency that required memory for specific experiences. In addition, other arms were never baited, and rats were to learn across trials not to enter these arms at all. The latter capacity is another example of "reference memory" emphasizing the fixed nature of the stimulus–response associations for these arms. After initial training of all animals to high levels of performance on both components of the task, half

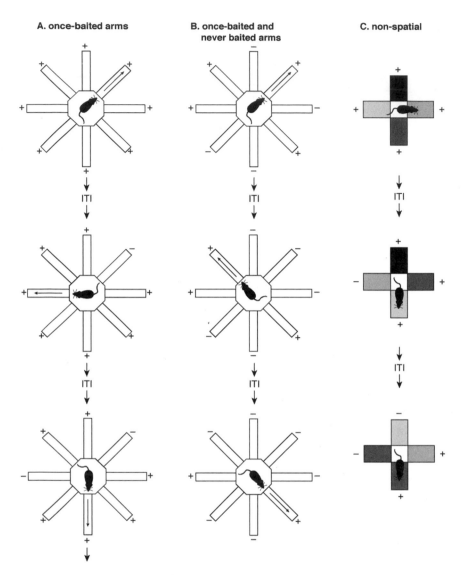

A. once-baited arms **B. once-baited and never baited arms** **C. non-spatial**

Figure 5–5. Three variations of the radial maze task. *A:* All maze arms are baited once, and the rat must visit each without a repetition. *B:* Only half the arms are baited once and the other half are never baited. Rats learn to visit each baited arm once per trial and never to visit the unbaited arms. *C:* The nonspatial version of the task. Each arm has a different surface on the floor, and the arms are interchanged randomly between trials. Rats learn to visit each cue once per trial.

the animals had the hippocampus disconnected by transection of a major fiber bundle called the fornix. Subsequently in postoperative testing, normal animals continued to perform at very high levels on both the components of the task. By contrast, rats with hippocampal disconnections performed less well than normals from the outset of postoperative testing on both components of the task, but improved rapidly on their reference memory choices. However, they never performed better than chance even with extended training on the arms that required memory for specific experiences.

Olton's proposal was seen as in direct conflict with the cognitive mapping notion, and many succeeding experiments provided support for one or the other proposal. Olton's hypothesis provided the better explanation of one of the early and persistent complexities of data on spatial discrimination, reversal learning, and alternation. Early studies found that hippocampal damage generally does not prevent learning of a simple spatial discrimination on a Y- or T-maze. O'Keefe and Nadel were quick to point out that this maze problem can be solved in two ways, by orienting for a left or right turn or by going to the place of reward. In their view, the hippocampus mediates the place strategy but not the orientation strategy, so that when deprived of hippocampal function the rats have an alternative solution and hence are unimpaired. However, an equally frequent result in the early studies is that rats with hippocampal damage are impaired at spatial reversal learning and are unable to learn to alternate left and right arm selections in Y- or T-mazes, and can show the clear dissociation between intact spatial discrimination and impaired alternation in the same T-maze apparatus outfitted with different types of choice points. It might well be that rats find it easy to adopt an orientation strategy in spatial discrimination, but strongly favor a place strategy in reversal learning and have to use a place strategy in delayed alternation. But it is not the nature of the spatial cues that differentiates these alternatives among these tasks. Rather, it is the demand to use the same cues in different ways for each task that is the critical factor. Olton's memory dichotomy accounts for these results more directly, in that only reference memory is required for the spatial choice never rewarded, but memory for the most recent experience is required for the alternation of choices.

Another line of evidence strongly favoring Olton's theory consisted of experiments extending the role of the hippocampus to memory for specific experiences in the radial maze guided by nonspatial stimuli. The structure of the task was generally the same as in the previous tests of spatial working memory. Each of multiple maze arms was baited just once and perfect performance was measured as the ability of the rat to obtain all the rewards by entering each arm only one time. For the nonspatial version of this task, however, they created a four-arm maze in which the walls and floor of each arm were covered by a distinct set of tactile and visual cues, and distant cues were eliminated by covering the arms with a translucent gauze (Fig. 5–5C). Furthermore, after each arm entry the rat was briefly confined to the central platform while the arms were rearranged to eliminate any consistent arm positions or their configuration. Thus, the rats had to remember entered arms by their distinctive internal (intramaze) cues and ignore any spatial cues about the locations of the arms. After initial preoperative acquisition, normal rats continued to perform the task well but rats with fornix transections failed to reacquire the task even with extended retraining, despite the nonspatial nature of this variant of the task.

The findings on these two theories of hippocampal function leave us in a quandary. O'Keefe and Nadel's theory predicts impairment on any task that requires the use of spatial cues in a cognitive map. It is not entirely clear that performance on the radial maze requires cognitive mapping. But the same spatial stimuli guide performance on both the episodic memory and reference memory versions of the task (Fig. 5–5B). So, the cognitive mapping view would not predict a difference in role of the hippocampus in the two versions of the task. On the other hand, the pattern of deficits on the radial maze tasks indicates that memory for specific prior episodes is critical, and not a demand for the use of spatial cues per se. At the same time, the Morris water maze task is clearly a "reference" memory task. Learning this task requires hippocampal function, a finding that cannot be explained by Olton's hypothesis. Clearly these two theories each capture a critical aspect of hippocampal functioning. However, another fundamental formulation must be pursued to account for both sets of findings. The following section diverges from these maze studies and reconsiders the properties of declarative memory that emerged from studies on human amnesia. Subsequently I return to the findings from the maze studies, as well as other experiments, and offer a reconciliation of the findings within the framework of properties of declarative memory.

Convergence on the relational account of hippocampal function in memory

As discussed in the preceding chapter, characterizations of memory functions of the medial temporal lobe in humans focus on declarative memory, the memory for everyday facts and events that can be brought to conscious recollection and can be expressed in a variety of venues. An approach to investigating this kind of memory can be obtained through a deeper consideration of the fundamental features of declarative memory. First, consider the notion that declarative memory is a combination of "event" or episodic memory and "fact" or semantic memory. How do these two kinds of memory combine to compose declarative memory? We acquire our declarative memories through everyday personal experiences, and in humans the ability to retain and recall these "episodic" memories is highly dependent on the hippocampus. But the full scope of hippocampal involvement also extends to semantic memory, the body of general knowledge about the world that is accrued from linking multiple experiences that share some of the same information. For example, a typical episodic memory might involve recalling the specific events and places surrounding the meeting of a long-lost cousin. Your general knowledge about the relationships of people that compose your family tree and other facts about the history of your family come in great part from a synthesis of the representations of many meetings with relatives and other episodes in which family personalities or events are observed or discussed. Similarly, our episodic memory mediates the capacity to remember a sequence of events, places passed, and turns taken while walking across a city, and a synthesis of many such representations provides general knowledge about the spatial layout of the city.

Second, consider the nature of declarative memory expression. Declarative memory has been characterized as available to conscious recollection and subject to verbal reflection or other explicit means of expression. By contrast, procedural memory has been characterized as the nonconscious acquisition of a bias or adaptation that is typically revealed only by implicit or indirect measures of memory. Thus, declarative memory for both the episodic and semantic information is special in that one can access and express declarative memories via various routes and these memories can be used to solve novel problems by making inferences from memory. For example, even without ever explicitly studying your family tree and its history, one can infer indirect relationships, or the sequence of central events in the family history, from the set of episodic memories about your family. Similarly, without ever studying the map of a city, one can make navigational inferences from the synthesis of many episodic memories of previous routes taken.

These descriptions present a formidable challenge for the study of declarative memory in animals. We do not have the means for identifying episodic memory or monitoring conscious recollection in animals; the very existence of consciousness in animals is a matter of debate. An assessment of verbal reflection is, of course, out of the question, and it is not otherwise obvious how to assess episodic and semantic memory or evaluate "explicit" memory expression in animals. However, these aspects of memory may in fact be accessible if we consider further characterizations that have been offered to distinguish declarative and procedural memory. To the extent that these descriptions do not rely on consciousness or verbal expression, they might be operationalized for experimental analysis in animals.

To this end, in 1984 Cohen offered descriptions that could be helpful toward the goal of operationalizing fundamental properties of declarative memory. He suggested that "a declarative code permits the ability to *compare and contrast* information from different processes or processing systems; and it enables the ability to *make inferences* from and generalizations across facts derived from multiple processing sources. Such a common declarative code thereby provides the basis for access to facts acquired during the course of experiences and for conscious recollection of the learning experiences themselves" (p. 97, italics added). Conversely, procedural learning was characterized as the acquisition of specific skills, adaptations, and biases and that such "procedural knowledge is tied to and expressible only through activation of the particular processing structures or procedures engaged by the learning tasks" (p. 96).

Two distinctions revealed in these characterizations have been employed during development of assessments of declarative and procedural memory that may be applicable to animal studies. First, declarative memory is distinguished by its role in comparing and contrasting distinct memories, whereas procedural memory involves the facilitation of particular routines for which no such comparisons are executed. Second, declarative memory is distinguished by its capacity to support inferential use of memories in novel situations, whereas procedural memory only supports alterations in performance that can be characterized as rerunning more smoothly the neural processes by which they were initially acquired.

These distinctions, plus consideration of the nature of episodic and semantic memory as described in humans, can be extended to make contact with the broad literature on hippocampal function in animals, resulting in a proposal for the representational mechanisms that might underlie declarative memory. Based on a consideration of these characteristics of declarative memory, Eichenbaum and Cohen suggested that the hippocampal system supports a *relational representation* of memories. Furthermore, a critical property of the hippocampal-dependent memory system is its *representational flexibility*, a quality that permits inferential use of memories in novel situations. According to this view, the hippocampal system mediates the organization of memories into what may be thought of as a "memory space."

This theory has been elaborated to make contact with several of the key observations of the theories of memory described earlier.

Within the relational memory theory, the memory space is constructed by an interleaving of episodic memories into a semantic structure in which memories are connected by their common elements. In this scheme the major components of a memory space are the representations of memories as sequences of events that compose specific experiences, that is, distinct episodic memories. Episodic memories, then, are interleaved into the memory space by shared events within related memories. Thus, the construction of family trees and layouts of cities are built up from linking together many episodic memories for specific encounters with family members and for specific trips through a city.

Furthermore, such a memory space supports the kind of comparing and contrasting among memories that allows flexible and inferential use of memories. Within the memory space scheme these capacities are generated by the structure of the relational representation. When one element of the network is activated by a retrieval cue, all memories that contain that item and are sufficiently strongly associated will be activated, including elements of those memories that are elements of yet other related episodic representations. Consequently, memories that are only indirectly associated with the originally activated element would also be activated. Such a process would support the recovery of memories in a variety of contexts outside the learning situation and would permit the expression of memories via various pathways of behavioral output.

Conversely, according to the relational memory account, hippocampal-*independent* memories involve *individual representations*; such memories are isolated in that they are encoded only within the brain modules in which perceptual or motor processing is engaged during learning. These individual representations are *inflexible* in that they can be revealed only through reactivation of those modules within the restrictive range of stimuli and situations in which the original learning occurred. One might expect individual representations to support the acquisition of task procedures that are performed habitually across training trials. Individual representations should also support the acquisition of specific information that does not require comparison and consequent relational representation.

The combination of relational representation (a consequence of processing comparisons among memories) and representational flexibility (a quality of relational representation that permits inferential expression of memories) suggests an information processing scheme that might underlie declarative memory in humans and animals as well. Most important, this description of the nature of declarative memory is testable in animals.

Testing the relational memory theory

Large-scale networks for family trees and city layouts are but two examples of the kind of memory space proposed to be mediated by the hippocampus. Within this view, a broad range of such networks can be created, with their central organizing principle the linkage of episodic memories by their common events and places, and a consequent capacity to move among related memories within the network. These properties of declarative memory suggest an approach for the development of animal models. Thus, a way to study the development of a memory space from overlapping experiences, and to make inferences from the network knowledge, is to train subjects on multiple distinct experiences that share common elements and then test whether these experiences have been linked in memory to solve new problems. One can conceive of this approach as applied to various domains relevant to the lives of animals, from knowledge about spatial relations among stimuli in an environment, to categorizations of foods, to learned organizations of odor or visual stimuli or social relationships.

In the remainder of this section some of the evidence supporting the relational account of hippocampal memory function is elaborated. The first set of experiments reexamines discrimination learning, showing once more that learning performance may be severely impaired or completely intact depending on performance demands, showing how a critical demand for relational processing leads to different behavioral outcomes. The second set of experiments examines directly the role of the hippocampus in flexible memory representations and the expression of memory by novel uses of previously acquired knowledge.

The importance of linking multiple distinct experiences

A critical aspect of the relational theory is the interleaving of multiple experiences that share information into a larger network of memories. Therefore, it can be expected that the hippocampus will play a critical role in learning in situations where the task has a strong demand to synthesize multiple overlapping experiences. One such case involves spatial learning, similar to the example of the learning of routes through a city, but involving rats and the Morris water maze task. As described before, in the conventional version of this task, rats learn to escape from submersion in a pool by swimming toward a platform located just underneath the surface. Importantly, training in the conventional version of the task involves an intermixing of four different kinds of trial episodes that differ in the starting point of the swim (see Fig. 5–4A). Focusing on this task demand, the relational memory account offers a straightforward accounting of the pattern of deficits and situations where intact spatial learning is observed. Releasing the rats into the water at different starting points on successive trials strongly encourages the subjects to compare their views along the swim paths as they pass the positions of extramaze stimuli, forcing the animal to consider its relation to the positions of the cues across trials. Indeed, it is difficult to imagine how the task could be solved without synthesizing the information acquired during the different swim episodes into a representation of spatial relations among cues, allowing them to disentangle otherwise conflicting associations of the separate views seen from each starting point. Under these conditions of strong demands to interleave the different types of episodes, animals with hippocampal damage typically fail to acquire the task.

The importance of the demand for interleaving four different types of trial episodes was demonstrated in an experiment that explored acquisition of the water maze when this requirement was eliminated. This experiment used a version of the task where rats were released into the maze from a constant start position on each trial. Initially, animals were trained to approach a visible black-and-white striped platform. Then the visibility of the platform was gradually diminished using a series of training stages that involved a large, visible, white platform, then smaller platforms, and finally sinking the platform below the water surface. With this gradual training procedure, rats with fornix transections learned to approach the platform directly, although they were slower to acquire the response at each phase of training (Fig. 5–6A). In addition, their final escape latencies were slightly higher than those of intact rats, due to an increased tendency for "near misses," trials on which they passed nearby the platform without touching it and forcing them to circle back. But, in contrast to the standard version of this task, animals with hippocampal damage were able to learn the location of the escape platform.

Both sets of rats were using the same extramaze cues to guide performance, as indicated by the results from the standard "transfer" test in which the escape platform is removed and the swimming pattern of the rats is observed for a fixed period. Both normal rats and rats with hippocampal damage swam near the former location of the platform, indicating that they could identify the place of escape by the same set of available extramaze cues rather than solely by the approach trajectory. After several probe tests, these rats were to learn a novel escape location using multiple starting points. Rats with hippocampal damage failed completely. The success of rats with hippocampal damage on the constant start version of the task, contrasted with their failure on the standard, variable

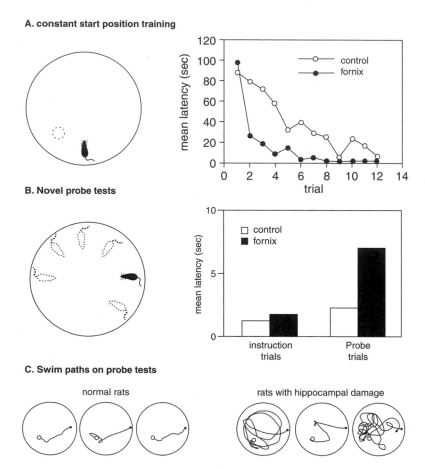

A. constant start position training

B. Novel probe tests

C. Swim paths on probe tests

normal rats

rats with hippocampal damage

Figure 5–6. Place learning in the water maze. *A:* In the constant start version of this task, the rat always begins from the same location near the escape platform. Note that rats with hippocampal damage (fornix lesions) learn the task more slowly than normal rats, but eventually succeed. *B:* Navigation from novel starting locations. Six novel starting locations were used in the probe testing trials that were intermixed among repetitions of the instruction trial. *C:* Example swim paths for individual normal control rats and rats with hippocampal damage on the probe trial that began from the "east" start location (see black rat in *B*) (data fom Eichenbaum et al., 1990).

start version, indicating that it was not the use of distal spatial cues *per se*, but rather other factors governing how these cues were used that determined the critical involvement of the hippocampus. Rather, the cognitive demand that invoked critical hippocampal function was the requirement to interleave information from multiple experiences on different escape paths taken across trials.

The flexible and inferential expression of spatial memories

Were there differences in the way in which rats with hippocampal damage and normal rats learned and represented the task? This question was addressed by using a series of probe tests, each involving an alteration of the cues or starting points, intermixed within a series of repetitions of the instruction trial. One of the probe tests demonstrated a particularly striking dissociation between the two groups of rats. In this test, the platform was left in its normal place but the start position was moved to various novel locations. When the start position was the same as that used during instruction trials, both normal rats and rats with hippocampal damage had short escape latencies (Fig. 5–6B). On the critical probe trials with novel starting positions, normal rats also swam directly to the platform regardless of the starting position. By contrast, rats with hippocampal damage rarely swam directly to the escape platform and sometimes went far astray, subsequently having abnormally long average escape latencies on these probe trials. This striking deficit in rats with hippocampal damage was demonstrated by a close examination of their individual swim trajectories (Fig. 5–6C). All the normal rats nearly always swam directly to the platform regardless of their starting point. But rats with hippocampal damage swam in various directions, occasionally leading them straight to the platform, but more often in the wrong direction, and they sometimes never found the platform in this highly familiar environment. The observation of a severe deficit in using spatial information acquired successfully to navigate from novel starting points constitutes strong evidence indicating the importance of the hippocampus in the flexible and inferential expression of spatial memories.

Extending the role of the hippocampus in relational representation and representational flexibility to nonspatial learning and memory

The preceding set of experiments provides compelling evidence that the hippocampus plays an important role in spatial learning by supporting the interleaving of multiple overlapping experiences and in using the resulting organized spatial representation to navigate from new locations. Now we consider whether this accounting applies globally to nonspatial as well as spatial memory organizations. One study that examined this issue directly explored the role of the hippocampus in learning an organization of odor stimuli, and in flexible and inferential expression of this organization. This study compared normal rats and rats with selective damage to the hippocampus on their ability to learn a set of odor problems and to interleave their representations of these problems to support novel inferential judgments about them.

To accomplish this an odor-guided version of the so-called paired associate task was developed for rodents, and this task extended the learning requirement to include multiple stimulus–stimulus associations with overlapping stimulus elements (Fig. 5–7). The task was especially designed to take advantage of the superb abilities of rats to learn about odors, and to exploit their natural food foraging behaviors. The stimuli were common household spices, such as oregano, garlic, etc. These stimuli were mixed into ordinary playground sand and presented in small plastic cups. Rewards were a highly preferred sweetened cereal (Froot Loops) buried under the sand. Prior to formal testing the animals were exposed to cups of sand with buried cereal, and rapidly learned to forage through the sand to find the rewards.

Animals were initially trained to associate pairs of odor stimuli with one another. For brevity, the initial pairs will be called A-B and X-Y, where each letter corresponds to a different odor. Each trial was composed of an initial presentation of one of two sample stimuli, A or X. Then that stimulus was removed and the pair of choice odors, B and Y, was presented (Fig. 5–7A). The rule for the choice was as follows: If A was the sample, then B should be selected to obtain a reward; if X was presented, Y contained the reward. Animals were trained on repetitions of these two types of trials (A-B and X-Y) until they achieved a criterion of 80% correct choices. Then they were trained on a second set of paired associates, and this time each association involved an element that overlapped with one of those in the previous pairings, B-C and Y-Z. So now the sample stimuli were B or Y, and the choice stimuli were always C and Z. This problem was also trained to the 80% correct criterion. Then they were trained with all four problems (A-B, X-Y, B-C, and Y-Z) intermixed (Fig. 5–7B). Normal rats learned each set of paired associates rapidly, and hippocampal damage did not affect acquisition rate on either of the two training sets or their combination. It is important to recognize that correct response for each pairing can be learned independently for each problem. That is, unlike the situation with the water maze described before, the solution to each problem does not interfere with solutions to any of the other problems. Therefore, it was not expected that damage to the hippocampus would affect the ability to acquire these problems. However, it was expected that normal rats and rats with hippocampus damage would form qualitative different representations of the problems, and this was examined next.

Following successful acquisition of all the paired associates, subjects were given probe tests to determine whether they organized their repre-

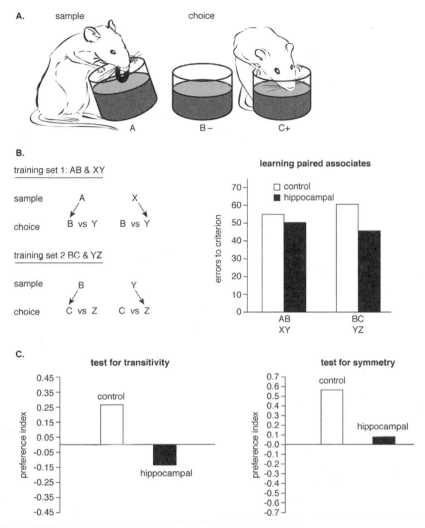

Figure 5–7. Paired associate task. *A:* Illustration of a rat performing the sample and choice trials of the task. *B:* Odors presented in the sample and choice trials in each training set (left) and performance of rats in learning each set. *C:* Performance on the probe tests for transitivity and symmetry. The preference index was calculated as the ratio of the difference in times spent (transitivity) or choice (symmetry) in digging between the two cups and that for the sum on the same measure for the two cups (data from Bunsey and Eichenbaum, 1996).

sentations of the four odor pairs into an efficient scheme that interleaved overlapping odors pairs, or simply learned each problem independently. In the preceding scheme, representations of the pairs A-B and B-C could be organized into a larger network, A-B-C, and similarly X-Y and Y-Z could be organized into X-Y-Z. Two kinds of probe tests were presented to examine whether these larger network representations were formed, and to assess their flexibility.

One test assessed the capacity for "transitive inference," the ability to make a judgment about two odors that are only indirectly related by another, not presented item. In this scheme, note that odor A and odor C were never presented together but can be indirectly related via their shared associate B. Similarly, X and Z are indirectly related via odor Y. In a critical test for transitivity, subjects were presented with trials using the same sample-choice format with trials on A-C and X-Z. However, in these tests no reward was provided, and the time spent foraging in the two choice cups was compared as a measure of their recognition of the appropriate relations between indirectly associated elements. Normal rats also showed strong transitivity, reflected in a preference for odors indirectly associated with the presented sample (Fig. 5–7C). By contrast, rats with selective hippocampal lesions were severely impaired, showing no evidence of transitivity.

The other probe involved a test for "symmetry" of the learned associations, the ability to recognize related pairings regardless of the order in which the items are presented. In this scheme, the subjects were asked to recognize appropriate pairings in the reverse order of that used in training on the second set of problems. Again, the sample-choice format was used, but the pairings were C-B and Z-Y. In the symmetry test, normal rats again showed the appropriate preference in the direction of the symmetrical association. By contrast, rats with hippocampal lesions again were severely impaired, showing no significant capacity for symmetry (Fig. 5–7C). The combined findings show that rats with hippocampal damage can learn even complex associations, such as those in the odor paired associates. But unlike normal animals, they do not interleave the distinct experiences according to their overlapping elements to form a larger network representation that supports inferential and flexible expression of their memories.

A case of naturalistic learning, and natural inferential memory expression

Extending the range of our study of hippocampal involvement in associative learning, the role of the hippocampal region has also been assessed using a type of social olfactory learning and memory, called the social transmission of food preferences. This test is based on observations of rat social behavior in the wild. Rats form large social communities and send out "foragers" to explore for food sources. When forager rats return to the nest, they inform others of new foods by carrying the odor of a new

food on their breath. Subsequently, the other rats to whom this information is conveyed seek out that same food. This form of social learning is
interpreted within the heuristic that a food recently consumed by the forager is safe, and thus transmitting this information is adaptive in rat social groups.

This behavior can be easily adapted to a formal laboratory test by des-
ignating "demonstrator" (forager) and "observer" (subject) rats, and
reproducing the elements of the foraging and social communication events
(Fig. 5–8). Initially, the demonstrator rat is given rat chow tainted with a
food spice, such as cinnamon or chocolate powder. Then the demonstrator is placed in the home cage of the subject for several minutes, during

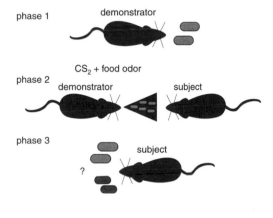

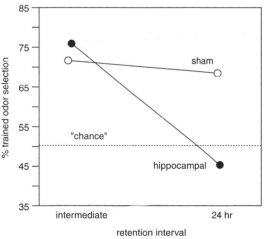

Figure 5–8. The social transmission of food preferences task.
Top: Protocol for the task. *Bottom:* Performance of intact rats
(open circles) and rats with selective hippocampal lesions (filled
circles) in immediate and 1-day
retention tests (data from Bunsey
and Eichenbaum, 1995).

which the two animals socially interact. Then the demonstrator is removed, and the subject must remember the food odor for a variable period. Finally, the subject is presented with two food cups, one with rat chow tainted with the same odor as presented to the demonstrator and the other cup with another food odor that may be equally familiar or novel to the subject. Learning is demonstrated as an increase in the probability that the observer will later select that same food as the demonstrator had eaten over other foods.

Previous investigations of this behavior in normal rats has shown that the mechanism underlying this learning involves an association between two odors present in the demonstrator rat's breath, the odor of the recently eaten food and a natural odorous constituent of rat's breath, carbon disulfide. These studies have shown that exposing the subject to the distinctive food odor alone, or to carbon disulfide alone, have no effect on later food preference. However, exposure to the combination of these two odors using a "surrogate rat," a cotton ball saturated with carbon disulfide, substitutes well for the social interaction in producing the appropriate learned food preference. Thus, the shift in food choice cannot be attributed to mere familiarity with the food odor. Rather, the conclusion from these studies is that the formation of a specific association between the food odor and carbon disulfide, in the absence of any primary reinforcement, is both necessary and sufficient to support the shift in food selection.

Social transmission of food preferences provides a strong example of declarative-like learning in the natural behavior of rats. Learning involves the formation of a specific stimulus–stimulus association in a single training episode. Furthermore, this paradigm provides one of the best examples of a natural form of "inferential" expression of the memory. Thus, note that the training experience involves a social encounter without any feeding, during which the subject is exposed to an arbitrary stimulus and another natural stimulus that acts as a reinforcer. By contrast, the memory testing situation is nonsocial, and involves food selection choices without the presence of the same stimulus that reinforced learning the new food odor. This aspect of the task, expression of memory in a situation very different from the learning event, is strongly consistent with the declarative property of representational flexibility.

The role of the hippocampus has been investigated using this task, assessing both immediate memory and delayed memory for social exposure to the odor of a novel food. The behavior of rats with hippocampal damage during the social encounter is entirely normal. In the memory test, normal rats showed a strong selection preference for the trained food odor, and this memory was robust when tested immediately and after a 1-day retention period (see Fig. 5–8). By contrast, rats with selective damage to the hippocampus showed intact immediate memory, but their performance fell to chance level of food choices within 24 hours. The observation of intact immediate memory, similar to the pattern of spared short-term memory in human amnesics, indicates that the hippocampus is not required for perceptual, motivational, or behavioral components of the social learning or the ability to express the learned food choice preferences. But the hippocampus is required for long-term expression of the memory in a situation that is far outside the learning context.

Summing up

There is a long and mixed history of attempts to model amnesia in animals. Efforts in both monkeys and rats were largely unsuccessful owing to the poor choice of memory tests and the lack of realization that there are different forms of memory, only one of which depends on the medial temporal lobe. However, there have now been many successful demonstrations of the characteristics of human amnesia in both monkeys and rats. In monkeys, major advances were made with the advent of the delayed nonmatch to sample test that provided a novel test of recognition memory. The results using this test plus those of a set of related tests showed that medial temporal lobe damage similar to that in H.M. results in a remarkably similar pattern of impaired and spared memory abilities. In rats, major advances were made following the realization that much of the ambiguity in the pattern of effects of hippocampal damage could be explained by distinctions between impairments in spatial memory versus spared nonspatial memory, and between memory-specific recent experiences versus spared learning guided by habits or dispositions of specific stimuli. However, experiments in support of each of these two accounts are in apparent conflict.

The combined results from both these accounts, and across many other experiments, provide compelling evidence for a comprehensive account of the cognitive mechanisms of declarative memory. Various kinds of learning, spatial and nonspatial, simple and complex, can be accomplished independent of the hippocampus in animals, as indeed is the case in human amnesic patients as well. However, the hippocampus is required to link together the representations of overlapping experiences into a relational representation, and supports the flexible and inferential expression of indirect associations among items within the larger organization of linked memories. This hippocampal function applies across many situations, including navigation within spatial organizations, and nonspatial organizations of specific stimuli (e.g., odors) in logical schemes or in natural social behavior. The next chapter explores the nature of the neural code that accomplishes this networking function of the hippocampus.

READINGS

Cohen, N.J. 1984. Preserved learning capacity in amnesia: Evidence for multiple memory systems. In *The Neuropsychology of Memory*, N. Butters, and L.R. Squire (Eds.). New York: Guilford Press, pp. 83–103.

Cohen, N.J., and Eichenbaum, H. 1993. *Memory, Amnesia, and the Hippocampal System*. Cambridge: MIT Press.

Eichenbaum, H. 1997. Declarative memory: Insights from cognitive neurobiology. *Annu. Rev. Psychol.* 48:547–572.

Mishkin, M,, and Petri, H.L. 1984. Memories and habits: Some implications for the analysis of learning and retention. In *The Neuropsychology of Memory*, N. Butters, and L.R. Squire (Eds.). New York: Guilford Press, pp. 287–296.

Morris, R.G.M., Garrud, P., Rawlins, J.P, and O'Keefe, J. 1982. Place navigation impaired in rats with hippocampal lesions. *Nature* 297:681–683.

O'Keefe, J.A., and Nadel, L. 1978. *The Hippocampus as a Cognitive Map*. New York: Oxford University Press.

Olton, D.S., Becker, J.T., and Handlemann, G.E. 1979. Hippocampus, space, and memory. *Brain Behav. Sci.* 2:313–365.

Squire, L. 1992. Memory and the hippocampus: A synthesis from findings with rats, monkeys, and humans. *Psycho. Rev.* 99(2): 195–231.

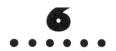

Windows into
the Workings of Memory

STUDY QUESTIONS

What is brain imaging, and how can it be used to study human memory?

What are the characteristics of memory processing that activate the medial temporal lobe in normal human subjects?

What are place cells?

What is the full characterization of events that are encoded by hippocampal neuron firing patterns?

What is a "memory space," and how might it be constructed by the properties of hippocampal neuron firing patterns?

So far this review of our understanding of hippocampal function in memory has focused predominantly on studies of amnesia in humans and on the effects of hippocampal damage in animals. In the present chapter, complementary evidence is presented from other related approaches. These approaches involve monitoring the ongoing operation of the human hippocampus and related brain structures during memory performance, providing a virtual "window" into the inner workings of the normal brain. This is accomplished at two levels of analysis: by using functional neuroimaging methods in normal humans and by recording the activity patterns of single neurons in animals.

With regard to the functional imaging studies, there are now multiple sophisticated methods that are employed, particularly positron emission tomography (PET) and functional magnetic resonance imaging (fMRI). It is beyond the scope of this text to discuss the details of these methodologies, except to say that both involve measurements of blood flow and brain oxygen consumption, which provide good reflections of the level of activation of a brain area encompassing several thousand neurons over a second-to-second time scale. By telling us when, for example, the medial temporal area becomes active, functional neuroimaging studies in humans can inform us about the aspects or kinds of memory in which the hippocampal system is and is not involved, providing a way to assess its functional role.

Single cell recording studies in animals provide an even closer look at the inner workings of the hippocampus. This method involves monitoring the action potentials of individual neurons and so allows a major increase in resolution of cellular activity within different parts of the medial temporal area, and even allows us to distinguish particular types of neurons within a specific brain structure. Also, this method has a greater resolution in time, allowing us to capture millisecond-to-millisecond computations by the fundamental elements of neural processing. Thus, these two approaches have complementary strengths and limitations. The strength of functional imaging is that it allows the simultaneous examination of the entire system, but at only a gross level that tells us which structures are activated to major shifts in task demands. Single cell recording methods allow us to monitor only one part of the system at any time, but offer insights into the fundamental coding properties of the units of neural computation.

Functional neuroimaging studies of the human hippocampal system

Early attempts to observe hippocampal activation in PET or fMRI during one or another memory performance were largely disappointing. Scannning during the study of materials such as word lists, and other tasks for which memory depends on hippocampal function, failed to show increased activation over nonmemory processing of the same materials. However, this turns out to be an artifact of the procedures in analysis of brain images. All imaging techniques involve a *comparison* of activation levels between two conditions, an experimental and a control condition. In memory studies, the experimental condition involves the critical memory demand under study, for example, memorizing word lists. The control condition involves the same perceptual and cognitive demands, except without the critical memory demand. In the word list example, the control might be reading words without having to remember them. The areas associated with memory processing *per se* are defined operationally as those brain regions where the activation level is greater in the experimental condition than in the control condition. However, the evidence described previously, as well as other physiological data that are described later, indicate that the hippocampus is always active in encoding new information for declarative memory. In the example, the control condition where subjects merely read words may invoke quite substantial hippocampal activation associated with remembering the experience of reading the word list. More generally, there is virtually no condition where memory processing is expected to be altogether absent. Thus, the failure to find activation associated with memory in the early studies may be attributed to the lack of a substantial difference in the activations associated during the memory condition (e.g., studying a word list) and apparent nonmemory activities for which memory processing was nevertheless invoked (reading a word list).

Since those early studies, another generation of experiments has taken the issue of control conditions into consideration and in recent years has shown that the human hippocampal system can be seen in action during various memory performances and the results of these studies correspond well to those of the studies of amnesia. Thus, the findings from functional brain imaging generally support the distinction between declarative and procedural memory, and they provide new details on the nature of events that activate the medial temporal area. The following section explores these characteristics of medial temporal activation.

The medial temporal area is involved in "global" information processing

Consider first the range of to-be-remembered materials over which the medial temporal area operates. Studies of patients with bilateral damage to the medial temporal area have shown that amnesia is a *global* memory deficit. As discussed in Chapter 4, amnesic patients have a memory impairment that crosses between different learning materials and sensory modalities, encompassing verbal and nonverbal, spatial and nonspatial materials, regardless of whether they are presented visually, auditorily, etc., indicating that the role of this region in memory is, likewise, *non*specific with regard to material and modality. However, other studies involving patients with *unilateral* damage, that is, involving damage only to the left or right medial temporal lobe region, have shown clear material-specific memory impairments: Verbal memory performance is selectively compromised after *left* medial temporal lobe damage, and nonverbal memory performance is selectively compromised after *right* temporal lobe damage. In other words, there is a *laterality* in the critical medial temporal lobe contribution to memory, corresponding to the different types of learning materials. Furthermore, the nature of processing for which the hemispheres are specialized follows the well-known laterality for nonmemory processing of verbal versus nonverbal materials assigned to the left and right hemispheres, respectively. How well do the findings from functional imaging studies of memory correspond to this picture from studies of amnesia?

Across a variety of functional imaging studies one can see both the globalness of medial temporal processing, considering both hemispheres, and also the material-specificity of left versus right hemisphere processing. Looking across the range of studies that have reported medial temporal activation, one sees that a range of stimulus materials can engage this system. Thus, ignoring the particular hemisphere in which activation occurs, activation in the medial temporal lobe has been reported for words, objects, scenes, faces, and spatial routes, landmarks, or locations. In addition, in studies that compared different classes of materials, clear hemispheric specialization has been seen. The results generally indicate greater left than right activation for words, and greater right than left activation for novel faces or objects. Accordingly, with regard to the scope of the materials processed by the medial temporal lobe, there is good concordance of the functional imaging and the data from studies on amnesia.

Next we consider several general findings on the types of memory processing that have consistently activated the medial temporal area across multiple studies. These include activation by the simple presentation of novel stimulus information, activation by the processing of new stimulus associations, and activation associated with explicit, conscious recollection.

Activation of the medial temporal region
by the presentation of novel information

There are now several lines of evidence that have suggested medial temporal lobe involvement in specific aspects of cognitive processing, although some of these are not identical to dimensions that are featured in accounts of amnesia. However, it is important to keep in mind that functional imaging studies are likely to reveal the initial stages of memory processing when the medial temporal area becomes involved, even in situations where its involvement may not be critical to that particular type of processing. A good example involves several reports of engagement of the medial temporal region by the mere presentation of novel information. These studies have found greater activation for the processing of *novel* as compared to *familiar* pictures of complex scenes or objects. In one study, subjects viewed magazine photos of scenes in alternating blocks of trials that included either a series of different scenes, each presented once, or just one scene that was presented repeatedly as a control. Subjects were instructed to study the scenes so they might be able to recognize them later, and they were scanned during this study phase. Greater activation was seen in the medial temporal region for the novel scenes in the experimental condition compared to the single repeated scene in the control condition. In perhaps the most striking example of a novelty detection effect, the right hippocampus was selectively activated by the presentation of novel visual noise patterns, that is, a series of random dot patterns, compared to the presentation of the same patterns a second time (Fig. 6–1A).

These findings have led some investigators to propose that the medial temporal region may be involved in novelty detection per se. However, as you will see later, the medial temporal region is activated also by familiar material under circumstances where the subject is making recognition judgments. So, clearly the detection of novelty *per se* is not the primary function revealed in activation by novel stimuli. Rather, an effect of stimulus novelty on medial temporal activation makes good sense as a reflection of the kind of processing that would underlie declarative memories of the many pictures. The presentation of a brand new scene every few seconds should invoke considerable declarative memory processing as the hippocampus is involved in encoding the information within scenes and the sequence of constantly changing scenes. By contrast, the control condition that involves repeated presentations of a single unchanging scene, minimizes this processing demand. Therefore, the comparison of these two conditions is likely to reveal the differential activation for maximal and minimal processing of new information.

Medial temporal activation associated with processing stimulus associations

The data just described suggest that the hippocampus always becomes engaged when new material is presented, but may become more activated to the extent that processing relations among elements within or across scenes is strongly demanded by the materials or the task. This view could account for why the early studies failed to find medial temporal activation when subjects were presented with highly familiar stimuli such as word lists, as compared to other manipulations of the same materials that also invoke memory processing. The studies that focused on the presentation of several changing scenes as compared to the same unchanging scene may have revealed a difference in the amount of hippocampal activation de-

A. novel visual "noise"

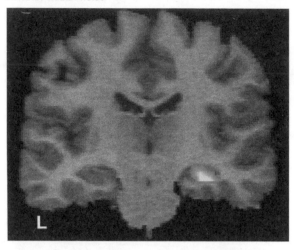

B. the combination of time-specific and personally relevant memory

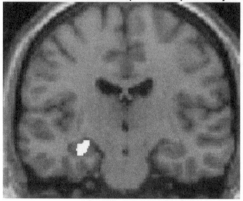

Figure 6–1. Functional imaging of the human hippocampus. *A:* Activation of the right hippocampus during viewing of novel as contrasted with familiar visual noise patterns (from Martin, 1999). *B:* Activation of the left hippocampus during recall of memories that are both temporally specific and personally relevant (from Maguire and Mummery, 1999).

manded by the differential requirement for processing information within and across items that would be encoded in memory.

Consistent with this expectation the strongest support for the medial temporal region activation in processing information across scenes for explicit memory comes from a study by Henke and colleagues in which subjects were shown a series of pictures, each of which showed a person and a house (either the interior or the exterior) simultaneously. Subjects were required to judge if the person was likely to be the inhabitant or a visitor to that house, based on their appearance and that of the house. For example, one pair of pictures showed an elegant lady and an equally elegant sitting room that would constitute an appropriate match. Another example showed a disheveled man and a large mansion, representing an unlikely match. Thus, while the task did not directly demand the subjects to associate the two images, the nature of the judgment encouraged them to make an association between the person and the house. As a control, subjects were shown other pairs of pictures and requested to make separate decisions about the person's gender (male or female?) and view of the house (exterior or interior?). This test requirement encouraged the subjects to encode the house and person separately.

Greater medial temporal activation was observed when the subjects were encouraged to associate the person and the house than when they encoded the same kinds of items separately. These findings suggest that it is not merely the processing of novel pictures that activates the hippocampus. If this were so, one would expect the same level of activation for similarly novel pictures of people and houses. Instead, the findings support the view that the medial temporal region is more activated when there is a greater demand for learning associations or relations between items in single learning episodes, as compared with processing the items separately.

In a related study, Maguire and Mummery examined the activation of medial temporal structures during recollection of different types of materials. They found a large network of brain areas activated during different types of recall associated with different aspects of real-world memory, including whether the memory occurred at a particular time or instead involved time-independent factual information, or was personally relevant or instead involved general knowledge of public events. They found a striking and specific activation of the left hippocampus when what subjects recollected was a combination of personally relevant and specific in time (Fig. 6–1B).

Medial temporal activation associated with conscious recollection

More directly related to declarative memory, other studies have considered whether the medial temporal lobe region is disproportionately engaged in explicit memory, that is, in conscious recollection. In one experiment, subjects first studied word lists and then their memory was later tested in different ways during scanning. At testing, subjects were given word stems and asked to complete the stems either with the first word that came to mind, just as in a typical repetition priming experiment (see Chapter 4), or with a word from the study list, to engage conscious recollection, or with the first word that came to mind that was *not* on the study list, as a baseline condition where the subject stared at a cross-hair on the screen. Medial temporal activation was found for the condition that involved conscious recollection, as compared to either the priming condition, which involved implicit memory instructions, or the baseline condition.

Other studies have related medial temporal activation to successful retrieval of previously stored information, that is, success in the effortful reactivation of stored representations. In one such study, subjects listened to two lists of words prior to being in the scanner. For one list, subjects were to decide whether each word was said by a male or female speaker. This condition was employed to encourage processing at the level of perceptual features of the words and to deemphasize encoding the semantic or conceptual content in the words. For the other list, the subjects had to decide whether each word referred to a living or nonliving thing, in order to encourage conceptual or semantic encoding over perceptual encoding. Subjects were subsequently tested for recognition memory while being scanned, in a series of test blocks that assessed memory separately for perceptually encoded and semantically encoded words.

Greater medial temporal lobe activation was observed for test blocks that involved words from the semantically encoded list compared to the perceptually encoded list. The fact that there was a higher rate of successful recall of semantically encoded words compared to perceptually encoded words suggested that increased medial temporal activation for semantically encoded words was a consequence of the role of this region in successful recall, that is, in successfully gaining access to some memory representation. This connection was seen more formally as a strong positive correlation across subjects and conditions between test performance and medial temporal lobe activation.

Another line of studies has shown that the medial temporal region is activated when subjects are involved in effortful retrieval and manipulation of retrieved geographical information. In these studies experienced London taxi drivers were scanned as they were requested to retrieve information about routes around London. Greater activation of medial temporal structures was seen during recall of route information than during recall of famous landmarks, movie plot lines, or movie scenes. In another study subjects learned to navigate around in a virtual reality environment. Subjects were then scanned while they made judgments about the appearance or relative position of particular places in the environment compared to a control condition involving scrambled versions of the same stimuli. Medial temporal activation was observed bilaterally for both conditions that tested memory of the learned places compared to the control condition.

These functional brain imaging studies indicate that the medial temporal region becomes activated whenever new, complex material is presented. Furthermore, these results indicate that the medial temporal region is maximally activated when processing this material demands encoding new associations or relations among separate items in specific memory episodes. In addition, the medial temporal area is similarly invoked during the act of explicit memory retrieval, that is, during conscious recollection. These findings are entirely consistent with the observations on the pattern of impaired and spared capacities in human amnesia, and thus demonstrate a close correspondence of the data from two different approaches. Furthermore, the combination of activations during both episodic learning and conscious recollection indicates that the medial temporal area is involved similarly in encoding and retrieval phases of declarative memory.

The representation of experience in the activity
of networks of hippocampal neurons

The foregoing characterizations of the effects of damage to the hippocampal region (in Chapters 4 and 5), and of activation of the hippocampal region in humans, suggest that its fundamental role is in encoding rich episodic information and conscious and flexible memory expression. What kind of neural representation within the hippocampus would support this functional role? As described in the preceding chapter, on a conceptual level, the form of such a representation might be constituted as a large network that encodes episodic memories and links these memories via their shared features. Can such a scheme be confirmed and elaborated by observations on the elements of the hippocampus, that is, in the firing patterns of single hippocampal neurons?

While any conclusions about the nature of firing patterns in the hippocampus is still quite preliminary, there is an emerging body of data consistent with this scheme. A wealth of evidence indicates that hippocampal neurons encode a broad variety of information, including all modalities of perceptual input as well as behavioral actions, and cognitive operations. In addition, hippocampal neurons seem especially tuned to relevant conjunctions among features that reflect unique episodic information, rather than simple perceptual or motor features. Moreover, hippocampal neural activity is particularly sensitive to modifications with experience such that alterations in the meaning of items or their relationships result in major changes in cellular firing patterns. Combined, these observations provide a bridge to current characterizations of declarative memory being accessible by many routes of expression, including literally one's verbal declarations about the contents of prior experiences. I begin with a conceptual scheme that could accomplish the coding of episodic information and the linking of this information into a larger network or memory space. Then I review the observations from studies on the firing patterns of hippocampal neurons that support this scheme.

A scheme for hippocampal representation in declarative memory

The evidence from both studies on human and animal amnesia and from brain imaging studies on humans points to an important role for the hippocampus in encoding complex information that contributes to our memory for personal experiences, that is, episodic memories, and for our ability to synthesize this episodic information into our body of world knowledge, fact or semantic memory. It is well known that the hippocampus receives information from virtually all sensory domains as well as other information about our internal states and our own behaviors (see Chapter 9). In addition, the hippocampus is remarkable for the extent of interconnectivity among the principal cells in its major processing areas. Also, the studies on hippocampal plasticity outlined in Chapter 3 have indicated that hippocampal neurons are particularly good at encoding conjunctions of diverse inputs. This combination of observations suggests a scheme in which subsets of hippocampal neurons could act as small networks for encoding episodic memories and for linking them together into larger networks that could support the properties of declarative memory.

An outline of such a scheme is presented in Fig. 6–2. The scheme proposes three types or levels of coding by single hippocampal neurons. At the lowest level in this scheme, each hippocampal cell encodes a highly complex set of sensory and other information that composes a single behavioral "event." A single event is brief in its scope, akin to a single photographic snapshot that would include information about any salient stimuli, ongoing behavior, and the location or background in which the event occurred. In this scheme, single hippocampal neurons are viewed as capable of encoding the conjunction of all of this information that composes a single event captured in a brief moment of time.

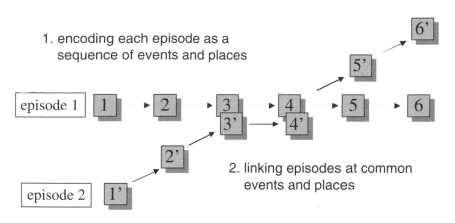

Figure 6–2. Schematic model of a simple "memory space." Events include ongoing behavior and location information, as indicated by individual numbered boxes. Episodes are composed of a sequence of event representations. The memory space is composed of a set of episodes linked by common, nodal events.

In addition, at the second level of this scheme, the activities of a set of hippocampal cells that are activated in sequence during a particular episode are preserved. This may be accomplished by cells whose plasticity properties can incorporate features of two or more sequential events, thus providing a mechanism for tying together the individual representations of multiple events. This combination of a set of sequential individual event codings and the codings that link multiple event sequences constitute the complete representation of a single episodic memory.

Finally, at the third level of this scheme, it is proposed that there are other "nodal" hippocampal cells that encode features that are common across multiple episodes. According to this account, these cells receive strong inputs from some information about specific stimuli, behaviors, or location or other contextual information that is a salient element among otherwise distinct experiences. This feature could include a common critical stimulus to be remembered across different types of training trials, a common response one made to various stimuli in different trials, or a common location where different experiences occurred.

The combination of these three functional prototypes of hippocampal cells provides the fundamental elements of a "memory space" that could support the properties of declarative memory. The event cells would capture unique combinations of behavioral and location information that would mark specific episodes. The cells that encode sequences of multiple events could allow the recovery of entire episodes. The nodal cells could provide a bridge between episodic representations that could support the capacity for flexible and inferential memory expression by linking together indirectly information obtained across distinct episodes. What is the evidence that hippocampal cells have the properties of these prototypical units? A review of the story of efforts to characterize hippocampal neuron activity provides strong support for this model and insights into the workings of memory processing within the hippocampus.

Early observations on the firing patterns of hippocampal neurons

Following on the advent of technologies for recording the extracellular spike activity in behaving animals, several investigators began to explore the firing patterns of the large pyramidal cells in the hippocampus of rats. Electrophysiological techniques allowed these investigators to make the recordings in awake and behaving animals, providing the opportunity to correlate neuronal activations with stimulus events and motor patterns during a broad variety of behaviors, including learning. The expectations of investigators in these explorations were marked by caution. James Ranck, Jr., as he pioneered the earliest recording of hippocampal neurons in behaving animals, worried that cells in a brain structure located so many synapses from sensory input and motor output would have firing activity significant only as part of a large network; he suspected that neural firing patterns in response to external stimuli or behavioral output would be uninterpretable. But this clearly turned out not to be the case. Quite the opposite—hippocampal neuronal activity is well correlated with a very broad variety of stimuli and behavioral events, with the activity of cells "mirroring" virtually all the combinations of stimulus and behavioral events in any situation. Thus, identifying the scope and nature of information processing by hippocampal neurons has proved a formidable challenge, not because of the paucity of responses they might have evoked, but because of their variety, their complexity, and their plasticity in response to change.

In Ranck's landmark 1973 paper, he described a large number of behavioral correlates of hippocampal neuronal activity. His categorization included cells that fired associated with specific orienting behaviors, approach movements, or cessation of movement, and with consummatory behaviors (feeding and drinking) or the mismatch of expected consummatory event (e.g., the absence of water when it is usually found). At the same time, John O'Keefe was also recording from hippocampal cells in rats exploring open environment. His observations on hippocampal cellular activity led him to a different conclusion—rather than neuronal activity reflecting ongoing behaviors, O'Keefe and his colleague John Dostrovsky made the remarkable and historic discovery that hippocampal cells fire associated with locations the animal occupies at least as much as with the ongoing behavioral events. Ranck noted the possibility that his findings might be characterized in terms of the spatial specificity of firing patterns, and for some period the "behavioral" correlates of hippocampal firing patterns were largely overwhelmed with excitement about the spatial coding properties of these cells. This led to a period when considerable attention was given to the spatial properties of hippocampal neuronal activity, within the framework of the cognitive map theory of O'Keefe and Nadel, as introduced in the preceding chapter.

What are place cells? Do they compose a "cognitive map"?

The existence of location-specific neural activity in hippocampal neurons has been confirmed in many systematic studies. The common observation is that pyramidal neurons of the CA1 and CA3 fields of the hippocampus fire at high rates when the animal is in a particular location in the environment and fire little or not at all when the animal is located in other places. This observation led to the conclusion that each hippocampal cell has a distinct "place field," or area of the environment associated with high firing rate. Many current studies of place cells involve computerized tracking of the animal's position continuously in space, and automated means of determining the firing rate of the neuron associated with a matrix of locations. These studies show that many hippocampal cells have spatially specific activity that can be observed in many behavioral situations. A particularly clear example comes from a simple protocol where a rat forages for small food pellets distributed randomly throughout an open field. The rat continuously searches in all directions for extended periods (Fig. 6–3A). In this situation many hippocampal cells fire at a high rate only when the rat crosses a particular area in the environment (the place field), regardless of the rat's orientation within the environment. Once established, place fields can be very stable, and have been observed to show the same spatial firing pattern for months. However, the probability of firing of place cells is highly variable, in that sometimes the rate exceeds 100/sec on a pass through the field. Yet, on other passes, the cell may not fire at all, such that the average firing rate within the place field is typi-

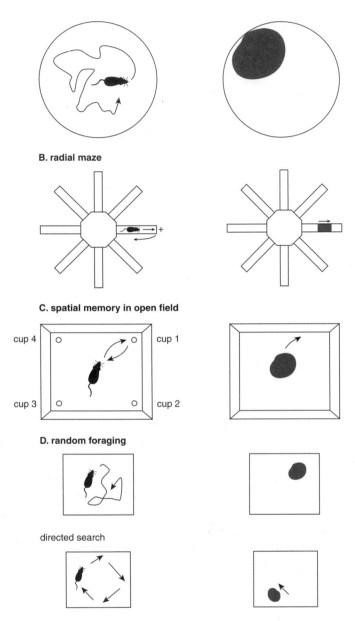

A. random foraging in open field

B. radial maze

C. spatial memory in open field

cup 4   cup 1

cup 3   cup 2

D. random foraging

directed search

Figure 6–3. Four different protocols used to map hippocampal place fields. For each protocol, the task is illustrated on the left. On the right is a mapping of an example place field (filled area), the location in the environment where the cell increased firing rate of the cell. Directional place fields are indicated by an arrow showing the direction of movement associated with increased firing.

cally about 10/sec. This variability portends that factors other than the location of the animal *per se* determine the activity of these cells.

In their initial report, O'Keefe and Dostrovsky realized immediately the potential significance of this neural correlate, and suggested that the hippocampus might subserve the creation and utilization of cognitive maps that animals use to navigate their environment, just as Tolman proposed in his efforts to characterize maze learning capacities in animals. In support of this view, O'Keefe later reviewed the existing findings on hippocampal place cells, focusing on the number and types of stimulus features in the environment that were encoded by place cells. He concluded that "a place cell is a cell which constructs the notion of a place in the environment by connecting together several multisensory inputs each of which can be perceived when the animal is in a particular part of the environment" (O'Keefe, 1979, p. 425). He supported this characterization by showing that the location-specific firing of most hippocampal neurons is controlled by the global configuration of the distant salient stimuli, and that any substantial subset of the spatial cues is sufficient to support spatially specific activity in some cells. More recent studies have shown that while some cells encode all of the available sensory cues, the location-specific activity of most hippocampal neurons is controlled by a subset of the spatial stimuli. Therefore, the overall representation of space is a composite of many partial representations where each cell encodes the spatial relations between a few of the cues.

The view that hippocampal cells encode spatial position is a critical feature of O'Keefe and Nadel's cognitive mapping hypothesis. The concept of hippocampal spatial representation that has emerged from these findings, illustrated in Fig. 6–4, is that the hippocampus contains a map-like representation of space. At a conceptual level, the map constitutes a coordinate grid, instantiated by intrinsic connections among hippocampal neurons. During investigation of a novel environment, representations of the relevant environmental stimuli are associated with appropriate spatial coordinate points. The resulting map is Cartesian in that it provides metric representations of distances and angles between the relevant stimuli. At the physiological level, a place cell reflects the occurrence of the rat at a particular coordinate position within the map. Thus, implicit in this model is the assumption that place fields can be considered "pointers" within a unified map, such that either every cell contains information about all of the cues or that cells representing subsets of the cues are all linked and bound by the global coordinate framework. O'Keefe and Nadel's central notion then is that the hippocampus constructs a facsimile of the environment, including the salient environmental cues.

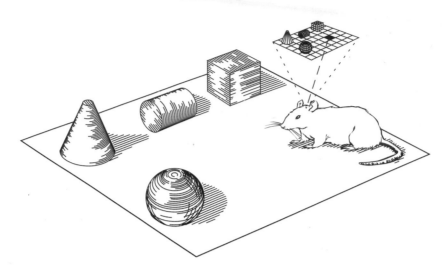

Figure 6–4. A schematic illustration of how an environment is mapped in the hippocampus, according to the cognitive mapping hypothesis (from Eichenbaum et al., 1999).

Despite the attractive features of a cognitive map in the hippocampus, there is little in the way of evidence that hippocampal cells act as elements of a cohesive map of the environment. Indeed, in contrast to this view, there is no topographical relationship between place cells in the hippocampus and locations in space. Furthermore, in many situations individual place cells are simultaneously controlled by different cues in the environment. So, while the existence of place cells as encoding location-specific sensory information is now widely accepted, there is no strong evidence that these place representations are elements of a cohesive map of space. Instead, a strong possibility is that place cells represent familiar places as complex contextual information rather than as coordinates of a map. Additional evidence that place cell activity is strongly influenced by nonspatial factors suggests that location-specific activity may reflect the encoding of the places where important events happen.

Hippocampal cells encode actions in places

Do hippocampal place cells encode only the location of the animal? Even in his earliest description of place cells O'Keefe reported that the spatial activity of hippocampal neurons was influenced by more than just the location of the animal in the environment. Indeed, the preliminary study by O'Keefe and Dostrovsky emphasized that all the place cells fired only when the rat was facing a particular direction. O'Keefe's subsequent full analysis reported several variables in addition to location that determined place cell firing rate, including orientation, how long the rat was in the place field, and the elicitation of particular behaviors such as eating, grooming, and exploratory sniffing. Motion- and behavior-related correlates were the focus of Ranck's analysis of hippocampal firing properties, in which he described cells that fired primarily as a rat was involved in orientation, approach to particular objects or goals, consummatory movements, or cessation of movement.

Several studies have now demonstrated that place cell firing is strongly influenced by movement direction and speed. Indeed, as rats perform in maze tasks, such as the radial maze, the majority of place cells in rats running on a radial maze fired almost entirely when the animal was running outward or returning inward on the maze arms (see Fig. 6–3B), and the firing rate was somewhat higher when the rat was running with greater speed. This finding is not dependent on the structure of the maze itself, but rather on the movement patterrns of the rat in the task. For example, in one study rats were required to begin each trial at the center of the open rectangular environment, and then could approach any of the four corners to obtain a reward. Subsequently they had to return to the center and then approach a different corner to obtain another reward, etc. The majority of place cells fired differentially according to the direction the rat was moving (see Fig. 6–3C). In addition, most place cells were also tuned for the speed of movement, and in many of these cells there was an optimal movement speed such that the cell fired at lower rates for both slower and faster movements through the place field. Also, the majority of the place cells fired differentially depending on the angle of the turn taken during movements. The activity of most cells was best described not so much in terms of spatial parameters but simply as firing at a particular time during the trip to or from a particular goal.

A critical role for the animal's behavior, as much as the nature of cues available or the shape of the apparatus, was most directly demonstrated in a study that involved training rats in two different versions of the same task (see Fig. 6–3D). In one version the rats were initially trained to forage in an open environment for tiny food pellets distributed in random locations, causing the rats to move in all directions throughout the environment. In the second version of the task, the same rats were subsequently trained to find food only at four specific locations in the same open field that were repeatedly baited. Consistent with other descriptions of place cells of rats performing the random foraging task, in this situation the place cells were generally nondirectional, that is, fired similarly regardless of the direction of the animal's movement through the place field. By contrast, when the rats approached a small number of repeated reward locations, most of the cells (even the same cells) were directional, that is, fired only during the approach to, or the departure from, a particular location. These findings are distinct from the conventional characterization of place cells as localized with respect to static cues in the environment, and show that the ongoing behavior, defined as direction of movement, can strongly influence cell activity.

Furthermore, these findings show that, even in the identical apparatus, place cells can exhibit a specific movement correlate depending on whether the task makes particular movement direction patterns significant to the structure of the task. Thus, in this context, the cells are not well characterized as place cells, because their activity does not reliably predict the animal's location. Rather, these cells seem to encode a particular relevant action in a particular place. This conclusion opens up the possibility that hippocampal cells may also encode other variables, including stimuli, behaviors, or other events that have no particular identity in location.

Hippocampal neurons encode nonspatial stimuli and events

As noted previously, even the earliest studies on hippocampal activity in animals exploring open environment included some cells that appeared to have nonspatial firing correlates. Consistent with these early findings, several investigators who have intentionally looked for event-related neural activity have demonstrated firing patterns of hippocampal neurons related to nonspatial stimuli and events. In most of these studies, as in the earliest place cell studies, the relevant stimuli and behaviors were confounded with spatial location in that each event is associated with the animal's presence in one place. Nevertheless, these studies show that nonspatial stimuli and events can be a necessary component of cellular activation, and a recent study provides compelling evidence of nonspatial firing patterns that occur independent of the animal's spatial location.

Among the first findings of nonspatial correlates of hippocampal cellular activity were observations that hippocampal neurons fire associated with the development of a Pavlovian conditioned eyeblink, even when the animal was restrained throughout the training session. In addition, several studies have shown hippocampal neural activity associated with stimulus sampling in rats performing learned sensory discriminations or delayed matching or nonmatching to sample tasks. Notably in all these tasks other individual hippocampal cells exhibited striking responses associated with various behaviors including approach to the relevant discriminative stimuli or the reward. Indeed, the activity of the population of hippocampal cells could be characterized as a set of neurons firing selectively at each phase of the task.

Perhaps the most striking of these studies is a series of experiments by Sam Deadwyler and his colleagues, who have studied the firing properties of single hippocampal neurons and neuronal ensembles in rats performing delayed matching and nonmatching to sample in a discrete trials version of the task where the cues were left and right positions of two response bars. On each trial one bar was extended into the apparatus and pressed by the animal to obtain an initial reward. During the delay period the bar was withdrawn and the animal had to nose poke at a port on the opposite side of the apparatus. Finally both bars were extended into the apparatus and the animal could press the matching or nonmatching bar to obtain a second reward. In Deadwyler's analysis of single hippocampal cells, many of the neurons fired during the sample or match responses or upon the delivery of the reward, or combinations of these events. Many of these cells fired differentially depending on the left–right position of the bar pressed, or whether the response was correct or an error. In addition, many individual cells fired during the delay period, but their activity did not predict the position of the correct response.

Deadwyler and colleagues' characterization of the activity of ensembles of cells recorded at several locations in the hippocampus focused on a statistical analysis that could extract patterns of covariances among the cells associated with different task events. These analyses showed that specific task parameters accounted for most of the overall variance in ensemble activity. The major components corresponded to encoding of the sample versus choice phase of the task regardless of bar position, encoding of the spatial position of the lever independent of task phase, encoding of left versus right error responses, and encoding of the sample position during the sample and choice phase. The encoding of lever position may be regarded as a spatial mapping. However, the coding of task phase cut across locations where the rat was positioned, and the coding of the sample position lingered into the choice phase when the rat was at the opposite bar on correct trials. Thus, while all the correlates of these cells can be considered "spatial" in various ways, a considerable amount of the variance in ensemble activity was not associated strictly with the animal's location but rather with the encoding of task-relevant spatial information.

Analyses of the firing properties of hippocampal neurons have been extended to studies on the primate hippocampal region. In general the evidence for pure place-specific activity is poor, although sensory-evoked neural activity is often modulated by a variety of spatial variables. In humans, visually evoked responses of hippocampal neurons have also been observed, and a substantial fraction of these cells fired on the sight of a particular word or face stimulus or during execution of task-relevant key press responses. In one recent study, Itzak Fried and his colleagues characterized the responses of hippocampal neurons in human subjects performing a recognition memory task with face and visual-object cues. Again a substantial number of cells responded to the stimuli, and individual cells had activity that differentiated faces from objects, or distinguished facial gender or expression, or new versus familiar faces and objects. The largest fraction of cells differentiated combinations of these features. Some of the cells had a specific pattern of responsiveness across all of these parameters.

Some studies have been directly aimed at dissociating spatial and non-spatial firing patterns of hippocampal neurons by requiring animals to perform the same tasks using identical cues located at different locations in the environment. A particularly compelling study involved olfactory cues that were moved systematically among locations within a static environment, and provided unambiguous evidence of place-independent nonspatial hippocampal activity. Rats were trained to perform an odor-guided delayed nonmatch to sample task at multiple locations on a large open field (Fig. 6–5A). The stimuli were plastic cups that contained playground sand scented with one of nine common odors (e.g., coffee, cinnamon, etc.). On each trial one cup was placed randomly at any of nine locations on the open field. Whenever the odor differed from that on the previous trial (i.e., was a nonmatch) a Froot Loop was buried in the sand, and the rat would dig for the reward. Whenever the odor was the same as that on the previous trial (i.e., was a match) no Froot Loop was buried and the rat would turn away. The firing rate of hippocampal cells was assessed during the approach to the cups, focusing on the last second of the approach during which the animal arrived at the cup and generated its response. Firing rates were statistically compared across the set of odors, the set of locations, and match–nonmatch conditions.

About two-thirds of hippocampal cells fired in association with one or more of these variables during the task. About one-third of the active cells' firing was not differentiated by the location of the cup, and about one-third of the active cells demonstrated some spatial component of firing. Some of the nonspatial cells were activated during the approach to any of the odor cups at any of the nine locations. Other cells fired differentially across the odor set (Fig. 6–5B), or between match and nonmatch conditions, or some combination of these variables and the approach. Only a small proportion of the location-selective cells fired associated only with the position of the cup (Fig. 6–5C). For the majority of cells, their activity was conjointly associated with the position where the cup was pre-

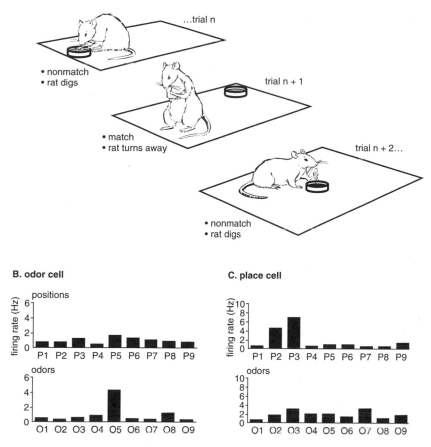

A. delayed non-match to sample task

...trial n

• nonmatch
• rat digs

trial n + 1

• match
• rat turns away

trial n + 2...

• nonmatch
• rat digs

B. odor cell

C. place cell

Figure 6–5. Delayed nonmatching to sample test where the location of trials varies randomly. *A:* On those trials when the odor is different from that presented on the preceding trial (i.e., a nonmatch) the rat can dig in the scented food cup for a buried reward. On those trials when the odor is the same as that on the preceding trial (i.e., a match), there is no reward and the rat turns away. *B:* Example of a cell that fires associated with trials when odor 5 (O5) was presented but not when other odors were presented. The activity of this cell did not distinguish the locations where the trial was performed or the match–nonmatch status of the odor. *C:* Example of a cell that fired when trials were performed at adjacent locations P2-P3, but not when the trial was performed at other locations. The activity of this cell did not distinguish between different odors or their match–nonmatch status (data from Wood et al., 1999).

sented, the odor, the status of the odor as a match or nonmatch, and many of the cells fired at some point as the animal approached any cup. These results show that the activity of fully half of the activated cells acted completely independent of location, and most of the location-specific cells involved more than purely spatial features of the task. In addition, while some cells encoded particular odors or places, the activity of most cells was associated with one of the many potential conjunctions of odors, places, approach movements, and match–nonmatch events. These data indicate that, when important stimuli move unpredictably within an environment, a segment of the hippocampal population encodes the regularities of these stimuli without coding of the global topography. Combined with the other findings described before, these data provide compelling evidence that hippocampal cells can encode purely nonspatial information that is relevant at many locations in the environment.

The hippocampal network mediates a "memory space"

The preceding review both confirms the existence of location-specific activity of hippocampal neurons, and suggests that place cells are parts of a neural representation that is both less than, and more than, a map of space. The representation is less than a map because it is clear that place cells individually and independently encode pieces and patches of an environment without acting as part of a full mapping. The representation is also more than a map because spatial codings are modulated by relevant nonspatial task variables and hippocampal cells encode nonspatial stimuli and events. How can the impressive location-specific activity be reconciled within a larger framework of memory representation? The properties of hippocampal firing patterns are entirely consistent with the memory space scheme proposed earlier in this chapter.

To place the properties of hippocampal firing patterns in the context of this scheme, let us review the firing patterns of hippocampal cells in rats performing two prototypical tasks, a spatial task similar to the radial maze task, and an odor-guided memory task. Begin with the data from rats performing the spatial memory task in a large arena (see Fig. 6–3C). Many of the cells can be described as place cells having a place field in a particular portion of the arena, with their activity modulated by several movement parameters such that the cells fire maximally when the rat is moving at a particular speed, in a particular direction, and when the rat is turning in one particular angle. One cell, whose firing patterns are depicted in Fig. 6–3C, can be described as a cell with a place field near the center of the arena, and its activity is modulated by several movement parameters: It fires maximally when the rat is moving at a moderate speed, when the rat is moving "north," and when the rat is turning slightly to the right. Alternatively, however, virtually all of the activity of this cell can be characterized more simply as firing when the rat initiates its approach to cup 1. Most cells recorded as rats performed this task could similarly be described by a complex combination of place, direction, and turning angle, or could be at least as well described by when the cell fired during movements toward, or in return from, a particular reward cup. Furthermore, the population of hippocampal neurons contains cells that fire at virtually every point in the path to and from each of the cups (Fig. 6–6A). So one can best describe the full data set as a network of neurons each of which encodes one fragment of the approach and return from each reward cup. Of course, within the memory space framework outlined previously, the hippocampal network representation contains a subset of cells that represents distinct events, each defined by a specific location and a specific set of movement attributes, linked to encode a particular kind of trial episode, defined as the approach to and return from a particular goal location.

Now let us expand the same kind of characterization to hippocampal cellular activity in rats performing the odor-guided tasks such as those described earlier, with the additional insight into how "secondary" nonspatial firing properties are accommodated into hippocampal spatial activity (Fig. 6–6B). As animals perform these tasks individual cells activate at vir-

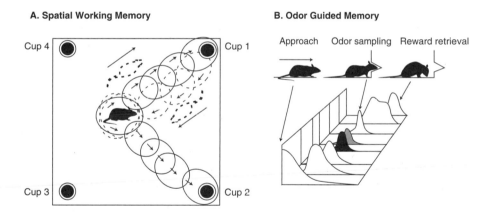

Figure 6–6. Temporal organization of hippocampal neuronal activity. *A:* Schematic illustration of firing patterns of a set of cells as the rat performs a spatial memory test. Different cells fire at each successive moment as the rat approaches each cup and returns. Note that each cell has a place field and directional firing preference associated with a particular segment of a particular outward-bound or inward-bound episode. *B:* Schematic illustration of firing patterns of a set of cells as the rat performs an odor discrimination task. Different cells fire at each successive moment as the rat approaches the odor ports, samples the odors, and retrieves the reward, and other behaviors. Some cells fire on all trials, others fire only if a particular odor is presented (data from Eichenbaum et al., 1999).

tually every instant of the task, defined as time-locked neural activity to identifiable stimulus and behavioral events. Individual cells in animals performing the odor-guided nonmatch to sample task fired at different times associated with the approach to the odor sampling port, during the odor sampling period, and during the discriminative response and reward period. Thus, overall hippocampal activity in this situation, like that in the spatial task described before, can be described as a network of cells that encode each event that characterizes each type of discrimination trial episode.

In addition, in both spatial and odor tasks, some of the hippocampal cells showed considerable specificity for particular locations of approach or odors sampled, whereas other cells fired on every trial for different directions of movement and different types of odor trials. This observation leads to an additional characterization of how hippocampal cells are "tuned" to brief segments of behavioral episodes. Let us first consider the cells that show the greatest specificity for particular conjunctions or relations among stimuli or events. Prominent examples include conjunctions or relations between the places and actions that occur in those places, or between sequences of odors. A similar characterization can be offered to describe the data from the odor-guided delayed nonmatch to sample task where the trials were performed at different locations on an open field. Some cells associated only with particular conjunctions of events, places, or both, and virtually every possible conjunction was represented. These most selective cells might be thought of as reflecting ever more rare variations of events.

Now let us consider the cells that fired consistently on different types of trials in spatial and odor tasks. Indeed, many of these cells fired associated with locations or events that were common across all the different types of trials within a task. In the spatial task, some cells fired whenever the animal's path crossed a particular place regardless of what cup was being approached or left behind. In the odor tasks, some cells fired during a particular common behavioral event, for example, during the approach movement regardless of spatial location, and others fired on all match or nonmatch trials. In the task where the odor test was performed at multiple locations some cells fired on all trials at a particular location regardless of the current odor or type of trial. These cells might be thought of as the "nodal" cells introduced in the scheme presented in Figure 6–2, the cells that encode intersections among the episodes that have in common a particular place or a particular stimulus or behavior. Of course, the full range of cells extends continuously from the most common nodal point cells to the most highly specific cells. From this perspective, "pure" place cells (ones that are location specific and have no other quality) are one of the more common nodal correlates, whereas the highly combinatorial cells represent events that occurred only a few times in a session.

Evidence of episodic-like representations in the hippocampus

More direct evidence of coding for information specific to particular types of episodes comes from another experiment where hippocampal cells fire differentially even in situations where the overt behavioral events and the locations in which they occur are identical between multiple types of experience. In this experiment rats performed a spatial alternation task, a simple version of one of Olton's episodic memory tasks, performed in a T-maze. Each trial commenced when the rat traversed the stem of the T and then selected either the left- or the right-choice arm (Fig. 6–7A). To alternate successfully the rats were required to distinguish between their left-turn and right-turn experiences and to use their memory for the most recent previous experience to guide the current choice. Different hippocampal cells fired as the rats passed through the sequence of locations within the maze during each trial. Most important, the firing patterns of many of the cells depended on whether the rat was in the midst of a left- or right-turn episode, even when the rat was on the stem of the T and running similarly on both types of trials—minor variations in the animal's speed, direction of movement, or position within areas on the stem did not account for the different firing patterns on left-turn and right-turn trials (Fig. 6–7B). Other cells fired when the rat was at the same point in the stem on either trial type. Thus, the hippocampus encoded both the left-turn and right-turn experiences using distinct representations, and included elements that could link them by their common features. In each of these experiments, the representations of event sequences, linked by codings of their common events and places, could constitute the substrate of a network of episodic memories.

Elaboration of a general scheme for memory representation by the hippocampus

There are three central aspects of this novel characterization of the firing properties of hippocampal neurons in animals performing a broad range of learning and memory tasks. First, cellular activity can be described as a sequence of temporally and spatially defined events that constitute each trial. Second, some cells show a very high degree of specialization, such as the approach to a particular odor at a particular place only when it is

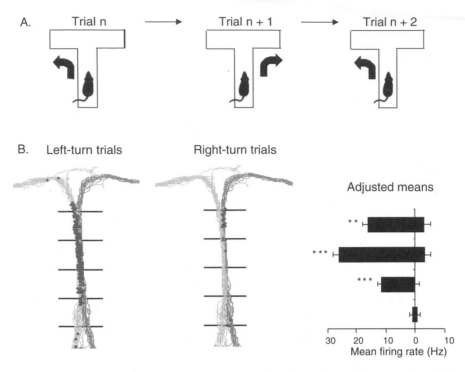

Figure 6–7. T-maze alternation. *A:* Illustration of trials in this task. On each trial the rat must remember the previous episode and then turn in the opposite direction. *B:* Example of a hippocampal cell that was active when the rat is traversing the stem section of a T-maze while performing the spatial alternation task. This cell fired almost exclusively during left-turn trials. In the left and middle panels, the paths taken by the animals on the central stem are plotted for left-turn trials (light gray) and for right-turn trials (dark gray). The locations of the rat when individual spikes occurred are indicated by dots for left-turn trials (left panel), and then right-turn trials (middle panel). In the right panel, the mean firing rate of the cell for each of four sectors of the maze, adjusted for variations in firing associated with other behavioral factors, is shown separately for left-turn trials (left bars) and right-turn trials (right bars). (significant differences: ** $p<.01$, *** $p<.001$) (data from Wood et al., 2000).

on a nonmatch trial. Third, other cells are activated on different kinds of trials, and the activity of some reflects the common places animals pass through and behavioral actions they take on all such trials. One hypothesis that may account for these three aspects of the firing patterns is that, when the animal enters a novel situation, the activity of the hippocampal neural network reflects specific ongoing behavioral episodes. As more and more experiences are accumulated within that overall situation, common locations, stimuli, and actions are reflected in enhanced firing by cells that initially are active during the relevant parts of episodes. Eventually the hippocampal network encodes the organization of related episodes, including both the frequent elements common across many similar events, and rare conjunctions of elements that define infrequent episodes in the task. This view of hippocampal representation puts the hippocampus squarely as central to episodic memory but also assigns its purpose in identifying and organizing events into a general memory organization that relates events to one another.

How might such hippocampal episodic codings and organizational processing serve the global declarative memory function of the hippocampus? The present considerations provide support for a working hypothesis about a common organization of spatial and nonspatial memories in the hippocampus. According to this view, individual hippocampal neurons encode all manner of conjunctions and relations among combinations of perceptually independent cues. The domain of relations captured within hippocampal codings is broad, indeed may involve virtually any conceivable dimension by which stimuli can be related through experience. Furthermore, hippocampal representations include behavioral actions as well as stimuli, internal stimuli (e.g., hunger, fear) as well as exteroceptive stimuli.

Consider the example of T-maze performance. In this situation distinct subsets of hippocampal neurons are active during either of the two trial types (left-turn and right-turn), and some cells are active at least to some extent on both. Thus, a way to view these findings is that specific networks of cells encode the sequence of places passed through, as well as the direction of running, motivation, etc., for each trial type, as if the composite of these firings were a videoclip of that type of trial. In addition, the cells that fire similarly on both trial types contribute representations of the "overlap" in the different codings, presumably by sharing subsets of the overall set of relevant cues. This creates a framework that extends the set of stimuli and actions represented in the network, and it constrains the nature of the network organization by the accommodation of both types of trial representations into a single larger framework for the entire task (Fig. 6–8).

The same scheme can be extended to account for the development of spatial memory representations for an environment. The findings just summarized, and other studies, indicate that hippocampal place cells encode small portions of space, or, more specifically, the spatial relations among subsets of the environmental cues. How can one build a representation of the environment that would support the important spatial navigation functions of the hippocampus? Suppose the environment as a whole is not rep-

T-maze Alternation

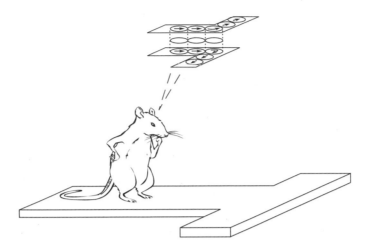

Figure 6–8. Idealized firing patterns of sets of hippocampal neurons that form separate network representations of left-turn and right-turn trials, and cells that represent the overlapping spatial information that links the two representations into a larger "memory space."

resented explicitly by a "map" in the hippocampus. Rather, spatial memory could be mediated as the byproduct of a large set of overlapping representations of specific subsets of the environmental stimuli. Within this view, during a sequence of episodes in which the animal explores the environment, individual hippocampal cells encode relative distances between small sets of cues, as well as the distance from the subject to those cues as they were experienced from a particular perspective or set of perspectives during different paths taken through the environment. Furthermore, each cell encodes only a subset of the available cues, and different cells encode overlapping combinations of those cues. The "map" of space, then, is constituted as a large collection of cue conjunctions that overlap so as to constrain the spatial relations among all the cues, and to provide a framework for moving among the cues.

A simplified version of this model is illustrated in Figure 6–9A. In this illustration, each cell is conceived as encoding only two cues in terms of their spatial separation and the distance of the animal from each of them as experienced in a separate episode. Furthermore, different cells encode overlapping pairs of cues, such that an organization of the cues emerges within the hippocampal population. To the extent that these overlapping codings constrain the overall population code, the network hippocampal

A. Representation of space

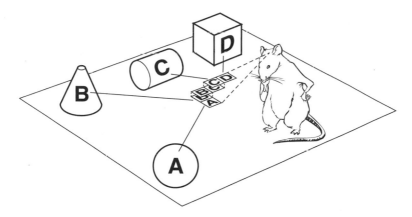

B. Representation of paired associates

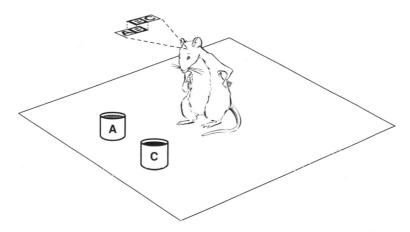

Figure 6–9. Memory space models: *A:* For the representation of space, separate "episodes" composed of distinct views of AB, then BC, then CD, are linked. *B:* For the representation of the paired associates task, separate episodes composed of each stimulus pairing (AB and BC) are linked to support inferential memory expression of B versus C.

representation crudely approximates the relative topography among all the codings. In this example, the topography of the network representation of stimuli A–D is constrained to form an L-shape, like the topography of the actual stimuli. Furthermore, this model can be envisioned as sufficient to support "navigation" among the cues in the sense that it can begin with any particular cue and know how to proceed to any other one by generating the entire set of representations. In the example, one can conceive of activation of each pair-wise coding as also exciting adjacent copings that share overlapping elements. We will call this conception the "memory space" model because it describes a network of associative connections among related stimuli. The model is "spatial" only in the sense that the specific representations are based on spatial relations. However, the links between representational elements are based on associative strengths, not on metric distance or angle representations.

Now imagine that precisely the same kind of hippocampal representation supports entirely nonspatial learning dependent on the hippocampus. A particularly good example of this learning that involves overlapping representations of nonspatial stimulus items comes from the study of transitivity in paired associate learning in rats. In the study described in Chapter 5, intact rats were trained on sets of overlapping odor associations, and demonstrated the capacity to infer relations among indirectly related items. For example, after they had learned that stimulus A was associated with stimulus B, and B was associated with C, they could infer that A was associated with C. This task directly demonstrates that rats can represent overlapping stimulus associations, and that these associations become linked to support inferential judgments. Furthermore, the capacity to build the overlapping associations into a network representation that supports inferential judgments depends on the hippocampus. In our conceptual model of the "memory space" for this task, distinct sets of hippocampal neurons might encode each pairwise trained cue relationship (Fig. 6–9B). Because of the structure of the learning task, these codings would necessarily provide a set of overlapping representations. Assuming the different representations that contain the shared item C are each activated by presentation of C in any one of them, it would be expected that the representation of the entire odor series (A–C) would be activated to support the inferential choice among nonadjacent items B and C.

Within this overall conceptual framework, three guiding principles can account for both spatial and nonspatial memory dependent on the hippocampus: (1) discrete subsets of cues and actions are encoded by hippocampal cells in terms of appropriate relations among the items; (2) the contents of these representations overlap to generate a higher-order framework or "memory space"; (3) animals can conceptually "navigate" this memory space stepping across learned associations to make indirect novel associations or other inferential judgments among items in the memory space. From this view, the key properties of spatial memory performance are particularly powerful examples of a memory space in operation. For example, the capabilities for taking "shortcuts" and "roundabout routes," types of spatial inference outlined by Tolman as defining properties of a cognitive map, can be accomplished within such a memory space without performing metric calculations of exact distances or angles. Rather, they are reflections of inferential memory expression within a constrained framework of associations.

These considerations serve to show how the spatial and nonspatial firing properties of hippocampal neurons might be reconciled. Furthermore, the "memory space" model offers insights into how the hippocampus serves its global role in declarative memory, by mediating the establishment of a relational representation among items in memory. Finally, this model shows how such a relational representation can mediate the capacity for flexible, inferential expression of memory from nonspatial as well as spatial organizations. These considerations provide a preliminary, yet clear, view of how "cognitive" memory is accomplished by the brain.

Summing up

Studies using brain imaging techniques complement the findings on human amnesia showing a critical role for the medial temporal lobe in declarative memory. These studies have shown that the medial temporal region is activated for a broad range of materials, and shows the laterality of hemispheric differences in verbal versus nonverbal information processing observed throughout the cortex. In addition, the medial temporal area is activated when a large amount of novel information is being processed, by the processing of new stimulus associations, and associated with explicit, conscious recollection.

In addition, further insights into the neural coding mechanisms of declarative memory have been made through observations on the firing properties of hippocampal neurons in behaving animals. Many cells fire selectively when an animal is in a familiar location in its environment, showing that remembered locations are an important component of the information coded by hippocampal neurons. In addition, hippocampal neurons are activated by nonspatial stimuli and their activity is associated with behavioral events. Some cells fire only when the animal is in a particular place and is engaged in a particular behavior or is presented with a particular stimulus. These cells encode combinations of places and behaviors that define specific events within learning episodes. Furthermore, the sequential activations of sets of these cells could be used to represent the sequences of events in episodic memories.

Other hippocampal cells fire associated with a spatial or nonspatial feature that is common across multiple related learning episodes. These cells could be used to link the representations of distinct experiences together within a larger organization of memories, called a "memory space." This perspective on observations on hippocampal neuron firing patterns offers clear insights into the structure of relational representations that support the properties of declarative memory.

READINGS

Amaral, D.G., and Petersen, S., Eds. 1999. Functional imaging of the human hippocampus. A special issue of *Hippocampus* 9(1).

Eichenbaum, H., Dudchencko, P., Wood, E., Shapiro, M., and Tanila, H. 1999. The hippocampus, memory, and place cells: Is it spatial memory or a memory space? *Neuron* 23: 209–226.

Henke, K., Buck, A., Weber, B., and Wieser, H.G. 1997. Human hippocampus establishes associations in memory. *Hippocampus* 7:249–256.

Muller, R.U. 1996. A quarter of a century of place cells. *Neuron*, 17: 813–822.

O'Keefe, J.A. 1979. A review of hippocampal place cells. *Prog. Neurobiol.* 13:419–439.

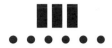

COMPARTMENTALIZATION:
CORTICAL MODULES AND
MULTIPLE MEMORY SYSTEMS

There are two parts to the story on the compartmentalization of memory in the brain. The first part is a continuation on the theme of cortical localization, with regard to both its information processing functions and memory *per se*. Enormous progress has been made in identifying functional modules within the cerebral cortex, and in showing how memory is compartmentalized within the same cortical areas that subserve specific perceptual, motor, or cognitive functions. The second story is a continuation of the revelations about different kinds of memory introduced in the last section of this book. That review focused on distinctions between "cognitive" memory and other noncognitive forms of memory, and characterized some fundamental aspects of the mechanisms and neural coding scheme that subserve cognitive memory. This part expands the notion of multiple memory systems and considers compartmentalization both within the cognitive memory system and other memory systems.

Localization of memory in the cerebral cortex

The early neurologists and physiologists characterized the cerebral cortex into a large set of sensory processing areas, identified with regions within the posterior cortex, and motor processing areas, mainly in the anterior cortex. Pavlov had just succeeded famously in identifying a conditioned reflex, showing that a very simple kind of memory could be reduced to the association between an arbitrary stimulus and a similarly arbitrary response. Combining these findings, a prevalent view was that associations were instantiated within specific circuits that connected sensory and/or motor representations in the cortex.

• 171

Guided by this view, Karl Lashley pioneered the effort to localize stimulus–response associations to specific sensory–motor connections. He surveyed the entire cerebral cortex, attempting quite directly to disconnect the critical sensory-to-motor connections by knife cuts between posterior sensory and anterior motor cortical areas (Fig. III–1). In later studies the damage went further, and involved removing portions of the cortex from virtually all areas and to varying extent in different animals. He then trained rats on a set of maze problems that were progressively more difficult and compared the severity of subsequent learning deficits with the location and extent of cortical damage. In other studies he examined the effect of the disconnections or lesions on retention of previously learned maze problems.

Lashley found that maze performance was not affected, and therefore that maze memories were not stored in any single location or in any particular pathway within or between sensory and motor areas. While not rejecting the idea of cortical localization of function in general, Lashley concluded that one also cannot view memories as stored in switchboard-like fashion within specific circuits or locations; instead he argued that memories were diffusely distributed in the brain.

At about the same time that Lashley left the field with the issue of localization unresolved, the Canadian psychologist Donald Hebb provided a possible reconciliation of the stimulus–response (S-R) and antilocalization views. In his classic 1949 monograph, Hebb recognized both the "switchboard" and cognitive theories, and argued that the eventual explanation of mental phenomena would have to incorporate plasticity of neural transmission mechanisms that lead from sensory excitation to motor responses. But to expand beyond a simple "habit" mechanism, Hebb proposed the notion of "cell assemblies," diffuse circuits of connected neurons that develop to represent specific percepts and concepts. These as-

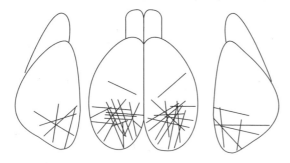

Figure III-1. Composite diagram showing top and lateral views of the rat brain indicating long axes of lesions that separated cortical areas. None of these lesions produced a substantial effect on learning ability (from Lashley, 1929).

semblies could involve diffuse circuits within a brain area, and indeed might involve sets of cell assemblies across multiple areas. His proposal retained the idea that structural changes in specific synapses would make lasting memory possible. But rather than relying on a single stimulus-to-response circuit to mediate any memory, Hebb emphasized some kind of reverberatory activity among a network of many cells, outlasting the learning event and leading to a stabilization of the cooperative activity of cells in that cell assembly. He suggested that short-term memory could be maintained within the reverberatory activity of such circuits, but long-term memory would require the ability to reinstantiate the activity within cell assemblies through changes in the connectivity of the elements and the particular pathways among them excited during learning. This view incorporated both the specificity of functions of connections in the cortex, and the distribution of global functions across cortical areas. This part reviews further advances in our understanding of how memory is compartmentalized in cell assemblies throughout the cortex.

Multiple memory systems

The findings on H.M. and other amnesic patients made it clear that structures in the medial temporal lobe including the hippocampus mediate one type of memory function, declarative memory. Conversely, these findings showed that other brain areas are sufficient to mediate other nondeclarative memory functions. What is the full extent of the declarative memory system? What are the types of nondeclarative memory and what brain systems support them? It turns out the story on the declarative and nondeclarative memory systems focuses not on the issue of cortical localization previously discussed. Rather, the story on multiple memory systems involves brain systems in which widespread areas of the cortex feed into, and are influenced by, different subcortical areas. Thus, the multiple memory systems story should be viewed as a set of parallel, functionally dedicated memory systems each of which stems from and involves cortical processing plus a separate stream of subcortical processing. After a consideration of the modular organization of the cortex, this part of the book also considers the number and nature of memory systems in the brain. I expand on the considerations of the medial temporal lobe system, to outline the entire brain system in which the hippocampus operates to support declarative memory. A review of other memory systems follows, outlining both the brain pathways and characteristics of the different forms of nondeclarative memory.

READINGS

Hebb, D.O. 1949. *The Organization of Behavior*. New York: Wiley.

Lashley, K.S. 1929. *Brain Mechanisms and Intelligence: A Quantitative Study of Injuries to the Brain*. New York: Dover (1963 edition).

7

• • • • • •

The Cerebral Cortex
and Memory

STUDY QUESTIONS

What is the functional organization of the cerebral cortex?

Is the organization of the cortex fixed during the course of development?

Is the organization of the cortex fixed in adulthood?

How are ordinary memories encoded by neurons in the cerebral cortex?

Franz Joseph Gall was the first to propose a detailed formulation of cortical specialization in which distinct types of memory are imbedded within the functional domains of different cortical areas (see Chapter 1). Although Gall's phrenology was justifiably discredited (for reasons described in Chapter 1), it turns out that the notion that cerebral cortex is made up of multiple, functionally distinct processing regions has proven correct. Also correct is Gall's notion that memory is integrally tied to these various processing systems. As will become apparent, memory is both a necessary part and an obligatory product of the ongoing processing activities of areas of the cerebral cortex.

This chapter begins with a brief summary of the evidence regarding functional specialization of the cortex. Then the role of experience in shaping the responses of neurons in various cortical areas is reviewed. There are striking commonalities in the forms of plasticity observed across cortical areas and among different types of experiential modifications. These commonalities provide the basis for the subsequent outline of general rules for how memories are represented in the cortex and, more specifically, how memory is embedded in the various networks, a fundamental part of these networks in operation.

Cortical localization

Parallel with the discoveries on functional distinctions in cortical areas, in 1909 Korbinian Brodman provided the first architectonic map of the cerebral cortex, a parcellation in which cortical areas were subdivided based on cell types and their laminar organization (Fig. 7–1). Several subsequent mappings of the human and animal cortex followed, and there was (and still is) disagreement about the number and types of areas, and about their evolutionary origins. From the outset, it was expected that the micro-anatomical differences among these areas would provide the substrate for, and therefore have been seen as reflecting, functional differences. These original observations have been extensively supplemented by further anatomical techniques, including histochemistry and connectional studies, as well as by physiological techniques, including recording and stimulation studies. The latter have provided substantially greater resolution of the anatomical divisions and, perhaps more important, given us a greater understanding of the functional distinctions among these areas in a number of species. In addition, functional neuroimaging, using positron emis-

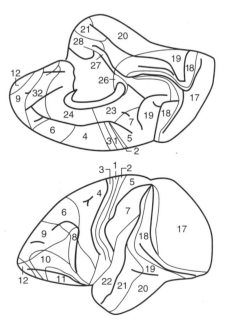

Figure 7–1. Brodman's (1909) cytoarchitectonic map of the macaque monkey cortex.

sion tomography (PET) and functional magnetic resonance imaging (fMRI), has provided strong confirmation of the functional specialization of different cortical regions. These techniques have permitted detailed mapping of the functionally distinct cortical areas specialized from processing highly specific types of information processing.

Summarizing this still unfolding story about the functional specializations of cortex is well beyond the scope of this book. Indeed, it is the subject of various books or texts in cognitive neuroscience and cognitive neuropsychology. However, a few very general principles should be committed to mind for the present purposes. First, the cortex can roughly be divided into posterior fields that are involved in perceptual processing and anterior areas that are involved in motor processing (Fig. 7–2). Second, in the posterior cortex, most of the fields are divided by sensory modality. Third, the fields in both the anterior and posterior cortex involve processing hierarchies. In the anterior cortex, there is the primary motor area just in front of the central sulcus, where the muscles of the body are mapped out in a topographic organization, with adjacent areas of cortex representing muscle groups in adjacent areas of the body. The primary motor cortex is the origin of a progression of projections to higher-order processing areas that are involved in the sequencing and organization of response output and, more generally, in the planning, executing, and withholding of goal-directed behaviors.

In the posterior cortex there are distinct primary areas for each sensory modality. Each of these is characterized by cells that respond to stimulation within a small circumscribed spatial region of the sensory field, known as a receptive field, and respond preferentially to other specific trigger features of the stimulus. The receptive fields and other trigger features

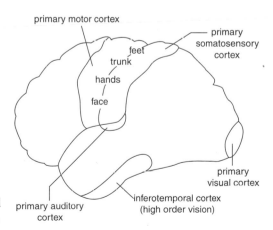

Figure 7–2. Some of the functional areas of the human cerebral cortex.

are organized in a topographic map of the sensory field and of other relevant sensory dimensions, such that adjacent neurons represent contiguous parts of the field and closely related dimensions of the trigger features. For each sensory modality these primary areas are the origins of a hierarchy of specialized processing regions leading to more and more complex perceptual areas. Eventually, some of these streams of sensory processing are combined in multimodal cortical areas, which in turn project to the supramodal processing areas in frontal, temporal, and parietal cortices.

The intertwining of information processing and memory storage in the visual cortex

To appreciate how memory is integrally related to specific cortical processors a specific example of functional specialization and memory representation in cortex will be considered in some detail. The obvious choice for this example is vision, because its functional properties and its cortical substrates have been so extensively studied. There exist more than 30 functionally distinct visual fields that encompass a large proportion of the primate brain. These different visual areas follow a complicated combination of parallel and sequential pathways that are organized hierarchically into several stages of processing. At the earliest processing stages, distinct areas are involved in identification of basic properties of visual stimuli such as their orientation, spatial frequency, speed, color, and location in the visual world. At the highest levels of visual cortex, distinct areas are responsible for localization of salient stimuli in visual space and categorization of visual stimuli according to their meaning. An example from the lowest and highest levels, and the characteristics of memory representation at both levels, are discussed next.

The primary visual cortex can alter its functional organization in response to the competition of input activities

The early visual cortical areas are particularly well characterized. The first stage of visual cortical processing involves a "topographic" representation of simple visual features. In this representational scheme small groups of neighboring cells have the same receptive fields, or areas of the visual world in which they are responsive to visual stimuli. The best understood of these areas is primary visual cortex, where cells of the input layer respond to small spots of light in highly restricted receptive fields. Neighboring principal cells in other layers respond to stable or moving contrast edges with similarly small receptive fields. Furthermore, cells with these response properties are organized topographically along two dimensions. One dimension corresponds to a preference for activation by the ipsilateral (same side of the head) or contralateral (opposite side) eye—this is called the ocular dominance property of these cells. The other dimension, which applies to cells that respond to edges of light, corresponds to preferences for an optimal orientation of the contrasting edge (Fig. 7–3). The cells are arranged in columns, such that through the depths of the cortical layers, neurons have very similar properties in ocular dominance and orientation selectivity. Ipsilateral and contralateral ocular dominance columns alternate, and orientation columns are arranged in a systematic sequence. The combination of a full set of ocular dominance and orientation columns that represent the same small receptive field area is known as a "hypercolumn." Sets of such modules are organized systematically to provide a full representation of the contralateral visual field for each hemisphere.

The linkage between memory and perceptual processing involves the experience-driven tuning and modification of the cells in this organized network—a rewiring of the cells in the network and of the maps they form. The tuning and modification of cortical processing networks by experience was first observed in the primary visual cortex associated with development in young animals. The classic studies by David Hubel and Torsten Wiesel showed that response properties of primary visual cortex neurons are plastic, that is, modifiable by experience, during a "critical period" of the first 4 weeks of life. They found that closure of one eye during this period in kittens resulted in a shift in ocular dominance of all

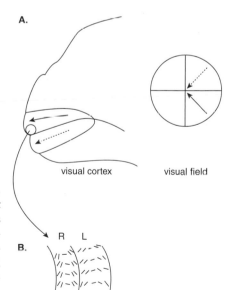

Figure 7–3. Map of primary visual cortex. *A:* Areas on the medial surface of the left visual cortex sensitive to parts of the arrows designated in the right visual vield. *B:* Expansion of the circled area in *A* showing orientation selectivities indicated by slanted lines and right (R) and left (L) ocular dominance stripes.

cells toward a preference for the active eye. Similarly, restricting exposure in kittens to stimuli with only certain orientations of visual contrast (e.g., only vertical or only horizontal) during the critical period resulted in a shift of all cells toward selectivity for the trained orientation. Such manipulations are not nearly so effective in producing tuning of visual cortex after this early critical period ends, a finding that led most investigators to conclude that cortical organization becomes fixed in adulthood.

There are indications that the reorganization of sensory maps, as well as the normal initial organizing of sensory maps, arises from a competition of activity among different inputs to each cell. Some of the earliest and most impressive evidence for competitive mechanisms underlying cortical organization, and reorganization, came from studies of the optic tectum in frogs. In frogs, the major projection of the retina arrives in the part of the midbrain known as the optic tectum, the highest visual area of the frog brain. This projection is entirely crossed such that all of the fibers from the left eye arrive in the right tectum and *vice versa* (Fig. 7–4A). This pattern of connections can be visualized by injecting a radioactively labeled amino acid into one eye and then observing the transport of radioactivity into the synapses of the optic tectum.

Studies of plasticity in this system exploited the regenerative capacities of the frog nervous system to examine the effects of additional abnormal inputs to the optic tectum. The manipulation in this study was to add a third eye to the head of the frog embryo. At this time the partially developed eyes are only protruding bulges on the head. But, as the animals mature, the retinal elements develop optic nerves that innervate one or the other optic tectum of the host brain. Amazingly, in each of these animals, the topographic pattern of the synapses making these connections was dramatically altered from the normal monocular input pattern, such that in three-eyed frogs there were periodic bands of input from the two eyes innervating half of one tectum (Fig. 7–4B). Thus, inputs from the additional eye mapped onto one or the other tectum along with those from the natural eye. Moreover, in each case, the competition of inputs from two eyes elicited a pattern of ocular dominance stripes essentially the same as that observed in mammals with naturally occurring binocular inputs to each side of the cortex.

Is this peculiar phenomenon restricted to the lowly frog? Not at all. In mammals, normally the retina sends inputs to major targets in the brain stem areas known as the superior colliculus and the lateral geniculate nucleus of the thalamus. Concurrently, the cochlea normally sends auditory inputs to the medial geniculate nucleus of the thalamus. In a landmark experiment on newborn ferrets, the retina of one eye was prevented from

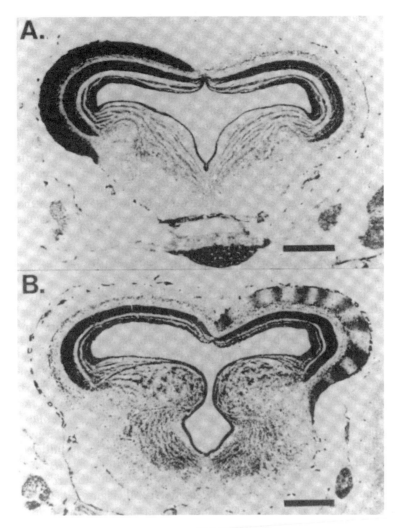

Figure 7–4. Reorganization of the frog optic tectum (top layers in frontal section of the frog brain) *A:* Black area on left side (right hemisphere) indicates deposition of radioactive amino acids transported following an injection into the right eye. This shows that the normal projection is entirely contralateral. *B:* Pattern of transport in a frog with a third eye transplanted near the normal right eye. The left optic tectum (on right) receives alternating zones of input from both eyes (from Constantine-Paton and Law, 1982).

sending its normal inputs to the brain stem by transecting the optic nerve, and the normal inputs to the medial geniculate were severed. Subsequently, the retinal projections innervated the disconnected medial geniculate nucleus, resulting in visual responses being observed in normally auditory parts of the thalamus and the auditory cortex. Furthermore, a visual map developed in auditory cortex and it involved an organized topographic map in which the two-dimensional visual fields were mapped precisely onto the cortical area that normally holds a one-dimensional representation of auditory frequencies. These findings indicate that the competitive activities of inputs are sufficient to determine the general aspects of cortical organization. Thus, the pattern of cortical reorganization after sensory deprivation is no different from that by which the processing system becomes organized during development.

The adult cortex also shows plastic changes in response to altered input activity

Is this kind of plasticity observed only in the developing brain? Or is plasticity associated with a competition among inputs a property of the mature brain as well? One way in which the plasticity of the adult cortex has been explored is by creating small and selective damage to a part of the normal inputs to the cortex and subsequently examining the effects of this deprivation of input on the area of cortex that had previously received those inputs.

There is now considerable evidence that such selective deprivation of inputs produces a reorganization in the adult visual cortex. In the most sophisticated of these experiments, a laser light was used to produce a very small lesion of the retina that deprives animals of a small area of the visual field. This lesion initially produces a correspondingly small area of silent primary visual cortex. However, after a 2-month recovery period, the topography of the cortex is reorganized such that the formerly disconnected zone becomes responsive to neighboring parts of the visual field (Fig. 7–5). Also, whereas *complete* recovery requires a prolonged period, some cells at the border of the deafferented area become responsive to stimulation of intact visual field areas within hours of the lesion.

A parallel pattern of reorganization follows selective deafferentation of other primary cortical areas in the adult cerebral cortex. For example, in the monkey primary somatosensory (touch) cortex, the normal representation of the hand is extremely orderly, involving a systematic mapping of sequential finger surfaces. When the nerve innervating the surface of some of the fingers was cut, the cortical region normally representing these areas was initially unresponsive. However, after several months this cortical area became responsive to stimulation of neighboring regions of the palm and to intact portions of remaining fingers. In other studies where the input from one finger was eliminated, the area that had been disconnected became responsive to stimulation of the neighboring fingers and the palm.

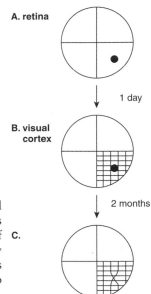

A. retina

1 day

B. visual cortex

2 months

C.

Figure 7–5. Reorganization of visual cortex after a small retinal lesion. *A:* Initially a very small area of damage is created in a spot on the retina. *B:* This results in loss of responsiveness in the corresponding area of the primary visual cortex, determined the next day. *C:* After 2 months of recovery, that region of cortex becomes responsive to visual stimulation in the adjacent areas of the retina.

A similar pattern of results in seen in the reorganization of rat motor cortex representation when a single whisker is eliminated—the disconnected area becomes responsive to stimulation of the neighboring intact whiskers.

Similar results have been obtained in studies on the primary auditory cortex. In this system the cochlea, or inner ear, is normally organized such that successive parts of its surface area are responsive to sequential frequencies of sound. Furthermore, the auditory cortex is topographically organized in a sequence of frequency bands that receive inputs from adjacent areas of the cochlea, similar to the topographic organization in the visual cortex. In these studies a restricted area of the cochlea was lesioned, such that a single frequency band of the auditory cortex representation was deprived of its normal input. Initially, cells in this band became silent to normal levels of stimulation, although they were responsive to louder stimuli. After a month of recovery, these cells became fully responsive to tones in the frequencies neighboring that lost after the lesion.

All of these phenomena speak to the integral role of real-world experience in the basic processing functions of these various cortical systems. Experience shapes the operation of these systems, altering the mapping of the sensory and motor world by primary sensory and motor cortices. Thus, a record of experience is embedded in these networks. A fundamental aspect of these networks in operation involves the competition among inputs to dominate the activity of, and representation in, cortical areas.

Cortical reorganization also occurs as a result of learning

Are these dramatic changes in cortical organization limited to drastic alterations or disconnection of inputs? Do similar changes occur during "real" learning, and, if so, are such changes of sufficient magnitude to be observable after the typically brief and subtle experiences of real-life learning? It is now clear that reorganizations of primary cortical areas indeed do occur as a consequence of conventional learning experiences.

An early report of learning-related reorganization in the visual cortex came from an experiment where young kittens were outfitted with special goggles that could be used to present each eye separately with a vertically or horizontally oriented set of lines. The kittens were trained to avoid a forearm shock by moving the arm to a particular position when signaled by an oriented visual grating presented to one eye. A visual grating of the opposite orientation was presented to the other eye, and its presentation was not associated with shock. Following several weeks of training, recordings were made in the forearm area of the somatosensory cortex, and cells were examined for both tactile and visual responsiveness. In trained animals a large number of cells showed selective visual responses to the training cues. Presentations of the oriented visual stimuli in the correspondingly stimulated eyes produced robust responses in the forelimb area of the somatosensory cortex that represented the shocked arm, whereas presentation of other line orientations were relatively ineffective. These studies showed that cortical areas that are normally responsive only to tactile stimulation could, through training, become activated by visual stimuli. Furthermore, the acquired visual responsiveness is closely related to the significance of the association between an arbitrary visual stimulus and tactile stimulation.

Since that time, a number of studies have now shown changes in cortical responses following Pavlovian conditioning. Among the most elegant of these demonstrations come from experiments by Norman Weinberger and his colleagues, showing shifts in the tuning curves of auditory cortical cells following training in tone-cued classical conditioning. Initially, recordings were taken from a single auditory cortex neuron of an anesthetized guinea pig, and its frequency tuning curve fully characterized (Fig. 7–6). Then a nonoptimal frequency was selected as the conditioning stimulus and its presentation was paired repeatedly with foot shocks, which typically produce unconditioned pupillary dilation responses. Following several pairings of the tone and shock, presentation of the tone alone produced a pupillary conditioned response that reflects an expectancy of the shock.

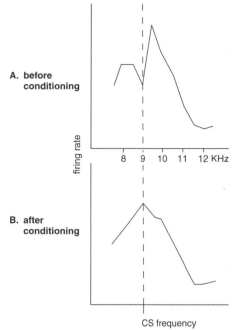

Figure 7–6. Learning related firing pattern in an auditory cortex neuron. *A:* The tuning curve for an auditory cortex neuron before classical conditioning indicates an optimal response at about 9.5 KHz. *B:* After conditioning with a 9 Khz tone as the conditioning stimulus (CS), the cell shifts its tuning curve to be most responsive at the CS frequency and less responsive at the preconditioning optimum (data from Weinberger, 1993).

After this training the frequency tuning curve of the cell was again characterized. The typical finding was that auditory cortex neurons showed enhanced responses to the initially nonoptimal tone frequency, and reduced responses to other frequencies including the former best frequency of the cell. When the training involved a discrimination between one tone associated with shock and another not paired with shock, responses to the tone associated with shock increased, whereas those to the other tone decreased, as did the responses to other frequencies including the cell's former best frequency. These effects developed in just a few conditioning trials and were long-lasting. Indeed, the magnitude of the novel response grew over the hour after training and was maintained at least 24 hours, for as long as observations could be made. Overall, these changes in the response distribution across the population of auditory cells indicate a general shift in the topographic map. The map would shift strongly toward greater representation of the task-relevant frequency at the expense of other frequencies in the audible spectrum—a pattern of results markedly similar to results from the sensory deprivation experiments in various developing and adult cortical areas.

Similar enhancements of tuning of auditory cortical cells toward relevant conditioning frequencies have also been observed in monkeys. In monkeys who were trained to discriminate small frequency differences, it was found that the monkeys' performance improved progressively over a period of several weeks. In subsequent recordings, changes were found in the size of the auditory cortex representation of the task-relevant frequencies, the sharpness of tuning to these frequencies, and the latencies of cellular responses—all were greater than those of untrained frequencies or of all frequencies in untrained animals. Furthermore, the changes in area of the cortical representation were correlated with the improvement in task performance.

In parallel studies on tactile discrimination learning, monkeys were trained to hold a joystick while a 20 Hz vibration was applied to a small area of a single finger. To obtain rewards the monkey had to release the stick whenever the stimulations were presented at any of several higher frequencies. After months of training the animals, the investigators recorded cellular responses in the primary somatosensory cortex and found that the hand representation in the stimulated finger area was more complex, and had increased in size severalfold, and receptive fields were substantially increased in overlap (Fig. 7–7). These expansions of the stimulated area occurred at the expense of other parts of the finger representation, similar to the findings on auditory responses after training. Using a different task that required monkeys to discriminate the roughness of tactile stimuli presented to varying loci on the finger, the receptive fields in the somatosensory cortex were *reduced*, unlike the preceding findings, although the overall area of the finger representation was, as in the preceding study, increased greatly to take over regions previously unresponsive to these stimuli. Thus, the overall size of the network of neu-

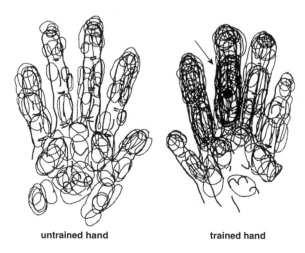

untrained hand   **trained hand**

Figure 7–7. Receptive fields of somatosensory neurons in a monkey's hand before training, and then after training where tactile stimulation was presented in the area indicated by the black circle. Note the large number of overlapping receptive fields after training (arrow) (from Recanzone and Merzenich, 1991).

rons was increased, as was the resolution for detection of fine differences in somatosensory input.

How do higher areas of cortex respond to learning?

At higher levels of sensory processing, the relevant cortical areas are involved in more complex distinctions, and, accordingly, the cells in these areas have more complex response properties that appear to arise from combinations of inputs from the lower levels. One of these areas that has been extensively studied is the inferotemporal cortex (IT). IT is the highest-order cortical visual processing area, whose function is the identification of objects by their visual qualities—and this area is thought to be the site of long-term storage of memory about visual objects. This section reviews the role of IT as indicated mainly by studies of the effects of damage to this area, then describes the normal sensory response properties of IT cells. A discussion of the nature of memory coding by IT cells follows.

Damage to inferotemporal cortex in humans results in visual agnosia, a selective deficit in visual object recognition, and this area has been observed to be activated in various PET or fMRI studies of neurologically intact individuals performing tasks requiring visual object recognition. Damage to inferotemporal cortex in monkeys produces a complex visual impairment. Unlike damage to early visual cortical areas, there is no blindness as a result of IT damage—monkeys with damage to this area have normal thresholds and acuity of visual detection. However, their capacity for visual discrimination is impaired whether the discriminative stimuli involve color, brightness, two-dimensional patterns, or three-dimensional objects, and the deficit is exacerbated when the stimuli are perceptually similar or the number of stimuli to discriminate is large. The deficit in monkeys with IT damage may result from the loss of "perceptual constancy," that is, loss of the ability to recognize a target stimulus across changes in many perceptual qualities including retinal location, rotation, size, color, or contrast, as revealed in studies showing an exception to the generality of an impairment on difficult discrimination problems. Monkeys with inferotemporal lesions perform surprisingly well on mirror-image or inverted stimulus problems, which normal monkeys find rather difficult because of their tendency to see the stimuli as identical in form. It appears that the lesion of the inferotemporal cortex eliminates the appearance of similiarity among mirror-image and inverted stimuli, making this aspect of discrimination less of a problem for monkeys with such lesions.

IT cortex receives information from earlier stages in the ventral visual stream that, when combined, permit it to compute the three-dimensional form of objects. Accordingly, neurons in inferotemporal cortex respond exclusively to visual stimuli and are responsive to whole objects positioned almost anywhere within the visual fields. These cells respond best to the presentation of two- and three-dimensional objects, or to some aspect of visual color or form. Many of these cells respond similarly to a particular stimulus regardless of its size, degree of contrast from the background, or details of its form, location in the visual field, or motion.

The selectivity of IT cells is sometimes highly specific. For example, the first explorations of IT described a cell that responded best to the silhouette of a monkey's hand. Other cells responded to the shape of a banana or a toilet brush (used to clean monkey cages). Studies have concluded that some of these responses to complex stimuli can be reduced to more elemental, albeit still somewhat complicated, forms. Perhaps most widely studied are IT cells that respond best to faces, a finding that has been replicated and studied extensively in a number of laboratories. The responses of these cells are relatively invariant to size, color, contrast, and position. Some cells respond to particular features of faces, but others respond selectively to a particular face orientation, or decrease firing rate when parts of the face are eliminated or scrambled. Some of these cells have selective responses to face identity, that is, to a particular person, and the selectivity of these responses is maintained across a variety of stimulus transformations.

Neurons in inferotemporal cortex change their firing patterns in accordance with their recent past history. The initial evidence for this came from studies of short-term or working memory. In the standard delayed match to sample task typically used to study short-term memory, an animal is presented with a sample cue, followed by a memory delay during which that sample has to be remembered. Then one or more choice stimuli are presented and the animal is required to respond depending on whether the choice cue is the same as the sample (a match) or not (a nonmatch). Joaquin Fuster and his colleagues performed the first studies in which cortical neurons were recorded in monkeys performing this task. They characterized the responses of cells in the inferotemporal cortex following presentations of the sample and choice cues, and during the delay period. In one version of their task the monkey was presented with a color cue and was required to retain it for up to 20 seconds prior to the choice. They identified cells that fired differentially to specific colors of the sample and choice. Some of these cells maintained high levels of activity during the memory delay, and this activity was specific to the sample cue.

In another version of the task, compound stimuli with both color and pattern information were presented as samples. When one particular pattern was presented, the color dimension had to be remembered. When other patterns were presented, the pattern information had to be remembered. Some inferotemporal cells responded selectively to a color or pattern, and the activity of many of these responses was strongly modulated by the relevant memory dimension. In a subsequent study, Fuster found that the magnitude of the enhancing effect was correlated with the animal's response latency.

Other studies have revealed that many inferotemporal cells show suppressed responses to repeated stimuli, and suggested that this phenomenon may provide signals for short-term memory. In the earliest observations of this phenomenon, Malcolm Brown and his colleagues found that inferotemporal cells showed suppressed stimulus-selective responses to stimulus repetition in monkeys performing a delayed matching task where stimuli were reused repeatedly across trials. More recently, Earl Miller and his colleagues have reported multiple correlates of short-term memory in the inferotemporal cortex. They elaborated the delayed match to sample task to include multiple choice cues, and the monkey was required to restrain from making a behavioral response until the matching choice appeared. Their initial main finding was that inferotemporal cells showed suppressed responses on repetition of the sample cue as choice. These responses were maintained across intervening items, but were reset between trials, except for a general decrement in responses across the entire session. A few cells showed the opposite response, an enhancement for matching choice stimuli. In addition, delay firing was observed in some cells, but this activity ceased upon presentation of any subsequent stimulus.

In subsequent studies, the task was changed so that the intervening nonmatch choice stimuli repeated prior to representation of the sample as a choice. In this situation the proportions of inferotemporal responses changed such that many cells showed suppression for any repeated stimulus, whether it was a repetition of the sample or of a nonmatching intervening stimulus. However, now a much larger proportion of cells showed match enhancement responses, and these were observed only for repetition of the sample cue. This pattern of findings was interpreted as evidence for a combination of memory mechanisms within the inferotemporal cortex. Match suppression was viewed as a passive consequence of stimulus repetition such that it occurs whether or not the stimulus had to be remembered. On the other hand, match enhancement was viewed as reflecting the continued processing of a stimulus to maintain a memory. Sustained firing could also be used to bridge a memory delay, but it appears this mechanism cannot be maintained through interfering stimuli by the inferotemporal cortex.

Other studies on inferotemporal cortex have revealed activity patterns that reflect long-lasting stimulus associations. An early study inadvertently found a capacity for cross-modal associations in IT neurons of animals performing a visual discrimination task. In this experiment, monkeys were trained to discriminate four different visual patterns, including a plus sign, a triangle, a square, and a circle. Before presentation of each of those stimuli, a brief tone signaled the monkey to fixate its eyes on the central position of the visual display in anticipation of the visual stimulus onset. To the surprise of the investigators, a third of the visually responsive inferotemporal neurons fired after the onset of the tone at long latencies, and continued to fire after the onset of the visual stimulus. At that point the cells either increased firing rate if the optimal cue was presented, or ceased firing if a different stimulus was presented.

In a study explicitly designed to evaluate such "associative" neuronal responses, Miyashita and his colleagues examined responses of inferotemporal neurons to 24 fractal stimulus patterns. These stimuli were arbitrarily paired such that on each trial one stimulus of a pair was presented as a sample cue, and after a delay period was followed by a choice between the assigned paired cue and one of the other stimuli. After acquisition of this paired associate task over a series of training sessions, two different associative correlates were observed in the firing of these neurons. "Pair-coding" neurons fired maximally for the two cues that were paired associates, more so than for any other cues (Fig. 7–8 top). "Pair-recall" neurons increased firing rate during the delay period following presentation of the associate of the optimal cue (Fig. 7–8 bottom). This study made clear that the preferences of inferotemporal neurons for specific objects can be permanently modified to incorporate a preference for the objects associated with them during learning.

Taken together, these findings suggest that in the course of processing, cortical neurons are sensitive to both short-term and long-term contingencies of the items they are called upon to handle. Here too, then, memory becomes an integral part of the normal operation of these cortical processing systems, as experience continues to shape the nature of processing that is performed.

Summing up

The cerebral cortex is subdivided first into major zones called the frontal, parietal, occipital, and temporal lobes. Within these are a multitude of functionally specific areas segregated into motor, specific sensory modal-

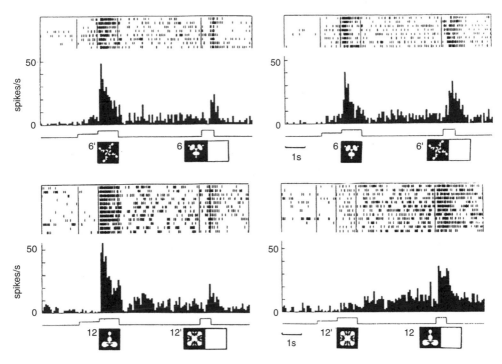

Figure 7–8. Two types of firing patterns that reflect the paired association. *Top:* A "pair-coding" neuron that fired for both associated stimuli. *Bottom:* A "pair-recall neuron" that fired when one of the cues was presented, or in anticipation of that cue predicted by its associated stimulus (from Sakai et al., 1994).

ities, and "association areas" that mediate higher-order functions that often involve a combination of modalities. The general organization of early stages of cortical processing involve systematic topographies of specific sensory or motor features onto the cortical surface. In higher stages of processing these systematic topographies are lost. All cortical areas, both in development and in adulthood, demonstrate considerable plasticity in the form of alterations in the size and topographic organization of cortical areas corresponding to increases or decreases in the activity of inputs to these areas.

The cortical code for memory involves the plasticity of the inherent information processing attributes of the cortex. Sometimes the broad variety of cellular memory correlates in the cortex seems almost as large as the number of studies that report them. However, these diverse findings can be consolidated by thinking about memory as encoded within the cortex in two general ways, each of which involves a modification of the normal sensory processing function of the cells in these areas. First, memory is reflected in the capacity of cortical cells to shift or modulate the responses evoked by the stimuli that drive them. This kind of memory coding is observed as an increment (or enhancement) or as a decrement (or suppression) of sensory responsiveness. A combination of incremental and decremental changes could be integrated to shift a tuning curve, and many of such coordinated tuning-curve shifts could account for the expansion or shrinkage of parts of the overall sensory representation within a cortical area. These response biases can be held briefly, as observed in working memory tasks, or permanently, as observed in an increased resolution within the cortical maps for a relevant stimulus dimension. In working memory tasks, enhanced responses could amount to an attentional "filter" that generates a bias in signals that generate the selection of choice stimuli. Suppressed responses could reflect a kind of subthreshold sustained activation, that is, "primed" neural activity that subsequently requires less processing to identify the familiar stimulus, and this would appear as less activation of the cells required to reidentify a familiar stimulus.

Second, memory is encoded in the capacity of cortical cells to sustain or reactivate their normal sensory responses in the absence of the stimulus ordinarily required to evoke the representation. This type of coding can be observed in firing patterns maintained during the delay in working memory tasks, providing a confirmation of Hebb's "reverberating circuit" notion. In addition, the capacity of cortical cells to regenerate item-specific firing patterns when cued by an associated event seems to confirm Hebb's model of complex memories as "phase sequences" involving replays of linked stimulus representations.

These observations serve to emphasize a fundamental theme, that memory should be conceived as intimately intertwined with information processing in the cortex, indeed so much so that the "memory" and "information processing" are inherently indistinguishable. One understanding of this view holds that memory is nothing more or less than the plastic properties of specific cortical information processings. Another equally valid point of view holds that all cortical information processing inherently involves adaptations to stimulus regularities and contingencies, and/or storage of the information processed. By either view, the mechanisms of the cerebral cortex involve a combination of information processing and memory to constitute neural networks that contain the structure of our knowledge about the world. The memory code is thus both constrained by and revealed in acquired biases in evoked activity patterns and in the ability to recreate those knowledge representations.

READINGS

Constantine-Paton, M., and Law, M.I. 1982. The development of maps and stripes in the brain. *Sci. Am.* 247: 62–70.

Fuster, J.M. 1995. *Memory in the Cerebral Cortex: An Empirical Approach to Neural Networks in the Human and Nonhuman Primate.* Cambridge: MIT Press.

Gilbert, C.D. 1992. Horizontal integration and cortical dynamics. *Neuron* 9: 1–13.

Gross, C.G. 1992. Representation of visual stimuli in inferior temporal cortex. *Phil. Trans. R. Soc. Lond. B* 335: 3–10.

Kaas, J.H. 1995. The reorganization of sensory and motor maps in adult mammals. In *The Cognitive Neurosciences*, M.S. Gazzaniga (Ed.). Cambridge: MIT Press, pp. 51–71.

Kandel, E.R., and Schwartz, J.H. 1985. *Principles of Neural Science,* 2nd edition. New York: Elsevier.

Merznich, M.M., Recanzone, G.H., Jenkins, W.M., and Grajski, K.A. 1990. Adaptive mechanisms in cortical networks underlying cortical contributions to learning and nondeclarative memory. In *The Brain,* Cold Spring Harbor Press: Cold Spring Harbor Symposium LV, pp. 873–887.

Miyashita, Y. 1993. Inferior temporal cortex: Where visual perception meets memory. *Annu. Rev. Neurosci.* 16:245–263.

Perrett, D.I., Mistlin, A.J., and Chitty, A.J. 1987. Visual neurones responsive to faces. *T.I.N.S.* 10: 358–364.

Tanaka, K. 1993. Neuronal mechanisms of object recognition. *Science* 262: 685–688.

Weinberger, N.M. 1995. Retuning the brain by fear conditioning. In *The Cognitive Neurosciences*, M.S. Gazzaniga (Ed.). Cambridge: MIT Press, pp. 1071–1089.

8
• • • • • • •

Multiple Memory Systems
in the Brain

STUDY QUESTIONS

What are "behaviorism" and "cognitivism"?

What strategies do rats use in maze learning?

What is a double dissociation, and why does it allow powerful conclusions about functional assignments of brain areas?

What functional dissociations characterize the existence of multiple independent memory systems in both rats and humans?

Much of the thinking and research about the nature of cognitive processes in memory, specifically the "behaviorist" versus "cognitivist" debate, proceeded independently of the explorations on cortical localization. Picking up from where we left off in Part II, the evidence from Tolman's work showing capacities that exceeded the predictions of the behaviorist position did not end the debate. Rather, the evidence simply inspired more sophisticated additions to the behaviorists' construction of the internal representation of habit. The debate became focused on the central issue of whether rats acquire maze problems by learning specific turning "responses" or by developing an expectancy of the "place" of reward.

The issue was addressed using a simple T-maze apparatus where "response" versus "place" strategies could be directly compared by operational definitions (Fig. 8–1A). The basic task involves the rat beginning each trial at the base of the T and being rewarded at the end of only one

A.

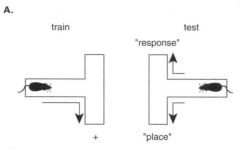

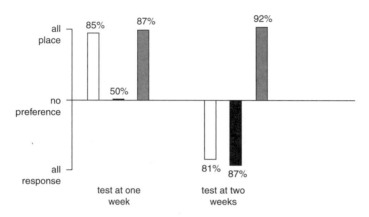

Figure 8–1. Place versus response learning. *A:* Initially rats were trained in the T-maze to turn right in order to obtain a food reward in a particular place. In a subsequent probe test the maze was rotated 180 degrees and then rats were run a single trial to determine if they chose the same right turn "response" or instead chose to go to the same "place." *B:* Probe test performance when given a placebo or lidocaine in the hippocampus or striatum. When tested after 1 week of training most normal control rats chose the "place" strategy, whereas after 2 weeks of training most chose the response strategy. Inactivation of the hippocampus abolished the place strategy at 1 week, but had no effect on selection of the response strategy at 2 weeks. Inactivation of the striatum did not affect selection of the place strategy at 1 week, but at 2 weeks abolished the response strategy and returned the rats to the place strategy. Open bars = placebo; black bars = hippocampus; shaded bars = striatum (data from Packard and McGaugh, 1996).

arm, for example, the one reached by a right turn. The accountings of what was learned in this situation differ strongly by the two theoretical approaches. According to behaviorist theory, learning involves acquisition of the reinforced right-turn response. By contrast, according to Tolman's account, learning involves the acquisition of a cognitive map of the envi-

ronment and the expectancy that food was to be found at a particular location in the test room. The critical test involved effectively rotating the
T by exactly 180 degrees, so that the choice arms still end at the same two
loci (albeit which arms reach those loci are now exchanged), and the start
point would now be at the opposite end of the room. Behaviorists would
predict that a rat would continue to make the previously reinforced right-
turn response at the choice point, leading it to a different goal location
than that where the food was provided during training. By contrast, Tolman's account predicts that the rat would switch to a left-turn in order to
arrive at the expected location of food in the same place in the room where
it was originally rewarded.

Many experiments ensued, with mixed results indicating that place
learning was more often favored but that there were conditions under
which response learning was preferred, and the nature of the available cues
was the primary determining factor for the differences in the results. In
general, whenever there was salient extramaze visual stimulation that differentiated one goal location from the other, a place representation pre-
dominated; and whenever such differential extramaze cues were absent,
the response strategy would predominate. Such a pattern of results did
not, of course, declare a "winner" in the place-versus-response debate. Instead, these results suggested that both types of representation are available to the rat, and that it might use either one under conditions of different salient cues or response demands.

Tolman himself was conciliatory in his explicit suggestion that "there
is more than one kind of learning." He offered that different theories and
laws might all have some validity for some types of learning. He suggested
the possibility of both stimulus-response and cognitive map representations, and elaborated variations on each. He also suggested a distinct form
of learning for emotional dispositions for stimuli, calling these *cathexes*,
similar to Main de Biran's sensitive memory. Tolman did not consider
whether these different types of learning were mediated by different brain
pathways. But it turns out that different types of learning do exist, that
they follow different rules, and that they are supported by different brain
mechanisms.

A most elegant demonstration of such a conclusion was recently provided by Mark Packard and James McGaugh, 50 years after the classic
Tolman studies. In Packard and McGaugh's experiment, rats were trained
for a week on the T-maze task, then given the rotated-maze probe trial.
Then they were trained for another week with the maze in its original orientation, and then finally presented with an additional probe trial. Packard
and McGaugh found that normal rats initially adopted a place represen-

tation, as reflected in their strong preference for the place of the previous goal during the first probe trial. However, after the additional week of overtraining, normal rats switched, now adopting a response strategy on the final probe test. So, under these training circumstances, rats developed both strategies successively. Their initial acquisition was guided by the development of a cognitive map, but subsequent overtraining led to development of the response "habit."

But Packard and McGaugh's experiment went beyond merely showing that the same rats can use both learning strategies. In addition to the behavioral testing, Packard and McGaugh also examined whether different brain systems supported these different types of representation. Prior to training, all animals had been implanted with indwelling needles that allowed injection on the probe tests of a local anesthetic, which would silence all the cells in a local area for several minutes, or saline placebo directly and locally into one of two brain structures, the hippocampus or the striatum. The choice of these particular brain structures follows from work conducted in the 50 years intervening between Tolman's and Packard and McGaugh's work, particularly the work on human amnesia that so conclusively ties the hippocampus to certain aspects of memory, to be described in subsequent sections of this chapter.

The results on normal animals described previously were from those subjects that were injected with placebo on both probe tests (Fig. 8–1B). The effects of the anesthetic were striking and different depending on when and where the drug was infused. On the first probe trial after only 1 week of training, animals that were injected with anesthetic into the striatum behaved just as control subjects had—they were predominantly "place" learners, indicating the place representation did not depend on the striatum. In striking contrast, the animals that had been injected with anesthetic into the hippocampus showed no preference at all, indicating that they relied on their hippocampus for the place representation, and that this was the only representation normally available at that stage of learning. On the second probe test after 2 weeks of training, a different pattern emerged. Whereas control subjects had by now acquired the response strategy, animals given an anesthetic in the striatum lost the turning response and instead showed a striking opposite preference for the place strategy. Animals given an injection of anesthetic into the hippocampus maintained their response strategy.

A clear picture of the evolution of multiple memory representations emerges when these data are combined. Animals normally develop an initial place representation that is mediated by the hippocampus, and no turning-response representation has developed in this initial period. With over-training, a turning-response representation that is mediated by the striatum is acquired, and indeed predominates over the hippocampal place representation. The latter is not, however, lost—it can be "uncovered" by inactivating the striatum and suppressing the turning-response strategy. Why in particular the hippocampus and striatum might serve these particular roles in memory is discussed extensively later. For now, these findings offer compelling evidence that elements of both the behaviorist and the cognitive map views were right: There are distinct types of memory for place and response, and they are distinguished by their performance characteristics as well as by the brain pathways that support them.

The power of "double dissociation"

The Packard and McGaugh experiment demonstrates the power of the neuropsychological approach in providing compelling evidence both for the existence of two different kinds of learning and for the mediation of different forms of memory by distinct memory systems. Of course, the existence of the hippocampal memory system, and many of its characteristics, was well known long before the Packard and McGaugh study, as outlined in detail in Chapters 4 and 5. And the Packard and McGaugh study was not the first to reveal a role for the caudate nucleus and other parts of the striatum in response learning. But most of the experiments that preceded Packard and McGaugh were based on investigations of only one brain structure in a particular experiment. Although many of these studies, as outlined in the previous chapters, have provided compelling evidence of high specificity in the functional contribution of one brain structure, it is generally agreed that the strongest evidence of differential roles of particular brain structures comes from a design called "double dissociation." In this experimental design, the object is to demonstrate that damage to brain structure A, but not structure B, results in impairment on task X, but not task Y, while damage to brain structure B and not structure A results in impairment on task Y and not task X. Such a design shows, at the same time, that both loci of damage are effective in altering behavior, and both structures play a selective role. The Packard and McGaugh study is a particularly good example of the success of the strategy of double dissociation. This strategy has been extended in several other studies on memory, and the results reveal the existence of and some of the critical brain structures participating in, distinct memory systems.

An anatomical framework for parallel memory systems in the brain

The studies to be described in the remainder of this chapter are examples of research guided by the view that distinct types of memory processing are mediated by distinct functional systems of the brain. A general, anatomically based framework for some of the major memory systems has emerged from this research. A preliminary outline is presented here to provide a framework for discussing the hypotheses and results of the dissociation experiments that follow. In subsequent chapters, greater detail on the anatomical circuits of each pathway is provided.

An outline of some of the most prominent memory pathways currently under investigation is provided in Fig. 8–2. In this scheme, the origin of each of the memory systems is the vast expanse of the cerebral cortex, focusing in particular on the highest stages of the several distinct sensory and motor processing hierarchies, the cortical association areas. As discussed in Chapter 7, each of these areas is responsible for both perceptual, motor, or cognitive processing and for memory of the same domain of information. The cerebral cortex then provides major inputs to each of three main pathways of processing related to distinct memory functions. One pathway, already discussed in part in Chapters 4 and 5, is to the hippocampus via the parahippocampal region. In addition, the main output of hippocampal and parahippocampal processing is back to the cortical areas, the sites of storage and consolidation of long-term declarative memories. As we have seen, this pathway supports the relational organization

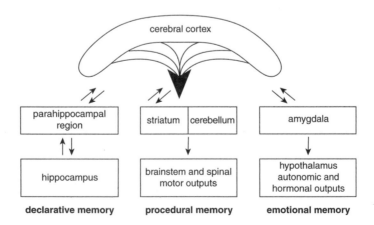

Figure 8–2. Schematic diagram of pathways for the three major "memory systems" discussed in this chapter plus other pathways and modules that are introduced later.

of cortical representations and representational flexibility in declarative memory expression. Further details on the operation of this entire system are discussed in detail in Chapter 9, and its contribution to memory consolidation is considered in Chapter 12.

Two other main pathways highlighted here involve cortical inputs to specific subcortical targets as critical nodal points in processing leading to direct output effectors. One of these systems involves the striatum as a nodal stage in the association of sensory and motor cortical information with voluntary behavioral responses via the brain stem motor system. Another component of this system involves the cerebellum. The putative involvement of these pathways in the acquisition of specific behavioral responses has led many researchers to consider this system as specialized for habit or skill memory, examples of "procedural memory." This hypothesis is tested in the experiment described below in this chapter, and is considered in more detail in Chapter 10.

The other system involves the amygdala as a nodal stage in the association of exteroceptive sensory inputs to emotional outputs effected via the hypothalamic–pituitary axis and autonomic nervous system. The putative involvement of this pathway in such processing functions has led many investigators to consider this system as specialized for "emotional memory." This hypothesis is treated in experiments described below in this chapter and in Chapter 11.

The goal of the remainder of this chapter is to provide a preliminary characterization of the roles of these systems, and in particular to show how they operate differently in the acquisition of different types of memory for the same materials. The comparisons I describe are some of the most striking examples of the success of the double dissociation approach in demonstrating and defining distinct memory systems. The first experiment described involves a "triple dissociation" of memory functions in rats. This study reveals three different patterns of sparing and impairment of memory following damage to three different brain structures. Then two studies are described that involve double dissociations of memory functions in humans with specific types of brain damage. Taken together, the findings suggest a similar set of memory functions supported by homologous brain areas in animals and humans.

Distinct memory functions and brain areas supporting radial maze performance in rats

One of the most striking dissociations among memory functions supported by separate brain structures comes from studies by Normal White and his colleagues. These studies involved multiple experiments in which separate groups of rats were trained on three different versions of the spatial radial maze task. Each version of the task used the same maze, the same general spatial cues and approach responses, and the same food rewards. But the stimulus and reward contingencies of each task differed, each focusing on a different kind of memory processing demand. For each task, performance was compared across three separate groups of rats operated to disrupt the hippocampal system, the amygdala, or the striatum. In addition, different methods of brain damage were compared. Hippocampal system disruption was accomplished by either a fornix transection, which disconnects the hippocampus from important subcortical areas, or by direct lesion of the hippocampus. The effects of these kinds of damage were compared to different methods for direct damage to the amygdala and the striatum.

One test was the conventional version of the radial maze task (Fig. 8–3A). In this version of the task, an eight-arm maze was placed in the midst of a variety of stimuli around the testing room, providing animals with the opportunity to encode the spatial relations among these stimuli as spatial cues. On every daily trial, a food reward was placed at the end of each of the eight maze arms, and the animal was released from the center and was allowed to retrieve the rewards. Optimal performance would entail entering each arm only once, and subsequently avoiding already visited arms in favor of the remaining unvisited arms. The central memory demand of this task was characterized as a "win–shift" rule; such a rule emphasizes memory for each particular daily episode with specific maze arms. Also, the task requires "flexible" use of memory by using the approach into previously rewarded locations to guide the selection of other new arms to visit (see Chapter 5). Accordingly, it was expected that performance on this task would require the hippocampal system.

It was found that normal animals learned the task readily, improving from nearly chance performance (four errors out of their first eight arm choices) on the initial training trial to an average of fewer than half an error by the end of training. Consistent with expectations, damage to the hippocampus resulted in an impairment on this version of the radial maze task. Compared to normal animals, rats with hippocampal damage made more errors by entering previously visited maze arms. Even after extended training, hippocampal-damaged rats continued to make substantially more errors than controls. By contrast, amygdala and striatum lesions had no effect on task performance. Indeed, the group of animals with amygdala lesions performed at least as well as the controls.

A. win-shift

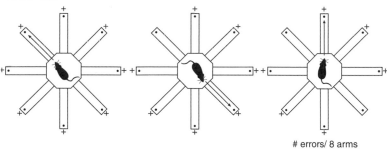

errors/ 8 arms

B. win-stay

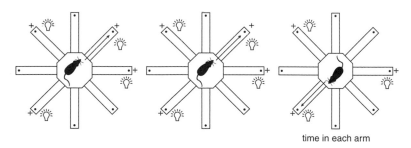

time in each arm

C. conditioned place preference

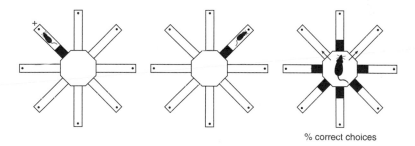

% correct choices

Figure 8–3. Illustrations of example trials in different variants of the radial arm maze task. For each, the measure of performance is indicated below the N + 2 trial. + = rewarded arm (from descriptions in McDonald and White, 1993).

The second test involved a variant of the same radial maze task (Fig. 8–3B). In this version, the maze was surrounded by a curtain, and lamps were used to cue particular maze arms. On the first trial of each daily training session, four arbitrarily selected arms were illuminated and baited with food, whereas the other four arms were dark and had no food. When a lit arm was entered for the first time, that arm was rebaited, so the animal could return to the arm for a second reward. Subsequently that lamp in that particular arm was turned off and no more food was provided at that arm. Thus, here the task was characterized by a "win–stay" rule in which animals could approach any lit arm at any time and could even re-execute the approach to a particular arm for reward one time in each daily trial. This version of the task minimized the availability of spatial cues, and indeed associated rewards with different sets of locations across days. Thus, the task emphasized the approach to a specific cue (a light) across all trials and made no demand to remember particular trial episodes. Also, this version of the task did not require flexible expression of memory under conditions different than original learning—memory was expressed in choice selections during repetitions of the learning trials. Therefore, performance was not expected to rely upon the hippocampus. Furthermore, following learning, the expression of the acquired approach responses is not sensitive to manipulations of the reward level, indicating the task is mediated by stimulus–response habits, rather than by the stimulus–reward association. For these and additional reasons to be made clearer later, performance on the win–stay task was expected to rely on the striatum.

Results showed that normal control subjects learned the appropriate behavioral response to approach the lit arms gradually over several training sessions. In the first few sessions they selected lit arms on only 50% of the trials, but, by the end of 24 sessions, they performed at about 80% correct. Consistent with expectations, animals with striatal damage were impaired, barely exceeding chance performance even with extended training. By contrast, animals with hippocampal damage succeeded in learning and even outperformed the control subjects in learning rate. Animals with amygdala lesions were unimpaired, learning the task at a normal rate.

The third test involved yet another variant of the radial maze task in which animals were separately conditioned to be attracted to one maze arm and habituated to another arm (Fig. 8–3C). In this version, the maze was surrounded by a curtain to diminish the salience of spatial cues. Six of the maze arms were blocked off to make them inaccessible, and one of the remaining two arms was illuminated by proximal lamps, whereas the other was only dimly illuminated. After a preliminary session in which rats could explore both available arms, conditioning proceeded with daily exposures to one of the two arms. For each rat, either the lit or the dark arm was associated with food by confining the animal in that arm for 30 minutes with a large amount of food on four separate trials. On another four trials, the same animal was confined for the same period of time to the other arm, but with no food. Thus, in half of the rats, the lit arm was associated with food availability and the dark arm was not; for the other half of the rats the opposite association was conditioned. In a final test session, no food was placed in the maze and access to both the lit and dark arms was allowed. The amount of time spent in each arm for a 20-minute session was recorded to measure the preference for each of the two arms. This version of the radial maze task emphasized the strong and separate associations between food reward or absence of reward with a particular maze arm defined by a salient nonspatial cue. This task minimized the availability of spatial relations among stimuli. Also, because the same lit and dark arms used during training were re-presented in testing, the task did not require flexible expression of memory under conditions substantially different than original conditioning. Thus, it was not expected that the hippocampal system would be critical to learning. Also, no overt approach response was required during initial learning, minimizing the involvement of learning specific behavioral responses. For these and additional reasons to be discussed later, learning would seem to depend on memory processes associated with emotional conditioning that is expected to depend upon the amygdala.

It was found that normal animals showed a strong preference for the arm associated with food, typically spending 50%–100% more time in the maze arm in which they had been fed compared to the arm where no food was previously provided. Consistent with expectations, rats with amygdala damage showed no conditioned preference for the cue arm associated with food. By contrast, rats with hippocampal or striatal damage showed robust conditioned cue preferences. Despite their lesions, they performed at least as well as intact animals.

The results of this study confirmed all of the findings described earlier, showing that selective ablation of the hippocampus disturbs a form of episodic memory, that selective ablation of the striatum disturbs response or habit learning, and that selective ablation of the amygdala disturbs a conditioned emotional preference.

Double dissociation of memory systems in humans

Studies on human patients provide another potential source for the possibility of double dissociations among the functional memory systems. Studies on humans can extend the dissociations described so far to the distinction between declarative memory, as it is defined in humans, and different forms of nondeclarative or implicit memory, and can reveal significant similarities in the memory dissociations across species. The following sections summarize the findings of two recent studies that have compared different patient populations on a variety of learning and memory paradigms. Despite some potentially important differences across studies in the nature of the disorders represented in these patients, there are strong similarities across studies in the overall pattern of findings. In each study, the learning and memory capacities of amnesic patients with damage to the medial temporal lobe were compared with the capacities of "nonamnesic" patients, that is, humans with brain pathologies not producing the classic amnesic syndrome discussed in Chapter 4. Also, in each study, the performance of these patient groups was compared on standard tests of declarative memory for the learning materials used in each of the tests. The resulting double dissociations in human patients with various memory disorders provide especially compelling evidence for the existence of multiple parallel memory systems in the brain.

There have been no fully parallel triple dissociation experiments performed on humans. However, in the next sections of this chapter, two double dissociation experiments are described—one study compares the abilities of amnesic subjects to the performance of patients with damage to the striatum, and the other study compares the abilities of amnesics to those of patients with damage to the amygdala.

Procedural (habit) learning and declarative memory

One example of a double dissociation involves the analysis of an unusual form of habit learning. Barbara Knowlton and her colleagues studied patients in the early stages of Parkinson's disease, associated with degeneration of neurons in a part of the brain stem (the substantia nigra) resulting in a major loss of input to the striatum, and a set of amnesic patients with hippocampal damage or damage elsewhere in that memory system. Subjects were trained in a probabilistic classification learning task formatted as a "weather prediction" game. The task involved predicting one of two outcomes (rain or shine) based on cues from a set of cards. On each trial, one to three cards from a deck of four were presented. Each card was associated with the sunshine outcome only probabilistically (Fig. 8–4A) and the outcome with multiple cards was associated with the conjoint probabilities of the cards presented in any configuration. After presentation of the cards for each trial, the subject was forced to choose be-

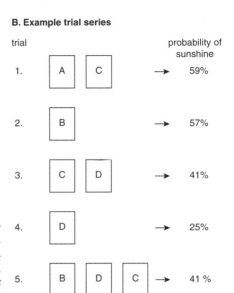

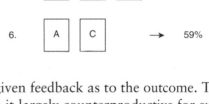

Figure 8–4. The "weather prediction" probabalistic learning task. *A:* The four stimulus cards and their individual assigned associations with the outcome "sunshine." A–D stand for distinct complex stimulus patterns. *B:* An example of a series of trials and the average probability of sunshine for each. Note a repeat of the same stimulus pair on trials 1 and 6.

tween rain and shine, and was then given feedback as to the outcome. The probabilistic nature of the task made it largely counterproductive for subjects to attempt to recall specific previous trials, because repetition of any particular configuration of the cues could lead to different outcomes. In the example set of trials shown in Fig. 8–4B, when presented with the pattern shown on trial 6, subjects might remember their response to the same pattern on trial 1—but the outcome on the current trial need not be the same as on that first trial, leading to confusion. Instead, the most useful information to be learned concerned the probability associated with particular cues and combinations of cues, acquired gradually across trials much as conventional motor habits or skills are acquired.

Over the initial block of 50 trials, normal subjects gradually improved from pure guessing (50% correct) to about 70% correct, a level consistent with the optimal probability of accuracy in this task. However, the patients with Parkinson's disease failed to show significant learning, and the failure was particularly evident in those patients with more severe Parkinsonian symptoms. By contrast, amnesic patients were successful in learning the task, achieving levels of accuracy not different from those of controls by the end of the 50-trial block.

Subsequent to training on the weather prediction task, these subjects were debriefed with a set of multiple-choice questions about the types of stimulus materials and nature of the task. Normal subjects and those with Parkinson's disease performed very well in recalling the task events. But the amnesic subjects were severely impaired, performing near the chance level of 25% correct. These findings demonstrate a clear double dissociation, with habit learning disrupted by striatal damage and declarative memory for the learning events impaired in amnesia, providing further evidence for the view that different forms of memory are represented for the identical learning materials within parallel and separable brain systems.

Declarative memory and emotional memory

Another double dissociation in the literature on amnesia involves the analysis of a type of emotional conditioning. Antonio Damasio and his colleagues studied three patients with selective damage to the hippocampus or amygdala. One patient suffered from Urbach-Wiethe disease, a rare disorder resulting in selective bilateral calcification of the tissue of the amygdala, sparing the adjacent hippocampus. Another patient experienced multiple cardiac arrests and associated transient hypoxia and ischemia that resulted in selective bilateral hippocampal atrophy, sparing the neighboring amygdala. The third patient suffered herpes simplex encephalitis resulting in bilateral damage to both the amygdala and hippocampus.

This study focused on a form of classical conditioning involving an association between a neutral stimulus and a loud sound that produces a set of autonomic nervous system responses (Fig. 8–5A). All subjects were conditioned twice, once in the visual modality where the conditioning stimulus (CS+) was a simple colored slide, and then again in the auditory modality where the CS+ was a pure tone. Subjects were initially habituated to the CS+ as well as to several other stimuli in the same modality (different colors or different tones) that would be presented as CS− stimuli. Subsequently, during conditioning, the CSs were presented in random order for 2 seconds each. Each presentation of the CS+ was terminated with the unconditioned stimulus (US), a loud boat horn that was sounded briefly. The loud horn produced a set of involuntary emotional responses, including sweating that was measured through electrical recordings of skin conductance.

Normal control subjects showed skin conductance changes to the US, and robust conditioning to the CS+, with smaller responses to the CS−

A. conditioning protocol

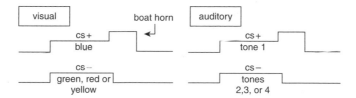

B. declarative memory questions

1. How many colors?
2. Name the colors.
3. How many colors were followed by the horn?
4. Name the colors followed by the horn.

Figure 8–5. Protocols for emotional conditioning and declarative memory. *A:* The protocols for visual and auditory classical conditioning. *B:* The questions asked in the post-training interview.

stimuli (Fig. 8–6). The patient with selective amygdala damage showed normal unconditioned skin conductance responses to the US, but failed to develop conditioned responses to the CS+ stimuli. By contrast, the patient with selective hippocampal damage showed robust skin conductance changes to the US and normal conditioning to the CS+ stimuli. This pa-

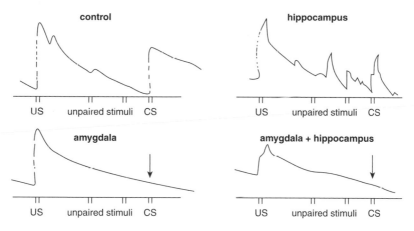

Figure 8–6. Skin conductance responses to the boat horn unconditioned stimulus (US) followed by responses to the unpaired stimuli and the conditioning stimulus (CS). Note that all subjects show strong unconditioned responses to the US. Controls also show a strong conditioned skin conductance response to the CS but not to the unpaired stimuli. The subject with hippocampus damage only shows a strong response to the CS and some generalization to the unpaired stimuli. Subjects with amygdala damage did not acquire a response to the CS (from Bechera et al., 1995).

tient also showed responsiveness to the CS− stimuli, but clearly differentiated these from the CS+ stimuli. The subject with combined amygdala and hippocampal damage failed to condition, even though he responded to the US.

After the conditioning sessions, the subjects were debriefed with several questions about the stimuli and their relationships (see Fig. 8–5B). Control subjects and the patient with selective amygdala damage answered most of these questions correctly, but both patients with hippocampal damage were severely impaired in recollecting the task events. These findings demonstrate a clear double dissociation, with a form of emotional conditioning disrupted by amygdala damage and declarative memory for the learning situation impaired by hippocampal damage. The finding that these different forms of memory for the identical stimuli and associations are differentially affected by localized brain damage further supports the notion of multiple memory systems.

Summing up

Combining the results of the studies presented in this chapter permits some critical nodal points for memory processing to be identified, and these functional assignments are similar across species. These multiple dissociations show that the hippocampal region mediates memory for adoption of the "place" strategy in a T-maze and expression of episodic memories in rats, and memory for facts and events in humans. These dissociation studies show additionally that the striatum plays a critical role in the learning of habitual behavioral responses as reflected in the "response" strategy in a T-maze and stimulus–approach learning in the radial maze by rats and in probabilistic cue–response associations in humans. Furthermore, these studies have provided compelling evidence that the amygdala is critical to emotional learning, as reflected in the acquisition of cue preferences in rats and conditioned emotional responses in humans. Across all these experiments, a salient theme is that these different forms of memory, even for the identical learning materials, are mediated largely independently and in parallel.

Note that although particular nodal brain loci are claimed critical to particular forms of memory, we should not think of these particular brain structures as "black boxes" that contain and perform different types of memory in isolation. Specific brain structures, including (but not restricted to) the hippocampus, the striatum, and the amygdala, are key centers for processing one of the many streams of the flow of cortical information outward to other brain systems. Because these particular structures are central "bottlenecks" for particular pathways, and because each is part of only one of the main functional pathways, these structures become loci of critical and selective processing for that type of memory. Thus, one should be wary of viewing the hippocampus as "the" center for relational or declarative memory. Rather, it is only one (albeit crucial) part of that memory system, but perhaps the only part that is not shared in the pathways for other memory systems. A similar characterization fits for the striatum and for the amygdala. Further details on the circuitry and functional properties of those two memory systems follow in the next three chapters.

READINGS

Bechera, A., Tranel, D., Hanna, D., Adolphs, R., Rockland, C., and Damasio, A.R. 1995. Double dissociation of conditioning and declarative knowledge relative to the amygdala and hippocampus in humans. *Science*, 269: 1115–1118.

Knowlton, B.J., Mangels, J.A., and Squire, L.R. 1996. A neostriatal habit learning system in humans. *Science*, 273: 1399–1401.

McDonald, R.J., and White, N.M. 1993. A triple dissociation of memory systems: Hippocampus, amygdala, and dorsal striatum. *Behav. Neurosci.*, 107: 3–22.

Packard, M.G., Hirsh, R., and White, N.M. 1989. Differential effects of fornix and caudate nucleus lesions on two radial maze tasks: Evidence for multiple memory systems. *Neurosci* 9: 1465–1472.

Packard, M.G., and McGaugh, J.L. 1996. Inactivation of hippocampus or caudate nucleus with lidocaine differentially affects expression of place and response learning. *Neurobiol. Learn. Mem.* 65: 65–72.

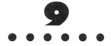

A Brain System for Declarative Memory

STUDY QUESTIONS

What are the main components of the declarative memory system, and what are the subcomponents of each of them?

What is the general pattern of connectivity among the main components of the system and within each of the main components?

What is the evidence for a selective and independent role for the parahippocampal region in the persistence of representations in intermediate-term memory?

What is the evidence for a separate and selective role for the hippocampus itself in the organization of memories into a relational representation?

How is information differentially encoded in the parahippocampal region versus the hippocampus?

So far the discussion of declarative memory has considered the role of the entire medial temporal lobe region, or the hippocampus specifically, making little distinction between anatomically separate components of this area of the brain. However, the hippocampus is many synapses from sensory inputs and motor outputs, and so its contribution must be considered in the context of how the hippocampus performs its functions within the larger system of brain structures of which it is a part. Indeed, the hippocampus is only one of several structures that compose the full brain system that mediates declarative memory. The aims of this chapter are to identify the main components of this system, to outline the anatomical pathways by which information flows through the system, and to characterize the functional contributions of its different components.

Anatomical characterization of the hippocampal memory system

The *declarative memory system* is composed of three major components: the cerebral cortex; the parahippocampal region, which serves as a convergence center for neocortical inputs and mediates two-way communication between cortical association areas and the hippocampus; and the hippocampus itself. Figure 9–1 illustrates the multiple areas of the cerebral cortex that are involved in this system, and shows the basic anatomical connections between the several neocortical areas that provide specific per-

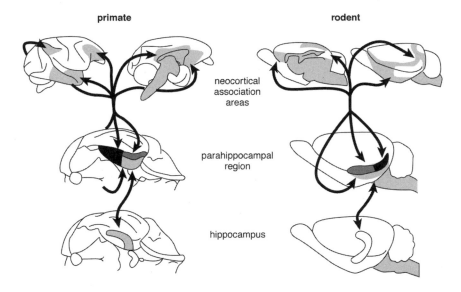

primate   rodent

neocortical
association
areas

parahippocampal
region

hippocampus

Figure 9–1. The anatomy of the hippocampal memory system. In both monkeys and rats the origins of specific information to the hippocampus include virtually every neocortical association area. Each of these neocortical areas projects to one or more subdivisions of the parahippocampal region, which includes the perirhinal cortex, the parahippocampal (or postrhinal) cortex, and the entorhinal cortex. The subdivisions of the parahippocampal region are interconnected and send major projections to multiple subdivisions of the hippocampus itself. Thus, the parahippocampal region serves as a convergence site for cortical input and mediates the distribution of cortical afferents to the hippocampus. The outcomes of hippocampal processing are directed back to the parahippocampal region, and the outputs of that region are directed in turn back to the same areas of the cerebral cortex that were the source of inputs to this region (from Eichenbaum, 2000).

ceptual and motor information to the relevant medial temporal lobe areas, and are the main recipients of the outputs of processing by structures within the medial temporal area. The diagram also shows the location of the components of this system that lie within the medial temporal area. In the terminology suggested by Menno Witter and his colleagues, the large collection of structures within the medial temporal lobe that participate in this system are consolidated into two functional components, the *hippocampus* and the *parahippocampal region*. This diagram also indicates the flow of information among the three major components of the system, highlighting the similarity of the main pathways in monkeys and rats.

The flow of information within the hippocampal memory system

The major pathways of the hippocampal memory system connect the system's three main components, with one set of bidirectional connections between the cortex and the parahippocampal region and another set of bidirectional connections between the parahippocampal region and the hippocampus. This three-stage, two-way communication scheme provides both the basic framework of information flow through the system and strong limitations on how the system works. In this anatomical scheme the cortex provides specific information to the medial temporal lobe structures, this information is manipulated in two stages, and the product of these manipulations is targeted to influence the same cortical areas that provided the original inputs. The message one should take from these anatomical facts is that the role of the medial temporal lobe is to enhance the storage of, change the organization of, or otherwise modify the nature of cortical representations. The next sections provide an overview of the anatomy of each of the main components of the system and outline the main pathways of communication between them.

Areas of the cerebral cortex that interact with the medial temporal lobe

Only highly preprocessed sensory information reaches the medial temporal lobe structures, but these inputs come from virtually all higher-order cortical processing areas. Thus, the larger scheme in which perceptual information reaches the medial temporal lobe is as follows: Sensory information enters the primary cortical areas, then passes through multiple secondary and tertiary stages of sensory processing that are segregated for each sensory modality, as discussed in Chapter 7. The highest areas for each sensory modality then project to the association areas, multimodal areas in the prefrontal parietal, and temporal lobes, as well as the cortex on the midline called the cingulate area. A somewhat similar hierarchy exists for stages of processing in the motor cortical areas, which also ultimately project to association areas in the cingulate and prefrontal cortex. The functional role of these areas differs, but for each that role involves a very high order form of sensory, motor, emotional, or cognitive processing that includes and supersedes specific sensory modalities of the information these areas receive. For example, the association areas of the parietal lobe process spatial information about visual and other sensory inputs, and association areas of the temporal lobe process are involved in object identification from information from multiple sensory modalities. The precise function of prefrontal and cingulate areas is less well understood, but may involve a combination of information about the significance of stimuli, the rules of tasks, and plans for task solutions. The outputs of these areas are the source of inputs to the parahippocampal region.

The parahippocampal region

The parahippocampal region comprises three distinct and adjacent cortical zones, the entorhinal cortex, the perirhinal cortex, and the parahippocampal cortex (as it is called in monkeys, or postrhinal cortex as it is called in rats; (see Fig. 9–1)). Each of these areas can be characterized as receiving input from multiple neocortical association areas and thus constitutes an important convergence site for neocortical input to the hippocampus.

The input connections to the parahippocampal region arise in virtually all the higher-order association areas, including several parts of the prefrontal cortex, parietal cortex, temporal cortex, as well as olfactory cortex in both monkeys and rats. A major similarity of the perirhinal and parahippocampal (postrhinal) areas is that both heavily project to parts of the entorhinal cortex. These areas connect with subdivisions of the hippocampus and also have major projections back to the same neocortical areas that provided the major inputs.

The cortical inputs to the parahippocampal region demonstrate a systematic organization, but one that is unlike the precise topographies that characterize the primary sensory and motor cortical areas (see Chapter 7). Instead, these projections involve large and overlapping zones of projection, an organization of "topographical gradients." Individual cortical association and olfactory areas project differentially along the parahippocampal region. Generally, inputs from more anterior cortical areas, the ones from olfactory, anterior cingulate, and frontal areas, terminate within anterior parts of the perirhinal and lateral part of the entorhinal cortex.

Conversely, inputs from more posterior cortical areas, the ones from parietal and temporal areas, terminate in more posterior parts of the perirhinal, parahippocampal (postrhinal), and lateral entorhinal cortex. In monkeys, the overwhelming input to perirhinal cortex is from visual association areas, whereas in rats there is a more even distribution of inputs from all the ventral temporal association areas. Olfactory inputs to all areas of the parahippocampal region are more prominent in rats than monkeys. These differences largely reflect species differences in the distribution of cortical specializations, for example, differences across species in the amount of cortical area devoted to vision. The perirhinal and parahippocampal (postrhinal) areas, in turn, project heavily onto entorhinal cortex, providing about two-thirds of their cortical input, and contribute to the inputs to the hippocampus itself. There are also major connections between the perirhinal and parahippocampal (postrhinal) cortex. Therefore, these three areas are viewed as highly interconnected cortical zones that, as a whole, accumulate and send cortical information to the hippocampus.

The hippocampus

The hippocampus is composed of several subfields that are distinguished according to the types and layout of cells, and the anatomical connections of these cells. These subfields include an area called Ammon's horn (composed of two main subdivisions called CA1 and CA3) , the dentate gyrus, and the subiculum (Fig. 9–2A). The hippocampus is connected to other brain areas via two main bidirectional routes. One of these routes is via a major axon bundle called the fornix, which carries input and output connections with the hippocampus and several subcortical areas. This connection pathway supports multiple modulatory influences on the hippocampus, including attentional controls that tell the hippocampus when to become activated and rhythmic controls that pace its processing cycles. The other route of communication for the hippocampus is via the parahippocampal region. This route, by contrast to the fornix pathway, supports specific informational inputs to the hippocampus from a variety of cortical areas as well as outputs from the hippocampus to these same cortical areas.

There are two main routes by which the parahippocampal area projects into the hippocampus; these are characterized here as the "long" and "short" routes (see Fig. 9–2B). The long route is the so-called trisynaptic circuit, which begins with the perforant path, composed of axons of the entorhinal cortex that penetrate the hippocampal fissure to invade the dentate gyrus. The perforant path originates in superficial cells of the entorhinal and perirhinal cortices, and the projection into the dentate gyrus

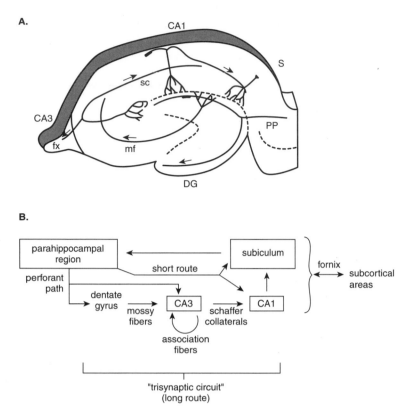

Figure 9–2. Pathways within the hippocampus. *A:* A hippocampal slice indicating the anatomical positions of the major areas and pathways. DG = dentate gyrus; fx = fornix; mf = mossy fibers; sc = Schaffer collaterals; pp = perforant path; S = subiculum. *B:* A flow diagram of the major pathways through subdivisions of the hippocampus, including the several known "loops" between these areas. The traditional "trisynaptic circuit" is the lower "loop" proceeding successively from the parahippocampal region, to the dentate gyrus, to CA3, to CA1, to the subiculum, and then back to the parahippocampal region. The short route involves direct connections between the parahippocampal region and CA1 plus subiculum.

involves well-organized but coarse topographic gradients. These projections pervade the superficial layer of granule cells in the dentate gyrus and on the apical dendrites of pyramidal cells in CA3. Then the dentate granule cells, via the mossy fibers, project to the proximal dendrites of CA3 cells in Ammon's horn. Next, the CA3 pyramids give rise to a large number of collateral outputs: First, some of these axons terminate on other CA3 cells broadly in the hippocampus, via the so-called association fibers.

Second, the CA3 pyramidal cells give rise to the earliest projection out of the hippocampus via the fornix to subcortical areas. Third, CA3 pyramids also give rise to the Schaffer collateral system that provides the major long-route input to the pyramidal cells of CA1. CA1 pyramidal cells project broadly onto cells in the subiculum. The short route of communication involves direct input from the deep layer cells of the parahippocampal cortex to the subiculum and to CA1. The organization of these inputs is essentially the same as that of the entorhinal–dentate inputs.

The return circuit out of the hippocampus begins with the subiculum giving rise to major subcortical and cortical outputs of the hippocampus. The subcortical projection is through the fornix and into multiple subcortical areas (other fibers of the fornix carry subcortical inputs into all the subfields of the hippocampus). The cortical projections, involving outputs of both CA1 and the subiculum, project primarily to deep layers of the entorhinal cortex, completing the parahippocampal–hippocampal loops. These projections follow the same topographic arrangement as the input connections.

Next, the deep pyramidal cells of entorhinal and perirhinal cortex project to the same cortical areas from which inputs originated. In addition, part of the prefrontal cortex receives a direct projection from the CA1. Thus, the cortical recipients of parahippocampal output include the polymodal association areas of the frontal, cingulate, and temporal areas, and the unimodal higher cortical areas in the piriform (olfactory) cortex and neocortex. The organization of these projections follows that of the input organization: More anterior parts of the parahippocampal region project to anterior cortical areas and more posterior parahippocampal areas to more posterior cortical sites.

These anatomical details provide the framework for understanding the functional roles of each of the major components of the system. The cortical association areas provide specific information to the parahippocampal region and hippocampus and in turn are influenced by the outputs of processing in these areas. Notably, in this scheme the parahippocampal region has prominent bidirectional connections with the cortex, and so could support some aspects of memory function on its own even without the contribution of the hippocampus—this possibility is explored in the next section. In addition, the hippocampus depends on two kinds of connections, the general modulatory connections with subcortical areas through the fornix and the specific informational connections with cortical areas. As you will see, both kinds of connections are important to its contribution.

Functional distinctions between the components
of the medial temporal lobe

There is now substantial evidence that the major components of the hippocampal memory system contribute differentially to overall memory functions of the system. Here evidence is presented indicating two sequential functions corresponding to the parahippocampal region and the hippocampus. First, it is argued that the parahippocampal region by itself mediates the representation of isolated items and can hold these representations in a memory "buffer" for periods of at least several minutes. This "intermediate-term memory" function bridges the gap between the very brief period of immediate (or short-term) memory and the potentially permanent (or long-term) memory store. Second, it is argued that during this intermediate period, the hippocampus itself mediates comparing and relating these individual representations to other memory representations, creating or modifying the overall memory organization according to the relevant relations between the items and the structure of any already established memory organization that involves those items. The combination of these two processing functions constitutes *declarative memory* as it has been characterized in previous chapters.

Although these two processing functions are seen as supported independently, they normally function interactively, with relational memory processing by the hippocampus operating on new items being held in the intermediate-term store in the parahippocampal region. The intermediate storage function is accomplished at the earlier stage of parahippocampal processing, which contains a full set of input and output connections with neocortical areas, as described earlier. Thus, even without a functional hippocampus, one might expect that the parahippocampal region may be able to support intermediate-term memory for individual items. By contrast, the hippocampus itself interacts with the neocortex only via the parahippocampal region, so one might expect that damage to the parahippocampal region would eliminate any relational processing contribution of the hippocampus. Thus, the intermediate-term storage of single items does not require the relational memory processing function, but relational memory processing depends on the intermediate-term store. This sequential stage model is entirely consistent with the known anatomy of the system.

Further supporting evidence comes from observations concerning the behavioral physiology of the parahippocampal region and the hippocampus. Consistent with the functional distinction proposed earlier, neural activity within the parahippocampal region reflects encoding of individual items and intermediate-term storage for specific items, whereas activity in the hippocampus involves highly specific conjunctions of behavioral events and place where they occur, sequences of information in episodic memories, and extraction of information that is common across episodes, as described in Chapter 6.

In the following sections of this chapter other relevant findings are presented, offering specific comparisons between the parahippocampal region and hippocampus both in their critical functional roles and in their information coding properties. The memory functions assigned to these two regions are seen as reflecting the separation between two general aspects of memory dependent on the medial temporal lobe. First, there is an aspect of this function in which information is held for some period of time that outlasts a single experience. This aspect of medial temporal function is reflected by evidence showing that this region is critical in very rapid acquisition of information and in persistence of memory representations bridging the gap between short-term and long-term memory. Capacities for rapid acquisition and intermediate-term memory persistence are evident in a broad range of human memory tasks and are particularly prominent in the studies on simple recognition in monkeys and rats. Second, there is an aspect of medial temporal function by which this region is involved in aspects of memory organization and expression that mediate the fundamental properties of declarative memory in humans and that are particularly evident in studies on relational learning in rats. In the next sections, it is argued that the parahippocampal region is more critical to the persistence functions of the medial temporal region, whereas the hippocampus is more critical to the organizational functions of this region.

The parahippocampal region and intermediate-term memory

The persistence properties of declarative memory have been studied extensively in animals using the simple recognition memory test known as delayed nonmatch to sample (DNMS), introduced in Chapter 5 (see Fig. 5–1C). Reiterating briefly here, in the original development of this task for monkeys, the subject is presented with a novel "sample" object and rewarded for displacing it. Then, after a variable memory delay, two objects are presented, one identical to the sample and the other a novel one. In this choice phase, the monkey is rewarded for selecting the novel, nonmatching object. The nonmatching rule is easily learned because monkeys are naturally attracted to novel objects. More to the point, the delayed nonmatch to sample task is ideal for measuring the persistence of memory representations for single, isolated stimuli. Indeed, to the extent that memory performance can be related specifically to variations in the length of the memory delay, it would seem that this task selectively assesses the persistence of memories as supported by medial temporal lobe structures.

Following on the initial successful studies showing that large medial temporal lobe ablations produce severe deficits on long delay performance in DNMS, this assay was used to determine which specific structures within the temporal lobe are critical. In H.M. the entire medial temporal lobe region was removed, including the amygdala, the hippocampus, and the immediately surrounding cortex. The ability to produce selective ablations of each of these structures within the monkey allowed the investigation of the role of each of these structures individually.

One part of the story about which there is general agreement is that the amygdala is not critical to the kind of memory modeled by these tasks. A surgical method was developed that allowed selective ablation of the amygdala, including virtually all of its nuclei, without damaging the surrounding cortical areas. Circumscribed lesions of the amygdala had no effect on performance on tasks for which larger medial temporal ablation produces a deficit, specifically DNMS (Fig. 9–3A), as well as retention of object discriminations and concurrent object discrimination.

The other obvious structure that was implicated in the early neuropsychological studies of human amnesia was the hippocampus. Its specific role, independent of the surrounding cortex, has been examined in several ways, including different means for ablating the hippocampus itself and transecting the fornix, the major fiber bundle connecting the hippocampus with subcortical areas. Given the focus on the hippocampus in studies on human amnesia, it came as somewhat of a surprise that the deficit following hippocampal damage or fornix transection is modest compared to that of medial temporal lobe ablation. Monkeys with damage to the hippocampus involving less damage to the surrounding parahippocampal cortical region were less severely impaired than those with full medial temporal ablations (see Fig. 9–3A). Moreover, monkeys with selective hippocampal ablations or fornix transections either show a reliable but small deficit, or perform fully normally (Fig. 9–3A,B) on the conventional DNMS task with delays as long as 2 minutes or sample lists as long as 10 items. In perhaps the most challenging version of the DNMS task, Elizabeth Murray and Mortimer Mishkin presented monkeys with a list of 40 sample objects at 30-second intervals. Subsequently, choice tests were presented in the reverse order at 30-second intervals, so that the effective memory delays spanned from 30 seconds to 40 minutes, and the longest delay was filled with all of the other testing. Under these difficult conditions normal monkeys showed very good performance up to 5 minute delays, with a smooth dropping in performance to about 60% correct at de-

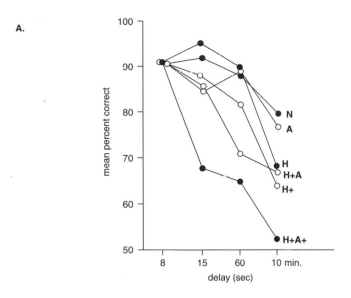

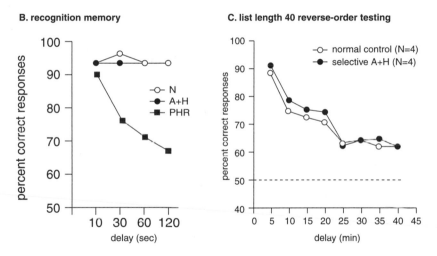

Figure 9–3. Performance of monkeys with different medial temporal lesions on delayed nonmatch to sample (DNMS). *A:* Comparison of the effects of different lesions from one series of studies. N = normal controls; A = amygdala; H = hippocampus; H+ = hippocampus plus a part of the surrounding parahippocampal region; H + A = hippocampus plus part of surrounding cortex and amygdala; H+A+ includes the hippocampus, amygdala, and most of the parahippocampal region (data from Alvarez et al., 1995; Zola-Morgan et al., 1989). *B:* Comparison of the performance on DNMS in another series of studies in normal monkeys (N) with that of monkeys with lesions of the amygdala plus hippocampus and no cortical damage (A + H) or of the parahippocampal region (PHR). *C:* Performance on a variant in which a list of 40 items is tested in the reverse order of their presentation (data from Murray and Mishkin, 1998).

lays over 20 minutes (Fig. 9–3C). Monkeys with ablations of the hippocampus (as well as the amygdala) showed a virtually identical pattern of performance.

These findings of modest or no effect of selective hippocampal damage contrasted sharply with data from contemporaneous studies that examined the role of the cortical areas immediately surrounding the hippocampus and amygdala. Damage to the combined perirhinal, parahippocampal, and entorhinal cortex produces a very severe deficit on the acquisition, long delay, and sample-list performance of DNMS (Fig. 9–3B, see also Fig. 9–3A H+A+), as well as on retention of object discriminations and concurrent object discrimination, and on the acquisition and long delay performance of the tactual version of DNMS. Furthermore, there was no impairment on pattern discrimination. The severity of the impairment was at least as much as that of the original combined medial temporal lobe ablation that involved the hippocampus, amygdala, and surrounding cortex. Indeed, to achieve the learning criterion with short delays on DNMS, monkeys with damage to the perirhinal and entorhinal cortex required remedial training with repetition of the sample trial. Finally, there appears to be a hierarchy of importance of distinct areas within this region. Perirhinal damage produces the greatest deficit, parahippocampal lesions less effect, and entorhinal lesions produce a significant, yet lesser effect.

The evidence from studies on rats supports this basic pattern of findings. In one series of studies on rats, a variant of the delayed nonmatch to sample task, called continuous delayed nonmatch to sample (cDNM), was developed (Fig. 9–4A). This task employed odor cues and involved a stimulus presentation protocol suitable for characterizing neural firing patterns to single memory stimuli as well as behavioral responses in accordance with the nonmatch memory contingency. On each trial, one of a large set of odors was presented with the contingency that a response to the odor was rewarded only if that odor was different from (i.e., a nonmatch with) the immediately preceding one. Rats were trained initially with a very brief interval between odor presentations. Subsequently, the interstimulus interval was manipulated to vary the retention delay, allowing an assessment of the persistence of memory as in the earlier studies on monkeys.

An initial experiment compared the effects of selective ablation of the parahippocampal region versus a fornix transection that selectively disrupted hippocampal function. Normal rats acquired the task within approximately 150 trials and neither of the lesion groups was impaired on

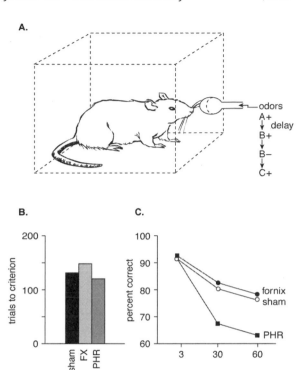

Figure 9–4. The continuous delayed nonmatch to sample (cDNM) task. *A:* A single odor is presented on each trial when the rat inserts its snout into a port on the wall. The sequence of odors (A, B, C) is random, and each is associated with reward if it is different from (a nonmatch with) the one that precedes it. *B:* Acquisition of the cDNM task with short delays by SHAM rats (that is, with surgeries involving no brain damage), rats with fornix transections (FX), and rats with lesions of the perirhinal and entorhinal cortex (PHR). *C:* Performance on short and long delays (data from Otto and Eichenbaum, 1992).

acquisition (Fig. 9–4B). Subsequent testing of memory across various delays showed that intact rats performed at a level of 90% or better at the shortest delay, with performance gradually declining as the retention interval was increased (Fig. 9–4C). Rats with damage to the parahippocampal region also showed good retention at the shortest delay, but their performance declined abnormally rapidly across delays, showing a severe deficit within 1 min. By contrast, rats with fornix lesions performed identically to normal rats across delays, showing intact performance at the short delay and the normal gradual memory decay as a function of increasing delay. These findings indicated that neither the parahippocampal region nor hippocampus is critical for perception of the odor cues, for acquisition of the nonmatch rule, or for short-term retention of odors. However, the parahippocampal region was shown to be critical for mediating a memory representation that persists beyond immediate memory in rats, as it is in monkeys. Furthermore, we may infer from these results that through its direct, reciprocal connections with the cortex, the parahippocampal region is sufficient to mediate the persistence of single-item memories independent of hippocampal processing.

Electrophysiological studies of the parahippocampal region

Using the odor-guided cDNM task in electrophysiological studies of rats, the response properties of neurons in the parahippocampal region and in the hippocampus have been examined. In the studies of the parahippocampal region, the firing patterns of cells were examined associated with three critical aspects of odor coding (Fig. 9–5). First, firing during the period when rats were sampling the odor cues was compared across all the odors presented in order to assess the extent to which odors were selectively encoded. Second, firing during the memory delay was assessed to determine the capacity of these areas for maintaining an odor memory representation in the absence of the stimulus. The focus on delay activity was particularly for the end of the delay period, immediately preceding the initiation of the subsequent odor presentation. At this time, the overt behavior of the animal is consistent across trials—the rat is approaching the stimulus port, in the absence of an odor cue—allowing one to determine if neural activity varies as a function of the memory for the identity of the preceding sample cue just before the recognition judgment must be made. Third, firing during odor sampling was also examined comparing activity

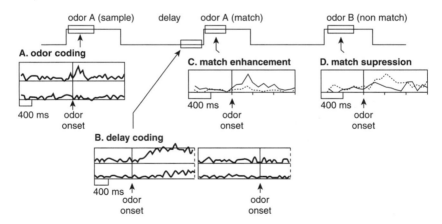

Figure 9–5. Firing patterns of cells in the parahippocampal region during analysis periods in the continuous delayed nonmatch to sample (cDNM) task. *A:* A cell in the entorhinal cortex that shows odor selective responses in the sensory period of the cDNM task. Top panel: strongest response to an odor; bottom panel: weakest response. *B:* A cell in the entorhinal cortex that showed a selective response and sustained selective firing during the delay. Top panel: strongest response to an odor; bottom panel: weakest response. *C:* A "match enhancement" cell that showed a greater response when the odor was a match (solid line) than when it was a nonmatch (dotted line). *D:* A "match suppression" cell that showed a greater response when the odor was a nonmatch (dotted line) than when it was a match (solid line) (data from Young et al., 1997).

levels when a stimulus was a match and when the same stimulus was a nonmatch, to determine the capacity of cells to signal the outcome of the comparison of the preceding and current odor.

A substantial proportion of cells in each of the subdivisions of the parahippocampal region fired during the odor sampling or delay periods. Many cells encoded the identity of the odor cues during the odor sampling period (Fig. 9–5A). Some of these cells fired selectively or differentially to odors at odor onset and ceased firing when odor sampling was concluded, much as one would expect of a sensory neuron. Other cells showed striking odor-specific activity at the end of the memory delay period, indicating some form of intermediate-term storage that was still available just before the choice phase of the trials regardless of the length of the delay. Some of these cells fired during odor sampling and then throughout the delay period, such as the example shown in Figure 9–5B.

Another set of cells showed selective activity that reflected the match and nonmatch qualities of the odor cues during the choice phase. Some of these cells, called "match enhancement cells," fired at a higher rate when the rat was sampling a repeated (matching) odor, and this differential response was largest for the most preferred odor for that cell (Fig. 9–5C). Other cells, called "match suppression cells," fired at a higher rate when the rat was sampling a different odor than the one on the previous trial (i.e., a nonmatch), and this differential response was largest for the most preferred odor for that cell (Fig. 9–5D).

Taken together, neurons in the parahippocampal region have all the properties required to support recognition performance. They encode specific odors, hold these representations (either by maintaining their activity or by regenerating activity) during an extended delay period during which an intact parahippocampal region is required, and they detect match versus nonmatch qualities of the presented choice odors.

In the studies of hippocampus itself, CA1 pyramidal neurons of rats were recorded in animals performing the same cDNM task. A large proportion of hippocampal cells could be activated in association with virtually every identifiable behavioral event in the task. A substantial subset of CA1 cells was selectively active during the odor sampling period, and the activity of some of these hippocampal cells reflected the "match" or "nonmatch" relationship critical to performance in this task. By contrast with the cells in the parahippocampal region, however, no hippocampal cells fired in association with the sampling of a particular odor or with particular combinations of odors that composed specific matching comparisons. Rather, hippocampal cellular activity reflected all comparisons with the same outcome. This finding is entirely consistent with the results of the lesion studies. It appears that the hippocampus itself is *not* involved in the encoding and storage of representations for *specific items* in this task.

Findings from recording studies of monkeys are entirely consistent with the observations of hippocampal system activity in rats. Malcolm Brown and his colleagues first compared the firing properties of neurons in the cortical area surrounding the hippocampus versus the hippocampus itself in monkeys performing a delayed matching task guided by complex visual pattern cues. The cortical cells showed stimulus-specific decrements in response (match suppression) when the choice stimulus was a repetition of the sample, but no such responses were observed in the hippocampus itself. In subsequent studies, Brown and colleagues confirmed that a large percentage of cells in the perirhinal cortex demonstrated match suppression responses. They showed evidence of three different types of recognition-related decremental responses in those cells. Some cells, called "novelty neurons," fired only on the first presentation of a novel visual pattern, and did not recover for at least 24 hours. Other cells, called "familiarity neurons," did not decrement on the choice phase of the first trial in which the stimulus appeared, but showed reduced responses on all subsequent presentations. Yet other cells, called "recency neurons," showed match suppression only on the choice phase of each trial when a particular stimulus appeared, but recovered fully when the same cue was presented as a sample on a subsequent trial. Brown has argued that all of these recognition-related firing patterns coexist, and may serve different roles in visual recognition. Importantly, no stimulus-specific match suppression responses were observed in the hippocampus in any of his studies.

Other recent studies have provided evidence of intermediate-term memory processing by the parahippocampal region in monkeys performing a more complex delayed matching to sample task. Earl Miller, Robert Desimone and their colleagues trained monkeys to perform a variant of delayed matching to sample, where a pattern cue was presented as the "sample," and, followed by several choice stimuli, the monkey had to respond only to the matching choice stimulus. In these studies, cells in the perirhinal cortex of monkeys showed selective responses to the visual cues. Some cells fired persistently during the initial part of the delay, but ceased firing when the first choice item was presented. In a version of the task where each choice stimulus was presented only once per trial, the predominant observation was "match suppression," where many cells fired less to the matching choice item. In another version of the task, where incorrect (nonmatching) choice items were presented repeatedly, forcing the animal to attend to the designated sample cue, a substantial number of "match enhancement" cells were also observed.

Wendy Suzuki and her colleagues employed the same task to study the firing properties of neurons in the entorhinal cortex of monkeys. They found a fraction of entorhinal cells that fired selectively to specific visual cues. In addition, unlike perirhinal cells in the monkey but like cells throughout the parahippocampal region in the rat, neurons in the entorhinal cortex fired throughout each of the delay periods between the sample stimulus and each of the choice items. Finally, entorhinal neuronal activity also reflected the match and nonmatch qualities of the choice stimulus, by showing match suppression and match enhancement responses.

The role of the hippocampus and parahippocampal region in relational memory

The parahippocampal region plays a more critical role in some forms of simple recognition memory than the hippocampus itself. Indeed, some researchers have suggested that the parahippocampal region plays a more critical role than the hippocampus for a broad range of memory tasks, at least as tested in monkeys. However, as seen in Chapters 4 and 5, studies of memory in humans and animals indicate that the hippocampus itself does play a critical role in some types of memory, and recent studies have extended this role even to other forms of recognition memory. The role of the hippocampus is seen most clearly in tasks that emphasize the representational properties of declarative memory rather than the temporal properties. It turns out that the heavy reliance of primate work on the DNMS task has led to emphasis in that literature on the temporal characteristics of the hippocampal memory system and has therefore focused attention on the role of the parahippocampal region, which has the ability to maintain a persistent intermediate-term memory representation. Work on amnesia in humans and rats, by contrast, has explored a variety of tasks that call upon the special representational characteristics of the hippocampal memory system, namely the ability to perform relational memory processing, which depends critically on the hippocampus itself. To clarify this point, we turn now to one further set of results in which the ability to learn the relations among items is challenged in rats with selective damage either to the parahippocampal region or to hippocampus (following transection of the fornix).

In Chapter 5, evidence was presented that the hippocampus plays a critical role in transitive associations in the representation of multiple paired associates. A more ambitious test of the role of the hippocampus was provided in an experiment that examined the capacity for learning and remembering large and structured odor memory organizations and the ability for representational flexibility. This experiment involved the development of a task that required animals to learn an orderly hierarchy of odor representations, and then tested their ability to make transitive inference judgments. The task was based on a test Piaget pioneered to assess human cognitive development. In tests of this type in human children, subjects are initially presented with a set of *premises*, such as "the blue rod is longer than the red rod" and "the red rod is longer than the green rod." Then the children are asked whether they can make an inference that the blue rod is longer than the green rod. The capacity for inferential judgment in this test is interpreted as prima facie evidence of the representation of orderly relations; moreover, it is the kind of relational representation structure that we attribute to the hippocampal memory system.

In the study on rats, the stimuli were different scents added to sand-filled cups in which the animals dug to find buried rewards (Fig. 9–6A), similar to the paired associates task described in Chapter 5. Initially the animals were trained on a series of two-item odor discriminations called premise pairs that collectively included five different odors (e.g., A+ versus B−, B+ versus C−, C+ versus D−, D+ versus E−, where + or − refers to which item is rewarded; see Figure 9–6B). Animals were initially trained on the series of premise pairs using a trial-blocking method that introduced the pairs and their correct responses gradually. Ultimately, however, they were presented with premise pairs in random order. Learning could occur by representing each of the discriminations individually or they could instead be represented within an orderly hierarchy that includes all five items.

To examine which of the representations was actually employed by the animals, they were given probe tests derived from two pairs of nonadjacent elements (Fig. 9–6B). When presented with the probe pair B versus D, two nonadjacent and non-end elements, consistently choosing B provides unambiguous evidence for transitive inference. B and D have never been presented together, and judging between them requires knowledge about their indirect relations via a representation of the missing item C. The other probe involved items A and E. Note that in this pairing correct choices could be entirely guided by the independent reinforcement histories of these elements individually, because choices of A during premise training were always rewarded and choices of E were never rewarded. Thus, the combination of the probe tests B versus D and A versus E provided a powerful assessment of capacities for making novel judgments guided by inferential expression of the orderly organization or by reward history of the individual elements, respectively.

After achieving solid performance on the premise pairs, probe trials containing the critical B versus D problem and the control A versus E prob-

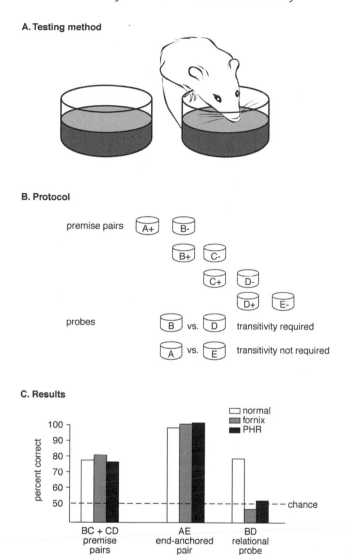

Figure 9–6. The transitive inference task. *A:* Illustration of a rat and the odor stimuli presented on a trial. *B:* Odor pairs presented on training (premise pairs) and transitive inference on control testing (probes). *C:* Average performance on inner premise pairs, on the control probe AE, and on the transitive inference test BD (data from Dusek and Eichenbaum, 1997).

lem were presented intermingled with repetitions of the premise pairs. On these probe trials, animals were rewarded for the "correct" (transitive) selection, in order to avoid dissuading them from making transitive choices and to maintain performance on the probe trials. To minimize new learning of the B versus D problem, probes were presented only twice per test session and were widely spaced among repetitions of premise pairs. In addition, to test for possible contamination by new learning of the B versus D problem, all animals were subsequently tested for their ability to learn about new odor cues presented in the probe test format.

The performance of normal rats was compared to that of rats with fornix transection, preventing the normal operation of the hippocampus, and rats with ablation of perirhinal and entorhinal cortices. Both normal rats and rats with fornix transections or parahippocampal ablation achieved criterion performance on each training phase very rapidly. In addition, all rats readily reached criterion with randomly presented premise pairs in an equivalent number of trials. In probe testing, all rats continued to perform well on the premise pairs during the test sessions, and in particular performed at about 80% correct on the "inner" pairs BC and CD (Fig. 9–6C). Also, all rats performed extremely well on the A versus E trials, which can be solved without a transitive judgment.

On the critical B versus D probe test, normal subjects demonstrated robust transitive inference. Their performance on B versus D trials significantly exceeded chance level and was not different from their performance on premise pairs that included items B and D (the B versus C and C versus D pairs; see Fig. 9–6C). In striking contrast, the rats with either type of hippocampal damage performed no better than chance on the BD probe—their performance on the B versus D problem was much lower than that on the premise pairs that included B and D, and on the other novel probe (AE), and much worse than the performance of normal animals on this test of transitivity.

A further analysis of transitivity examined performance on the very first presentation of the B versus D pair, which may be considered a "pure" test of inferential responding uncontaminated by food reinforcements given on repeated probe trials. Of the normal subjects, 88% chose correctly on the first B versus D probe, whereas only 50% of the rats with either type of hippocampal damage were successful on the initial B versus D judgment. Thus, by several measures, the data strongly indicate that rats with hippocampal damage have no capacity for transitive inference, despite their having learned each of the premise problems as well as normal subjects.

Most important for our considerations of anatomical distinctions within the hippocampal region, in this challenging test of relational memory, transection of the fornix and ablation of the parahippocampal region produced equivalent full-blown impairments. These findings strongly implicate the common structure compromised by these disconnections, the hippocampus itself, as playing the critical role in the representational properties of declarative memory. Furthermore, this pattern of findings is quite different than the selective effect of parahippocampal damage, and not hippocampal damage or fornix transection, on delayed nonmatch to sample. Thus, whereas the parahippocampal region can mediate sustained representations for single items without hippocampal involvement, the hippocampus itself is required for the organization of memories required to perform the relational task.

Differential activation of the parahippocampal region and hippocampus

Two recent studies, one in rats and the other in humans, provide further evidence consistent with the notion that the parahippocampal region and hippocampus are differentially activated in different types of memory processing. One study involved an extension of Brown and colleagues' examination of *c-fos* (a marker for gene expression) activation in the hippocampal region. In this study they presented rats with computer images of novel and familiar object stimuli, and compared responses to changes in the familiarity of particular stimuli or the familiarity of stimulus arrangements. To initiate each trial the rat placed its nose into an observing hole that stabilized the position of its eyes. Then two images were presented in the extreme left and right visual fields; because the visual circuitry of the rat involves a nearly complete hemispheric crossing of the most lateral parts of the visual fields, these images would be expected to drive neurons primarily in the opposite hemisphere. In each case a familiar image was presented to one visual field and a novel image was presented to the other— the key variable in this study was the nature of the images. For some animals the images involved pictures of single objects, whereas in other animals the images involved novel and familiar spatial arrangements of the same three objects. When the images involved single stimuli, the perirhinal cortex showed greater *c-fos* activation in the perirhinal cortex on the side that viewed novel as compared to familiar pictures. No differential activation was observed for single stimuli in the hippocampus. By contrast, when the images involved arrangements of multiple stimuli, hippocampal subdivisions (as well as the postrhinal cortex) showed greater *c-fos* activation for novel as compared to familiar stimulus arrangements. In this condition, no differential activation was observed in the perirhinal cortex.

The other recent study, performed by John Gabrieli and his colleagues, involved an examination of human brain activation using fMRI associated with the presentation of novel pictures. This study also involved two conditions. In one condition, subjects were presented with a series of novel pictures of indoor and outdoor scenes or line drawings. In this condition, the parahippocampal region was activated but the hippocampus itself was not. In the other condition, prior to scanning, subjects were presented with, and asked to remember, a set of line drawings of common objects and animals, or the names of these items. Then, during scanning, the subjects were presented with the names of the drawings they had seen, or with the drawings of the items whose names they had previously seen, respectively. In this condition, a subdivision of the hippocampus (specifically, the subiculum) was activated when the items were accurately remembered, whereas no activation was observed in the parahippocampal region. This study provided evidence in human subjects of a dissociation of memory processing functions in the hippocampal region.

Furthermore, the evidence from both of these studies can be viewed within the framework outlined here based on single neuron recordings and lesion experiments in animals. In both rats and humans, the parahippocampal region is activated during the perception and encoding of novel pictures. This could reflect the activity of neurons in the parahippocampal region associated with recognition of specific single items, as observed in rats and monkeys. These activation findings complement the observations of selective deficits in recognition memory for single items in rats and monkeys with parahippocampal damage. Furthermore, in rats the hippocampus itself is activated when memory processing involves the identification of novel arrangements of multiple items. In humans the hippocampus is activated when memory processing involves the identification of a word from a picture or vice versa. Both of these types of processing are likely to invoke the processing of relationships between items in memory, consistent with the role of the hippocampus in relational processing.

Summing up

The findings we have discussed speak to the roles of the parahippocampal region and the hippocampus in realizing the persistence and organizational properties, respectively, of hippocampal-dependent memory processing. But how do these components provide their separate functions within the declarative memory system, and how do they interact to produce declarative memory? To address this question, this chapter concludes with a model for successive stages of memory processing within the entire declarative memory system.

Prior to processing by the medial temporal lobe, neocortical areas create specific perceptual representations that can be sustained briefly within those processing areas. Such memory traces are able to support perceptual matchings between current and stored representations, and can support performance in short-term recognition, consistent with the observed sparing of working memory even in severe amnesia.

At the first stage of processing within the medial temporal lobe, perceptual codings from the neocortical processors reach the parahippocampal region, where functionally distinct representations of the to-be-remembered events converge prior to processing in the hippocampal formation itself. In the parahippocampal region, specific information is encoded, and neural activity representing that information is sustained, persisting through considerable interference and intervening processing. Furthermore, the parahippocampal region is capable of processing the matchings between current representations and the contents of the intermediate-term store. This processing appears to be sufficient to support delayed nonmatch to sample performance in the absence of normal function of the hippocampus.

At the final stage of declarative processing, the hippocampus enters the picture, *not* to maintain a memory representation of single sensory cues, but rather to process comparisons among the various current stimuli and events and between current stimuli and representations of previous stimuli and events, presumably those maintained at earlier levels of this system. Hippocampal processing appears to be quite different from the perceptual matching taking place in cortical areas. Thus, hippocampal processing relies on cortical inputs and presumably will exert its effects by modifying those inputs or by making connections among those cortical areas. In recognition memory, the hippocampus processes comparisons between current and previous stimuli as well as rich episodic and contextual information that goes beyond the strict perceptual properties on which cortical matchings are based; this may in some cases make a distinctive contribution to intermediate-term memory. Moreover, when the requirements of the task go beyond what can be accomplished by sensory matching processes, requiring comparisons among experiences with items and the flexible expression of memories, the entire system contributes critically to a distinctly new capacity for declarative memory representation.

Putting together the results of the studies presented here, a preliminary picture of the processes that mediate declarative memory emerges. It appears that the parahippocampal region contributes to declarative memory by "buffering" specific representations that can be accessed and manipulated by the hippocampus. Then the hippocampus represents the critical relations among the items and other event information held by the parahippocampal region, and indeed has access to the much larger organization of item representations in cortical association areas via the parahippocampal region. We presume the full relational memory organization comes about through multiple iterations of cortical input to the parahippocampal region and temporary storage there. This might be followed by hippocampus-mediated relational processing that adds to, or restructures, interconnections among parahippocampal and cortical representations. Over extended time periods, new experiences that bear on the established organization reactivate established representations as well as add new ones, and these are processed together by this hippocampal circuit to weave the new information into the established relational network. Precisely because this network is so extensive and systematically interconnected, access to items via novel routes and in novel experiences is not only possible but also occurs continuously as we express memories to guide almost every aspect of daily life. These interactions, by feeding back and forth, can go on for a significant period, and may be reinstated repeatedly by experiences that bear partial similarity to the learning event. This repetitive processing could contribute to the consolidation of memories over very long periods. The larger issue of memory consolidation itself is considered in Chapter 12.

READINGS

Amaral, D.G., and Witter, M.P. 1995. Hippocampal formation. In *The Rat Nervous System*, 2nd edition. G. Pacinos, (Ed.). San Diego: Academic Press, pp. 443–493.

Brown, M.W., and Xiang, J.Z. 1998. Recognition memory: Neuronal substrates of the judgement of prior occurrence. *Prog. Neurobiol.* 55:149–189.

Burwell, R.D., Witter, M.P., and Amaral, D.G. 1995. Perirhinal and postrhinal cortices in the rat: A review of the neuroanatomical literature and comparison with findings from the monkey brain. *Hippocampus* 5:390–408.

Dusek J.A., and Eichenbaum, H. 1997. The hippocampus and memory for orderly stimulus relations. *Proc. Nat. Acad. Sci. U.S.A.* 94:7109–7114.

Eichenbaum, H., Otto, T., and Cohen, N.J. 1994. Two functional components of the hippocampal memory system. *Brain Behav. Sci.* 17:449–518.

Miller, E.K., Li, L., and Desimone, R. 1991. A neural mechanism for working and recognition memory in inferior temporal cortex. *Science* 254: 1377–1379.

Suzuki, W.A., Miller. E.A., and Desimone, R. 1997. Object and place memory in the macaque entorhinal cortex. *J. Neurophysiol.* 78: 1062–1081.

Witter, M.P., Groenewegen, J.J., Lopes da Silva, F.H., and Lohman, A.H.M. 1989. Functional organization of the extrinsic and intrinsic circuitry of the parahippocampal region. *Prog. Neurobiol.* 33:162–243.

Young, B.J., Otto, T., Fox, G.D., and Eichenbaum, H. 1997. Memory representation within the parahippocampal region. *J. Neurosc.* 17: 5183–5195.

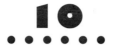

A Brain System for
Procedural Memory

STUDY QUESTIONS

What are the basic types of procedural memory?

What are the major anatomical subsystems involved in procedural memory?

What is the role of the striatum in habit learning?

What is the role of the cerebellum in conditioning?

What is the role of the motor cortex in learning?

Procedural memory. It's a term I use when I coach baseball to 10-year olds. I tell them each time they use the correct form in throwing a ball, and in swinging a bat, they strengthen the program for that correct movement. And, conversely, each time they do it wrong, they strengthen that incorrect style to the detriment of their overall performance. Some coaches call it "muscle memory." But while that term gets closer to the observable behavioral output, we know the memory for such complicated coordination is not stored in the muscles. It is stored in the nervous system, and in particular in a complicated brain system that plans and executes coordinated motor programs or procedures. From playing a sport to the act of reading aloud this manuscript and writing notes on its content, an endless array of coordinated behaviors we execute in everyday life are the product of *procedural memory*, the habits and skills that our motor system has acquired and built into its very circuitry. Other than in such painful circumstances as trying to learn a new skill in adulthood, we typically take procedural memory for granted. It goes on seamlessly and unconsciously. Yet, while development of these procedural memories is a prominent part of our childhood—as we learn to write and to ride a bicycle—they are never fully complete. Instead, procedural memories are continuously modified by experience and tuned by repeated practice throughout life.

From the perspective of the study of motor systems, a number of investigators have separated procedural memory into two general types. One type involves the acquisition of habits and skills, the capacity for a very broad variety of stereotyped and unconscious behavioral repertoires. These can involve a simple refinement of particular repeated motor patterns and extend to the learning of long action sequences in response to highly complex stimuli. These abilities reflect both the acquisition of general skills (writing, piano playing, etc.) and the unique elements of personal style and tempo in the expression of these behaviors.

The other type of procedural memory involves specific sensory-to-motor adaptations, that is, adjustments of reflexes, such as changing the force exerted to compensate for a new load, or acquisition of conditioned reflexes that involve novel motor responses to a new sensory contingency, as characterize many instances of Pavlovian conditioning described earlier. An analysis of the brain systems that support these two types of unconscious learning is the focus of this chapter.

Overview of brain anatomy relevant to procedural memory

The anatomy of brain systems that mediate procedural memory is highly complex and only partly understood, so only a few parts of these pathways that support different aspects of procedural memory are sketched here. At the top level of these various circuits is the primary motor cortex, a cortical area that is critically involved in directing the force and flow of muscle contractions generated by neural controls at the level of the spinal cord. An additional neighboring critical structure is the premotor cortex, which plays a central role in the preparation for movement and in the coordination of movements on the two sides of the body, as well as the sequencing of motor coordination over time. These cortical motor areas work in close concert with two major subcortical structures, the *striatum* and the *cerebellum* (Fig. 10–1). Each of these subcortical structures forms the nodal point in a major circuit "loop" that begins with downward projections from the cortex and ends in a route from the thalamus back to the cortex. However, there are important differences between these two subsystems with regard to the specific sources of cortical input and output, and the connections with the brain stem and the spinal cord.

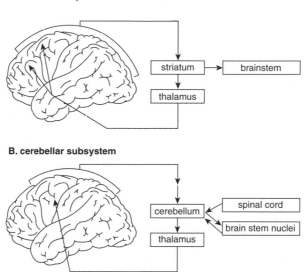

Figure 10–1. Two major motor system pathways. *A:* Connections from virtually every cortical area are sent to the basal ganglia. The major output of this subsystem is through the thalamus back to the frontal cortex. *B:* Connections from frontal and parietal cortical areas indirectly reach the cerebellum, which interacts directly with the spinal cord and brain stem motor and sensory nuclei. This system also has outputs via the thalamus back to parts of the frontal cortex.

The striatum is the combination of the anatomically distinct caudate nucleus and putamen. It works together with other components of the so-called basal ganglia, and is the focus of most of the recording and lesion studies on procedural memory in this subsystem. The striatum receives its cortical inputs from the entire cerebral cortex, and these projections are capable of activity-dependent changes in responsiveness. These projections are topographically organized into divergent and convergent projections into modules within the striatum that could sort and associate somatosensory and motor representations. The striatum projects mainly to other components of the basal ganglia and to the thalamus, which project back to both the premotor and motor cortex, and the prefrontal association cortex. Notably, there are minimal projections of this circuit to the brain stem motor nuclei and none to the spinal motor apparatus.

This pattern of anatomical connectivity suggests that the striatum is not involved directly in controlling the details of motor output. Instead, the connections to premotor and prefrontal cortex suggest that the cortical–striatal loop contributes to higher motor functions including, many researchers believe, the planning and execution of complex motor sequences. When the striatum is considered together with the anatomical connections between parts of the striatum and the brain structures involved in motivation and emotion, the suggestion has arisen that the striatum may be involved more generally in the planning and execution of goal-oriented behavior.

The cerebellum is a distinctive structure, remarkable particularly for the regularities of its internal circuitry. It has several subdivisions associated with different sensory and motor functions. The cerebellum receives cortical input from a much more restricted cortical area than the striatum, including only the strictly sensory and motor areas projecting via brain stem nuclei into the lateral part of the cerebellar cortex. Like the striatal subsystem, the cerebellum has a thalamic output route to the cerebral cortex, although the cortical target is also more restricted than that of the striatum, limited to motor and premotor cortex. In addition, the cerebellum receives somatic sensory inputs directly from the spinal cord and has major bidirectional connections with brain stem nuclei associated with spinal cord functions. Based on these connections, and on behavioral and electrophysiological data to be discussed later in this chapter, the cerebellum is believed to more directly contribute to the execution of movement details, and to the acquisition of conditioned reflexes and body adjustments to changing environmental inputs.

The striatal habit subsystem

In the preceding chapter, the striatal habit system was introduced via experiments that dissociated this system from the hippocampal and amygdala memory systems. Those experiments provided evidence indicating a role for the striatum in the acquisition of specific stimulus–response associations, as contrasted with declarative memory and emotional memory functions of the hippocampal and amygdala systems, respectively. Here the role of the striatum in habit acquisition is further elaborated, considering further the nature and scope of learning mediated by this system.

One early study illustrates the scope of memory mediated by this system and shows a particularly striking dissociation between regions within the striatum that control approach behavior conditioned by different cues. In this study, thirsty rats with lesions of the posterior-ventral or ventral-lateral regions of the striatum were trained to approach a water spout over several days. Subsequently, they were given foot shocks in the same chamber in the presence of a conditioning cue, which was either a light or an odor. The animals were tested later for their latency to approach the water spout when the conditioning cue was present versus when it was absent. Animals with lesions of the posterior-ventral striatum failed to show discriminative avoidance of the light cue, but showed good avoidance of the olfactory cue. Conversely, animals with ventral-lateral striatal lesions failed to show discriminative avoidance of the olfactory cue, but showed good avoidance of the light cue.

It was clear from the early studies, taken together, that the scope of striatal involvement is not limited to a particular sensory or motivational modality, or to a particular type of response output. The studies by Packard, McDonald, and their colleagues outlined in Chapter 8 indicate that the striatum is also essential for learning that involves acquisition of a consistent approach response to a specific stimulus. How broadly does this characterization apply to the larger body of data on lesions of the striatum in animals? In addition to the dissociation of hippocampal and striatal involvement in radial maze learning described Chapter 8, other studies by the same investigators have provided parallel data on versions of the aversively motivated water maze task. For example, in one study rats with hippocampal or striatal damage were trained on two variants of the Morris water maze task (see Chapter 5) that used the same stimuli but involved different stimulus–response demands. In both tasks, the animals were always presented with two rubber balls distinguished by different visual patterns as the learning cues. One of the cues was attached to a stable submerged platform on which the animals could climb in order to escape swimming, and the other cue was anchored to a thin pedestal that could not be mounted.

In the "visual discrimination" task variant, the positions of the cues varied, but the cue with a particular visual pattern was always mounted to the escape platform (Fig. 10–2A); here, the animal had to ignore the locations of previous escapes and consistently approach a particular visual pattern. Conversely, in the "place learning" task variant, the escape platform was always located in the same place in the maze, but the visual pattern on the cue above it varied randomly (Fig. 10–2B). In this version of the task, the animal had to ignore the visual pattern and swim consistently to a particular location defined by extramaze stimuli.

The results of this study indicated a clear double dissociation of hippocampal and striatal memory functions. Animals with hippocampal damage failed to acquire the place learning variant of the task (Fig. 10–2A), performing hardly better than chance (four correct choices out of each block of eight trials) over several training sessions. By contrast, rats with lesions of the striatum succeeded in learning to approach the correct location of the escape platform by the fourth training block, just like nor-

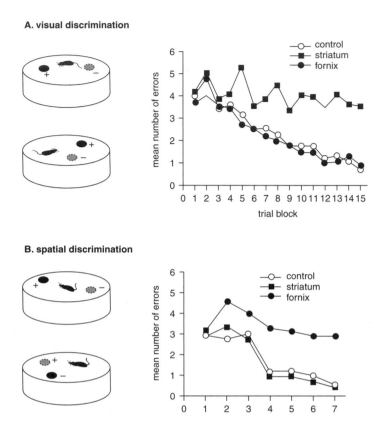

Figure 10–2. Visual or spatial discrimination in the water maze. *A:* In the visual discrimination version, the stimuli varied in location, and the escape platform was always identified by one visual cue (+) and not the other (−). *B:* In the spatial discrimination version, the same two stimuli were employed, but the escape platform was always in the same location regardless of which stimulus was nearby (data from Packard and McGaugh, 1992).

mal rats. The results were precisely the opposite on the visual discrimination task variant. Animals with striatal lesions performed at chance levels over many training blocks, whereas rats with hippocampal damage, like normal rats, gradually acquired the pattern discrimination over the course of training (Fig. 10–2B).

In another study, rats with hippocampal or striatal damage were trained on the visible platform version of the water maze task in which, from multiple starting points, they were to approach a platform that was visible above the surface of the water, always at the same location (Fig. 10–3A). Subsequently, the visible platform was replaced with a submerged plat-

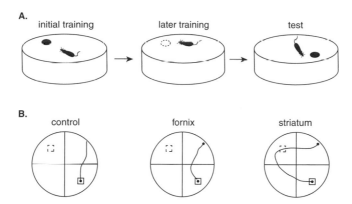

Figure 10–3. Visual versus spatial learning in the water maze. *A:* Stages of training, involving initial training with a fixed visible platform, continued training with a submerged platform at the same location (as well as further training with the visible platform at that locus), and finally testing with the visible platform moved to a new location. *B:* Examples of swim paths on the first test trial in which the escape platform was moved from its original location (dotted square) to a new locus and made visible (filled circle in square) (data from McDonald and White, 1994).

form in the same location for a single block of trials. Then, training continued with repetitions of multiple trial blocks with the visible platform, and a single trial block with the submerged platform. Finally, the visible platform was moved to a new location, and the rats were tested in a single block of trials.

All rats quickly learned to swim to the visible platform. On the first test with the submerged platform after initial training, escape latencies were elevated for all groups. On subsequent trials with the submerged platform, normal rats and rats with striatum lesions quickly learned to approach the correct escape location with shorter latencies, approximating the performance level they had achieved with the visible platform. By contrast, rats with hippocampal damage failed to improve on the submerged platform trials, consistent with their well-described deficits in place learning in the water maze. When the visible platform was moved to a new location, normal rats followed the obvious visible cue and swam to it despite its novel location (Fig. 10–3B). Rats with hippocampal damage behaved similarly, swimming directly to the visible platform as well. By contrast, rats with lesions of the striatum did not swim immediately to the visible platform, but instead swam directly to its previous location and only subsequently to the visible platform at its new site. This finding indicates that the initial successful performance in rats with striatal damage was guided primarily by learning the location of escape. Normal rats demonstrated they were capable of either learning strategy, whereas rats with hippocampal damage were guided primarily by the visual cues. This pattern of results is entirely consistent with the earlier described comparisons of hippocampal and striatal lesions. Furthermore, these data parallel those from the T-maze place-versus-response study of Packard and McGaugh. They reveal that in water maze learning too, even when initial learning performance is equivalent among animals with distinct brain damage, the representational strategies may differ qualitatively as revealed in subsequent probe tests.

These double dissociations of striatal versus hippocampal function followed on earlier studies showing a special role for the striatum in "egocentric" localization, the kind of representation that would mediate learning left or right turns in a T-maze, as illustrated in the Packard and McGaugh experiment described in Chapter 8. Raymond Kesner and his colleagues performed a study that shows compellingly the striatum's role in egocentric as opposed to "allocentric" localization, the ability to locate items in space regardless of the positions relative to the subject, exemplified in water maze learning.

In one of their experiments, a group of rats was trained on the standard eight-arm radial maze task, in which they were required to remember each of the arms they had visited based on their allocentric location in the room. The same rats were also trained in a different maze on a variant of the task in which they began each trial on an arbitrarily selected arm and were required to subsequently select an egocentrically defined adjacent arm. Rats with striatal lesions performed well on the standard radial maze (allocentric) task, but they could not learn the adjacent arm (egocentric) task (Fig. 10–4). In a second experiment, rats were trained on two tasks on different radial mazes. In a place learning (allocentric) task, only one arm of an eight-arm maze was consistently baited, and the rat began each trial from any of the remaining arms chosen at random. In a right–left discrimination (egocentric) task, the animal began each trial in the central area of the maze and two randomly chosen adjacent arms were indicated for a choice. The rat had to choose only the left (or, for other rats, the right) of the two arms regardless of its absolute location. Here, too, rats with striatal lesions performed well on the place learning task but did not learn the right–left discrimination task (Fig. 10–4).

These findings, combined with those of several other similar studies, suggest that the deficit following striatal damage can be characterized as an impairment in generating behavioral responses toward important environmental stimuli. The deficit extends to both approach and avoid-

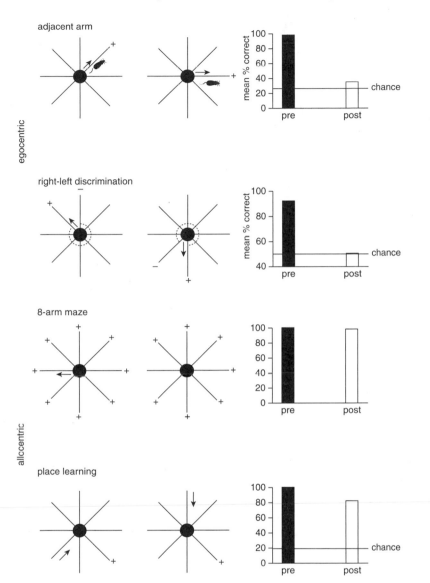

Figure 10–4. Pre- and postoperative performance of rats with striatal lesions on egocentric and allocentric spatial tasks. For each task two successive example trials are illustrated. + = rewarded arm; − = nonrewarded arm; arrow indicates beginning of run on a trial.

ance responses and to both egocentric spatial and nonspatial stimuli. However, it is likely that the deficits in egocentric localization and stimulus–response learning in animals with striatal damage may reflect only a subset of the forms of behavioral sequence acquisition mediated by the striatum.

The striatal habit subsystem: studies on human patients with striatal damage

In Chapter 8, it was shown that patients with striatal dysfunction associated with Parkinson's disease are impaired in probabilistic learning in a weather prediction task. This deficit is just one aspect of the deficit in habit learning in patients with striatal damage. Indeed, the deficit in probabilistic learning is among a number of findings in the clinical literature that raise questions about the scope of learning and memory impairments following striatal damage; more specifically, about whether deficits are limited to habit or motor skill learning or whether, instead, they extend to all domains of skill learning. The weather prediction results can be seen as entirely consistent with the findings in animals with striatal damage indicating an impairment in learning to generate one particular response among many to a complex stimulus, except that here patients were impaired in learning to generate a variety of specific responses to the appropriate sets of complex stimuli. This section considers other findings from the clinical literature. The findings described here demonstrate that this correspondence between the animal and human clinical literatures is strong and extensive.

Patients who have been studied in order to examine the role of the striatum in learning and memory come mainly from two etiologies, Parkinson's disease and Huntington's disease. Both disorders lead to profound motor deficits. In Parkinson's disease, patients suffer from tremor, rigidity, and akinesia (inability to move) following substantial cell death in other parts of the basal ganglia and the resultant depletion of dopamine, a major neurotransmitter in the striatum. Huntington's disease is characterized by primary degeneration of the striatum, and these patients exhibit irregularities in their movement patterns (athetosis and chorea). In addition to the motor deficits, some patients with Parkinson's disease also suffer from depression or dementia, and patients with Huntington's disease always progressively develop dementia. Furthermore, drug treatments administered to these patients, such as L-dopa for Parkinson's disease, have cognitive consequences. Thus, work with such patients aimed at characterizing the role of the striatum in memory is somewhat more complicated than the animal work.

Notwithstanding those limitations, both types of patients exhibit deficits on motor skill learning tasks. In one experiment, subjects were required to maintain contact of a handheld stylus with a target metal disk revolving on a turntable—this task is called rotary pursuit. Normal subjects showed robust learning over repeated practice sessions on this often-studied task, increasing the amount of time they maintained contact with the target. However, patients with Huntington's disease showed virtually no learning. To control for the possible effects on learning of differences in baseline motor performance due to the motor deficits associated with Huntington's disease, the speed of the turntable rotation was manipulated to equate the patients' initial performance to that of control subjects. Equating initial levels did not reduce the learning deficit; indeed, even when initial performance was adjusted to be better than that of normal subjects, the patients with Huntington's disease still failed to show learning.

The motor learning deficit in patients with Huntington's disease and patients with Parkinson's disease extends to unconscious learning in a task called the serial reaction time test. In this task, one of a number of different locations on a computer screen is flashed on each trial and the subject is to press the button corresponding to that location. Unbeknownst to the subject, the locations are flashed in a particular repeating order. For example, in one such item a 12-item fixed sequence involves each of the four locations flashed three times in a particular order. During the course of repetitions, implicit learning of the sequence is revealed in reductions in the subjects' average reaction time to respond to a given item within repeating sequences. Conversely, their reaction times are slower in a transfer test where subjects are presented with randomly ordered items. Several reports have indicated deficits in learning on this task in patients with Parkinson's disease or Huntington's disease, suggesting that tasks requiring memory for and sequencing of responses tap into the selective functions of the human striatum.

Functional brain imaging studies have provided another way to explore the role of the striatum in learning and memory in humans, with results paralleling closely the results of the patient studies just described. Increases in striatal activation have been seen in association with learning of finger movement sequences and with learning in the serial reaction time tasks. More recently, activation has been documented in the striatum in the more perceptual and cognitively based skill learning tasks used in other patient studies of striatal function, including probabilistic classification in the weather prediction task and other skill learning tasks. Taken together, these results indicate that the role of the striatum in habit or skill learning extends beyond the motor domain, encompassing a variety of performances that all involve multiple input or response options and that all show gradual, incremental learning across trials. The number of neuropsychological and functional imaging studies of striatal function is growing very rapidly, offering promise of clarifying the striatum's contribution to human learning and memory.

Learning-related neural activity in the striatum

Recent neurophysiological studies have provided converging evidence for the involvement of the striatum in programming stimulus–response sequences. These studies have characterized striatal neurons as anticipating movements, and have suggested that striatal activity might be associated with the relation between behavioral contexts and responses. Work by Wolfram Schultz and his colleagues has revealed striatal neural activity associated with the expectation of predictable environmental events in monkeys performing conditional responses. In one experiment, such activity was found using a variant of the delayed response task where delayed go and no-go responses were conditioned by visual stimuli. Neuronal activity sustained during the delay period reflected anticipation of either the active arm movement or of withholding that movement. A variety of cellular responses has been seen, including task-dependent anticipatory activity and activity related to the expectation and reception of reward. These findings have led Schultz to suggest that the striatum incorporates knowledge about the behavioral context of the task to plan behavioral responses.

Other studies, focusing on striatal interneurons that are tonically active, have led to a similar conclusion. Ann Graybiel and her colleagues identified a substantial population of tonically active neurons in the striatum that became responsive to an auditory cue only when the cue acquired predictive value for subsequent delivery of a reward. These cells did not respond to primary rewards, but did establish cued responses in expectation of a reward and maintained those conditioned responses for weeks. The conditioned responses were entirely dependent on dopamine inputs from the substantia nigra. Selective depletion of dopamine cells in the substantia nigra, another major part of this system that sends inputs to the striatum, resulted in a reduction of the cued responses of tonically active striatal neurons, to the same level as observed prior to conditioning. Subsequent systemic administration of a dopamine receptor agonist reinstated conditioned responses of these striatal cells. Based on these findings, Graybiel emphasized the role of limbic reward-related inputs via the substantia nigra in mediating the establishment of context-dependent striatal activity participating in the selection and execution of learned behavioral repertoires.

In addition to these observations on simple and conditional motor responses, there are data indicating a prominent role for the striatum during spatial sequencing behavior. In one study monkeys were trained to fixate a central location and encode a sequence of spatial target illuminations, then visually orient to and subsequently reach toward each target in order (Fig. 10–5A). Many striatal neurons responded to the visual instruction stimuli during central fixation or during the saccade or arm move-

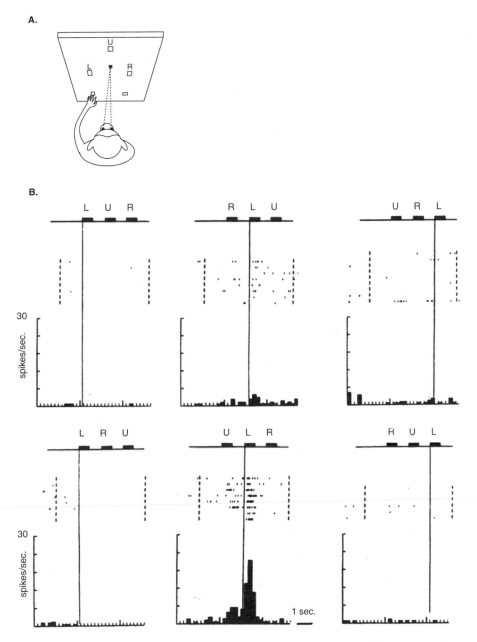

Figure 10–5. Striatal neural activity during sequence memory. A: Task protocol. On each trial the animal begins the trial by fixating its eyes at the fixation point (FP). This results in a sequence of brief illuminations of targets at right (R), left (L), and upward (U) positions in a particular order that is reproduced in eye and arm movements. B: Example of a striatal neuron that fired upon presentation of the L cue, only when in the ULR sequence (data from Kermadi and Joseph, 1995).

ment. Furthermore, the responses of a substantial proportion of these cells were highly dependent on the sequential order of the targets, responding only to a particular visual cue if it was in a particular position in the three-item sequence (Fig. 10–5B). None of the cells showed sustained activity after the target instructions, but rather the cells fired in anticipation of each item in the sequence, consistent with the view that the striatum participates with other structures in the anticipation of sequential behaviors to be performed.

Summarizing the role of the striatum in habit learning

The findings from different approaches to understanding the role of the striatum converge well, leading to the suggestion that the striatum plays a critical role in habit learning, particularly in tasks involving the learning of response sequences to specific stimuli. The necessary circuitry exists in the striatum for cortical sensory input and direct motor outputs to mediate the association of both simple and highly complex stimuli with specific behavioral outputs. Furthermore, there are clear striatal pathways for, and well-documented influences of, reward signals capable of enhancing the associations of stimuli and responses. The striatum represents a broad variety of cues, motor responses, and rewards, although in the spatial domain its role is limited to egocentric knowledge. There are both direct output pathways for control of voluntary behavior and feedback pathways to the cerebral cortex, particularly the prefrontal cortex, that could mediate complex sequencing and planning. Current research seeks to determine whether the system works to resolve competition among competing input or response options, or to permit manipulation of or shifting among representations of these input/response options, or to learn and execute the desired input–output mappings. It is clear that the striatum is a key element in a pathway for sequence learning and other aspects of habit learning involving the acquisition of stereotyped and unconscious behavioral repertoires. This procedural learning pathway is independent of the earlier described circuits for declarative memory and for emotional memory.

The cerebellum and motor conditioning

The cerebellum has long been considered a brain structure closely involved in motor control and motor learning. Experimental investigations into the role of the cerebellum in motor learning have focused on its highly organized circuitry and emphasized its mechanisms for reflex adaptations. The circuitry involves a complex set of connections among several nuclei in the brain stem. Here some of the details of that circuitry are introduced, allowing insights into the precise mechanisms of plasticity that underlie procedural memory supported within this system.

This relevant circuitry involves both the cerebellar cortex and underlying deep nuclei, plus several other specific nuclei in the brain stem (Fig. 10–6A). The principal cells of the cerebellar cortex are the Purkinje cells, which send entirely inhibitory inputs to the deep nuclei. These cells receive

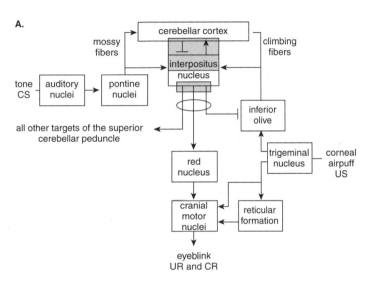

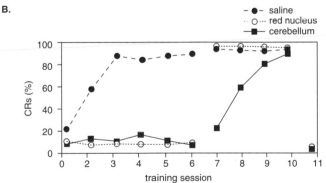

Figure 10–6. A: Schematic diagram of the essential brain circuitry that mediates classical conditioning of the eyeblink response. B: Effects of muscimol on conditioned reflex eyeblinks (CR). All groups received injections prior to training on sessions 1–6, not on sessions 7–10, and all groups received muscimol on session 11 (data from Krupa et al., 1993).

two excitatory inputs, from the mossy fibers and the climbing fibers. The mossy fibers constitute the major afferent input. They originate from several brain stem nuclei that represent the spinocerebellar inputs, and they influence Purkinje cells indirectly through clusters of cerebellar granule cells that lie beneath. The granule cells originate the parallel fibers, the set of axons that run several millimeters along the long axis of the cerebellar folia. The parallel fibers make their excitatory connections onto the dendrites of a row of Purkinje cells, all oriented perpendicular to the parallel fibers.

There is considerable convergence of sensory inputs both at the level of the granule cells and onto Purkinkje cells. The other excitatory input, the climbing fibers, originates in the inferior olivary nucleus of the medulla. These axons rise within the cerebellar cortex and wrap around the Purkinje cell soma and dendrites, making numerous excitatory synaptic contacts. Each Purkinje cell receives input from only one climbing fiber, but these inputs have a powerful influence over the Purkinje cells, resulting in an all-or-none influence over the activity of Purkinje cells. Furthermore, coactivity of mossy and climbing fibers results in a long-term depression (LTD) of the mossy fiber synapse that is thought to play a central role in mediating the cerebellum contribution to motor learning. The cerebellum receives input from, and forms topographic representations of, the entire body surface. In addition, inputs from the vestibular, visual, and auditory areas are conveyed through other deep nuclei. The main outputs of the cerebellum to spinal motor mechanisms are through areas of the brain stem including the red nucleus and reticular formation, in addition to the upward going outputs to the premotor and motor cortex.

Eyeblink conditioning as an example of motor learning supported by the cerebellum

Considerable recent attention has focused on Pavlovian eyeblink conditioning as a model learning paradigm in which to study the role of the cerebellum. In this paradigm, rabbits are placed in restraining chambers where they can be presented with a well-controlled tone or light as the conditioning stimulus (CS), and a photoelectric device records eyeblinks. In classic *delay conditioning*, this stimulus lasts 250–1000 ms and coterminates with an airpuff or mild electrical shock to the eyelid (the unconditioned stimulus, or US) that produces the reflexive, unconditioned eyeblink (the UR). After several pairings of the CS and US, the rabbit begins to produce the eyeblink after onset of the CS and prior to presentation of the US. With more training, this conditioned response (CR) occurs somewhat earlier, and its timing becomes optimized so as to be maximal at the US onset, showing that not only is a CR acquired but also a timing of the CR is established.

Permanent lesions or reversible inactivation of one particular cerebellar nucleus, the interpositus nucleus, result in impairments in the acquisition and retention of classically conditioned eyeblink reflexes, without affecting reflexive eyeblinks (URs). Consistent with the role of gene expression and cellular changes that underlie learning (see Chapters 2 and 3), inhibition of protein synthesis in the interpositus nucleus prevents establishment of the conditioned reflex. The cerebellar cortex plays a more complicated role, revealed in disruption of the timing of conditioned eyeblink responses following cerebellar cortical lesions.

These and other observations have led Richard Thompson and his colleagues to propose a model of eyeblink conditioning that includes a central set of elements by which the CS input is sent via the brain stem pontine nuclei to the interpositus as well as to the cortex of the cerebellum (Fig. 10–6A). The US input is relayed by the trigeminal nucleus and inferior olive of the brain stem to the same cerebellar sites where the essential plasticity occurs. Outputs for the CR are then mediated by projections from the interpositus to the red nucleus, which projects to the accessory abducens motor nucleus, which also executes the UR via direct inputs from the trigeminal nucleus.

The evidence for involvement of these particular structures in different aspects of eyeblink conditioning is substantial. Studies by Joseph Steinmetz and colleagues using stimulation and recording techniques within the cerebellar circuit have shown that stimulation of the auditory pathway via the pontine nucleus can substitute for the tone CS in establishing the conditioned response. Similarly, the US pathway has been traced through the trigeminal nucleus to a circumscribed area in the dorsal accessory inferior olive, by showing that lesions of this area prevent the UR and stimulation of this area substitutes for the US.

Additional compelling data come from studies using reversible inactivations of particular areas during training. These studies showed that drug inactivation of the motor nuclei that are essential for production of the CR and UR prevented the elicitation of behavior during training. However, in trials immediately following removal of the inactivation, CRs appeared in full form, showing that the neural circuit that supports UR production is not critical for learning *per se*. A similar pattern of results was obtained with inactivation of the axons leaving the interpositus or their target in the red nucleus (Fig. 10–6B), showing that the final pathway for CR production is also not required to establish the memory trace.

By contrast, inactivation of the anterior interpositus nucleus and overlying cortex by drugs (muscimol, lidocaine) or temporary cooling did not affect reflexive blinking, yet resulted in failure of CR development during inactivation and the absence of savings in learning after removal of the inactivation (Fig. 10–6B). These results point to a small area of the anterior interpositus nucleus and overlying cerebellar cortex as the essential locus of plasticity. It is in this area, of course, where the interactions occur between the mossy and climbing fibers resulting in LTD, and the connections with the relevant outputs exist. Consistent with a view that this plasticity is essential, mice with gene knockouts resulting in deficient cerebellar LTD were impaired in eyeblink conditioning.

Recording studies have also been helpful, and are beginning to shed light on the nature of the neural coding in the cerebellar cortex and interpositus nucleus that mediates the conditioning. During the course of training, neurons in both areas developed increased firing to the CS. During subsequent extinction trials, during which the US was withheld while the CS was presented repeatedly, the CR gradually disappeared while interpositus cells ceased firing. By contrast the neural code remained in the activity of the cerebellar cortex long after extinction. These data support the view that the cortical and subcortical components of the cerebellum play somewhat different roles in maintaining and modulating this form of motor learning.

The hippocampus and eyeblink conditioning

An interesting contrast with the complex but circumscribed circuitry that supports standard eyeblink conditioning involves the larger set of brain structures that become involved with elaborations on this kind of motor learning. One particularly intriguing story involves the role of the hippocampus in an unusual kind of eyeblink conditioning called *trace conditioning*. Notably, the hippocampus is not required for the standard *delay conditioning* paradigm described so far. However, the hippocampus is required for the trace conditioning variant of the paradigm. In this version of the task, the conditioning stimulus (CS) involves a brief 100 ms tone followed by a silent 500 ms "trace" interval punctuated by the unconditioned stimulus (US). Rabbits develop conditioned responses (CRs) in this form of eyeblink conditioning, and hippocampal neurons also are active associated with the CS and US. This variant of eyeblink conditioning is sensitive to damage to the hippocampus. Thus, even though this form of learning does not fit the typical definitions of declarative or hippocampal-dependent memory, it is an example where the hippocampus is part of a larger circuit including the cerebellum in producing a form of reflex adaptation.

The extent of cerebellar involvement in procedural memory

Does the role of the cerebellum extend to other learning situations? The emerging evidence is that the cerebellum is involved in a broad scope of procedural learning. One of the most striking examples involves a demonstration of cerebellar plasticity in studies by William Greenough and his colleagues. In these studies rats were given "acrobatic" training by challenging them to acquire complex motor skills necessary to traverse a series of obstacles, involving moving over barriers and balancing on teeter-totters and tightropes. Rats with such training developed an increased volume of the parallel fiber layer in the cerebellar cortex, and increased number of synapses onto Purkinje cells without an increase in synaptic density. Control rats exercised in a running wheel without acrobatic training, having extensive motor activity without the requirement to acquire new motor skills. The cerebellum of these animals did not develop these characteristics of synaptogenesis. Instead, the cerebellum of control animals demonstrated increased blood vessel density associated with motor activity.

Evidence for the involvement of the cerebellum in procedural memory in humans

Studies on humans have shown that the scope of the cerebellum's role in habit or motor skill learning extends to classical conditioning in that species, and further to several other forms of motor adaptation. Patients with cerebellar damage are impaired in the acquisition of classically conditioned eyeblink responses and show other abnormalities of conditioned responses. In addition, patients with cerebellar damage are impaired in adaptation to lateral displacement of vision produced by prism glasses. When normal subjects first wear the prism glasses, their pointing to targets is typically off in a systematic way, but they gradually adapt and begin pointing correctly. When the glasses are subsequently removed, normal subjects' pointing is offset in the opposite direction and readapts to the normal matching. By contrast, patients with cerebellar damage show impaired adaptation. Patients with cerebellar damage are also impaired in skill learning tasks and in the serial reaction time test described earlier. Such patients have also been shown to be impaired at planning a sequence of actions in a problem-solving task. Functional imaging studies have documented decreases in cerebellar activation in association with learning of finger movement sequences, with learning in the sequential reaction time task, and with learning in drawing or tracking tasks.

By one view, virtually all skill learning tasks require motor adaptations, in which case the cerebellum may play its role in the execution of skill learning, that is, in the production of the learned responses, rather than the learning of movement sequences. Alternatively, the same results have been employed to suggest that the cerebellum plays a critical role in temporal sequencing itself. This conclusion follows from work with the serial reaction time task, in which cerebellar patients showed a sequence learning impairment not only in their reaction time performance but also in their explicit remembering of repeating sequences.

Other work on the cerebellum in humans has explored its possible role beyond the motor domain. Cerebellar activation was seen in the deep nuclei during sensory discrimination, and in the cortex during an attention demanding task without movement and during verb generation. In the verb generation task, subjects are presented with nouns (e.g., *ball*) and are to generate an appropriate verb (e.g., *throw*) for each one. Compared to a control condition in which subjects are just to repeat the nouns aloud, generating verbs to the same nouns resulted in activation of cerebellar cortex along with activation of dorsal frontal cortex. There are now a number of reports of cerebellar activation associated with frontal cortex activation in various tasks requiring search or selection among multiple response options or representations. This participation of cerebellum in nonmotor tasks, while initially surprising, is consistent with anatomical findings of cerebellar outputs to higher cortical areas. Moreover, the participation of such noncerebellar structures as the hippocampus, in humans as well as animals, in the trace variant of the cerebellum-dependent eyeblink conditioning task, further implicates the interaction of higher systems with essential cerebellar function.

The role of the motor cortex in procedural memory

The motor and premotor cortical areas mentioned at the outset of this chapter are involved in all the circuits for procedural learning, so it is likely that these areas participate in some important ways in virtually all types of adaptation and skill acquisition. This has been confirmed in various ways in studies of humans and of animals. Functional imaging studies have shown activation of the motor (and somatosensory) cortical areas during various examples of skill learning, such as learning a sequence of finger taps on a keyboard (see Chapter 4). Several studies in animals have reported evidence of expansion of the motor cortex representation associated with procedural learning. An increased number of synapses per neuron in motor cortex was found in rats who have learned complex motor skills in the "acrobat" task, and training-induced physiological changes in the cortical representation of reaching movements were found in the motor cortex of monkeys. Other studies in animals have shown other learning-dependent effects on the physiology of cells in the motor cortex. Pioneering studies by Charles Woody showed that cells in primary motor cortex demonstrated conditioning-dependent changes in activity and threshold in the eyeblink conditioning task. Considerable attention has focused on the development of long-term potentiation (LTP) and other cellular changes underlying alterations in excitability and in functional mappings of motor cortical cells as a function of learning (see Chapter 3).

Finally, the premotor areas may play a special role in conditional motor learning. This type of learning involves the acquisition of different motor responses to distinct stimulus conditions. Lesions of the premotor cortex in monkeys result in severe impairments in conditional motor learning tasks, but do not affect discrimination learning that involves only a single go/no-go response. Importantly, the other region especially important for conditional motor learning is the relay through the thalamus that brings striatal input to the frontal cortex. Parallel findings from neurophysiological studies confirm an important role for the premotor area in conditional motor learning. These studies involve recordings from single neurons in the premotor cortex of monkeys performing reaching or visual saccade tasks where distinct visual cues are associated with arbitrary arm or eye movement responses. The principal result of these studies is the appearance of visually evoked neural activity at the time when the correct conditional behavioral responses occur. These neurons did not respond to familiar and overlearned stimuli that signaled identical arm or eye movements. Many of these cells that developed responses during initial learning disappeared shortly after. These data suggest that the premotor cortex may be involved in the initial correct selection of responses associated with novel stimulus contingencies.

Summing up

The observations considered here indicate that procedural learning is mediated by a complex circuitry involving the motor cortical areas and two main subcortical loops, one through the striatum and another through the cerebellum. While we are still at a relatively early stage of understanding the brain circuits that support even the simpler forms of procedural learning, some distinctions are beginning to emerge. The motor cortex and surrounding premotor and somatosensory areas are involved in several forms of procedural learning. The striatum plays a critical role in habit learning, particularly in tasks involving the learning of specific responses or response sequences to specific stimuli. The critical circuitry includes cortical sensory input and direct motor outputs to mediate the association of stimuli with specific behavioral outputs. The role of the striatum is especially important in the acquisition of skills that require resolution of competition among multiple input or response options, particularly in tasks involving the learning of response sequences. This role becomes even more important in more "cognitive" tasks where temporal sequencing of information is involved. The cerebellum is critical to a variety of reflex adaptations that are played out in simple, direct form in conditioning situations, and may be fundamental parts of more complicated sequencing tasks. The critical anatomical components of this system involve brain stem sensory inputs and direct and indirect motor outputs, although connections with the cerebral cortex may be very important in the contribution of the cerebellum to higher aspects of learning. Timing is a critical aspect of the involvement of the cerebellum, and the fundamental contribution of the cerebellum may lie in its role in adjusting the timing of skeletal muscle movements in the course of adapting to new stimulus-response contingencies.

Whether the functional roles of the striatum and cerebellum in temporal sequencing are fundamentally the same, or are really quite different, is unclear. It is obvious that these areas have substantially different circuitries, and some studies have suggested dissociations in the functional roles of these systems. However, it is also clear that these structures, the motor cortex, and yet other structures not considered here, all modify their circuitries in the service of procedural memory. It is likely that the contributions of the two main subsystems, and other elements of motor systems in the brain, overlap in contributing to complex forms of procedural memory.

READINGS

Bloedel, J.R., Ebner, T.J., and Wise, S.P. (Eds.). *The Acquisition of Motor Behavior in Vertebrates*, Cambridge: MIT Press, pp. 289–302.

Cook, D., and Kesner, R.P. 1988. Caudate nucleus and memory for egocentric localization. *Behav. Neural Biol.* 49:332–343.

Graybiel, A.M. 1995. Building action repertoires: Memory and learning functions of the basal ganglia. *Curr. Opin. Neurobiol.* 5:733–741.

Houk, J.C., Davis, J.L., and Beiser, D.G. (Eds.). 1995. *Models of Information Processing in the Basal Ganglia.* Cambridge: MIT Press.

Byrne, J.H. 1997. The Cerebellum. Special Issues of *Learning and Memory* 3(6) & 3(7), Cold Spring Harbor Laboratory Press: Cold Spring Harbor, NY.

McDonald, R.J., and White, N.M. 1994. Parallel information processing in the water maze: Evidence for independent memory systems involving dorsal striatum and hippocampus. *Behav. Neural Biol.* 61:260–270.

Mink, J.W. 1996. The basal ganglia: Focused selection and inhibition of competing motor programs. *Prog. Neurobiol.* 50: 381–425.

Packard, M.G., and McGaugh, J.L. 1992. Double dissociation of fornix and caudate nucleus lesions on acquistion of two water maze tasks: Further evidence for multiple memory systems. *Behav. Neurosci.* 106:439–446.

Swanson, G. 1998. The Cerebellum—Development, Physiology and Plasticity. Special Issue of *Trends Cogn. Sci.* 2(9).

White, N.M. Mnemonic Functions of the Basal Ganglia.

Wise, S.P. 1996. The role of the basal ganglia in procedural memory. *The Neurosciences* 8:39–46.

Woodruf-pak, D.S. 1997. Classical conditioning. *Int. Rev. Neurobiol.* 41: 341–366.

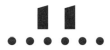

A Brain System for Emotional Memory

STUDY QUESTIONS

What is emotional memory?

What brain circuits mediate emotional expression and memory?

What circuitry in the amygdala makes it suited to play a central role in emotional perception, expression, and memory?

What is the range of emotional memories supported by this brain system?

One of my favorite memory experiences began when I entered an elevator in a busy downtown office building. I stepped in at the ground floor alone and pressed the button for the sixth floor where I had my upcoming appointment. At the second floor the elevator stopped for additional passengers. There were several, so I stepped to the back of the chamber to make room. The first passenger entering was a young woman who stopped just in front of me and turned around. I immediately noticed that she was wearing perfume, and it was a distantly familiar scent. As the next few seconds went by, I began to getting a great feeling of both familiarity and a sort of innocent sense of happiness. I found myself emotionally transported back to the "feeling" of high school. Within a few seconds, I began remembering girls I knew then, and then boys, too, classmates I hadn't thought of in many years. Finally, I fully recognized it—"Shalimar"—a perfume that was quite popular among teenagers in the early sixties. The latter specific recollections are run-of-the-mill declarative memories. But that initial "feeling of high school" was an example of emotional memory, an emotion evoked by a past association even before the conscious recollection of the experience that provoked it.

In this chapter our understanding of the brain pathways that mediate emotional experience and expression are reviewed. The early behavioral and anatomical studies identified specific brain areas, especially areas in the temporal lobe, that are involved in the appreciation of emotional cues and in the expression of emotional behaviors. Following this general review, I consider the current notion that some aspects of emotional memories involve a dedicated circuit of the brain that operates in parallel with other memory systems. In particular, it has been proposed that there is a specific memory system that mediates the learning and expression of emotional responses to stimuli of learned significance even in the absence of conscious memory for the events of the learning experience. Via this system, it is proposed, sometimes we can feel nervous or happy or scared at an image that evokes memory, even before, or independent of, our ability to declare the source of such feelings. This kind of learning is mediated by plasticity in components of the known pathways for emotional expression introduced earlier. Initially I consider the evidence for a specific system for the acquisition of learned fear, and then extend the review to consider whether the same brain system supports the acquisition and expression of a broad range of emotional associations.

The emergence of theories about brain pathways for emotional experience

The first theoretical proposal of a brain system for emotion was provided by James Papez in 1937. He postulated that sensory experiences took distinct pathways for "thought" and "feeling." The stream of thought, he proposed, involved channeling the sensory inputs from the thalamus to the wide expanse of the cerebral cortex on the lateral surface of the brain. The stream of feeling, he argued, followed a different path from the thalamus to the medial cortical areas known as the limbic lobe plus the neighboring hypothalamus. Based on gross anatomical evidence available at that time, Papez also speculated on the existence of a specific brain circuit for emotion (Fig. 11–1A). The system involves a *circular* sequence between several cortical and subcortical structures: The cingulate cortex, a major cortical division of the limbic lobe, connects to the hippocampal region. Then the hippocampus connects to an area of the hypothalamus called the mammilary bodies. Next the mammilary bodies connect to the anterior nuclei of the thalamus. These nuclei in turn project to the cingulate cortex, the beginning of the system, and so on around the circuit. Sensory in-

A. Papez circuit

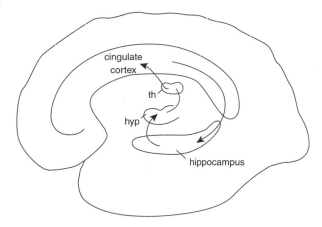

B. MacLean's limbic system

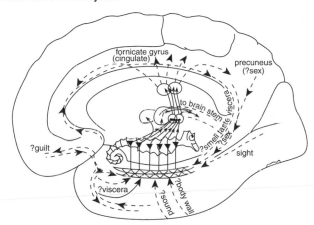

Figure 11–1. A: Pathway of the Papez circuit. *B:* Pathway of the limbic system as conceived by MacLean. In MacLean's illustration of the limbic system, the hippocampus is shown as a "seahorse" (hippocampus is Greek for seahorse). hyp = hypothalamus; th = thalamus.

puts from the posterior parts of the thalamus arrive into this circuit via either of two routes, either via inputs to the cingulate cortex from the lateral cortical areas that mediate the previously described "stream of thought" or from the posterior thalamus directly into the hypothalamus. Papez viewed the interactions between cortical and hypothalamic inputs as mediating the integration between cortical and subcortical processing of sensory inputs relevant to emotions. The outputs of this circuit course in two directions. One output is reflected by the cingulate cortex back to the stream of thought. The other output is via the hypothalamus to direct involuntary hormonal and autonomic nervous responses. The hormonal output route involves the release of stress hormones that activate the "fight or flight" response. The autonomic output route involves direct neural control over heart rate, blood pressure, and numerous other aspects of bodily regulation in the fight or flight response.

At around the same time, other evidence indicated a critical role for additional temporal lobe areas in emotion. In 1939 Kluver and Bucy described a syndrome of affective disorder following removal of the temporal lobe in monkeys. This disorder was characterized by "psychic blindness," which was observed mainly as a blunting of emotional reactions usually associated with fear of novel objects. Part of this disorder involved an impairment in object recognition known as agnosia. This part of the disorder is now associated with damage to the temporal cortex (see Chapter 7). Another part of the disorder, and the focus of this chapter, was the "taming" of these normally aggressive animals, as well as other abnormalities of social behavior. This part of the disorder has been attributed to the amygdala.

These distinct components of an emotional system in the brain were integrated into a more elaborate theoretical structure by Paul MacLean in 1949 (Fig. 11–1B). He combined the observations of Papez and Kluver and Bucy together with clinical observations on emotional disorders and electrophysiological evidence of internal organ sensory inputs to the hippocampus and other parts of the Papez circuit, arguing for the existence of a distinct "visceral brain," a system for regulation of internal organs. Using the full breadth of evidence from these various sources, MacLean expanded further on Papez's notion of distinct informational processing streams and on the anatomical components of the emotional system. He introduced the term "limbic system" as the anatomical designation of the emotional circuit and included within it Papez's circuit plus the amygdala, septum, and prefrontal cortex. MacLean proposed that the functional domain of this system encompassed all of emotional experience, from the role of lower brain stem structures in mediating instinctive and stereotyped behaviors, to that of the higher cortical areas in mediating real feelings.

Since then there have been numerous elaborations and modifications to the notion of the limbic system, and the boundaries of this system have become unclear. New anatomical evidence expanded the connections of the limbic system forward toward the frontal lobe and backward toward the midbrain. These interconnections are so strong that the anatomist

Walle Nauta proposed that we view this system as a continuum of structures throughout the entire brain. Interpretations about connections of the classic limbic structures has today become so intertwined with those of other brain systems such that today the term "limbic system" is somewhat outmoded. This and other evidence brought into question whether the specific components of the limbic system were correctly identified, and indeed whether one can circumscribe a complete and separate system for emotion. Nevertheless, more recent research has identified specific pathways within the classic limbic system as critical elements in emotional output. These are considered at some length next.

Pathways for emotional expression

Recent research has brought the focus on emotional memory specifically to pathways through the amygdala. This is justly deserved because the amygdala lies in a central position between cortical information processing, limbic circuitry, and hypothalamic outputs to the brain stem that mediate emotional responses. Thus, a brief summary of the organization of the amygdala, including its main inputs, intrinsic connections, and outputs is provided here (Fig. 11–2). The amygdala lies in the medial temporal

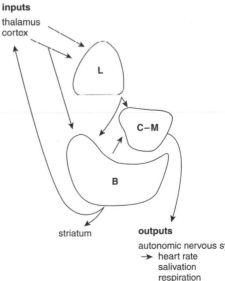

Figure 11–2. Schematic diagram of some major inputs, outputs, and intrinsic circuitry of the amygdala. L = lateral nucleus; C-M = centromedial nucleus; B = basal (or basolateral) nucleus.

lobe, just anterior to the hippocampus and surrounded by the parahippocampal cortical region. The amygdala involves a complex of many highly interconnected nuclei. The two most prominent major compartments are the group of nuclei that include the lateral nucleus and the basolateral complex, and the group of central and medial nuclei and their extensions. As it turns out, this division roughly corresponds to the major input and output sides of pathways of the amygdala. Thus, sensory inputs from the thalamus and cortex project mainly to the lateral and basolateral nuclei, whereas outputs of the amygdala to the cortex and subcortical areas originate mainly in the central and medial nuclei.

Several studies have shown that the amygdala receives widespread sensory inputs from the thalamus and cerebral cortex. These are derived largely from gustatory, thoracic–abdominal (vagus nerve inputs), and auditory thalamic nuclei, but not the main somatosensory, or visual thalamic nuclei. Cortical inputs are derived through the olfactory bulb and piriform (olfactory) cortex, plus higher-order sensory inputs from all sensory modalities via the entire cortex surrounding the rhinal sulcus (insular and perirhinal cortex). Joseph LeDoux and his colleagues have intensively studied auditory inputs, and have shown that the main locus of input involves a convergence of thalamic and cortical projections to the lateral nucleus. In addition, the medial prefrontal cortex and hippocampal regions, specifically the subiculum and entorhinal cortex, send substantial inputs to the lateral nucleus. Some inputs, however, arrive in other amygdala nuclei. In particular, some of the olfactory inputs arrive mainly in the cortical nuclei and the internal organ inputs arrive mainly in the central nuclei.

The intrinsic connectivity of amygdaloid nuclei is complex, and is characterized mainly by a distribution of connections from the lateral nucleus to the basal nuclear complex and central nucleus, which are also interconnected. Thus, whatever segregation of inputs may have been preserved at the input stage is likely lost within the amygdala where all the inputs are mixed.

The amygdala has several output pathways that direct a widespread influence of emotional expression. Amygdala outputs to the cortex are largely derived indirectly from several nuclei to components of the thalamus, in particular the mediodorsal nucleus. The basal nuclear complex sends direct outputs to several cortical areas, including the perirhinal, entorhinal, and prefrontal areas. In addition, the amygdala projects heavily to multiple basal forebrain areas that secondarily influence widespread cortical areas. Also, the basal amygdaloid nuclei project to components of the substantia nigra and striatum, and to the subiculum (a part of the hippocampus). Other subcortical targets of amygdala output are directed mainly from the central and medial nuclei to the substantia nigra, lateral hypothalamus, and to several brain stem motor, autonomic (vagus nerve), and endocrine effector areas. This complicated scheme of outputs supports a correspondingly broad range of emotional responses that are generated by direct electrical stimulation of amygdala and are observed in the syndrome of behaviors associated with emotional experience. High emotional states induce increases in heart rate and respiration, decreased salivation, urination and defecation, and increased vigilance and freezing.

These pathways are complicated, but the bottom line is that these anatomical facts tell us the amygdala is the recipient of multimodal information about both lower-order visceral structures of the body as well as the crude sensory inputs from thalamus and higher-order sensory information originating in the cortex. The internal connectivity within the amygdala combines these inputs. This conclusion about the inputs and synthesis of sensory information is supported by physiological studies showing that single neurons in the amygdala respond to complex multimodal, affectively significant stimuli. On the output side, the amygdala orchestrates an enormous range of influences on behavior. These include influences back to the thalamic and cortical areas that provided sensory input, plus direct influences onto other systems important for different forms of memory, specifically the striatum and hippocampal regions. In addition, there are direct outputs from the amygdala to the autonomic, endocrine, and motor systems that generate diverse aspects of emotional expression.

The amygdala and emotional expression

Following Kluver and Bucy's initial reports of the "blunting" of affect in monkeys with temporal lobe damage including the amygdala, several studies have shown that selective amygdala damage results in a syndrome characterized by decreases in responsivity to affective stimuli. After amygdalotomy, monkeys fail to respond differentially to a wide range of painful shock intensities, and are poor at temperature discrimination. These animals also fail to show classic "orienting responses" to unexpected salient noises or visual stimuli, which normally include changes in heart rate and respiration. These animals also have a diminished galvanic skin response, the change in skin resistance associated with sweating. Monkeys with amygdala damage also demonstrate diminished selectivity in feeding, diminished sensitivity to food deprivation, and depressed shifts in behavioral performance normally associated with changes to food reward magnitude or type of food reward. Parallel impairments in responsiveness to food reward alterations have been observed in rats with amygdala damage.

A study on the amnesic patient H.M., whose surgical damage to the medial temporal lobe included removal of the amygdala bilaterally, provides confirmation of the blunting of affective responsiveness in humans with amygdala damage, and offers some further insights into the nature of this disorder. In the clinical setting, H.M. was known not to complain about normally painful conditions including hemorrhoids, and did not produce a normal skin-resistance change to electrical stimulation. He also was noted to rarely mention being hungry even when his meals were delayed, but he otherwise ate in a normal manner when given a meal. These observations were followed up in a systematic study of H.M.'s responsiveness to pain and hunger. In this study H.M's responses to thermal stimulation were compared to those of control subjects and amnesic patients without amygdala damage. H.M. showed a diminished ability to discriminate painful stimulation. Most prominent was his failure to identify any of the thermal stimuli as "painful" no matter how intense they were. By comparison, other amnesic patients without amygdala damage did not show loss of pain discrimination and were as likely as normal subjects to label the stimuli as painful. So, it does not appear that H.M.'s impairment in pain perception was secondary to his memory deficit.

A further experiment to characterize H.M.'s appreciation of hunger involved an assessment of his reaction to eating multiple dinners. Initially H.M. was asked to rate his hunger on a scale of 0 to 100, with 0 identified as "famished" and 100 identified as "too full to eat another bite." Just before dinner, H.M. rated his hunger level as 50. He was served a full meal and again rated his hunger level as 50. After a short rest period filled with conversation, by prearrangement with a dietician, he was served another full dinner as if the first had not occurred. As expected, H.M. had forgotten eating dinner and began eating the second meal at his usual slow, steady pace. However, he stopped before completing the meal, leaving his salad and cake. When asked about his break, H.M. remarked that he couldn't decide which to eat, and upon prompting why, simply decided to eat the cake. Following this he also rated his hunger level at 50. When probed further why he had not fully completed the second meal, H.M. would only say he was "finished," but would not characterize himself as "full" or "stuffed." In a separate set of ratings taken before and after regular meals, both amnesic patients and normal controls consistently rated themselves as less hungry and thirsty after meals, but H.M. showed small and inconsistent changes in his hunger rating. These findings were interpreted as demonstrating that, while there is evidence of modest decrease in sensitivity, the major effect of his surgery was diminished ability to access information about his internal states. Because this impairment was not observed in other amnesic patients without involvement of the amygdala, H.M.'s deficit was attributed to amygdala damage per se.

More recent studies on the role of the human amygdala in the perception of affective stimuli have focused on responses to faces. Several studies have now shown that bilateral damage to the amygdala results in impaired recognition of emotional expressions in pictures of human faces. These studies assessed the recognition of various facial expressions by human subjects with unilateral or bilateral removal of the amygdala and by one subject (S.M.) with a rare disorder known as Urbach-Wiethe disease, which is associated with calcification of the amygdala sparing the neighboring cortex and hippocampus (this disorder is introduced in Chapter 8). S.M. showed a selective impairment in recognizing facial expressions of fear, surprise, and anger. Also, S.M. showed a deficit in the normal capacity for recognizing similarities among different emotions expressed by others. In contrast, S.M. showed no general deficits in language, memory, or perception. She was able to recognize familiar faces, even ones not seen in considerable time. Furthermore, S.M. did perceive fearful faces as expressing emotion, but refused to characterize the expression as fearful, leading the investigators to conclude she could perceive the facial expression but that it did not activate responses associated with fear. The observation of inability to appreciate emotional expression is remarkably similar to H.M.'s emotional perception deficit, but without the accompanying memory impairment.

These findings are consistent with electrophysiological data showing that neurons in the amygdala respond to faces in both monkeys and humans. In addition, a recent brain imaging study using fMRI showed that the amygdala is preferentially active in response to viewing fearful versus neutral faces, although some response to other facial expressions over that of neutral expressions was also observed. These data bring into focus the importance of the amygdala as a critical part of a specialized system for the analysis of affective information and for the expression of emotional output.

Evidence for a dedicated emotional memory system

How is memory for emotions different from declarative memory? Certainly we do consciously recall emotional experiences, so these clearly can be a part of our declarative memories. However, there is also substantial emerging evidence that some aspects or types of emotional memory are accomplished by a distinct brain system, parallel to the system for declarative memory—this is the subject of the remainder of this chapter.

In a classic case study of amnesia performed in 1911, a neurologist named Cleparede pricked the hand of an unsuspecting patient with

Korsakoff disease. Subsequently, she refused to shake Cleparede's hand, although she could not recall the painful incident. Later, Antonio Damasio and colleagues described intact affective learning in their amnesic patient Boswell. Even though he could not learn to recognize the hospital staff, he consistently claimed he liked those with whom he had repeated positive encounters over those with whom he had negative encounters. In another study, amnesic patients were presented with pictures and biographical descriptions of two individuals, one characterized positively and the other negatively. Normal subjects preferred the positively described individual, and based this on their recall of the biographical information. Amnesic patients could not recall the individual or descriptions, but showed a strong preference for the "good guy." These and other case studies show that memory for emotional aspects of experiences can indeed be dissociated from declarative memory for the same experiences in amnesic patients.

Other findings from studies on normal human subjects provide an additional line of evidence that affective memory can occur independently of declarative memory. Perhaps most prominent among examples of unconscious affective memory is the "mere exposure" effect described by Robert Zajonc and his colleagues. They found that exposure to words, faces, and other stimuli produced a preference for the familiar items, even if the stimuli were not explicitly remembered. In some of these studies, the stimuli were even presented subliminally, so that their presentation did not reach consciousness. Nevertheless, subjects subsequently showed a preference for the stimuli that they had briefly experienced. These findings reflect the operation of an emotional system in the brain that can perceive and store information that is not adequately salient to reach attention and engage the declarative memory system. Furthermore, the mere exposure effect may reflect the operation of the emotional memory system in normal subjects in the same way it does in amnesic subjects who have a compromised declarative memory system. The identification and analysis of the critical elements of the emotional memory system have now proceeded to an extent that a preliminary understanding of its operation is available.

A brain system for emotional memory

Many laboratories have studied a variety of forms of emotional memory, and have focused on somewhat different brain areas and circuits, as well as different aspects of motivation and emotion that affect learning mechanisms. This section reviews a few prominent examples of circuit analyses of the brain system for emotional expression.

Perhaps the best studied example of emotional memory involves the brain system that mediates Pavlovian fear conditioning as studied by Joseph

LeDoux and by Michael Davis and their colleagues. This research has focused on the specific elements of the pathways through the amygdala that support the learning of fearful responses to a simple auditory stimulus. The critical elements of the relevant amygdala pathways include auditory sensory inputs via the brain stem to circuits through the thalamus (Fig. 11–3A). Some of these auditory thalamic areas then project directly to the

A. pathway for fear conditioning

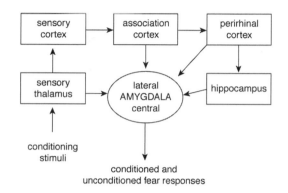

B. protocol

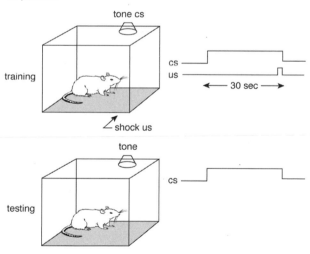

Figure 11–3. A: LeDoux's schematic diagram of a brain system for fear conditioning. Signals from the conditioned stimulus can reach the lateral amygdala at several stages of information processing. They converge in the lateral amygdala, which controls the output of conditioned responses. *B:* The procedure for fear conditioning. During training, rats are placed in a chamber where a tone is presented for several seconds punctuated by a brief foot shock. During testing the tone is presented again, and the amount of freezing, or other aspects of fear, are measured.

lateral amygdaloid nucleus. The other circuit involves auditory inputs to another part of the thalamus which projects to the primary auditory area of temporal cortex. This cortical area in turn projects to secondary temporal areas and the perirhinal cortex. These secondary auditory cortical areas are the source of cortical inputs to the amygdala, particularly the lateral and basolateral nuclei of this structure. Those areas of the amygdala project into the central nucleus, which is the source of outputs to subcortical areas controlling a broad range of fear-related behaviors, including autonomic and motor responses.

Learning to fear

LeDoux and colleagues have focused on the input side of these circuits. Their studies have examined the neuropsychology and neurophysiology of these structures in animals during the course of a simple tone-cued fear conditioning task (Fig. 11–3B). Rats are initially habituated to an operant chamber, then presented with multiple pairings of a prolonged pure tone terminating with a brief electric shock delivered through the floor of the cage. Subsequently, conditioned fear was assessed by measuring responses to the tone, including autonomic responses, such as changes in arterial pressure, and stereotypic behaviors, such as crouching or freezing. Unconditioned responses to the tone were evaluated by presenting other animals with unpaired tones and shocks. Under these conditions, the shocks produce the same set of autonomic and behavioral responses, but the tones do not acquire the capacity to evoke the responses.

Their initial experiments were aimed at identifying the critical input pathway to the amygdala. Animals with selective lesions in the lateral amygdala show dramatically reduced conditioned responses to the tone, both in the measures of autonomic and motor responses. Unconditioned responses consequent to unpaired presentations were not affected by this damage. Also, animals with damage to the adjacent striatum performed normally, showing anatomical specificity and confirming that the striatal system is not involved in emotional learning.

Subsequent efforts focused on identifying which of the two prominent auditory input pathways to the lateral amygdala was critical. Broad destruction of all auditory areas of the thalamus eliminated conditioned responses. However, selective ablation of either of the two prominent direct inputs to the lateral amygdala were individually ineffective. Lesions of the medial division of the medial geniculate, including all three nuclei that project directly to the lateral amygdala, *or* of the entire auditory cortex that projects to the amygdala did not reduce either the autonomic or freezing response. However, elimination of *both* of these inputs produced the full effect seen after lateral amygdala lesions. Thus, for this simple type of conditioning, either the direct thalamic input, which offers a crude identification of a sound, or the thalamocortical input pathway, which provides a sophisticated identification of auditory signal, is sufficient to mediate conditioning.

Additional experiments were aimed at another component of fear conditioning observed in these studies. After conditioning, when rats are replaced in the conditioning chamber, they begin to freeze even before the tone is presented. Thus, rats appear to condition both to the tone and to the environmental context in which tones and shock have previously been paired. This "contextual" fear conditioning is selective to the environment in which conditioning occurs. Furthermore, contextual fear conditioning can be dissociated from conditioning to the tone by presenting the conditioned tones in a different environment. Trained animals do not freeze prior to tone presentation in the unfamiliar environment, but do freeze when the tone is presented.

Moreover, contextual fear conditioning is mediated by a different pathway than tone-cued fear conditioning. To demonstrate this, the animals were trained on the standard version of the task, then their expression of memory was assessed both immediately after the rats were placed in the conditioning chamber and then subsequently in response to the tone. Amygdala lesions blocked conditioned freezing to both the context and the tone. By contrast, damage to the hippocampus selectively blocked contextual fear conditioning, sparing the conditioned response to the tone.

These data combined with the known anatomy of these brain structures demonstrate that the full set of circuits mediating fear conditioning in this task involves a set of parallel and serial pathways to the amygdala (see Fig. 11–3A). The most direct pathway is from areas within the auditory thalamus. A secondary path through the auditory thalamocortical circuit can also mediate tone-cued conditioning. Contextual fear conditioning involves a yet more indirect pathway by which multimodal information arrives in the hippocampus and is sent to the amygdala via the subiculum.

Additional studies by LeDoux and colleagues have elucidated the physiology of the neurons in the direct thalamic and thalamocortical auditory pathways to the amygdala. Cells in both the medial geniculate nuclei that project directly to the amygdala and in the thalamic nucleus that projects to the cortex demonstrate a variety of auditory responses. Finer auditory tuning was observed in the ventral medial geniculate than in areas that project directly to the amygdala. However, cells in the ventral nucleus responded only to auditory stimuli, whereas neurons in the medial geniculate nuclei that project to the amygdala also responded to foot shock stimulation. Furthermore, some amygdala-projecting cells that responded to somatosensory stimulation but not auditory stimulation showed potentiated responses to simultaneous presentation of both stimuli.

In the amygdala, cells in the lateral nucleus that receives thalamic input were responsive to auditory stimuli at both short (12–25 msec) and long (60–150 msec) latencies. Some cells had clear tuning curves, whereas others responded to a broad spectrum of sounds. Cells in the lateral amygdala could also be driven by electrical stimulation of the medial geniculate, and their responses were typically shorter than those in the basolateral amygdala. In addition, LeDoux and colleagues have provided several lines of evidence suggesting that direct medial geniculate–lateral amygdala inputs exhibit learning related plasticity, including evidence for alterations in synaptic efficacy (see Chapter 3). At the level of neuronal firing patterns, fear conditioning selectively enhances the short latency auditory responses of lateral amygdala neurons. Furthermore, some cells that were not responsive to tones prior to training showed postconditioning short latency responses.

The potentiation of startle by learned fear

Michael Davis and his colleagues have investigated a different form of fear conditioning, and have provided an extensive line of evidence that runs in parallel with LeDoux and colleagues' findings, and involves much of the same brain circuit (Fig. 11–4A). Davis's research focuses on a simple behavioral response known as startle, the jump or other sudden movement performed by animals and people in response to an unexpected salient stimulus such as a loud sound. Their examination of fear learning in this situation is derived from the observation that when animals or people are in a fearful state, the startle response is magnified, and so their fear conditioning paradigm is known as *fear-potentiated startle*. All of us have experienced this phenomenon, for example, when we jump at a sudden noise that occurs while listening to a scary story.

In the formal laboratory version of this task, animals are initially exposed to pairings of a light or a tone with foot shock. Subsequently, their startle reflex to a loud noise is evaluated in the presence or absence of the conditioned stimulus. When the conditioned light or tone is present, the startle reflex is considerably augmented (Fig. 11–4B). Potentiated acoustic startle does not occur if the animal is pre-exposed to *un*paired presentations of the light or tone and shock, and is thus as valid a measure of fear conditioned to the tone or light. The brain pathway for fear-potentiated startle contains many of the same elements of the amygdala circuit studied by LeDoux and colleagues (Fig. 11–4A). An important advantage of

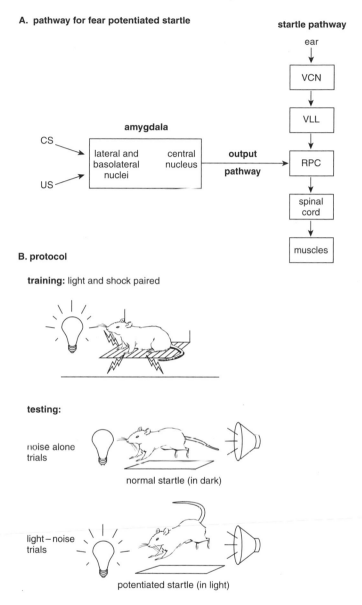

Figure 11–4. A: Davis's schematic diagram of a brain pathway that mediates the potentiation of the acoustic startle response. CS = conditioned stimulus; RPC = caudal nucleus of the pontine reticular area; VCN = ventral cochlear nucleus; VLL = ventral nucleus of the lateral leminiscus; US = unconditioned stimulus. *B:* The protocol for training and testing in fear potentiation of startle.

the fear-potentiated startle paradigm is that the startle response can be measured independently of the influence of conditioned fear, allowing a rigorous analysis of the effects of manipulations on the fear component of the task as distinct from the behavioral response (startle) per se.

Davis and colleagues have independently demonstrated the importance of the amygdala in fear conditioning, showing that lesions of the lateral or basal amygdala or the central amygdala nucleus prevent conditioning and abolish expression of previously learned acoustic startle responses. Correspondingly, they found that electrical stimulation of the amygdala enhances acoustic startle.

Furthermore, Davis and his colleagues have shown that N-methyl-D-aspartate (NMDA)-dependent plasticity (see Chapter 3) in the amygdala is critical for the development of fear conditioning, but not for the expression of already learned fear responses. Thus, application of the NMDA receptor blocker AP5 prior to training prevents conditioning, but similar treatment after conditioning or prior to testing has no effect on later expression of potentiated acoustic startle. To further address the possibility that NMDA receptors are directly involved in the expression of conditioned fear, rats were initially conditioned to fear a "primary" conditioned stimulus (CS) and then subsequently trained to fear a second stimulus paired with the primary CS. AP5 infused into the amygdala during the final "second-order" conditioning stage actually enhanced the fear expression to the previously conditioned primary CS while at the same time preventing the second-order conditioning. This finding strongly supports the conclusion that NMDA receptors are differentially involved in plasticity of startle but not in the performance of potentiated startle.

Davis and colleagues have also extended our understanding of the specific input and output pathways of fear conditioning. They found that ablation of the auditory thalamus blocks tone-cued fear-potentiated startle, sparing visually cued potentiated startle. However, ablation of the perirhinal cortex eliminates previous conditioning in either modality, suggesting that the cortical pathway through this area is normally predominant. Like LeDoux and colleagues, Davis has shown that tone-cued conditioning can be supported by the direct thalamic pathway as well.

Other studies of Davis and colleagues have focused on identifying the critical output circuitry for fear-potentiated startle. These studies have shown that interruption of the pathway from the amygdala via the ventral output pathway to caudal brain stem regions to the nucleus reticularis pontis oralis constitutes the critical circuit for expression of potentiated startle.

Is the amygdala part of a general system for emotional memory?

The notion that the amygdala is central to associating rewards, as well as fear, with stimuli has been traced to Lawrence Weiskrantz's observations in the 1950s on monkeys with amygdala lesions: ". . . the effect of amyg-dalectomy, it is suggested, is to make it difficult for reinforcing stimuli, whether positive or negative, to become established and recognized as such" (p. 390). Many amygdala neurons respond differentially to rewarded stimuli. Neurophysiological data showing strongly held reward-related responses, and their relation to unlearned reinforcing stimuli, have supported the view that the amygdala maintains neural representations of stimulus–reward associations. Thus, the notion that the amygdala plays a critical role in mediating stimulus–reward associations is widely held.

Yet, in studies on learning after damage to the amygdala, this notion has proven difficult to establish unambiguously in experimental analyses. Thus, the findings across a broad variety of learning tasks have indicated that amygdala lesions sometimes result in impairments in simple stimulus–reward learning tasks and sometimes do not. In addition, some studies have specifically contrasted the importance of the amygdala in appetitive and aversive learning. However, based on their experiment described in Chapter 9, McDonald and White suggested that the mixture of results may be explained by distinguishing cases where learning can be mediated by the establishment of stimulus–response associations even in the absence of normal stimulus–reward associations. Thus, in most simple conditioning and discrimination tasks, animals are rewarded for producing a specific behavior, for example, a choice and approach toward a particular stimulus. In such cases, they argue, two kinds of learning occur in parallel. In one type of learning, the positive reinforcer increases the likelihood of the behavioral response that preceded it—this is accomplished by brain systems that do not involve the amygdala. In particular, in McDonald and White's study of different forms of radial maze learning, animals with amygdala lesions normally acquired consistent approach responses to illuminated maze arms when specifically rewarded for such approach behaviors. In the other type of learning, the positive reinforcer enhances the attractive value of stimuli with which it is associated. In their study McDonald and White avoided the conditioning of habitual response by using a different training protocol (conditioned place preference) that involved simply feeding animals in an illuminated maze arm, with no requirement for an approach behavior. In this situation, amygdala lesions blocked the subsequent conditioned place preference. The distinction between stimulus–response and stimulus–reinforcer associations was made particularly compelling by the demonstration that striatal lesions had the opposite pattern of effects, blocking the learning of approach responses but not affecting the conditioned place preference.

Another behavioral paradigm that distinguished stimulus–reward from stimulus–response associations is "second-order conditioning," a procedure in which animals are first trained to associate a stimulus with reward, and then that stimulus is used as a reinforcer for subsequent conditioning. In an experiment by Barry Everitt and Trevor Robbins, thirsty rats were trained to associate a visual stimulus with their approach to a dispenser where they received water. Subsequently, they were trained to discriminate between two levers, one followed by the visual stimulus and an empty water dispenser, as a second-order reinforcer, and the other lever inactive. Normal animals pressed both levers somewhat, and much more on the lever associated with the second-order reinforcer. Amygdala lesions reduced responding on the lever associated with the second-order reinforcer to the same low level as that associated with the alternate lever. These findings are consistent with McDonald and White's proposal that simple stimulus–response learning is intact in animals with amygdala lesions, but they cannot differentially associate a specific lever with its acquired reinforcing properties. Similar results were obtained using second-order conditioning to a sexual reinforcer. Initially, male rats were allowed to interact sexually with a female in the presence of a visual stimulus (a light). Subsequently, the male rats were trained to bar press in the presence of the light. Normal animals bar press at high rates for this second-order reinforcer, and amygdala lesions reduced responding in that situation.

The same pattern of results has been obtained in experiments on monkeys. Amygdala lesions have no effect on traditional forms of simple discrimination learning. However, impairments have been observed in the acquisition of preferences to novel foods and when the animals must change responses to shifting reward contingencies. In addition, amygdala lesions interfere with the acquisition of a visual discrimination associated with a secondary auditory reinforcer. In an experiment performed by David Gaffan and his colleagues, intact monkeys were initially trained on visual discriminations in which the food reward was given along with an auditory stimulus. Following damage to the amygdala they were trained on new discrimination problems in which responses to one stimulus were followed by the second-order auditory reinforcer, and food reward was given only upon completion of the task. Amygdala damage severely retarded learning. In addition, disconnection of the amygdala from auditory input had the same effect, but disconnection of the amygdala from visual association cortex had no effect on this type of learning. These results confirm the findings on second-order conditioning in rats, and support the view that the effect of amygdala damage is to block the association between the primary reinforcer (food) and secondary reinforcer (auditory cue), but not the associations between the visual stimuli and the secondary reinforcer.

Additional evidence of the notion that the amygdala mediates stimulus–reward associations comes from an experiment performed by Raymond Kesner in which rats were presented with either one or seven pieces of food on different arms of a radial maze. After a delay period they could obtain an additional reward by choosing the arm with the larger reward. In this task, lesions of the basolateral nucleus had no effect, but lesions of the central nucleus produced a severe, delay-dependent deficit in memory for reward magnitude. This result confirms the role of the amygdala in affective discrimination and suggests a specific role for the central nucleus in this aspect of emotional learning.

Other experiments have also explored whether there are distinct pathways within or through the amygdala that support different types of stimulus-reinforcer learning. On the one hand, anatomical evidence indicates that the main sensory inputs to the amygdala arrive via the lateral, and to some extent the basolateral, nuclei, and that the main outputs are from the central nucleus. This suggests that damage to either set of nuclei would necessarily have similar effects on learning. However, there have been several reports that lesions within these amygdala nuclei have dissociable effects on performance in different tasks, making it tempting to speculate on the possibility that the minor inputs to all the amygdala nuclei, combined with the divergent output pathways, might support different forms of affective learning and memory.

The learning versus performance distinction

One final issue of importance to the analysis of the emotional memory system (as well as to the procedural memory system) is the extent to which one can distinguish the role of the amygdala and other structures in memory per se, as opposed to its role in emotional expression. This issue has most recently been brought to the forefront in comments by Larry Cahill and colleagues (1999), who have questioned the findings on the emotional memory system. In particular, they challenged the conclusion that lesions of the amygdala block conditioned fear responses, citing considerable evidence that indicates that amygdala lesions interfere with the expression of unconditioned as well as conditioned fear responses (see section on The amygdala and emotional expression). This suggests that the lesions affect performance functions of the amygdala but have no special role in blocking emotional memory. This alternative interpretation highlights the difficulty of identifying critical plasticity mechanisms within brain structures that are essential to performance functions involved in memory expression. However, two studies have addressed this criticism, with compelling results. One study, introduced previously, used the second-order conditioning test to show a sparing of a simple conditioned emotional response (fear-potentiated startle), in contrast to a total blocking of a second-order conditioned response. In a more recent study, Wallace and Rosen assessed freezing behavior of rats in contextual fear conditioning as well as unconditioned fear responses to a predator odor. Damage to the lateral amygdala using a toxin that selectively destroys cells in that region did not affect unconditioned freezing to the foot shocks, nor did this type of selective damage diminish unconditioned freezing to the predator odor. However, these lesions did produce an impairment in conditioned freezing. The combination of these studies, each involving the application of sophisticated behavioral and anatomical techniques, provides strong evidence favoring the view that a critical component of the emotional memory trace is formed in the amygdala.

Summing up

There is a distinct brain system that mediates the perception and appreciation of emotional stimuli as well as emotional expression. The system involves a complex set of cortical and subcortical areas in widespread areas of the brain. Recently, several studies have focused on the amygdala as a critical element of emotional perception and expression. The lateral and basolateral components of the amygdala receive both subcortical and cortical sensory inputs from both visceral and external stimuli. The central and basal nuclei send a broad range of outputs back to cortical areas, to subcortical areas involved in other memory systems and behavior, and to autonomic system and brain stem outputs for the expression of emotion through a variety of systems. Damage to the amygdala results in selective impairments in emotional perception and appreciation, as well as emotional expression in humans and animals.

There is substantial evidence that plasticity within this same brain system supports emotional memory in the absence of conscious recollection. The critical brain system involves pathways through the amygdala that are enhanced during emotional learning, leading to the appearance of emotional expression to previously neutral stimuli. This system mediates fear conditioning and the modulation of other behaviors by conditioned fear (e.g., fear-potentiated startle). The same system supports learned attractions, and there may be multiple distinct pathways through the system that support different aspects of learned emotional expression.

READINGS

Adolphs, R., Tranel, D., Damasio, H., and Damasio, A. 1994. Impaired recognition of emotion in facial expressions following bilateral damage to the human amygdala. *Nature*. 372:669–672.

Aggleton, J.P. (Ed.). 1992. *The Amygdala: Neurobiological Aspects of Emotion, Memory and Mental Dysfunction*. New York: Wiley-Liss.

Cahill, L., Weinberger, N., Roozendaal, B., and McGaugh, J.L. 1999. Is the amygdala a locus of conditioned fear? Some questions and caveats. *Neuron* 23: 227–228.

Damasio, A.R., Tranel, D., and Damasio, H. 1989. Amnesia caused by herpes simplex encephalitis, infarctions in basal forebrain, Alzheimer's disease and anoxia/ischemia. In *Handbook of Neuropsychology*, Vol. 3. F. Boller, and J. Grafman, (Eds.). Amsterdam: Elsevier.

Davis, M., Walker, D.L., and Lee Y. 1999. Neurophysiology and neuropharmacology of startle and its affective modulation. In *Startle Modification: Implications for Neuroscience, Cognitive Science, and Clinical Science*. M.E. Dawson, A.M. Schell, and A.H. Bohmelt, (Eds.). Cambridge University Press, pp. 95–113.

Gerwitz, J.C., and Davis, M. 1997. Second-order fear conditioning prevented by blocking NMDA receptors in the amygdala. *Nature* 388: 471–474.

Hebben, N., Corkin, S., Eichenbaum, H., and Shedlack, K. 1985. Diminished ability to interpret and report internal states after bilateral medial temporal resection: Case H.M. *Behav. Neurosci.* 99:1031–1039.

Kesner, R.P. 1992. Learning and memory in rats with an emphasis on the role of the amygdala. In *The Amygdala: Neurobiological Aspects of Emotion, Memory, and Mental Dysfunction*. J.P. Aggleton, (Ed.). New York: Wiley-Liss, pp. 379–399.

LeDoux, J. 1996. *The Emotional Brain*. New York: Simon & Schuster.

Wallace, K.J., and Rosen, J.B. 2001. Neurotoxic lesions of the lateral nucleus of the amygdala decrease conditioned fear but not unconditioned fear of a predator odor: Comparison with electrolytic lesions. *J. Neurosci.* 21:3619–3627.

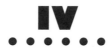

CONSOLIDATION:
THE FIXATION AND
REORGANIZATION OF MEMORIES

Memory consolidation is the name given to the hypothetical process or set of processes by which new memories make a transition from an initially labile state to become permanently fixed for the long term. As introduced in Chapter 1, the notion of consolidation was first proposed formally in 1900 by Muller and Pilzecker, to account for the decrement in human memory performance caused by the presentation of other material shortly after exposure to the to-be-remembered items. They suggested that this memory phenomenon reflected the disruption, by the intervening material, of physiological activity that fixes associations established during learning. Until those associations were fixed, or *consolidated*, memory would be susceptible to disruption. The connection between these experiments and the observation of retrograde amnesia following brain trauma—impairment of memories acquired prior to the trauma—was made shortly thereafter. Burnham proposed that consolidation involves a time-consuming "process of organization" of newly obtained memories through some combination of physical reorganization and psychological processes of repetition and association. Accordingly, he proposed that retrograde amnesia was a consequence of interrupted organizational processing, which must normally occur for a considerable period of time after learning. Other, more physiologically based conceptions followed. In particular, the notion that the physical reorganization involved networks of neurons interacting for long periods was captured prominently in Hebb's concept of reverberating activity by cell assemblies.

Reverberation may well contribute to consolidation processes that last several seconds or even minutes, and might mediate or facilitate cellular and molecular processes that are initiated by brain activity (see Chapters

2 and 3). But it is difficult to conceive that a substantial level of meaningful neural activity can be sustained independent of other brain activities for days or months-long consolidation processes indicated by the findings on retrograde amnesia described in Chapter 1. So, instead, it is commonly accepted that another kind of processing must support prolonged processes in consolidation. The following chapter considers the evidence that there are indeed two major stages or forms of consolidation.

.12.
• • • • • •

Two Distinct Stages of Memory Consolidation

STUDY QUESTIONS

What is memory consolidation? Are there different kinds of consolidation?

What are the steps in memory fixation? How is fixation modulated?

What memory system accomplishes the prolonged reorganization of memory following new experiences? What is the nature of that reorganization?

The term consolidation has been used in two ways in the memory literature. These two conceptions differ both in the presumed mechanisms that mediate consolidation and in the time scale of the relevant events. This difference has led to the view that there are two aspects of, or two kinds of consolidation, one that involves a *fixation* of memory within synapses over a period of minutes or hours, and another that involves a *reorganization* of memories that occurs over weeks to years.

Cellular events that mediate memory fixation

One approach to consolidation treats the phenomenon as a cascade of molecular and microstructural events by which short-term synaptic modifications lead to permanent changes in connectivity between neurons. These events are intended to capture the transition of memories from a short-term store to long-term memory, on a time scale of seconds and minutes. In principle these events can occur in any brain structure that participates in memory. Molecular events that mediate the formation of permanent structural changes associated with memory have been studied in a broad variety of invertebrate and mammalian brain structures that participate in memory.

The details of this work were described in Chapters 2 and 3. However, a few general points are reiterated and extended here. Studies on this conceptualization of consolidation focus on local network neural activity, that is, on highly integrated "cell assemblies," and on intracellular events that initiate nuclear transcription mechanisms for protein synthesis. The consolidation hypothesis received little attention in the twentieth century until the later 1940s, when studies showed that electrical currents applied to the head sufficient to produce overt convulsions (electroconvulsive shock; used successfully to treat psychiatric disorders such as major depression) produced a retrograde amnesia.

This finding led to many experiments that were aimed at determining the time course and features of memory lost following this treatment or various pharmacological treatments. For example, several studies showed that blockade of gene expression at the level of mRNA or protein synthesis did not affect learning but prevented later retention if the treatment was given shortly after learning but not if treatment was delayed by several minutes or hours. That is, these manipulations produce a temporally graded retrograde amnesia, similar in form if not time course to the observations of retrograde amnesia following head injury, brain damage, or disease. More recent studies on the molecular mechanisms of long-term potentiation have renewed the focus on protein synthesis as required for permanent physiological and microstructural alterations consequent both to long-term potentiation (LTP) or to learning. These studies have identified specific proteins, for example, CREB, the increased synthesis of which are seen as candidates for critical events in the formation of LTP and of permanent memory. Such cellular events begin immediately with the learning experience, but continue to unfold during the minutes and hours after learning. Treatments that disrupt the activity of cell assemblies and the molecular cascade leading to new protein synthesis are effective only within this relatively brief period, suggesting the time scale that characterizes this sense or this conception of memory consolidation.

The effort to identify specific molecules and the full cascade of molecular and cellular events that underlie memory fixation continues to be an area of considerable current research. One potentially important recent observation suggests that memory fixation processes may be labile for a period extending beyond several hours. Nader and colleagues trained rats in the fear conditioning protocol and then confirmed their memory as long as 14 days after. Then they infused a protein synthesis inhibitor into the amygdala either immediately or delayed following the retention test. If the infusion occurred shortly after the first retention test, subsequent memory in a second retention test was impaired. Delayed infusions had no effect on subsequent retention. The authors concluded that the first retention test "reactivated" the fear memory and that this reactivation was followed by a "reconsolidation" phase that requires protein synthesis. Currently, the generality and mechanism of the reconsolidation effect are under intense scrutiny.

Another major area of progress in understanding the short-term phase of consolidation has been in characterizing neural mechanisms that modulate the cellular processes of fixation. These discoveries are described next.

Modulation of memory fixation

James McGaugh and his colleagues observed that stimulant drugs could enhance the short-term process of memory consolidation. For example, they reported that the central stimulant picrotoxin given shortly after learning would facilitate later retention performance, but treatment several minutes after learning had no effect. This result, and many like it, showed that the neural information processing or molecular mechanisms of memory fixation could be influenced during a fixation period that extended for at least several minutes.

This situation provides an opportunity for events surrounding or following a learning experience to have some effect on the fixation or organization of memories. One of these modulatory influences that has been most studied is generated by the arousing nature of emotional experiences. Such experiences increase our attention toward particularly salient events, and can consequently increase the processing of memories for events as they occur during the emotional experiences, and indeed this has been shown to be the case. Another modulatory influence involves increments in memory processing that occur *even after the learning experience itself is completed*, and therefore can have their effects on subsequent retention, suggesting they operate on aspects of memory consolidation *per se*. This later influence of emotional arousal on the memory fixation is the main topic of this chapter.

Influencing memory by hormonal activation associated with emotional arousal

Stressful events that activate the sympathetic nervous system and pituitary–adrenal axis result in the release of epinephrine and glucocorticoids by the adrenal glands. These hormones have a variety of effects associated with the "flight or fight" response, including increased heart rate and blood pressure, diversion of blood flow to the brain and muscles, and mobilization of energy stores. There is now a wealth of evidence that another effect of this activation is to improve memory storage for experiences surrounding stress activation, and that the amygdala is critical to this influence on memory.

Investigations on the facilitation of memory by adrenal hormone activation in animals have largely focused on a step-through inhibitory avoidance task and post-training injections of drugs. In this task rats are initially placed in a small well-illuminated chamber that is attached to a larger, dimly lit area. When a door separating these chambers opens, the rat typically steps through to the larger compartment, where the floor is subsequently electrified. After a brief period of foot shocks the animal is allowed to escape back to the small chamber. In later tests of memory for this aversive experience, the animal is again placed into the small chamber and its latency to step through measured. Thus, the effect of training is to inhibit subsequent entry into the aversive compartment.

Many of the studies of memory modulation involve the systemic injection or brain infusion of drugs after the initial learning, with the common result that subsequent memory performance is altered. These effects typically depend on post-training drug administration within minutes after training, and have no effect if postponed for an hour or more. The post-training administration procedure eliminates the possibility that the drugs are altering perception, arousal, or motor performance during the learning experience. Conversely, this methodology, combined with the time-dependency of efficacy of the drug administration, provides strong evidence that neurochemical events strongly influence the consolidation of memories for several minutes after new learning.

There is now extensive evidence that administration of epinephrine (also called adrenaline) or adrenal glucocorticoids improves memory for inhibitory avoidance, and that these effects are mediated by the amygdala. In an elegant systematic series of studies, McGaugh, Larry Cahill, and their colleagues have provided a framework for the pathway by which these effects are exerted (Fig. 12–1). They have provided substantial and compelling evidence accumulated through a combination of behavioral analyses, selective lesions of parts of this system, and drugs that facilitate (agonists) or retard (antagonists) neurotransmitter receptors that are involved in the cascade of modulatory events that is generated by glucocorticoid release.

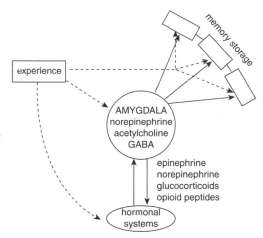

Figure 12–1. Schematic diagram of relationships between the amygdala and other systems, showing how the amygdala is influenced by hormonal systems and experience and can modulate memory storage in several memory systems.

According to their scheme, glucocorticoids released during stressful events, or administered by injection, can enter the blood brain barrier and influence receptors for this steroid in the brain directly. Epinephrine does not enter the blood brain barrier easily, however, and so it is likely that its effects are exerted via peripheral stimulation. This conclusion is supported by experiments showing that a β-adrenergic antagonist, a drug that blocks the β-subtype of epinephrine receptors, that does not pass the blood brain barrier blocks the memory-enhancing effects of epinephrine administration. The suspected target of peripheral epinephrine is β-adrenergic receptors on vagus nerve afferents that project to a brain stem area known as the nucleus of the solitary tract. This nucleus in turn projects into the amygdala where its afferents release norepinephrine (NE). This proposal is supported by studies showing that inactivation of the nucleus of the solitary tract by a local anesthetic blocks the effect of peripheral administration of epinephrine. In addition, other evidence shows that foot shock results in the release of NE within the amygdala. Furthermore, NE infused directly into the amygdala post-training enhances memory storage, and amygdala lesions or an NE antagonist infused into the amygdala block memory enhancement by peripheral epinephrine administration.

The effects of glucocorticoids on memory are remarkably similar to those of epinephrine. Peripheral treatment with glucocorticoids enhances memory, and this effect is blocked by lesions of outputs of the amygdala. The effect of glucocorticoids appears to be mediated selectively by the basolateral nucleus of the amygdala—a glucocorticoid receptor agonist infused into that nucleus, but not the central amygdala nucleus, enhances memory, and lesions of the basolateral nucleus, but not the central nucleus, block the memory-enhancing effects of glucocorticoids. Basolateral amygdala activation by glucocorticoids involves NE release, as shown by blockade of the effects of glucocorticoids by local infusion of a β-adrenergic antagonist. These responses of the amygdala are modulated by multiple other neurochemical systems. In particular, local infusions of agonists and antagonists of GABA (another neurotransmitter) and opioids (a type of neuromodulator) have demonstrated that these substances inhibit the release of NE in the amygdala and influence memory performance accordingly. In addition, other findings implicate a mechanism involving acetylcholine at a later synapse within the amygdala, providing yet another modulatory influence over this system.

Although most of the research on memory modulation involves the inhibitory avoidance task, consistent effects are observed on discrimination learning and maze learning tasks. In particular, one study has shown that these influences extend specifically to the types of memory mediated by the hippocampus and striatum. In this study, rats were trained on two different versions of the Morris water maze task, one in which learning was cued by a visible marker at the escape site, and the other where the platform was hidden (Fig. 12–2). In previous studies the same team had shown that learning the cued platform task depends on the striatum and learning the hidden platform task depends on the hippocampus. Animals were implanted bilaterally with cannuli in the striatum, hippocampus, or amygdala, then after recovery trained in a single session on one of the tasks. Post-training intrahippocampal infusions of d-amphetamine, which is an NE agonist, enhanced later retention on the spatial task, whereas intrastriatum infusions had no effect (Fig. 12–2A). Conversely, post-training intrastriatum infusions of d-amphetamine enhanced later retention on the cued task, whereas intrahippocampal infusions had no effect (Fig. 12–2B). Post-training intra-amygdala infusions of d-amphetamine enhanced retention on both tasks.

A follow-up study was conducted to examine whether the effect of amygdala infusions involved an influence on hippocampal and striatal mechanisms or whether the enhancement involved a direct involvement of the amygdala in performance. Animals were trained on the two versions of the task then given post-training injections of d-amphetamine into the amygdala, as in the first study. Then, prior to the retention testing, the amygdala was inactivated to eliminate the possibility that it was exerting a direct effect on retention performance. These inactivations did not block the enhancement effect, consistent with the view that the intra-amygdala infusions had exerted their effects via projections to the hippocampus and striatum.

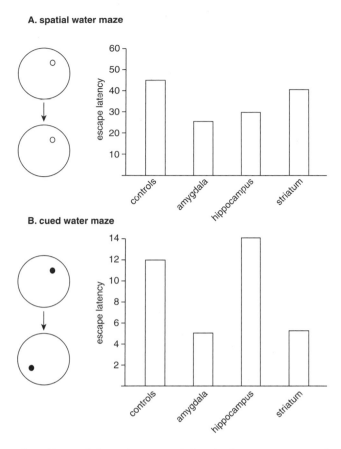

Figure 12–2. The effects of d-amphetamine infused after training into the amygdala, hippocampus, or striatum on water maze retention. A: The spatial water maze task, where the position of a hidden platform is constant. B: The cued water maze task, trials where the position of a visible platform is varied across trials (data from Packard et al., 1994).

The amygdala also plays a role in enhancing memory in humans

Studies on human subjects have provided additional evidence that emotional arousal can affect different forms of memory and that this effect is mediated by the amygdala. In a series of experiments, Larry Cahill and his colleagues have examined the influence of emotional content on declarative memory. Their test involves presentation of a series of slides and a narrative that tell a story about a mother and son involved in a traumatic accident, or a control story with neutral emotional content (Fig. 12–3A). The story had three parts. In the beginning and end parts the emotional and neutral stories are similar and are low in emotional content. In

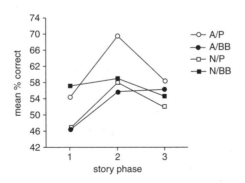

Narratives accompanying the slide presentation

	Neutral version	Arousal version
1.	A mother and her son are leaving home in the morning.	A mother and her son are leaving home in the morning.
2.	She is taking him to visit his father's workplace.	She is taking him to visit his father's workplace.
3.	The father is a laboratory technician at Victory Memorial hospital.	The father is a laboratory technician at Victory Memorial hospital.
4.	they check before crossing a busy road.	they check before crossing a busy road.
5.	While walking along, the boy sees some wrecked cars in a junkyard, which he finds interesting.	While crossing the road, the boy is caught in a terrible accident, which critically injures him.
6.	At the hospital, the staff are preparing for a practice disaster drill, which the boy will watch.	At the hospital, the staff prepares the emergency room, to which the boy is rushed.
7.	An image from a brain scan machine used in the drill attracts the boy's interest.	An image from a brain scan machine used in a trauma situation shows severe bleeding in the boy's brain.
8.	All morning long, a surgical team practiced the disaster drill procedures.	All morning long, a surgical team struggled to save the boy's life.
9.	Make-up artists were able to create realistic-looking injuries on actors for the drill.	Specialized surgeons were able to reattach the boy's severed feet.
10.	After the drill, while the father watched the boy, the mother left to phone her other child's preschool.	After the surgery, while the father stayed with the boy, the mother left to phone her other child's preschool.
11.	Running a little late, she phones the preschool to tell them she will soon pick up her child.	Feeling distraught, she phones the preschool to tell them she will soon pick up her child.
12.	Heading to pick up her child, she hails a taxi at the number 9 bus stop.	Heading to pick up her child, she hails a taxi at the number 9 bus stop.

Figure 12–3. The effects of arousal and a beta-blocker on story memory. *A:* Two versions of a story accompanied by slides. *B:* Performance on consistently neutral (phases 1 and 3; white background) and variable (phase 2; shaded background) components of the story. A/P = arousal story/ placebo treatment; A/BB = arousal story/ beta-blocker; N/P = neutral story/ placebo treatment; N/BB = neutral story/ beta-blocker (data from Cahill et al., 1994).

the middle section of the emotional story, the boy is critically injured and the events are depicted graphically; in the neutral story no accident occurs. In subsequent delayed memory testing, normal subjects show enhanced recall for the emotional component of the story, as compared to the parallel section of the neutral story (Fig. 12–3B). By contrast, subjects given a β-adrenergic antagonist (beta-blocker) showed no facilitation of declarative memory for the emotional component of the story, even though they rated that component of the story as strongly emotional and their memory performance on other parts of the story was fully normal. Performance on the neutral story was not affected by the beta-blocker, showing that there was no general effect of the drug on memory for the story. A subsequent study has now shown that an adrenergic agonist further enhances memory for the emotional component of the story.

The amygdala has been strongly implicated in the enhancement of memory for emotional events in humans. A patient with Urbach-Wiethe disease, the disorder that results in selective bilateral amygdala damage (see Chapter 8), was tested in the emotional story paradigm. Compared to control subjects this patient failed to show enhancement of memory for the emotional part of the story. The patient performed as well as controls on the initial neutral segment of the story, and rated the emotional material as affectively strong. In a complementary brain imaging study on normal human subjects, the amygdala was activated during the viewing of emotional material, and this activation was related to enhanced memory for that material. In different positron emission tomography (PET) scanning sessions, subjects viewed film clips that were strong or neutral in emotional content. The amount of PET activation in the amygdala was greater for the emotional than the neutral stories, and memory for this material was greater than for the neutral stories. Furthermore, the amount of amygdala activation was correlated with performance in a delayed test of memory for the material in the emotional films but not that in the neutral films.

Multiple emotional memory systems that involve the amygdala

Combining the findings across all the studies presented in this chapter, it is apparent that there are multiple influences of emotion on memory, and the nodal point in all these influences is the amygdala. It seems most likely that this confluence of emotional memory systems within the amygdala is a consequence of the convergent inputs and divergent outputs of this area of the brain. Thus, on the basis of the evidence presented here, it seems reasonable to suggest there are multiple emotional memory systems that involve the amygdala. One of these systems, or one set of systems, involves specific pathways for the attachment of perceptions to emotions, and to emotional output effectors. Another set of systems involves more general influences of emotional arousal on memory. One of these influences is mediated both by a neural pathway that increases memory processing during ongoing learning, whereas another influence involves a hormonal pathway for postlearning modulation of consolidation processes. These multiple aspects of emotional memory, and different types of emotional memory, are not incompatible. Instead, they could work largely in concert to acquire emotional responses and to mediate memory for associated information processed by other systems.

Brain systems that mediate prolonged processes in memory reorganization

The other conception of memory consolidation involves events above the level of cellular physiology; this kind of consolidation occurs at the brain systems level. The time scale of events involved in systems-level phenomena of consolidation are severalfold greater than that of the cellular fixation mechanisms. It appears that this kind of consolidation requires hours, days, months, or years, depending on the nature of the memory tested and the species tested. Indeed, it will be argued that this consolidation never ends completely, for reasons that are of considerable theoretical importance.

The notion of consolidation at the brain systems level, operating at this long time scale, is tied to the temporally graded retrograde amnesias discussed in Chapter 1, in which the susceptibility of recent memories to disruption extends over years. The neural processing that underlies this phenomenon is considered later in the chapter, addressing, along the way, various fundamental issues about consolidation. How long does this kind of consolidation go on? Precisely which brain structures are critical to mediate consolidation? Where are the memories stored after consolidation is complete? Are all kinds of memories subject to consolidation? How is the delay-dependent forgetting in anterograde amnesia related to this consolidation mechanism? Studies on both human amnesia and animal models of amnesia address different aspects of these issues, and provide an increasingly clear picture of the role of hippocampal involvement, and hippocampal–neocortical interaction, in consolidation.

Outlining the properties of this prolonged consolidation process is the focus of the remainder of this chapter. First, the literature on human retrograde amnesia is reviewed, including the methods used to test for retrograde amnesia in human subjects, the findings of temporally graded retrograde amnesia, and the identification of critical brain structures. Next, I review attempts to model retrograde amnesia in animals, again focusing on the testing methods, the findings of temporally graded memory loss, and on the critical brain structures. In addition, other relevant physiological findings are reviewed. Finally, conceptualizations of the information processing and circuitry critical to mechanisms of consolidation are considered, with the aim of combining the earlier discussed observations on the nature of memory representation in cortical and hippocampal areas with the phenomenology of consolidation.

The phenomenon of temporally graded retrograde amnesia

The main focus of studies on the long-term process of consolidation has been studies of amnesia following hippocampal system damage, and in particular the phenomenon of temporally graded retrograde amnesia. The conceptual linkage between the hippocampus and consolidation began with the earliest observations on the patient H.M. Scoville and Milner's report on H.M. focused on his disorder as a particularly good example of Ribot's law (see Chapter 1). They characterized his amnesia as a severe and selective impairment in "recent memory" in the face of spared remote memory capacities. Indeed, the dissociation in H.M. between impaired recent memories and intact remote memories was most striking. So far as could be ascertained by interviews with H.M. and his family, the retrograde memory loss dated back 2 years prior to the surgery, with remote memory seeming to be intact. More recent evaluations confirm that H.M.'s remote memory impairment is indeed temporally limited.

However, a large battery of tests of memory for public and personal events also extend the period of impairment back to 11 years prior to the surgery. These studies used several strategies to assess H.M.'s memory for material he was presumed to have acquired across the decades prior to his surgery. Some of these tests evaluated his memory for public events, including naming of tunes, verbal recognition of events, or identification of faces that became famous in a particular decade. For example, a test of recognition for famous events includes a series of questions about particularly important public events from the 1940s through the 1970s. H.M., whose surgery was performed in 1953, performed within the normal range of scores for questions about events that occurred in the 1940s, was borderline for events from the 1950s, and was clearly impaired on events from the 1960s onward.

A test for recognition of public scenes was included, in which pictures depicting important scenes from the 1940s to the 1980s were selected such that the famous event could not be deduced from the picture alone. Subjects were asked if they had seen the picture before and could identify the event, and then further questions were asked about details of the event depicted. H.M.'s content scores were deficient in all decades except the 1940s.

A method used to probe H.M.'s memory for personal events involved a test originally designed to access remote autobiographical memories. In this test, subjects were given concrete nouns and asked to relate them to some personally experienced event from any period in their life, and to describe when the event occurred. In addition, to assess the consistency of these memories, the test was readministered on another day. Normal subjects provided memories from throughout their life span, including especially the most recent time period. By contrast, the memories that H.M. retrieved to these cues all dated back to the age of 16 (i.e., 1942) or younger. Thus, he had no memories of the end of World War II or of his high school graduation (1947), or any other event onward. These data provided the strongest evidence that his retrograde amnesia extends back 11 years prior to his surgery. Note, however, that because this time frame corresponds with the onset of H.M.'s seizure disorder (that ultimately precipitated the surgery he received), there is the possibility that at least some of the loss of memories might be a result of compromised hippocampal function during the period prior to his surgery, that is, there might be a contribution here from a partial anterograde amnesia.

Subsequent studies on retrograde amnesia have provided confirmation of the phenomenon of temporally graded memory loss, in cases where the deficit is unambiguously a retrograde amnesia. For example, one line of studies with patients receiving electroconvulsive therapy for severe depression examined memory for television programs that were shown in a single viewing season. These patients were found to have a (temporary) retrograde amnesia extending back 1–3 years before the treatments. Other studies have shown temporally graded retrograde amnesia dating 10–20 years back from an anoxic or ischemic event.

In addition, in a recent study of temporally graded retrograde amnesia, Squire and his colleagues tied the severity of retrograde amnesia to the amount of damage to the medial temporal region. This study involved four patients who had become amnesic without other cognitive impairment following specific brain insult and who had, for unrelated reasons, subsequently died and come to autopsy involving histological analysis of the brain damage. Two patients developed moderately severe anterograde amnesia following a transient ischemic event. Both patients had a selective loss of cells in the CA1 field of the hippocampus, and had a very limited retrograde amnesia, extending only 1–2 years. Two other patients had more severe anterograde amnesia and more extensive retrograde amnesia extending back 15–25 years. The histopathological examination of these patients showed cell loss throughout the hippocampus and to some extent in entorhinal cortex as well. These studies further confirm that damage limited to the hippocampal region can result in temporally limited retrograde amnesia, and that the extent of the temporal gradient of retrograde amnesia might be associated with the anatomical extent of damage within the hippocampal region.

Recent studies by Squire and colleagues have also examined in detail whether the phenomenon of temporally graded retrograde amnesia extends to spatial memory. This study focused on a patient with extensive damage to the medial temporal lobe. The patient had lived in a neighborhood in California during the 1930s and 1940s, but had moved away and subsequently returned only occasionally. The patient's spatial memory for this period was evaluated by comparing his ability to construct routes between different locations in the community, as identified using archival maps of the areas from the relevant period. In addition, the patient's ability to plot alternative roundabout routes was examined, using tests where he was asked how to navigate among places when the major route between them was blocked. They also measured the patient's accuracy in pointing in the direction of major landmarks from an imagined position in the neighborhood. On all these tests, the patient scored as well as or better than a group of age-matched control subjects who had lived in the same area during the target period, and who had also subsequently moved away. By contrast, and unlike the control subjects, the patient failed completely in solving the same navigational problems based on knowledge about their current neighborhood. Thus, for this patient, the pattern of retrograde amnesia for spatial knowledge matched that of temporally graded nonspatial memory observed in previous studies in many amnesic patients.

Not all forms of retrograde amnesia are temporally graded, however. Thus, there are retrograde amnesias associated with a variety of etiologies in which gradients are flat, extending back to the earliest childhood memories. In addition, some researchers have argued that some retrograde amnesias show a pattern of memory loss characterized less by the age of the memories than by their nature. For example, in one study four patients with retrograde amnesia showed impairments in the ability to recall or recognize faces of people who had become famous in the news media dating back several decades. Some of these patients showed flat gradients of retrograde amnesia dating for all periods of their life span. A large number of cases of retrograde amnesia concluded that retrograde amnesia following medial temporal lobe damage affects memory for personal episodes more severely than semantic memory, and that this deficit in autobiographical memory extends back many years, and in many cases the entire life span.

It has been argued that flat gradients of retrograde amnesia, and particularly those involving autobiographical memory, occur only in cases where there is damage or suspected damage beyond the medial temporal lobe. Amnesia associated with Korsakoff syndrome, closed head injuries, seizure disorders, and certain other etiologies often include damage or cell loss in prefrontal cortex. This is important because damage to the prefrontal area is associated with disorders of "source memory," the ability to recall where and when information was acquired. Such an inability to identify the circumstances surrounding new learning might be expected to lead to a selective impairment in memory for personal experiences. In these cases, the content-selectivity of retrograde amnesia would *not* be related to hippocampal function.

Prospective studies of retrograde amnesia in animals

The relatively recent development of experimental protocols for studying retrograde amnesia in animals has been a major advance in understanding the role of brain structures in memory consolidation. The use of animals allows increased resolution of the anatomical structures under study. In addition, animal studies allow greater control over the learning experience prior to brain insult. Such prospective experiments can equalize the nature and extent of acquired information, and can precisely control when learning takes place before brain damage. There have now been several prospective studies of retrograde amnesia, using different species and different learning and memory protocols. The majority of these studies support the notion that damage to medial temporal structures results in a temporally graded retrograde amnesia. Nevertheless, this finding is not universal, and the severity and gradient of retrograde amnesia varies across studies with the species, types of tests, and locus of brain damage. The remainder of this section reviews a few of these studies that provide examples of the pattern of retrograde amnesia and the variety of memory tests employed.

Zola-Morgan and colleagues trained monkeys on a series of visual object discriminations at different times prior to ablation of the hippocampus and of some of the surrounding cortex. Animals were trained on 100 object discrimination problems, segregated into five 20-problem sets presented at 16, 12, 8, 4, or 2 weeks prior to the surgery. Each set of problems consisted of two problems per day, with each problem presented on 14 consecutive trials. Performance was typically very good in learning, averaging 88% correct on the last trial of all the problems. Two weeks after the surgery, memory was assessed for all 100 problems, with random order presentation of a single trial of each problem over 2 days of testing. Normal monkeys performed best at problems that had been learned in the 4 weeks just prior to the (sham) surgery, with significantly poorer performance on problems that had been learned earlier, thus showing the typical forgetting curve (Fig. 12–4A). Monkeys with hippocampal damage showed the opposite pattern, however. They were significantly impaired, and indeed performed poorest, for problems presented at the shortest interval prior to surgery. These monkeys were not impaired on problems presented 8–16 weeks before surgery. Accordingly, these findings document the existence of temporally graded retrograde amnesia, and hence the presumption of a consolidation deficit, in animals with damage limited to medial temporal lobe structures.

Several studies using rats and rabbits have also demonstrated temporally graded retrograde amnesia following damage to the hippocampal region. Winocur demonstrated temporally graded retrograde amnesia in rats using the social transmission of food preferences task described in Chapter 5. In this study, pairs of rats were housed together for 2 days, then one of the rats was fed rat chow mixed with either cinnamon or cocoa. Subsequent training involved reexposure of the fed rat to its cagemate for a 30-minute period. Then, either immediately, or after intervals varying between 2 and 10 days, rats were operated for lesions of the hippocampus, and were allowed to recover for 10 days. Thus, the retention interval varied between 10 and 20 days. Memory for the social learning of the food odor was tested by measuring the consumption of cinnamon-flavored versus cocoa-flavored chow in a preference test. Normal rats showed a striking preference for the trained odor that lasted at full strength for 15 days, with some subsequent forgetting on the 20-day test (Fig. 12–4B). Rats with hippocampal lesions were severely impaired when the interval between training and surgery was minimal, showing no significant preference for the odor trained soonest to the time of surgery. They showed some retention when the surgery was delayed to 2 days after training, and full recovery at longer training-to-surgery intervals. As in the experiment on monkeys described earlier, and as in human amnesia, the performance pattern after hippocampal damage was opposite to that seen in normal controls. Thus, whereas normal animals showed progressively poorer performance at progressively longer retention intervals, rats with hippocam-

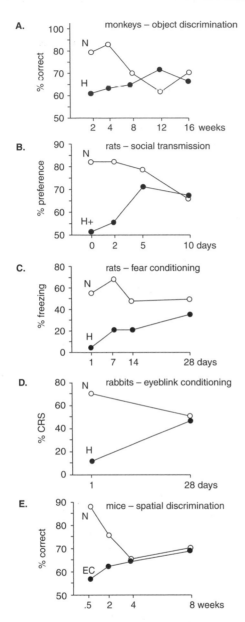

Figure 12–4. Several demonstrations of temporally graded retrograde memory impairments in animals following damage to the hippocampal region. *A:* Performance in normal (N) monkeys and that of monkeys with removal of the hippocampus plus some surrounding cortex (H+) on retention of 100 object discrimination problems learned at different times prior to surgery (data from Zola-Morgan and Squire, 1990). *B:* Performance of normal control rats (N) and rats with lesions of the hippocampus (H) on retention of the social transmission of food preference trained at different times prior to the surgery (data from Winocur, 1990). *C:* Performance of normal control rats (N) and rats with hippocampal lesions (H) on retention of contextual fear conditioning trained at different times prior to the surgery (data from Kim and Fanselow, 1992). *D:* Performance of normal control rabbits (N) and rabbits with hippocampal lesions (H) on retention of trace eyeblink conditioning performed at different times prior to the surgery (data from Kim et al., 1995). *E:* Performance of normal control mice (N) and mice with lesions of the entorhinal cortex (EC) on maze problems learned at different times prior to the surgery (data from Cho et al., 1993).

pal lesions performed better for learning that occurred at a more remote time.

Other evidence for temporally graded retrograde amnesia in rats comes from studies of contextual fear conditioning, a task described in Chapter 11. In a study by Fanselow and colleagues, like the one just described, animals were trained at different intervals prior to surgery. Then, all subjects were tested at a fixed interval postoperatively. Rats were placed in a conditioning chamber and presented a series of 15 tone-shock pairings in a single session. Hippocampal lesions were performed at 1–28 days after this training. Testing for conditioned fear associated with the shock was conducted separately for the context (the training chamber) and for the tone. To test for contextual fear, rats were placed back in the training chamber and freezing was measured for several minutes. To test for conditioned fear to the tone, animals were placed in a different chamber, and freezing during re-presentation of the tone was measured. As shown in Fig. 12–4C, normal rats exhibited substantial freezing across all retention intervals, indicating virtually no forgetting for the conditioned fear for both the context and the tone. By contrast, rats with hippocampal lesions showed impairment in contextual fear conditioning in a temporally graded way: They were severely impaired when the interval between training and surgery was 1 day, showing virtually no freezing in the familiar chamber; they showed some retention when the surgery occurred a week after training; and they demonstrated full retention when the surgery occurred a month after training. In addition, the retrograde amnesia was material specific in that rats with hippocampal damage showed fully normal retention of conditioned fear for the tone at all retention intervals.

A temporally graded retrograde amnesia has also been observed in rabbits trained on hippocampal-dependent trace (classical) conditioning, a task described in Chapter 10. Rabbits were trained using standard classical eyelid conditioning procedures for 100-trial-per-day sessions. On each trial, a 250 msec tone conditioning stimulus (CS) was followed by a 500 msec trace interval and then an airpuff unconditioned stimulus (US). Daily training continued until the rabbit elicited eyeblinks during the CS or trace interval on eight out of ten consecutive trials, requiring on average three to four training sessions. The rabbits then received hippocampal lesions, either 1 day or 1 month later. After a 7-day recovery period, all animals were tested for retention during retraining. As shown in Fig. 12–4D, normal rabbits showed complete savings of the conditioned eyeblink at both retention intervals. By contrast, rabbits given hippocampal lesions 1 day after training were severely impaired, exhibiting no retention of conditioning, and indeed were unable to acquire the task postoperatively. Nevertheless, when the surgery occurred 1 month after conditioning, rabbits were intact, showing as much savings as did control rabbits at both retention intervals.

Temporally graded retrograde amnesia has also been observed in mice and rats on spatial discrimination problems. In one study, mice were trained on a set of two-choice spatial discrimination problems using a radial maze. For each problem, the mouse was rewarded for selecting one of two adjacent maze arms, such that the same apparatus was used for multiple problems. Each problem was presented for 16 trials per day for 3–5 days, until the animals reached a performance criterion of 13 correct choices in a session. Training on successive problems was separated by 10 days. On the following day, animals were given ibotenic acid lesions of the entorhinal cortex, then allowed to recover for 10 days. Subsequent retention testing involved 16 trials on each problem presented concurrently on multiple problems. Control mice exhibited striking savings on problems presented 3 days prior to surgery, with significant forgetting at longer retention intervals (Fig. 12–5E). Mice with entorhinal lesions were severely impaired when the surgery had occurred 3 days after presentation of the problem, showing almost no retention at that interval, while some retention was observed when the surgery occurred 2 weeks after presentation of a problem, and normal retention was obtained for problems presented 4–8 weeks prior to surgery. Notably, as in the other studies presented, the patterns of performance across retention intervals for normal mice were the opposite of mice with damage to the entorhinal cortex.

A similar study using rats, run subsequently, replicated the main findings with entorhinal lesions, showing a severe retention deficit when the training-to-surgery interval was a few days, with better performance for more remotely acquired spatial discriminations and indeed normal performance for the longest interval. In addition, this study also examined the performance of animals given lesions of the parietal cortex at varying intervals after spatial discrimination training. In contrast to the pattern of findings on entorhinal lesions, rats with parietal lesions, though impaired, showed no sign of a temporal gradient. These data are consistent with the notion that the hippocampal region, but not parietal cortex, plays a role in the consolidation process.

There have also been failures to find retrograde amnesia following hippocampal damage, and reports of flat and not temporally graded deficits. These studies differ in the type of lesion and training, leaving open the critical parameters that determine the extent of the retrograde gradient in animals, as in humans. Notwithstanding the mixed results, the large number of successful demonstrations of temporally graded amnesia in animal models, using a compelling range of species and behavioral tests, adds to the conclusions from studies of human amnesia. At least some components of the hippocampal system play a critical role in consolidation of memory during the time after learning for at least some types of information.

Models of cortical–hippocampal
interactions in memory reorganization

There have been many theoretical proposals about the mechanisms of long-term consolidation. It is generally held that the final repository of long-term memories is the neocortex, and that hippocampal processing somehow facilitates, organizes, or otherwise mediates the creation of permanent memory representations in specific neocortical sites. The question to be addressed here is: What is the nature of the interaction of the hippocampal system with neocortical processors that permit memory storage and consolidation to occur?

Several models of hippocampal–cortical interactions have been proposed, including a number of computational models that implement various kinds of interactions that could occur. Two recent models that will be considered here focus on how the hippocampus could mediate a slow reorganization process.

Pablo Alvarez and Larry Squire offered a simple network model that highlighted several basic distinctions in the operating characteristics of the cerebral cortex and the hippocampus. They argued that the cerebral cortex was capable of storing an immense amount of information, but that cortical representations change slowly and incrementally. By contrast, the hippocampus had a limited storage capacity but recorded information rapidly through changing of synaptic weights using rapid LTP mechanisms. Their focus was to show how these properties instantiated within a simple neural network simulation could demonstrate key properties of consolidation.

The schematic diagram shown in Fig. 12–5A illustrates their model. The simulation contained two distinct cortical areas and a medial temporal lobe region (MTL). Each neural unit in these areas was connected to every other unit in other areas, and the connection strengths could be modified by a use-dependent competitive learning rule. The rate of change in connections between the MTL and cortex was designed to be rapid, but short-lasting, whereas the changes in connections between the two cortical areas was slow, but long-lasting. When new information was presented to the network that set up activations in each of the cortical areas, the MTL connections changed substantially and rapidly to represent the conjointly active units in the cortical areas, although very little permanent change had occurred in the cortical representations or their connection between them. Subsequently, when the MTL area was randomly activated, to simulate a subsequent consolidation event, the originally activated cortical input areas were reactivated, incrementally enhancing their connections.

A.

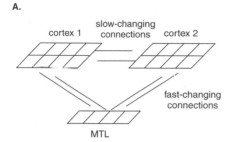

B.

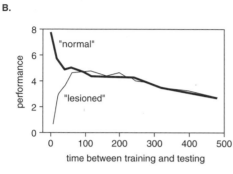

Figure 12–5. Alvarez and Squire's (1994) model of cortical–hippocampal interactions in consolidation. *A:* Conceptualization of the model. Eight units in two cortical areas and four in the medial temporal lobe (MTL) have different rates of change in connectivity. *B:* Performance of the intact model and the model with an MTL lesion on the capacity to excite units in one cortical area from the other in retention of associations acquired at different times prior to the surgery.

Memory performance of the model was assessed in terms of how well activation of one of the cortical representations could reinstate the associated representation in the other cortical area (Fig. 12–5B). The intact network showed strong performance in activating the associated representation shortly after learning, and showed some forgetting over time. By contrast, if the MTL was removed shortly after learning, memory performance was very poor, and the longer the period the MTL was left intact after learning, the stronger was the consequent memory performances. Accordingly, the model seemed to simulate the essential characteristics of memory consolidation.

Jay McClelland and his colleagues developed a more elaborate and larger-scale model, taking these ideas somewhat farther. In their model, cortical representations involved systematic organizations of related items in parallel, multidimensional hierarchies. They envisioned the operation of the cortex as identifying stimulus characteristics and sorting items into categories and subcategories within the large-scale organization. As an example, they considered the semantic network illustrated in Fig. 12–6A. In this network, birds and fish are characterized by a set of propositional properties, for example, a robin is an animal that has feathers and wings, is red, and can fly. They noted that elaborate parallel distributed networks can readily be trained on such sorting operations for a large set of ani-

A. propositional network

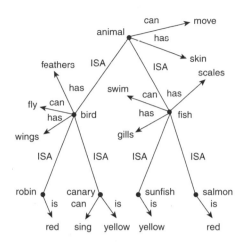

B. performance in new learning

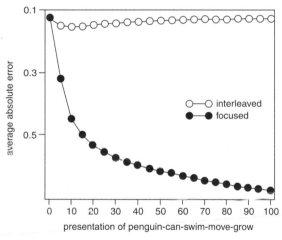

Figure 12–6. A semantic network used to train network models of the organization of propositional knowledge about living things. *A:* The propositional network which the model initially learned for the categorization of characteristics of fish and birds. ISA = is a. *B:* Overall categorization performance following either focused or interleaved training on a new item with characteristics of both birds and fish (penguins) (from McClelland et al., 1995).

mals according to these and similar characteristics. However, once a set of hierarchical organizations is established and stabilized, it is difficult to add new items smoothly, not because a network cannot be altered to include the new item by repetitive training—it will do so quite well. Rather, the problem is that such novel training causes changes in an already established network resulting, in turn, in catastrophic interference among the already existing items. New training alters a network to identify the new item, but such learning results in network modifications that interfere with the previously developed ability to correctly identify the old information. In the example network, catastrophic interference was illustrated by focused training on identification of a penguin, a bird that has some characteristics of other birds (e.g., wings) but also other characteristics of fish (can swim). The outcome of focused training was that network performance on overall categorization fell precipitously (Fig. 12–6B).

McClelland's solution to the problem of catastrophic interference was to add a new small network—a "hippocampus"—that could very rapidly acquire a representation of a new item, and then have this small network slowly and gradually "train" the large network. As a result, as in the Alvarez and Squire simulation, the synaptic weights in the hippocampal network changed rapidly, and that network sent its representation repetitively to the large—"cortical"—network. The cortical network modifications were slow and incremental. Also, in addition to the occasional input from the hippocampus, the cortical model was also repetitively exposed to the old materials it was built to represent, thereby resulting in an "interleaved learning" regimen that intermixed repetitions of old and new representations. This was key to the ability of the overall cortical network to be modified so as to incorporate new information without suffering from catastrophic interference. In the example, by contrast to focused training, such interleaved training led to successful preserved performance on all the categorizations (Fig. 12–6B).

Eventually, this process of interleaving produced an asymptotic state of the overall cortical representation, at which point it no longer benefited from hippocampal activations, and thus no longer depended upon the hippocampus. In this fashion, the model exhibited the critical features of consolidation. The duration of consolidation required would be expected to be indeterminate, depending on the nature and extent of new information to be obtained, as well as on any other new learning that must be incorporated during the course of consolidation of already stored information. Thus, consolidation should be conceived as a life-long evolution of cortical networks, one that only asymptotically approaches a state where more interleaving does not alter the network substantially. In this way, we can come to understand at least some of the mixed results regarding the duration and nature of temporal gradients in retrograde amnesia.

The nature of hippocampal representation and consolidation

How might information processing by the hippocampus support the reorganization of cortical information during a prolonged consolidation period? A further consideration of the nature of hippocampal representations discussed in Chapters 4–6, combined with our knowledge about cortical–hippocampal circuitry (Chapter 9), offers potential insights about the cortical–hippocampal interplay proposed to underlie memory consolidation. In the model of the hippocampal "memory space" developed in Chapters 5 and 6, the hippocampus was envisioned to represent learning episodes as a series of discrete events, each encoded within the activity of a single cell. Within the hippocampal memory space, some cells were characterized as encoding highly specific conjunctions or sequences of stimuli and actions that compose unique events that occurred in only one or a few learning episodes. Yet other cells were envisioned to encode "nodal" events, features of experience that are common across different episodes; these might mediate our capacity to link an ongoing event to previous episodes that share the nodal event.

In an extension of this model, Eichenbaum and colleagues suggested that the nodal codings could subserve the linking and interleaving processes of consolidation proposed by Alvarez and Squire and McClelland and his colleagues. According to this scheme, representations of discrete events and sequences of events within the hippocampus are conceived to occur within one or a few learning trials. Furthermore, "nodal" representations are conceived as developing in parallel with the variations in experience that occur across related learning episodes. Because of the very high level of interconnectivity of hippocampal pyramidal cells relative to that in all the cortical areas, the initial development of these nodal representations is envisioned as primarily within the hippocampus shortly after learning. Subsequent prolonged cortical memory consolidation involves the creation of the nodal properties within cortical cells, mediated through connections with the hippocampus and parahippocampal region.

Within this framework, memory reorganization may operate in two stages. The first stage involves interactions between the hippocampus and the parahippocampal region. Parahippocampal neurons receive direct inputs from many cortical areas, and so they would be expected to encode the configurations of stimuli to compose event representations and sequences based on simultaneity of these inputs alone. However, for some period immediately after learning, associations among the complex event representations within the parahippocampal region may depend upon the connections to and from the hippocampal cells that have encoded particular nodal events. At the same time, the feedback from the hippocampus to the parahippocampal cortex is envisioned to mediate the development of nodal representations within the parahippocampal region. This may occur by the hippocampus providing an indirect pathway that drives the coactivation of parahippocampal neurons, enhancing the connections within their intracortical network and producing nodal cell properties in parahippocampal neurons. Because parahippocampal neurons have an unusual capacity for prolonged firings following discrete events (see Chapter 9), cells in this region may rapidly support the coding of long event sequences through the interactions with the hippocampus. When long sequence and nodal properties have been acquired by parahippocampal cells, the memory can be considered to have consolidated there, in the sense that the memory abilities conferred by these cells would no longer require hippocampal feedback.

The second stage involves a similar interplay between the cortical association areas and the parahippocampal region. Initially, cortical associations are viewed to depend on the parahippocampal region to supply linkages between their representations. In addition, by simultaneously driving cells in cortical areas and activating their intracortical connections, these linkages would be expected to mediate the ultimate development of context and nodal properties in the cortical association areas. When this is accomplished the entire hippocampal circuit would no longer be necessary for the existence of event, long sequence, and nodal representations. Consistent with the proposal that the prolonged consolidation process occurs in stages involving first a reorganization within the parahippocampal region and then later in the cortex, human amnesics with damage extending into the parahippocampal region have a more extended retrograde amnesia than those with selective hippocampal damage.

The key aspects of this model involve the unusual associational structure of hippocampal anatomy that makes it the earliest site for arbitrary associations that underlie event, sequence, and nodal properties. At earliest stages of parahippocampal or neocortical processing, the range of associations and the speed of their formation may be much more limited. But they can mediate substantial development and reorganization of a memory space through the connections within the hippocampus initially. In this way the repeated invocation of hippocampal representations onto the cortex serves to reorganize cortical representations accommodating new information and new associations within the overall knowledge structure encoded there.

Summing up

There are two aspects of memory consolidation, one that involves molecular and cellular processes that support the *fixation* of memory within synapses over a period of minutes or hours, and another that involves interactions within the declarative memory system to support a *reorganization* of memories that occurs over weeks to years.

There is a cascade of molecular and microstructural events by which short-term synaptic modifications lead to permanent changes in connectivity between neurons, and this cascade is conserved across brain structures that participate in memory and across species in the phylogenetic scale. The fixation of memory can be halted or facilitated by postlearning treatments that interfere with the molecular/cellular cascade. There are also natural modulatory mechanisms that can facilitate fixation in the various memory systems of the mammalian brain. An important modulatory system involves the release of glucocorticoids and adrenergic mechanisms via the amygdala that can influence memory fixation in the declarative and habit systems in both animals and humans.

In addition, the declarative memory system mediates the prolonged reorganization of memories. This process has been identified in graded retrograde amnesia for declarative memories in both humans and animals. The nature of mechanisms within the declarative system is poorly understood. But current models propose that the role of the hippocampus is to rapidly store indices of cortical representations, and to slowly facilitate the interconnection of cortical representations by repeated two-way interactions between the cortex and hippocampus. Over a protracted period, these interactions ultimately result in an asymptotic level of reorganization and connections among cortical representations to incorporate new material into semantic knowledge.

READINGS

Alvarez, P., and Squire, L.R. 1994. Memory consolidation and the medial temporal lobe: A simple network model. *Proc. Natl. Acad. Sci. U.S.A.* 91: 7041–7045.

Cahill, L., and McGaugh, J.L. 1998. Mechanisms of emotional arousal and lasting declarative memory. *Trends Neurosci.* 21: 273–313.

McClelland, J.L., McNaughton, B.L., and O'Reilly, R.C. 1995. Why there are complementary learning systems in the hippocampus and neocortex: Insights from the successes and failures of connectionist models of learning and memory. *Psychol. Rev.* 102: 419–457.

McGaugh, J.L. 2000. Memory—a century of consolidation. *Science* 287: 248–251.

Nader, K., Schafe, G.E., and LeDoux, J.E. 2000. Fear memories require protein synthesis in the amygdala for reconsolidation after retrieval. *Nature* 406: 722–726.

.13.
• • • • • •

Working with Memory

STUDY QUESTIONS

What is working memory?

How does it differ from the mechanisms of declarative memory discussed so far?

What brain structures and systems support working memory?

What do we know about the anatomy and evolution of the prefrontal cortex?

What are the consequences of prefrontal damage in humans, in animals?

Do different parts of the prefrontal cortex have different functions?

What aspects of cognition and memory are encoded by prefrontal neurons?

The story of memory does not end with consolidation. Indeed, even after consolidation is completed, there is the issue of how we search for information during retrieval, as well as how new information becomes incorporated into the established organization during additional learning experiences. I think of cognitive processing that guides encoding and retrieval as "working-with-memory," the manipulation of information that is not memory per se, but handles our memory processing. While the entire cerebral cortex is involved in memory processing, the chief brain area that mediates these processes is the prefrontal cortex, the area in the frontal lobe whose functions are not fully understood but clearly involve strategic mechanisms of the sort that work with memory as a major part of its function.

The role of the prefrontal cortex is generally viewed as mediating "working memory," a concept akin to my notion of working with memory. Working memory involves a combination of storing new incoming information, plus some type of cognitive manipulation, during a brief period in consciousness. Consider a task in current common usage in memory research, called the "two-back" task. In this protocol, human subjects are presented with a string of stimuli (letters, words, or numbers). Their job is to say yes when the current item is the same as the one presented two back, that is, on the second trial previous to the current one. To succeed at this task one must create a buffer in memory that holds the last two items seen. Then when a new item is presented, one can match it to the first item in the buffer (the two-back item) and make a correct response. Then one must update the buffer by deleting that two-back item and adding in the current item, and so on.

We perform tasks that demand working memory in almost all of the activities of our conscious lives, from checking off the jobs accomplished in our morning routine, to keeping track of the flow of information in reading a text chapter, to solving the many complex problems we encounter during our work. Working memory is considered a form of declarative memory because this sort of processing goes on in consciousness and involves relational organization and inferential judgments, and is accessible to explicit forms of expression. However, our consideration of the short-term mechanisms of working memory here is also distinctly different from the mechanisms of long-term memory that have been the focus of this book so far (see also a discussion of short-term memory mechanisms of other cortical areas in Chapter 7).

Alan Baddeley and his colleagues first realized the importance of distinguishing the cognitive and storage processes in short-term memory, and replaced the concept of a unitary short-term memory with a multiple component conception of working memory. The multiple component model was inspired by findings from experiments in which they found an unexpected low degree of interference in the capacity for storing lists of visual patterns or word items when people performed cognitive tasks simultaneously. So, in their model of working memory they proposed the existence of a set of specialized subsystems that mediates the storage process, and a distinct "central executive" that controls the subsystems and performs the mental "work" of controlling the slave subsystems and forming strategies. Corresponding to the materials involved in Baddeley's studies, the model involved two distinct subsystems, a "visuospatial sketch pad" that could maintain nonverbal images and a "phonological loop" that mediated speech perception and subvocal rehearsal of verbal materials. These should be considered just examples of the full range of specialized subsystems available to the central executive.

Because this kind of conceptual model of working memory involves multiple types of cognitive processing combined with a range of stored material, it will come as no surprise that working memory relies on a widespread network of brain structures. Indeed, there is considerable evidence that the brain network for working memory is large and can be subdivided into a central executive with multiple subsystems. Considerable evidence points to the prefrontal cortex as the locus of the central executive, and to a variety of other cortical areas as the mediators of subsystem processes.

In this chapter, first, the anatomy of the prefrontal cortex is summarized. A review follows of the functional role of the prefrontal cortex, including a consideration of whether the prefrontal area is involved in memory *per se*, or other cognitive processes related to memory, and whether the expansive prefrontal area has specialized subdivisions between or within the hemispheres. Then the story is broadened to consider parcellation of functions and cooperation between the prefrontal cortex and other higher-order cortical areas. Finally, some of the main points made in earlier chapters are reviewed, with the aim of considering how the entire brain participates in ordinary learning and memory processing.

The anatomy of the prefrontal cortex

The assignment of the central executive function to the prefrontal cortex is supported by substantial anatomical data. The phenomenal expansion of the prefrontal area in primates and especially humans is impressively associated with the evolution of cognitive capacities (Fig. 13–1). The prefrontal cortex in humans is a diverse area, composed of several distinct subdivisions. There is considerable consensus on correspondences in monkeys with identified areas in the human prefrontal cortex. Although several anatomical areas have been characterized based on morphological appearance, most of the functional evidence has been related to four general regions. These include the medial, dorsolateral, ventrolateral, and orbital areas. Most of the attention with regard to working memory functions in monkeys and humans has focused on the dorsolateral and ventrolateral areas, and these areas are partially distinct in their connections with more posterior parts of the cerebral cortex. Each of the subdivisions receives input from a diverse set of rostral and causal cortical areas, and each has a distinctive input pattern.

In addition, prefrontal areas are characterized by considerable associative connections with other prefrontal areas. Nevertheless, despite this diversity and associativity with the prefrontal cortex, a few generalities

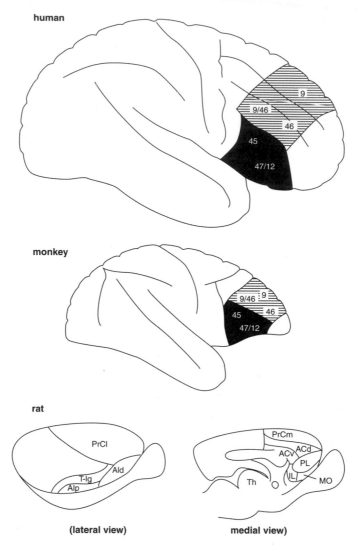

Figure 13–1. Designations of prefrontal areas in the human (top), monkey (middle), and rat (bottom; lateral and medial views). In the human and monkey, the designations are Brodman's areas. In the rat the designations are: AI = agranular insular; PrC = premotor; AC = anterior cingulate; PL = prelimbic; IL = infralimbic; MO = medial orbital; T-Ig = taste/granular insular; Th = thalamus; d = dorsal; l = lateral; m = medial; p = posterior; v = ventral.

have emerged about distinctions among prefrontal areas with regard to their inputs from posterior cortical areas. Thus, in general, the dorsolateral prefrontal area receives inputs mainly from medially and dorsolaterally located cortical areas that preferentially represent somatosensory and visuospatial information. Conversely, in general, the lateral prefrontal areas receive inputs mainly from ventrolateral and ventromedial cortical areas that represent auditory and visual pattern information. In particular, the differentiation of visuospatial input to the dorsolateral prefrontal area, and visual pattern input to the lateral prefrontal area has received considerable attention in studies on distinct working memory systems.

In rats there is also clear anatomical evidence for correspondences with some prefrontal regions in primates. However, the number of these areas is limited. And in particular, there is little evidence for the existence of rodent homologies for the dorsal and lateral convexity subdivisions of the prefrontal cortex prominent in views on working memory in primates and humans. Nevertheless, there is evidence that the medial and orbital areas in the rodent prefrontal cortex serve some of the general functions of working memory observed in primates.

The role of the prefrontal cortex in human memory function

Deficits in short-term or working memory can arise from a variety of disorders, including some associated with damage to multiple brain areas. Nevertheless, the greatest attention in behavioral studies has been accorded the prefrontal cortex, befitting its role as the putative "central executive" of working memory systems. However, prefrontal cortex function is a large issue, not limited to or even considered by some researchers as primarily an issue of memory processing, as suggested earlier. Rather, the role of the prefrontal cortex in human memory is differently viewed as only a part of its role in multiple higher cognitive functions including personality, affect, motor control, language, and problem solving.

Consistent with this view, in general, neuropsychological studies suggest that deficits in memory are secondary to an impairment in attention and problem-solving deficits. For example, one of the best studied and most profound impairments following prefrontal damage in humans is a deficit in the Wisconsin Card Sorting task. In this test, subjects are initially presented with four target items, playing cards each with a repeating pattern design that involves a unique combination of pattern color, shape, and number. Subsequently, the subjects are given a deck of similar cards and must sort the cards onto the target cards according to a criterion (color, shape, or number) the subject selects. The subject is given feedback with every choice, and must search for the correct sorting criterion. When the subject is sorting correctly, the experimenter shifts to a new criterion without warning and the subject must discover the new criterion.

This task contains an obvious working memory component, in that subjects must keep in mind the currently judged sorting criterion, and dispense with it and then select and maintain a new one. Patients with frontal lobe lesions are severely impaired on this task. However, the observed impairment in these patients is not that they forget the current sorting criterion. On the contrary, prefrontal patients have no difficulty learning the initial sorting criterion. Moreover, their disorder is that they subsequently *perseverate*, that is, continue to use a sorting criterion that is no longer operative. This pattern of findings is not consistent with the notion that the prefrontal cortex is specifically involved in the memory aspect of the task.

On the other hand, this does not mean that patients with prefrontal damage perform perfectly well in standard memory tasks. They do well at some, but not others. They perform normally in recall of stories or nonverbal diagrams. And they learn verbal paired associates as well as normal control subjects. These findings stand in marked contrast to the typically poor performance of amnesic subjects on the same paired associate learning tasks. By contrast, frontal patients perform poorly on other variants of memory tasks. For example, by contrast to their success in initial verbal paired associate learning, they are inordinately sensitive to proactive interference in learning paired associates composed of different pairings of the same target works. Frontal patients also perform poorly in "meta-memory," self-assessments of whether they feel they could recognize verbal memory items they cannot recall. Yet they perform just as well as normal subjects in the accuracy of recall of the same word items. Similarly, frontal patients do poorly in recalling the situation in which they learned correctly recalled materials. This deficit in "source memory" has been viewed as reflecting a deficit in memory for the context of learned items.

Another potentially related area of memory impairment in patients with prefrontal damage is a difficulty in remembering temporal order of recent events. In one study, patients were presented with a long series of cards in rapid succession, each card bearing two line drawings. Some cards also contained question marks, requiring the subject to indicate which of the two items had appeared more recently. In some cases both items had appeared earlier, but at different times in the sequence. In other cases one item has appeared before and the other item was new. Frontal patients could recognize the earlier-appearing items but could not identify their order. By contrast, patients with temporal lobe damage could identify the ordering of old items but showed impairments in recognizing new items, consistent with the typical pattern in amnesia. In another study, subjects were presented with a list of 15 words and were subsequently asked to reconstruct the order in which they appeared. Frontal patients performed poorly in replicating the presented order, but performed relatively well in recall and recognition of presented words. This pattern of deficits has led to the view that the fundamental deficit in humans with prefrontal damage is an inability to inhibit irrelevant information. Such a deficit could account straightforwardly for their difficulties on the Wisconsin Card Sorting and other tasks that require switching one's attention, and could underlie the impairments in source and meta-memory, as well as problem solving and temporal ordering, to the extent that performance on such tasks requires inhibiting irrelevant cognitive strategies.

The role of the prefrontal cortex in problem solving and memory in monkeys

Deficits in short-term memory following damage to the prefrontal cortex have been highlighted since the pioneering studies of Jacobsen and his colleagues in the 1930s. These studies focused on the delayed response task, a variant of the "shell game" in which the monkey views a reward being hidden under one of two plaques, then after a memory delay, must choose the location of the reward (see Fig. 5–1D). The specific demand for short-term memory was emphasized in an experiment where poor performance after prefrontal lesions was observed in delayed response, but not in a visual pattern discrimination task using the same stimuli.

Patricia Goldman-Rakic has shown that the deficit following damage to the dorsolateral prefrontal cortex is observed only when there is both a spatial and a memory component of the task. Other deficits in short-term memory, and sometimes in other types of learning, are observed after damage to different areas of the prefrontal cortex in monkeys. Most prominent among these are selective deficits associated with damage to three of the key areas of prefrontal cortex. Damage to the dorsolateral area produces a severe deficit in spatial delayed response and in the related spatial delayed alternation task where the food is hidden in the left and right locations on alternate trials. No deficits are observed on object alternation (choosing one of two objects on alternate trials), discrimination, or delayed nonmatch to sample, or a variety of other tasks with no spatial memory requirement. By contrast, damage to the lateral prefrontal cortex does not result in severe deficits in spatial delayed response or delayed alternation, but does produce severe impairments in object alternation and delayed nonmatch to sample. Damage to the orbital prefrontal area produces deficits in olfactory, taste, visual, and auditory discriminations and especially in discrimination reversal learning; orbital lesions also result in emotional disorders. These data are consistent with the heterogeneity of prefrontal connections, and with the proposal that areas of the prefrontal cortex may be distinct in the modality of information they process in memory.

More recent studies on the neuropsychology of prefrontal function in monkeys have expanded on these early findings, suggesting a broader role for the prefrontal cortex in cognition as observed in humans. For example, in one recent study by Angela Roberts and her colleagues, monkeys with lateral or orbital prefrontal lesions were trained on a variant of the attention switching tasks described before. In this experiment animals learned to discriminate compound visual stimuli each composed of a polygon and a curved line (Fig. 13–2). In the preliminary discrimination they

A.   compound discrimination

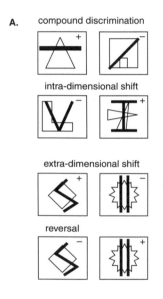

B.

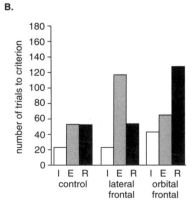

Figure 13–2. Attentional shift protocol. *A:* Examples of stimuli used in testing in each stage of training. The large polygon is the relevant dimension in all but the extradimensional shift and reversal conditions. *B:* Performance of monkeys with lateral or orbital prefrontal lesions on intradimensional shift (I), extradimensional shift (E), and reversal (R) conditions (data from Dias et al., 1996).

had to attend to one dimension (e.g., the polygon) and ignore the other (the line). Then they learned other discrimination problems: first, one involving an *intradimensional shift* (discrimination between new polygons, ignoring new lines); then one involving an *extradimensional shift* (discrimination between new lines, ignoring the new polygons; and, finally, a *reversal* of the last problem (where the reward assignments were switched for the same stimuli). Neither lesion affected performance on the intradimensional shift problem. Monkeys with lateral lesions were impaired on the extradimensional shift problem, but not on its reversal. Monkeys with orbital prefrontal lesions showed the opposite pattern—they were unimpaired on the extradimensional shift, but impaired on its reversal. These results indicate selective impairments after different prefrontal lesions not within the same visual modality, but associated with different cognitive demands. The lateral prefrontal region seems to be essential for switching the relevant visual perceptual dimension, whereas the orbital prefrontal area seems to be critical for reversing the affective association for the same stimuli.

Another recent study by Michael Petrides and his colleagues examined the capacity of monkeys with dorsolateral prefrontal lesions in working memory for temporal order. The key test for self-ordering involved presentations of three distinct objects on three successive trials each day. On the first trial all the objects were baited, and any could be selected to obtain a reward. After a 10-second delay the same objects were again presented with their positions randomized, and the initially selected item was not rebaited, so the subject was required to choose one of the remaining objects to obtain a second reward. On the third trial, the objects were again randomly rearranged, and the monkey had to select the remaining object. Monkeys with dorsolateral prefrontal lesions were impaired on this self-ordering task. They do no better when the same stimuli are presented one at a time during the first two trials, that is, when the stimuli are externally ordered. However, the same monkeys perform well on delayed object alternation (as observed following dorsolateral lesions in the above described studies), and a variant of the task showed that the central difference involved in the ordering task and delayed alternation is the number of stimuli that had to be remembered. In one more test, Petrides showed that the same monkeys could readily learn to appropriately select objects presented repeatedly in the same order, that is, in a task not requiring the monitoring of order in working memory. These findings demonstrate a strong parallel with the studies showing temporal ordering deficits in human patients with prefrontal damage, and suggest a common mechanism in strategic processing functions of the prefrontal area in humans and monkeys.

A similar role for the prefrontal cortex in rodents?

Other neuropsychological studies have provided parallel evidence of functionally heterogeneous areas in the prefrontal cortex of rats, suggesting these mechanisms of prefrontal function are common in mammalian evolution. Bryan Kolb reviewed the anatomical and behavioral evidence on rodent prefrontal areas, and concluded there are substantial similarities between rats and monkeys in the connections between the medial prefrontal area and spatial cortical areas, and between the orbital prefrontal area and subcortical limbic structures. The findings from neuropsychological investigations also suggest substantial similarities across species in the functions of these areas. Damage to the medial prefrontal area in rats results in deficits in spatial alternation, spatial working memory on the radial maze task, and impairments in the Morris water maze. These data indicate the rodent medial prefrontal area is involved in spatial memory performance similar to dorsolateral prefrontal involvement in spatial functions in monkeys. Notably, the poor performance in the water maze has been attributed to poor navigational strategies rather than memory *per se*, consistent with the findings from studies on human spatial working memory. A recent study showed that rats with medial prefrontal lesions normally acquired the water maze when trained from a single starting point, and accommodated successfully to finding the escape platform from a second location. However, they were impaired when the number of starting positions exceeded two, a finding reminiscent of Petrides's findings on object working memory in monkeys.

Also consistent with the findings on monkeys and humans, damage to the prefrontal cortex results in impairments in attention switching and temporal ordering. David Olton and colleagues trained rats to time each of two stimuli either independently or simultaneously by varying the rate at which they press a bar in anticipation of rewards delivered at different fixed intervals after each stimulus. Lesions of the prefrontal cortex severely disrupted performance on this task, consistent with an impairment in dividing or switching attention between two processing events. Hippocampal lesions do not impair performance on this divided attention task. In contrast, hippocampal lesions produce amnesia in a variant of the timing task where a gap is inserted in the timing procedure, whereas prefrontal lesions did not affect memory in the gap procedure. Thus, as in the previously described studies in monkeys, prefrontal damage results in a deficit in "executive" function, not memory, and hippocampal lesions result in the opposite pattern.

In addition, Raymond Kesner and colleagues have performed a series of experiments demonstrating that medial prefrontal lesions result in deficits in temporal ordering in rats. In experiments similar in design to those used with monkeys, rats were trained to enter arms on a radial maze to obtain rewards. On each trial, they were first allowed to visit each of four arms in a predetermined sequence for that day. Then they were give one of two types of memory tests. In the test for order they were presented with a choice of the first and second, or second and third, or third and fourth presented arms, with the contingency that another reward could be obtained in the arm that was presented earlier that day. Alternatively, they were presented with one of the arms that had been visited that day and another arm that was not presented in that trial. Animals were trained on the task preoperatively and retested after medial prefrontal lesions. They performed well on both tests preoperatively, but very poorly on the order test after surgery. They performed well when tested on recognition of the first arm presented on each day, but were impaired on subsequently presented arms. Thus, like monkeys with dorsolateral lesions, rats with medial prefrontal lesions are more severely impaired on order memory than on recognition. Unlike the monkeys in Petrides's study, the rats with medial prefrontal lesions remained impaired on order memory even when the same ordering was presented each day. However, the dissociation between order and recognition memory was more striking—these animals were completely unimpaired in recognizing repeatedly presented arms. In addition, Kolb documented several reports of medial prefrontal damage resulting in disruption of species-specific behavioral patterns including food hoarding, nest building, and maternal and sexual behavior. Kolb interpreted these findings as reflecting a general deficit in the temporal organization of behavioral sequences.

Several studies have demonstrated behavioral abnormalities in emotion and response inhibition after orbital prefrontal lesions in rats similar to those observed in monkeys. Furthermore, some studies have uncovered specific dissociations of function in medial and orbital lesions in rats similar to those seen in monkeys. Perhaps the most striking example comes from a double dissociation of the effects of selective prefrontal lesions on performance in spatial delayed alternation and olfactory discrimination. Preoperatively, all animals were trained on spatial delayed alternation in a standard Y-maze, and on a two-odor discrimination problem that involved a go/no-go response contingency (where the animal executed a response to one stimulus and inhibited that response to the other stimulus). Postoperatively, all animals were retrained on those tasks plus one more odor discrimination problem. Rats with medial prefrontal lesions were severely impaired on spatial delayed alternation, similar to the findings from several earlier studies, and were not impaired in retention or acquisition of odor discriminations (Fig. 13–3A). Rats with orbital prefrontal lesions showed the opposite pattern of effects, no deficit in reacquisition of the spatial delayed alternation, but severe impairment in both retention and acquisition of odor discriminations (Fig. 13–3B).

Subsequent analyses focused on the nature of the impairments and the perseverative tendencies in both tasks. In the spatial alternation task perseverative errors were measured as repetitive responses made during correction trials given following selection of the incorrect arm. This analysis showed that rats with medial prefrontal lesions made substantially more perseverative errors in the spatial alternation task than controls or rats with orbital prefrontal lesions. The analysis of perseveration in the odor discrimination task involved a replication of the previously described experiment, but with the addition of a symmetrical reward contingency by which animals were rewarded for correct go and no-go responses. Under these conditions intact rats showed relatively little overall bias toward go

A. spatial alteration

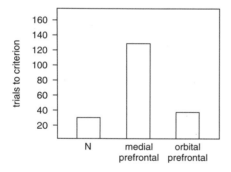

B. olfactory discrimination

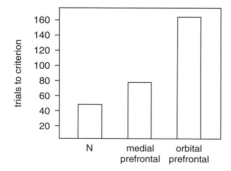

Figure 13–3. Double dissociation of areas of the rat prefrontal cortex. *A:* Performance of normal control rats (N) and rats with lesions of the medial prefrontal cortex or orbital prefrontal cortex on spatial delayed alternation. *B:* Performance of the same animals on a set of odor discrimination problems (data from Eichenbaum et al., 1983).

or no-go responses. Rats with orbital prefrontal lesions were again severely impaired, but the deficit was not attributable to a shift in their response bias. In addition, rats with orbital lesions showed an increased level of repetitive responses for both the go and no-go response types, showing that their impairment was associated with a general tendency to perseverate the last rewarded response. This pattern of findings shows that the different deficits associated with medial and orbital lesions can be characterized as modality-specific perseveration.

The scope of the deficit in olfactory guided learning following damage to the orbital prefrontal cortex in rodents has recently been extended by demonstrations of impairments in acquisition and performance of delayed nonmatch to sample, and conditional discrimination learning. In the odor-guided delayed nonmatch to sample task described in detail in Chapter 7, unlike hippocampal and parahippocampal cortical lesions, damage to the orbital prefrontal cortex results in a deficit in acquisition of the task even with brief memory delays. Conversely, unlike parahippocampal lesions, orbital prefrontal lesions resulted in no subsequent deficit in forgetting at extended delays. Rats with orbital prefrontal lesions were impaired, however, when the pool of repeating odor cues was reduced, that is, under conditions of increased inter-item interference. This pattern of results indicates once more that the effects of prefrontal and hippocampal lesions on performance in working memory tasks are quite different, and that the effects of prefrontal lesions are less attributable to a memory deficit *per se*, than to an impairment in strategic functions subject to interference.

Gordon Winocur reached a similar conclusion based on his studies that compared the effects of medial prefrontal and hippocampal lesions. Animals were tested on a delayed matching to sample task that required them to respond differentially to sample and choice lights that were of the same or different brightness. Normal rats performed the task very well and their accuracy declined only slightly as the memory delay was increased. Rats with prefrontal lesions were impaired at the matching judgment even with the shortest delay, but their accuracy declined over delays at the same rate as that of controls. By contrast, rats with hippocampal lesions performed normally at the shortest memory delay, whereas their performance across delays declined abnormally rapidly. These results suggested that the prefrontal cortex was essential to the working memory requirement for briefly remembering and matching the stimuli, whereas the hippocampus was essential to the maintenance of the stimulus representation.

Finally, Ian Whishaw and colleagues reported a severe impairment in conditional odor–tactile discrimination following orbital prefrontal lesions in rats. In this study rats were trained on a set of four discrimination problems between compound stimuli. The correct choice for each problem was a particular combination of two stimulus elements, although each element was individually equally often rewarded. The findings in this study parallel the findings from studies on humans and monkeys, showing that under conditions of high interference, the prefrontal cortex plays a critical role in learning stimulus–stimulus associations.

How information for working memory is encoded within the prefrontal cortex

In the early 1970s neurophysiologists began to study the activity of neurons in monkeys performing the delayed-response task. A large network of neurons was activated as animals performed each of the relevant task events. Some cells fired associated with presentation of the left or right cue in both the sample and choice periods, and subsequent work has shown that prefrontal neurons show considerable selectivity for visual and spatial properties of memory cues across a variety of working memory tasks. Moreover, many prefrontal neurons begin to fire upon presentation of the sample item or when it disappears, and many of these cells continued to fire throughout the ensuing delay period. These "delay cells" number half the recorded neurons in the prefrontal cortex and have received the most attention because they provided the first evidence of neuronal activity specifically involved in storing a short-term memory.

Recent studies have focused on the delay cells, using an oculomotor version of the delayed-response task developed by Goldman-Rakic and her colleagues (Fig. 13–4A). In this paradigm monkeys are trained to fixate a central spot on a display, and to maintain fixation while a target at one of eight locations is briefly illuminated. Following a delay period when the target must be remembered, the monkey then moved its eyes very rapidly (making what is called a "saccade") to the location of the former target to obtain a reward. In this variation of the delayed-response task, the prefrontal cortex is critical to memory, and this paradigm allowed a dissection of the topography of spatial memory in this cortical area. In a key experiment monkeys were trained to perform the task and then given small unilateral lesions of the dorsolateral prefrontal cortex. Subsequently, their performance was measured for each of the eight target locations, both in the memory task and in a simple task where the target stimulus was on at the time of the saccadic eye movement, eliminating the need for spatial memory. The lesions had no effect on eye movements in the nonmemory task, but resulted in poor delay-dependent performance within a spatially restricted region during the memory task. Furthermore, the deficit was re-

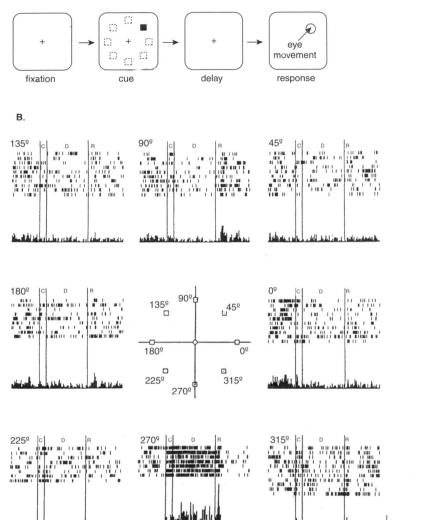

Figure 13–4. The oculomotor delayed-response task. *A:* The task protocol. Initially the animal fixates its eyes on a central cross-hair. Then a light flashes at one of eight positions, followed by a blank delay period when the animal must maintain fixated. Then, when the fixation cross-hairs turn off, the animal saccades to the locus where the cue was flashed. *B:* Responses of a prefrontal neuron during the cue (C), delay (D), and response (R) periods of the task when the cue was presented at different loci. Note selective response when the cue was at 270 degrees, and signs of inhibited activity when the cue was presented at 90 degrees (from Funahashi et al., 1989).

stricted to a portion of the contralateral visual field, and the magnitude of error in eye movements was minimal at short delays and greater at longer delays. These data provided the first evidence of a "mnemonic scotoma," a "blindness" in memory for a specific region of visual space.

Correspondingly, recordings made from prefrontal neurons in intact monkeys performing this task revealed that the majority of delay cells fired selectively while the animal was remembering a stimulus presented in a particular part of visual space (Fig. 13–4B). The average area of space where excitatory activity was observed was about 45 degrees, and most cells preferred the contralateral part of space, consistent with the findings in the lesion study. In addition, some cells showed distinct inhibitory activity for the direction opposite the preferred direction, suggesting a network mechanism for sharpening the spatial memory signal. Delay cells fired only on trials when a correct saccade was produced, indicating their activity reflected the maintenance of the spatial memory. Subsequent analyses showed that most of these cells maintained the memory of the target location, rather than firing in anticipation of the incipient response. To test this question directly, monkeys were trained in both the standard version of the task and an "antisaccade" version of the task where the monkey was required to move its eyes to the opposite location from where the spatial target had been illuminated. About 80% of the delay cells with directional activity fired during memory for a particular target stimulus location regardless of the direction of the subsequent response. The remaining 20% of the directional delay cells fired associated with the incipient direction of the saccade, indicating the prefrontal cortex also contains information about the intended response.

Reinforcing the view that the prefrontal cortex contains a specialized temporary store, Earl Miller and colleagues compared the capacity of prefrontal and temporal neurons in maintaining selective visual codings during the delay in monkeys performing a matching to sample task. A greater fraction of temporal cells showed selective responses to visual features, but the delay-related activity of these cells ceased abruptly when intervening stimuli were presented. Prefrontal cells that encoded specific visual features were not as prevalent, but these cells maintained elevated stimulus-specific activity throughout a delay filled with intervening stimuli.

A central current question about delay activity in the prefrontal cortex is whether there is regional parcellation of memory storage functions. Particularly striking evidence in favor of this view came from a study by Goldman-Rakic and colleagues in which monkeys were trained on two variants of the delayed-response task. One version was the standard oculomotor spatial delayed-response task, although only right and left target locations were employed. The other version was a visual pattern delayed-response task where one of two elaborate visual stimuli was presented at the central fixation point, and then after the delay the monkey was required to make a left or right saccade depending on which pattern was the sample cue. Neurons in the lateral prefrontal area were particularly responsive in the pattern delayed-response task, such that over three-quarters of the delay cells differentially fired associated with one visual cue. Some of these cells showed highly selective delay responses, such as cells that fired selectively associated with one of two faces, but did not differentiate two other visual patterns. The opposite result was obtained for cells in the dorsolateral prefrontal cortex, such that most delay cells fired selectively in the spatial task and not in the pattern task. The combination of these findings has been interpreted as strong support for the notion that there exist distinct working memory parcellations in the prefrontal cortex, one in the dorsolateral prefrontal area supporting spatial working memory and another in the lateral area supporting visual pattern working memory.

There are such considerable differences between working memory tasks used across species and in different laboratories that it is currently impossible to reach a conclusion about the nature of division of functions within the prefrontal cortex. Consistencies in the data across techniques and species implicate prefrontal processing as more "strategic" than "memory," even though there are also considerable data showing extensive intermixing of executive and storage functions in working memory. While a resolution of the functional mechanism of prefrontal cortex remains elusive, new studies on prefrontal neurons in monkeys performing novel working are providing insights that may supersede notions about division of function by modality or cognitive processing.

In one study Miller and his colleagues trained monkeys on a variant of the delayed matching to sample task in which subjects were shown a sample object stimulus at the central fixation point, then after a memory delay were shown that object plus another object choice at peripheral locations, then after another memory delay had to saccade to the location of the matching stimulus item (Fig. 13–5A). Thus, the monkeys had to remember two aspects of the sample object. During the initial delay they had to retain the visual content properties, or the "what" quality of the stimulus. Then in the second delay they had to retain the location where the object was again presented, that is, its "where" quality. Neurons in the lateral prefrontal area responded to the "what" and "where" qualities of objects. One example, shown in Fig. 13–5B (left), fired more to one particular object during the initial "what" delay. The example Fig. 13–5B

A. "what" then "where" task

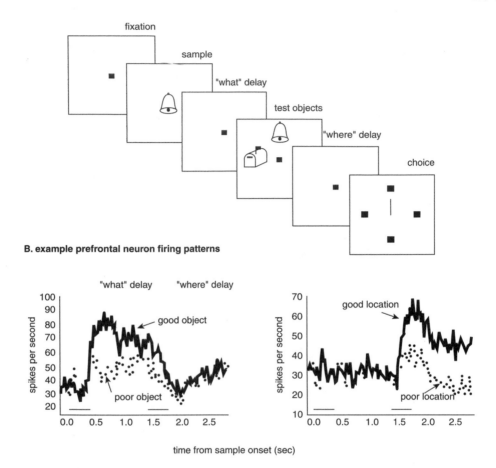

B. example prefrontal neuron firing patterns

time from sample onset (sec)

Figure 13–5. The "what" and "where" task. *A:* Sequence of trial stages in the protocol. After initial fixation, a sample stimulus is shown in the center. Then, after a delay, two choice stimuli are shown and the animal must saccade to the one that is the same as the sample. Then, following another delay, the animal must saccade to the location where the sample was last shown. *B:* Examples of object-tuned (left) and location-tuned (right) cells (from Rao et al., 1997).

(right) fired during the "where" delay more associated with location where the sample reappeared, regardless of which object was remembered. Yet other cells encoded both the "what" and "where" attributes, and fired either selectively both during the "what" and "where" delays, or fired maximally during the final delay associated with the combination of a particular object and a particular place it was presented. These data indicate that cells in the same area of the prefrontal cortex can represent both visual and spatial information when demanded by the task requirements.

The prefrontal cortex may also be especially suited to retrieving and utilizing representations of associations in memory. In another study, neurons in the prefrontal cortex were recorded in monkeys who were initially presented with a sample visual stimulus and then, after a delay, had to identify an arbitrarily paired stimulus associate from multiple choices. During the sample stimulus presentation, and partially into the memory delay, the activity of prefrontal neurons was selective for the characteristics of the sample stimulus. However, toward the end of the delay, and prior to presentation of the choice stimuli, prefrontal neurons altered their activity associated with the characteristics of the appropriate stimulus associate. These findings suggest that prefrontal neurons may have access to long-term stored representations of visual as well as spatial associations, and employ them in sequence following the demands of the task.

The prefrontal cortex is activated in humans performing working memory tasks

The emergence of brain imaging techniques has allowed investigators to examine the areas of cortex activated during working memory performance in human subjects. Among the first of these studies, John Jonides, Edward Smith, and their colleagues characterized areas of the human brain activated during a variant of the spatial delayed response task. In this task subjects fixated a central point on a computer monitor and were presented with three dots as target sample stimuli. Following a 3-second delay period, a circle marked one location on the screen where one of the targets had appeared, or another location. Thus, subjects had to remember a set of target locations and later identify a choice item as one of the set. The control task was similar, except that the three dots were presented only during the end of the delay then during the choice period when one of them was circled, so that responses were guided by perception not memory. The brain areas prominently activated by positron emission tomography (PET) included all the components of the working memory circuit outlined in monkeys, but all on the right side of the human brain. These included the dorsolateral prefrontal cortex, the posterior parietal area, plus parts of the occipital and premotor areas. Confirming these findings, a neighboring area of dorsolateral prefrontal cortex was activated in a functional magnetic resonance imaging (fMRI) study when subjects were required to identify repetitions of stimuli among a series of items presented at various spatial locations.

In humans, of course, one can examine the very same verbal and visuospatial working memory processes that were the focus of the Baddeley model, and indeed there is evidence for the existence of distinct areas that mediate the visuospatial sketch pad and the phonological loop. Tasks that require subjects to rehearse verbal material activate a part of the parietal cortex, whereas different parietal areas are activated during visuo-spatial processing. All tasks that require working memory activate prefrontal areas. In addition, parts of the prefrontal cortex are especially strongly activated when subjects are required to update verbal information, consistent with the putative role of this area as the central executive.

There is considerable agreement that different posterior cortical areas are activated during modality-specific working memory processing. On the other hand, there is considerable controversy over whether different kinds of processing are parcellated within the prefrontal cortex, and about the nature of parcellation. One study by Smith and colleagues, directly modeled after the work on monkeys, examined this issue with the "three-back" task designed to test working memory for spatial or verbal material. In both versions of the task, on a series of trials subjects fixate a central location and are presented with a series of letters at a peripheral site, with one letter presented each trial with blank presentations intervening (Fig. 13–6). In the spatial memory condition, on each trial the subject must identify whether the target on the current trial matches in location the item presented three trials back, and must ignore the identity of the letters. In the verbal memory condition, the subject, conversely, must identify whether the current letter matches the identity of the letter presented three trials back, ignoring the location of presentations. Thus, the stimulus presentations in both tasks are identical, but the memory demands differ according to a spatial or verbal rule. The findings indicated a clear dissociation of brain regions involved in the two tasks. In the spatial task there was more activation on the right hemisphere, and included both a posterior parietal and a prefrontal site of most prominent activation. Conversely, the verbal task activated primarily parietal and prefrontal areas in the left hemisphere. This dissociation is consistent with clinical observations of selective spatial and verbal working memory deficits following damage to the right and left prefrontal cortex, respectively.

A separate set of PET studies by Petrides and colleagues modeled after experiments on self-ordering and conditional learning in monkeys, examined whether these cognitive operations could be dissociated in human brain activations. In one of these studies, subjects either performed the self-ordering task described earlier, or a conditional visual-motor response task in which subjects had to point to a different design assigned to each

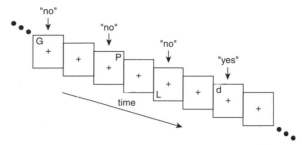

A. spatial memory condition

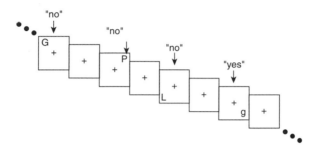

B. verbal memory condition

Figure 13–6. An example series of trials on each of two versions of the three-back task (from Jonides and Smith, 1997).

of a set of distinct color stimuli. Consistent with his studies on monkeys with selective prefrontal lesions, Petrides found that a middorsolateral part of the prefrontal cortex was selectively activated in the self-ordering task, whereas a premotor area was selectively activated in the conditional visual-motor task. In another study Petrides found that the same middorsolateral area is selectively activated in a verbal self-ordering task, showing the generality of function of this area over nonverbal and verbal stimulus materials. There was some degree of hemispheric lateralization consistent with the study described previously. In the nonverbal self-ordering task the right prefrontal area was differentially activated, whereas in the verbal task both hemispheres were equally activated.

In additional studies, Petrides and colleagues directly addressed potential distinctions between the dorsolateral and lateral areas of the human prefrontal cortex. These studies examined strategic retrieval from long-term memory for verbal and visuospatial materials. In the study on verbal strategic retrieval, Petrides scanned subjects performing different verbal recall tasks. In one task, subjects were required to recall a list of unrelated words, a task well acknowledged to depend on active retrieval mechanisms. To control specifically for strategic monitoring of the words that had been recalled, as opposed to the search in long-term memory *per se*, they compared the activation during word list retrieval with that during a control condition in which subjects produced correct responses in a previously well-learned verbal paired associate task. The latter task is much less demanding on active retrieval processes, but involves the same degree of self-monitoring. They found that indeed the left dorsolateral area was equally activated in both tasks, but the lateral prefrontal area was more activated in the list retrieval task. In the study on visuospatial strategic retrieval, subjects were trained to touch each of a set of displayed boxes on a screen, with each box touched as a nearby indicator light was illuminated. The sequence of indicated boxes was the same on each trial, so subjects reduced their reaction times over the course of training. This initially involved implicit learning, because the subjects could not generate the sequence explicitly. However, explicit training was then given by requiring subjects to touch each box in anticipation of the indicator.

Following training on this condition the subjects were scanned in both conditions of the task. Activity in the right lateral prefrontal area was greater in the explicit condition than in the implicit condition, consistent with the interpretation that only the explicit sequencing required active retrieval of the stored sequence. The combination of all these findings led Petrides to propose that the prefrontal cortex is parcellated, not according to different stimulus materials as Goldman-Rakic has argued, but rather according to the cognitive processing demands. Petrides argues that both verbal and nonverbal strategic ordering processes are reflected in selective activation of the dorsolateral prefrontal cortex, whereas strategic retrieval from long-term memory for both verbal and nonverbal materials selectively activates the lateral prefrontal cortical area. Notably, however, there are clear hemispheric differences in Petrides's findings on verbal and visuospatial materials, consistent with the proposal of Smith and colleagues. On the other hand, there are also considerable data showing hemispheric differences in the prefrontal cortex based on cognitive demands associated with long-term memory encoding and retrieval processes, such that encoding in episodic memory for various materials is associated with enhanced activity in the left prefrontal cortex, whereas retrieval of various materials is associated with enhanced activity on the right side.

A recent meta-analysis of a large number of studies using brain imaging techniques to characterize prefrontal activation in working memory has generally sided with Petrides's view of parcellation by cognitive functions. In his analysis Adrian Owen found that spatial working memory tasks can activate either the dorsolateral or lateral prefrontal region, such that the lateral region was activated when the task demanded retention of one or a few items, whereas the dorsolateral region was activated when the subject was required to constantly monitor and manipulate a series of ongoing spatial locations. A generally similar pattern was found across studies on visual working memory. Tasks that required subjects only to retain visual pattern information over a delay did not activate the dorsolateral area, whereas tasks that required constant monitoring and updating did. Overall, Owen concluded that the dorsolateral region is activated when the demand for continuous monitoring is high regardless of the materials to be remembered.

The orchestration of memory: Parcellation of functions among cortical areas

While the prefrontal cortex plays a critical and central role in working with memory, a role akin to that of an orchestra conductor, there are also other players in the orchestra distributed in other areas of the cerebral cortex. Two recent studies have promoted the view that different cognitive demands contribute to a distribution of functional activations among cortical areas during working memory performance in humans.

Jonathan Cohen and colleagues used variants of the "*n*-back" task combined with rapid fMRI scans to compare regional activations as a function of differing demands for executive control in managing memory load versus maintenance over time. They trained subjects to match verbal stimuli to items presented previously under four different conditions. These included comparisons to items either one, two, or three items back, and a zero-back condition where a particular stimulus was identified whenever it was presented. Scans were made during and just after the stimulus presentation, and repeatedly during the 10-second delay between trials. Areas in both the left prefrontal cortex and posterior visual areas were activated, but the extent of activation differed under the controlled conditions (Fig. 13–7). Prefrontal cortex activation was maximal under high memory load conditions, that is in the two- and three-back tasks, and less so in the zero- and one-back tasks, and the level of activation was constant throughout the memory delay. Conversely, the visual areas were more activated late in the delay when the memory demand was highest, regardless of load. In addition the amount of activation in Broca's area was affected by both factors, with the greatest activation for the highest load at the longest memory delay. These data are consistent with the notion that working memory circuits are widespread in the cortex, and with the findings from earlier described neuropsychological studies across species showing that the pre-

A. prefrontal cortex and memory load

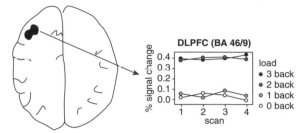

B. visual cortex and time

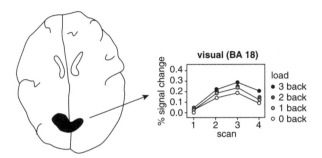

C.Broca's area and interaction of load and time

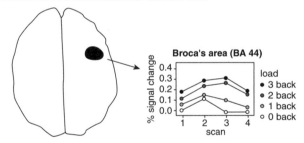

Figure 13–7. Activation of multiple brain areas during working memory. In each panel, the most activated brain area is shown, and the amount of activation is plotted over time during the memory delay and separately for the memory load zero, one, two, or three items. *A:* An area in the prefrontal cortex is activated more for higher memory load regardless of the delay. *B:* A visual area that is activated as the delay increased regardless of load. *C:* Broca's area is activated differentially associated with both the load and delay (data from Cohen et al., 1997).

frontal cortex is more involved in strategic processing associated with the number of items in memory, as opposed to storage of those items *per se*.

Another recent study by Courtney, Ungerleider, and their colleagues compared posterior and prefrontal cortical activations in humans performing a working task that required subjects to remember a face over a delay. They compared fMRI activations during presentations of face or visual "noise" stimulation, and during the memory delay between stimulus presentations. Responses of posterior and prefrontal cortical areas were characterized using complex statistical analyses aimed at three components of the task, transient nonselective visual responses, transient selective responses to faces, and sustained responses over the memory delay. They found that posterior visual cortical areas showed primarily transient nonselective or selective visual responses, whereas prefrontal areas exhibited strong delay responses plus face selectivity. Furthermore, the extent to which these factors activated areas throughout the cortex was graded, with the most posterior area responsive only nonselectively and without delay, and the most rostral prefrontal areas most responsive to delay with face selectivity. These findings again are consistent with the notion of widespread networks for working memory, with graded contributions of processing functions throughout the network.

In addition, recent studies of the firing patterns of single neurons in monkeys and rats have contributed to the view of a parcellation of functions in the prefrontal and posterior cortical areas during working memory. Miller and colleagues' studies on monkeys performing the visually cued working memory task described in Chapter 8 found that a greater proportion of cells in the lateral prefrontal region showed sustained responses during the delay, and conveyed more information about the match–nonmatch status of the test stimuli compared to perirhinal cortex. By contrast, more neurons in the perirhinal cortex and inferotemporal cortex show greater stimulus selectivity. Notably, in this task the memory delay was filled with interpolated material, which put a strong demand on working memory. By contrast, a study by Miyashita and Chang involved a visual recognition task where the memory delay was not filled with interpolated material, and they found that a large fraction of temporal neurons show sustained stimulus-specific delay activity. Similarly, in rats performing the continuous delayed nonmatch to sample task described in Chapter 7, it was found that more cells in the orbitofrontal area exhibited stimulus-selective match enhancement or suppression, whereas more cells in the parahippocampal region exhibited sustained stimulus-specific activity during the delay. This pattern of findings suggests that the posterior cortical areas play a strong role in encoding and maintaining sustained stimulus representations, and that the prefrontal cortex consistently plays a critical role in acquiring and employing the task rules as well as a variable role in maintaining stimulus representations depending on the demand for working memory.

Summing up

The prefrontal cortex performs a critical role in "working-with-memory" in rodents, monkeys, and humans. Most investigators regard its role as critical to working memory, the capacity to hold items and manipulate them in consciousness. The prefrontal cortex is parcellated into several distinct areas that have different inputs and whose functions can be dissociated according to different modalities of stimulus processing. However, they share common higher-order function in working memory and strategic processing, reflected in perseveration and other common strategic disorders following damage to any of the subdivisions.

Correspondingly, prefrontal neurons encode all events during working memory task performance, and large numbers of prefrontal cells are involved in maintaining item memories for brief periods and in encoding stimuli and events in accordance with acquired task rules. Prefrontal subdivisions are highly connected with one another and with posterior areas of the cortex to operate as a complex and widespread network for conscious control over memory and other intellectual functions.

READINGS

Baddeley, A. 1996. The fractionation of working memory. *Proc. Natl. Acad. Sci.* 93:13468–13472.

Cohen, J.D., Perlstein, W.M., Braver, T.S., Nystrom, L.E., Noll, D.C., Jonides, J., and Smith, E.E. 1997. Temporal dynamics of brain activation during a working memory task. *Nature* 386: 604–607.

Courtney, S.M., Ungerleider, L.G., Kell, K., and Haxby, J.V. 1997. Transient and sustained activity in a distributed neural system for human working memory. *Nature* 386: 608–611.

Eichenbaum, H. 2000. A cortical-hippocampal system for declarative memory. *Nat. Rev. Neurosci.* 1:41–50.

Goldman-Rakic, P.S. 1996. The prefrontal landscape: Implications of functional architecture for understanding human mentation and the central executive. *Phil. Trans. R. Soc. Lond. Ser. B*, 351: 1445–1453.

Jonides, J., Rugg, M.D. (Ed.) and Smith, E.E. 1997. The architecture of working memory. In *Cognitive Neuroscience*, Hove East Sussex: Psychology Press, pp. 243–276.

Kolb, B. 1990. Prefrontal cortex. In *The Cerebral Cortex of the Rat*, B. Kolb and R.C. Tees (Eds.). Cambridge: MIT Press, pp. 437–458.

Miller, E. The prefrontal cortex and cognitive control. *Nat. Rev. Neurosci* 1:59–65.

Owen, A.M. 1997. The functional organization of working memory processes within human lateral frontal cortex: The contribution of functional neuroimaging. *Eur. J. Neurosci.* 9:1329–1339.

Pandya, D.N., and Yeterian, E.H. 1996. Comparison of prefrontal architecture and connections. *Phil. Trans. R. Sec. Lond. B.* 351:1423–1432.

Roberts, A.C., Robbins, T.W., and Weiskrantz, L. (Eds.). 1996. Executive and cognitive functions of the prefrontal cortex. *Phil. Trans. Roy. Soc. Lond.* B351: 1387–1527.

Shimamura, A.P. 1995. Memory and frontal lobe function. In: *The Cognitive Neurosciences*, M.S. Gazzaniga (Ed.). Cambridge: MIT Press, pp. 803–813.

• • • • • •
Final Thoughts

Over a hundred years ago there was an amazing period of break-throughs in neuroscience, a Golden Era, in which major discoveries about the brain were made and during which the basic themes of memory research were generated. Recent decades have seen remarkable progress in clarifying questions raised in each of these themes, by elucidating the cellular bases for increased connectivity that underlies memory, by quali-fying the nature of different forms of cognition in memory, by showing how the different forms of memory are compartmentalized into distinct memory systems in the brain, and by providing an understanding of the processes that underlie memory consolidation. It should also be clear from this book that progress in understanding each of these themes is inter-twined, such that the elements that support alterations in connectivity and consolidation reflect a continuum of mechanisms and processes among the memory systems. Furthermore, the seamless experience of memory sug-gests that the different memory systems share information and work to-gether to mediate our sense of "autobiography," that is, the individuality of a lifetime of memories.

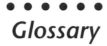

Glossary

Acetylcholine • One of the first discovered neurotransmitters, uses two major receptor subtypes, muscarinic and nicotinic.

Action potential • The active conduction of a depolarizing potential characteristic of axons. This potential is slower than electrotonic conduction but is faithful in magnitude over long distances. Its initiation and propagation involve an initial influx of sodium, then an outflow of potassium, and then a recovery period during which the cell is refractory to initiation of another action potential.

Adrenergic • Pertaining to the hormone adrenaline (also called epinephrine) or the neurotransmitter noradrenaline (norepinephrine). The two major subtypes of the neurotransmitter are α and β.

Agonist • A drug that facilitates or prolongs the action of a neurotransmitter, by enhancing its production, release, or persistence, or by triggering the receptors for that neurotransmitter.

Allocentric space • Position in the environment independent of the orientation or location of the subject.

Ammon's horn • A subdivision of the hippocampus that receives major inputs from the dentate gyrus and the parahippocampal region, and projects to the subiculum; composed of sequentially connected areas CA3 and CA1.

Amygdala • A complex set of nuclei located underneath the cortex and just anterior to the hippocampus in the temporal lobe. A critical component of the system for emotional learning and emotional expression, and for the modulation of memory consolidation by emotional state.

Antagonist • A drug that inhibits the action of a neurotransmitter, by retarding its production, release, or persistence, or by blocking the receptors for that neurotransmitter.

Anterior • Also called **rostral**. Toward the front of the brain.

Anterograde amnesia • Loss of the ability to acquire new information following head injury or brain damage.

AP5 • D-2-amino-5-phosphonovalerate. Selective and competitive antagonist of NMDA receptors.

Autonomic nervous system • Components of the peripheral nervous system that regulate various organs of the body including the heart, blood pressure, respiration, sweating, pupil dilation, digestion, and more.

Axon • The single long neuronal extension that conducts the action potential to the synapse.

Basal ganglia • Forebrain components of the extrapyramidal motor system that include the striatum.

Behavioral LTP • Changes in synaptic efficacy following and due to the formation of new memories.

Behaviorism • The view that all learned behaviors can be explained on the basis of elements of conditioned responses.

Bilateral • Pertaining to both sides of the brain.

Brain stem • Components of the brain that lie beneath the cortex and thalamus, typically in the midbrain or hindbrain.

Caudal • Towards thr rear of the brain.

Cell assembly • Hebb's notion of a local or diffuse circuit of connected neurons that develop to represent a specific percept and concepts.

Cerebellum • Major structure of the brain stem involved in motor control, a critical component of motor systems involved in conditioning of skeletal muscle responses. Major components include an outer cerebellar cortex composed of many folia and an inner complex of cerebellar nuclei.

Cerebral cortex • Structure on the outer surface of the brain, usually with six distinct layers, separated into major frontal, parietal, occipital, and temporal regions and many functionally distinct zones.

Classical conditioning (or conditioning) • The association of an arbitrary external stimulus (the conditioning stimulus, or CS) with another stimulus (the unconditioned stimulus, or US) that produces an unconditioned reflexive response (UR), resulting in the gradual acquisition of a conditioned response (CR) to the CS.

Cognitive map • A systematic representation of the topology of the physical environment.

Cognitivism • The view that the complexity of learned behavior requires consideration of capabilities for insight and planning, and cannot be explained by a combination of conditioned responses.

Conditioned reflex or conditioned response (CR) • Behavioral response arising from the association between an arbitrary external stimulus (the conditioned stimulus, or CS) and an unconditioned stimulus (US) that evokes a reflexive unconditioned response (UR).

Consolidation • The process by which initially labile memories become permanent and impervious to disruption. Separated into a molecular/celluar process of fixation of a memory trace that occurs for several minutes after learning, and a prolonged period of reorganization of memories mediated by interactions between structures of the declarative memory system.

Contralateral • Opposite side of the head or body. The alternative is ipsilateral, on the same side of the body.

Cortical column ● Functional and anatomical organization in the cortex by which closely connected and functionally similar cells are arranged vertically across layers into parallel columns. For example, in the primary visual cortex of higher mammals, there are alternating columns for ocular dominance and orientation selectivity.

"Cued" learning ● A term often used to describe learning guided by a single simple or complex stimulus, as contrasted with spatial learning that involves spatial relations among multiple cues. Synonymous with "nonspatial" learning.

Cytoarchitecture ● The types and arrangement of cells that characterize each brain area, and each distinct area of the cerebral cortex.

Deafferentation ● Disconnection of inputs.

Declarative memory ● Everyday memory for facts and events that are subject to conscious recollection and can be explicitly expressed in many ways outside the conditions of original learning. The combination of episodic and semantic memory.

Delay conditioning ● The standard version of classical conditioning where the conditioning stimulus (CS) is presented continuously until and through the presentation of the unconditioned stimulus (US).

Delayed alternation ● A task in which the subject must alternate between two conditions or stimuli to obtain rewards. In delayed spatial alternation, the subject alternates between two spatial directions or locations.

Delayed nonmatch to sample (DNMS) ● A task in which the subject must remember the identity of a stimulus across a delay period when no cues are present. Typically divided into three phases: a sample phase when the subject views the stimulus but cannot respond, a delay phase when the stimulus cannot be seen, and a choice phase when the subject must select an alternative stimulus to obtain a reward. Typical variants involve whether a small number of stimuli are used repeated across trials or unique stimuli are used on each trial, and the "delayed match to sample" version where during the choice phase the subject must select the sample stimulus and not the alternative to obtain the reward.

Delayed response ● A task in which the subject must remember the position of a reward across a delay period when no cues are present. Typically divided into three phases: a sample phase when the subject views the location of the reward but cannot respond, a delay phase when no spatial cues are provided to identify the reward location, and a choice phase when the subject is allowed to select the location of the hidden reward.

Dendrite ● One of several multiple fine processes that extend the neuron cell body that receives neural signals from other neurons.

Depolarization ● Change in the polarity of the cell membrane such that the inside of the cell becomes more positive relative to the outside, as compared to the resting state.

Discrimination learning ● Tasks in which the subject is presented with multiple (usually two) stimuli and must consistently select one of them and not the other to obtain a reward. Variants include simultaneous discrimination when all the stimuli are presented at the same time on each trial versus successive discrimination when only one stimulus is presented on each trial and the stimuli are presented in a random sequence.

Dorsal • Toward the top of the brain.

Double dissociation • The observation that damage to brain structure A, but not structure B, results in impairment on task X, but not task Y, while damage to brain structure B and not structure A results in impairment on task Y and not task X.

Effector • Brain structures that directly control muscle or hormonal responses.

Egocentric space • Position in the environment relative to the orientation and location of the body, e.g., left or right. Note the egocentric positions of fixed objects will change as the subject moves through space.

Electrotonic conduction • The passive conduction of a potential difference (depolarizing or hyperpolarizing) along any part of the neuron. It is fast but decremental, dissipating over a short distance.

Emotional memory • An unconsciously expressed, acquired aversion or attraction toward a previously arbitrary stimulus.

Entorhinal cortex • A subdivision of the parahippocampal region, the region closest to the hippocampus, which has the greatest connections with it.

Episodic memory • Representations of specific personal experiences that occur in a unique spatial and temporal context, typically involving the capacity to reexperience particular events in one's life by conscious recollection.

Excitatory postsynaptic potential (EPSP) • Depolarizing electrical potential created at the postsynaptic site of *excitatory synapses* as a result of neurotransmitter recognition, usually due to the influx of sodium.

Explicit memory • Memory expression based on conscious recollection involving direct efforts to access memories.

Exteroceptive • Reception of stimulus information from the external world.

Extramaze • Pertaining to the environment outside of a maze.

Fear conditioning • The acquired association between an arbitrary, conditioned, external stimulus and a natural, fear-producing, unconditioned stimulus. The most common example is the association between a tone and shock to the feet. Often categorized into "cued" fear conditioning, when the relevant conditioned stimulus is a punctate stimulus that has a close temporal association with the unconditioned stimulus (e.g., presentation of a tone just before the shock), and "contextual" fear conditioning, referring to acquired association between the static environmental context, typically the testing chamber, and the shock or other unconditioned stimulus.

Fear-potentiated startle • Magnification of the startle response when animals or people are in a fearful state.

Field EPSP • The summed excitatory postsynaptic potentials from many simultaneously activated synapses.

Fornix • A major axon bundle that connects the hippocampus with several subcortical areas including the hypothalamus, thalamus, septum, and brain stem. Likely carries nonspecific information that modulates the arousal and paces the processing rhythm of the hippocampus.

Gene expression • The cascade of molecular processes involving reading the DNA sequence, mediated via RNA, to direct new protein synthesis.

Go/no-go • A response modality in which subjects make an active movement (go) under one condition or to one stimulus, and make no response (no-go) under an alternative condition or to another stimulus.

Habit • An acquired and well-practiced response to a particular stimulus.

Habituation • The decrement in responsiveness to repeated sensory stimulation without reinforcement.

Hebb rule • Hebb proposed that increases in synaptic strength result from the combination of repeated activation of a presynaptic element and its participation in the success in firing the postsynaptic cell.

Hippocampus • Structure in the medial temporal lobe involved in declarative memory. Composed of distinct subdivisions, including Ammon's horn (CA1 and CA3), the dentate gyrus, and the subiculum.

H.M. • The patient who suffered a highly selective and severe global amnesia following bilateral removal of the medial temporal lobe region.

Hyperpolarization • Change in the polarity of the cell membrane such that the inside of the cell becomes more negative relative to the outside, as compared to the resting state.

Implicit memory • Unconscious changes in performance of a task as influenced by some previous experience, typically revealed by indirect measures such as changes in the speed of performance or in biases in choices made while reperforming a task.

Inferential memory expression • The capacity to deduce solutions to novel problems based on indirect relations among items retrieved from distinct memories.

Inferotemporal cortex • Cortical area of the lateral and inferior temporal lobe that is involved in higher-order visual pattern recognition.

Inhibitory postsynaptic potential (IPSP) • Hyperpolarizing electrical potential created at the postsynaptic site of *inhibitory synapses* as a result of neurotransmitter recognition, usually due to the influx of chloride.

Intermediate term memory • A period that follows short-term or working memory, but involves representations that are not yet permanently stored.

Intramaze • Pertaining to local stimuli available inside a maze.

Ionotropic receptor • Conventional neurotransmitter receptors found in postsynaptic elements that are transmitter-gated and allow charged molecules to flow briefly inducing the postsynaptic excitatory and inhibitory potentials.

Law of effect • Principle by which behaviors that lead to a positive reinforcement are more likely to reoccur under the same circumstances. Considered a formulation of the basis for strengthening stimulus–response connections.

Limbic system • The anatomical designation of the emotional circuit in the brain, including Papez's circuit (cingulate cortex, hippocampal region, mammillary bodies, thalamus) plus the amygdala, septum, and prefrontal cortex, and more recently the orbital frontal cortex and areas of the midbrain.

Localization • The view that specific psychological functions, or memories, can be identified with specific areas of the cortex or other parts of the brain.

Long-term depression (LTD) • Long-lasting decrease of synaptic transmission, that is, a permanent decrement in synaptic efficacy, resulting from lack of coincident presynaptic activation and generation of a postsynaptic action potential.

Long-term potentiation (LTP) • Long-lasting facilitation of synaptic transmission, that is, a permanent increase in synaptic efficacy, resulting from repeated activation of a presynaptic element and its participation in the success in firing the postsynaptic cell.

Medial temporal lobe • The area of the temporal lobe that lies nearest the midline, including the hippocampus, the amygdala, and the immediately surrounding cortex of the parahippocampal region.

Memory space • A large-scale neural network that organizes the codings for the sequences of events that compose episodic memories, and links these memories together by codings for common features among the episodic memories.

Metabotropic receptors • Receptors that are activated by transmitters or other molecules, but do not open channels and directly cause changes in the membrane potential, and instead produce other changes in the cell that can have lasting effects on its responsiveness.

Modulation of memory • Facilitation or retardation of memory fixation, mediated by hormones including a pathway through the amygdala.

Multiple memory systems • The notion that there are several at least partially distinct brain systems that mediate different forms of memory.

Neuromodulators • Molecules that influence the activity of synapses or the production of action potentials. These are often released at distant sites and act at metabotropic receptors.

Neuron doctrine • The hypothesis that the brain is composed of discrete nerve cells that communicate with one another via specialized connections (synapses).

Neuropsychological studies • Examinations that attempt to identify and characterize specific perceptual, cognitive, or behavioral effects of brain damage.

Neurotransmitter • Molecules that are released and recognized within a synapse to mediate changes in the potential of the postsynaptic cell.

Neurotrophins • Molecules that promote morphological change and increased connectivity.

NMDA • N-methyl-D-aspartate. A molecule that acts as a first messenger (neurotransmitter) that regulates the flow of Ca^{2+} into the cell membrane. Normally the NMDA receptor is blocked by magnesium (Mg^{2+}). However, NMDA receptors have the unusual property of being modulated by the voltage of the cell membrane such that when the membrane is depolarized the magnesium block is eliminated and Ca^{2+} can flow into the cell.

Nonsense syllable • A meaningless letter string composed of two consonants separated by a vowel (e.g., "ket," "poc," "baf").

Norepinephrine • An early discovered neurotransmitter. Uses two major subtypes of receptors, α and β. Also called noradrenaline.

Ocular dominance • Pertaining to the situation when a visual neuron is better stimulated by presentation of a stimulus from the ipsilateral or contralateral side of visual space.

Oculomotor • Pertaining to eye movement.

Orientation selectivity • Pertaining to the situation in primary visual neurons where cells are selectively responsive to the orientation (e.g., vertical, horizontal) of a contrast edge.

Paired associate learning • The acquisition of associations among arbitrarily paired stimuli. In humans, most commonly involves learning novel associations between unrelated works, (e.g., army-table, ball-elephant, etc). In animals, involves novel associations among perceptual stimuli that are not reinforcers.

Papez circuit • A set of structures proposed by James Papez to mediate emotion. The structures are connected in a circular arrangement and viewed to mediate the integration of external and visceral signals and expression.

Parahippocampal region • A set of cortical areas of the temporal lobe immediately surrounding the hippocampus. Includes the perirhinal cortex, the parahippocampal cortex (in monkeys, and called the postrhinal cortex in rats), and the entorhinal cortex. Connects the hippocampus with neocortical association areas.

Perirhinal cortex • A subdivision of the parahippocampal region in rats and monkeys.

Perseveration • Continuing or repetitive behavioral responses emitted when no longer appropriate or intruding from previous events into the current situation.

Place cell • A neuron, typically in the hippocampus, that is activated when the animal is in a particular location in its environment, most purely regardless of the direction of its orientation or the ongoing behavior.

Place learning • Acquisition of a maze or other spatial problem guided by the expectancy of reward at an absolute (allocentric) location.

Population spike • The summed waveform of action potentials from many simultaneously activated neurons.

Posterior • Also called *caudal*. Toward the back of the brain.

Postrhinal cortex • A subdivision of the parahippocampal region in rats, called the parahippocampal gyrus in monkeys.

Postsynaptic site • The specialization of the cell membrane of a dendrite, cell body, or presynaptic site for recognition of a neurotransmitter molecule. Contains neurotransmitter receptors specialized for one or more forms of a neurotransmitter and mechanisms for influx of specific ions as a result of recognition of the transmitter at the receptor.

Prefrontal cortex • A large region of the cerebral cortex that lies anterior to the primary motor cortex, composed of many subdivisions including premotor cortex, dorsolateral, medial, and orbital subdivisions.

Premotor cortex • A specific zone of the cerebral cortex that lies just anterior to the primary motor cortex and is involved in motor learning.

Presynaptic site • The specialization of the ending of the axon where the connection is made with another neuron, characteristically filled with synaptic vesicles that contain neurotransmitter molecules and molecular machinery for manufacture and packaging of neurotransmitter and special processes for release of vesicles and reuptake of the transmitter.

Procedural memory • A set of learning abilities that involves tuning and modifying the networks of many brain systems that support skilled performance.

Radial maze • A maze with a central platform and multiple (usually eight) arms radiating out in all directions, like spokes of a wheel. Typically the rat must traverse each arm to find rewards at the end of some or all arms.

Receptive field • The location of a stimulus for optimal activation of a neuronal response. For visual stimuli the receptive fields are locations in visual space. For auditory stimuli the receptive fields are frequencies of sounds. For touch the receptive fields are locations on the body surface.

Reference memory • Memory for items that have a constant significance across many episodes.

Reflex • Automatic, unconditioned behavioral or endocrine response to an external stimulus. Mediated by a reflex arc composed of sensory neurons that connect to motor neurons that connect to effectors (muscles or glands).

Refractory period • A brief time following the action potential when another cannot be initiated due to the imbalance of ionic concentrations.

Reinforcer • A stimulus of innate biological significance that can drive behavior. Common positive reinforcers include food, water, sex, and warmth. Common negative reinforcers include electrical shock or other forms of painful stimulation.

Relational representation • An organization of episodic memories according to common items among them, leading to the development and modification of semantic memory networks.

Representational flexibility • The capacity to compare and contrast memories in a relational representation, and to infer solutions to new problems as a result of such comparisons.

Response learning • Maze learning guided by the acquisition of specific stimulus–response (left and right turn) associations.

Resting potential • Normal potential of the cell membrane, usually negative on the inside relative to the outside.

Retrograde amnesia • Loss of information acquired prior to head injury or brain damage. Often *temporally graded*, such that information acquired remotely prior to the damage is preserved, whereas information acquired recently prior to the damage is lost.

Reverberatory activity • Regenerative activity in a neural circuit that could mediate the persistence of a representation.

Rostral • Also called *anterior*. Towards the front of the brain.

Savings • Retention of a memory measured as the decrease in amount of training on some occasion after learning required to reattain the originally successful level of learned performance.

Schema • An active organization of memories whose structure determines the framework in which new memories are added, and can be employed during remembering to reconstruct or infer the probable constituents of a memory and the order in which they occurred.

Second messenger • Intracellular signaling molecule that causes downstream effects in the molecular cascade of events that follows activation of membrane receptors by neurotransmitters (the "first" messenger).

Second-order conditioning • A procedure that begins with a trained association between an arbitrary stimulus, as a conditioned stimulus, and a primary reinforcer, such as food or shock, followed by training on the association between another arbitrary stimulus and the previous conditioned stimulus which now acts as a second-order reinforcer. For example, initially a tone and shock are associated, such that the tone now produces a fearful reaction. Then the tone can be used as a secondary reinforcer on second-order conditioning of a light–tone association.

Semantic memory • The body of one's world knowledge, the large-scale organization of memories not bound to any specific experience in which they were acquired.

Sensitization • The increment in responsiveness to sensory stimulation following other strong stimulation.

Septum • Subcortical structure of the forebrain that is interconnected with the hippocampus.

Somatosensory • Sensations of touch on the skin, including texture, pressure, heat, and pain.

Spatial learning • Learning guided by the use of spatial relations among external stimuli.

Spine • Protrusion of the postsynaptic element of dendrites.

Startle response • A jump or other sudden movement performed by animals and people in response to an unexpected salient stimulus such as a loud sound.

Stimulus–reinforcer (reward or punishment) association • The acquired attraction or aversion to a stimulus associated with a primary reinforcer, such as food reward or shock. The fundamental mechanism of emotional memory.

Stimulus–response (SR) association • The learned execution of a specific behavior following presentation of a particular stimulus, reinforced by positive or negative outcomes following the behavior.

Striatum • Subcortical structure of the forebrain, composed of the caudate and putamen, a component of the extrapyramidal motor system and critical to habit memory.

Subcortical • Brain structures that lie under the cerebral cortex, such as the thalamus, striatum, hippocampus, amygdala, and many other nuclei and axon tracts.

Subiculum • A subdivision of the hippocampus that receives major inputs from CA1 and the parahippocampal region, and projects to the parahippocampal region and through the fornix to subcortical areas.

Synapse • Specialization for communication between neurons composed of the end of an axon (called the presynaptic site) and its contact area (the postsynaptic site) on the dendrite, cell body, or presynaptic site of another neuron.

Topographic map • Continuous point-to-point correspondence of adjacent parameters of external stimuli (e.g., locations in visual space or on the body surface), and sensitivities of neurons in neighboring locations in a structure of the brain.

Trace conditioning • A nonstandard version of classical conditioning where the conditioning stimulus (CS) is brief and followed by a blank "trace" period prior to the presentation of the unconditioned stimulus (US).

Transitive inference • The capacity to deduce indirect relations among items that share a common feature and a set of logical rules. For example, if A>B and B>C, then A>C.

Trigger feature • The optimal quality of a stimulus for activation of a neuron. For example, for neurons in primary visual cortex, the trigger feature is a particular contrast orientation of an edge presented to one eye.

Trisynaptic circuit • The series of connections within the hippocampus from the entorhinal cortex to the dentate gyrus, then to field CA3, then to field CA1. Originally thought to be the main processing route through the hippocampus, but expanded by another stage in the circuit from CA1 to the subiculum and direct parahippocampal inputs to CA3 and CA1, and the subiculum.

Unilateral • Pertaining to one side of the brain.

Ventral • Toward the bottom of the brain.

Visual field • A part of the environment one can see, or in which a presented stimulus will cause a neuron to fire. The center and reference point of the visual fields is the fixation point, the locus in space where the eyes converge. All parts of the visual field are relative to the fixation point.

Visuospatial • Pertaining to the location in space of visual stimuli.

Water maze • Device developed by Richard Morris to test spatial memory. Made of a large (usually 2 meter) diameter swimming pool filled with tepid water made opaque with the addition of a milky powder. An escape platform is hidden at one location just beneath the surface of the water and cannot be seen. In the conventional version of the task the rat is released from one of four randomly selected starting points and must find its way to the escape platform guided by cues outside the maze.

Working memory • A combination of storing new incoming information, plus some type of cognitive manipulation, held over a brief period in consciousness. The same term was used by Olton to refer to memory for items that were useful on only a single trial; however, his definition confuses episodic memory and working memory as the contents of current consciousness.

• • • • • • •
References in Figure Captions

Alvarez, P., Zola-Morgan, S., and Squire, L.R. 1995 Damage limited to the hippocampal region produces long-lasting memory impairment in monkeys. *J. Neurosci.* 15:5 3796–3807.

Alvarez, P., and Squire, L.R. 1994. Memory consolidation and the medial temporal lobe: A simple network model. *Proc. Natl. Acad. Sci. U.S.A.* 91: 7041–7045.

Bear, M.F. 1996. A synaptic basis for memory storage in the cerebral cortex. *Proc. Natl. Acad. Sci. U.S.A.* 93: 13453–13459.

Bechera, A., Tranel, D., Hanna, D., Adolphs, R., Rockland, C., and Damasio, A.R. 1995. Double dissociation of conditioning and declarative knowledge relative to the amygdala and hippocampus in humans. *Science,* 269: 1115–1118.

Bliss, T.V.P., and Collingridge, G.L. 1993. A synaptic model of memory: Long-term potentiation in the hippocampus. *Nature* 361: 31–39.

Brodmann, K. 1909. *Vergleichen de Lokalisationslehre der Grosshirnrinde in irhen Prinzipien dargestellt auf Grund des Zellenbaues.* Leipzig: Barth.

Bunsey, M., and Eichenbaum, H. 1995. Selective damage to the hippocampal region blocks long term retention of a natural and nonspatial stimulus-stimulus association. *Hippocampus* 5: 546–556.

Bunsey, M., and Eichenbaum, H. 1996. Conservation of hippocampal memory function in rats and humans. *Nature* 379: 255–257.

Cahill, L., Prins, B., Weber, M., and McGaugh, J.L. 1994. β-adrenergic activation and memory for emotional events. *Nature* 371: 702–704.

Cho, Y.H., Beracochea, D., and Jaffard, R. 1993. Extended temporal gradient for the retrograde and anterograde amnesia produced by ibotenate entorhinal cortex lesions in mice. *J. Neurosci.* 13: 1759–1766.

Cohen, J.D., Perlstein, W.M., Braver, T.S., Nystrom, L.E., Noll, D.C., Jonides, J., and Smith, E.E. 1997. Temporal dynamics of brain activation during a working memory task. *Nature* 386: 604–607.

Constantine-Paton, M., and Law, M.I. 1982. The development of maps and stripes in the brain. *Sci. Am.* 247: 62–70.

Corkin, S., Amaral, D.G., Gonzalez, R.G., Johnson, K.A., and Hyman, B.T. 1997. H.M.'s medial temporal lobe lesion: Findings from magnetic resonance imaging. *J. Neurosci.* 17: 3964–3979.

Defelipe, J., and Jones, E.G. 1988. *Cajal on the Cerebral Cortex.* New York: Oxford University Press.

Dias, R., Robbins, T.W., and Roberts, A.C. 1996. Dissociation in prefrontal cortex of affective and attentional shifts. *Nature* 380: 69–72.

Dusek J.A., and Eichenbaum, H. 1997. The hippocampus and memory for orderly stimulus relations. *Proc. Natl. Acad. Sci. U.S.A.* 94: 7109–7114.

Eichenbaum, H, Clegg, R.A., Feeley, A. 1983. A re-examination of functional subdivisions of the rodent prefrontal cortex. *Exp. Neurol.* 79: 434–45l.

Eichenbaum, H., Stewart, C., and Morris, R.G.M. 1990. Hippocampal representation in spatial learning. *J. Neurosci.* 10: 331–339.

Eichenbaum, H., Dudchenko, P., Wood, E., Shapiro, M., and Tanila, H. 1999. The hippocampus, memory, and place cells: Is it spatial memory or memory space? *Neuron* 23: 1–20.

Eichenbaum, H. 2000. A cortical-hippocampal system for declarative memory. *Nat. Rev. Neurosci.* 1: 41–50.

Funahashi, S., Bruce, C.J., and Goldman-Rakic, P.S. 1989. Mnemonic coding of visual space in the monkey's dorsolateral prefronatl cortex. *J. Neurophysiol.* 61: 331–349.

Gabrieli, J.D.E., Milberg, W., Keane, M., and Corkin, S. 1990. Intact priming of patterns despite impaired memory. *Neuropsychologia* 28: 417–427.

Jonides, J., Rugg, M.D., and Smith, E.E. (Ed.). 1997. The architecture of working memory. In *Cognitive Neuroscience*, Hove East Sussex: Psychology Press, pp. 243–276.

Kermadi I., and Joseph, J.P. 1995. Activity in the caudate nucleus of monkey during spatial sequencing. *J. Neurophysiol.* 74: 911–933.

Kim, J.J., and Fanselow, M.S. 1992. Modality-specific retrograde amnesia of fear. *Science*, 256: 675–677.

Kim, J.J., Clark, R.E., and Thompson, R.F. 1995. Hippocamectomy impairs the memory of recently, but not remotely, aquired trace eyeblink conditioned responses. *Behav. Neurosci.* 109: 195–203.

Knowlton, B.J., Ramus, S., and Squire, L.R. 1992. Intact artificial grammar learning in amnesia. *Psychol. Sci.* 3:3 172–179.

Krupa, D.J., Thompson, J.K., and Thompsom, R.F. 1993. Localization of a memory trace in the mammalian brain. *Nature.* 260: 989—991.

Lashley, K.S. 1929. *Brain Mechanisms and Intelligence: A Quantitative Study of Injuries to the Brain.* New York: Dover (1963 edition).

Maguire, E.A., and Mummery, C.J. 1999. Differential modulation of a common memory retrieval network revealed by positron emission tomography. *Hippocampus,* 9: 54–61.

Martin, A. 1999. Automatic activation of the medial temporal lobe during encoding: Lateralized influences of meaning and novelty. *Hippocampus* 9: 62–70.

McClelland, J.L., McNaughton, B.L., and O'Reilly, R.C. 1995. Why there are complementary learning systems in the hippocampus and neocortex: Insights from the successes and failures of connectionist models of learning and memory. *Psychol. Rev.* 102: 419–457.

McDonald, R.J., and White, N.M. 1993. A triple dissociation of memory systems: Hippocampus, amygdala, and dorsal striatum. *Behav. Neurosci.* 107: 3–22.

McDonald, R.J., and White, N.M. 1994. Parallel information processing in the water maze: Evidence for independent memory systems involving dorsal striatum and hippocampus. *Behav. Neural Biol.* 61: 260–270.

Milner, B., Corkin, S., and Teuber, H.L. 1968. Further analysis of the hippocampal amnesic syndrome: 14- year followup study of H.M. *Neuropsychologia* 6: 215–234.

Morris, R.G.M., and Frey, U. 1997. Hippocampal synaptic plasticity: role in spatial learning or the automatic recording of attended experience? *Phil. Trans. R. Soc. Lond.* 352: 1489–1503.

Morris, R.G.M., Garrud, P., Rawlins, J.P, and O'Keefe, J. 1982. Place navigation impaired in rats with hippocampal lesions. *Nature* 297: 681–683.

Murray, E.A., and Mishkin, M. 1998. Object recognition and location memory in monkeys with excitotoxic lesions of the amygdala and hippocampus *J. Neurosci.* 18: 6568–6582.

Nicoll, R.A., Kauer, J.A., and Malenka, R.C. 1988. The current excitement in long-term potentiation. *Neuron* 1: 87–103.

Otto, T., and Eichenbaum, H. 1992. Complementary roles of orbital prefrontal cortex and the perirhinal-entorhinal cortices in an odor-guided delayed non-matching to sample task. *Behav. Neurosci.* 106: 763–776.

Packard, M.G., and McGaugh, J.L. 1992. Double dissociation of fornix and caudate nucleus lesions on acquistion of two water maze tasks: Further evidence for multiple memory systems. *Behav. Neurosci.* 106: 439–446.

Packard, M.G., and McGaugh, J.L. 1996. Inactivation of hippocampus or caudate nucleus with lidocaine differentially affects expression of place and response learning. *Neurobiol. Learn. Mem.* 65: 65–72.

Packard, M.G., Cahill, L., and McGaugh, J.L. 1994. Amygdala modulation of hippocampal-dependent and caudate nucleus-dependent memory processes. *Proc. Natl. Acad. Sci.* 91: 8477–8481.

Rao, S., C., R., G., and Miller, E.K. 1997. Integration of what and where in the primate prefrontal cortex. *Science* 276: 821–824.

Recanzone, G.H., and Merzenich, M.M. 1991. Alterations of the functional organization of primary somatosensory cortex following intracortical microstimulation or behavioral training. In *Memory: Organization and Locus of Change*, L.R. Squire, N.M. Weinberger, G. Lynch, and J.L. McGaugh, (Eds.). New York: Oxford University Press, pp. 217–238.

Rioult-Pedotti, M.-S., Feriedman, D., Hess, G., and Donoghue, J. 1998. Strengthening of horizontal cortical connections following skill learning. *Nat. Neurosci.* 1: 230–234.

Rogan, M.T., and LeDoux, J.E. 1995. LTP is accompanied by commensurate enhancement of auditory-evoked responses in a fear conditioning circuit. *Neuron* 15: 127–136.

Rogan, M.T., Staubli, U.V., and LeDoux, J.E. 1997. Fear conditioning induces associative long-term potentiation in the amygdala. *Nature* 390: 604–607.

Sakai, K., Naya, Y., Miyashita, Y. 1994. Neuronal tuning and associative mechanisms in form representation. *Learn. Mem.* 1: 83–105.

Squire, L.R. 1987. *Memory and Brain*. New York: Oxford University Press.

Warrington, E.K., and Weiskrantz, L. 1968. New method for testing long-term retention with special reference to amnesic patients. *Nature* 217: 972–974.

Weinberger, N.M. 1993. Learning-induced changes of auditory receptive fields. *Curr. Opin. Neurobiol.* 3: 570–577.

Winocur, G. 1990. Anterograde and retrograde amnesia in rats with dorsal hippocampal or dorsomedial thalamic lesions. *Behav. Brain Res.*, 38: 145–154.

Wood, E.R., Dudchenko, P.A., and Eichenbaum, H. 1999. The global record of memory in hippocampal neuronal activity. *Nature*, 397: 613–616.

Wood, E., Dudchenko, P., Robitsek, J.R., and Eichenbaum, H. 2000. Hippocampal neurons encode information about different types of memory episodes occurring in the same location. *Neuron* 27: 623–633.

Young, B.J., Otto, T., Fox, G.D., and Eichenbaum, H. 1997. Memory representation within the parahippocampal region. *J. Neurosci.*, 17: 5183–5195.

Zola-Morgan, S.M., and Squire, L.R. 1990. The primate hippocampal formation : Evidence for a time-limited role in memory storage. *Science* 250: 288–290.

Zola-Morgan, S., Squire, L.R., and Amaral, D.G. 1989. Lesions of the amygdala that spare adjacent cortical regions do not impair memory or exacerbate the impairment following lesions of the hippocampal formation. *J. Neurosci.* 9: 1922–1936.

Index

Page numbers followed by "f" indicate figures.

Accessory abducens motor nucleus, 253
Action potential, 36–37
  described, 31–33, 32f
  metabotropic receptors and, 45f, 46
  single cell recording of, 140
Adenosine triphosphate (ATP) in
  sensitization, 45
Adenyl cyclase in classical conditioning, 48
Adrenaline and fixation of memory, 288
β-Adrenergic receptors and fixation of
  memory, 289–90
  Cahill's experiments and, 291–93, 292f
Agnosia and emotional memory pathway, 264
"All-or-none" response, 37
"Allocentric" localization, 244
Alvarez, Pablo, 303–4, 304f
Alzheimer, Alois, 22
Alzheimer's disease, 23
D-2-Amino-5-phosphono-valerate (AP5)
  fear-potentiated startle and, 276
  long-term potentiation and
    blocking of, 71–72, 73f
    induction of, 59–62
α-Amino-hydroxy-5-methyl-4-
  isoxazolepropionate receptors
  in long-term potentiation, 59–62, 60f–61f
Ammon's horn, 217–19
Amnesia, 85–104
  animal models for, 105–38. *See also*
    Monkeys; Rats
  consolidation theme and, 21–22, 294–95
  electroconvulsive shock therapy and, 286
  emotional memory pathway and, 268–70
  H.M. research and, 87–92. *See also* H.M.
    (patient)
  prefrontal lobe lesions and, 316
  retrograde
    described, 21
    memory reorganization and, 295–98
    in monkeys, 111–12

prospective studies in animals of,
  298–302, 300f
spared learning abilities in, 92–98
nondeclarative memory
  characterization, 99–102
properties of declarative and
  procedural memory and, 98–99
d-Amphetamine and fixation of memory,
  290, 291f
Amygdala
  behavioral long-term potentiation and,
    67–69, 68f–69f
  Damasio's experiment and, 208–10, 209f
  in delayed nonmatch to sample task, 222,
    223f
  in emotional memory pathway, 265–69, 265f
    Cahill's experiments and, 291–93, 292f
  fear conditioning circuit in, 270–74, 271f
  fear-potentiated startle conditioning in,
    274–76, 275f
  in H.M.'s surgery, 88, 88f, 268–69
  hormonal activation and fixation of
    memory, 287–91, 289f, 291f
  as part of multiple memory systems,
    200–201, 200f
  White's triple dissociation test and, 203f,
    204
Anatomy
  of cerebellum, 238–40, 239f
  of functional cortical areas, 176–78, 177f
  of hippocampal memory system, 214–19,
    214f, 218f
  of neurons, 30–31, 30f
  of parahippocampal cortex, 214–19,
    214f, 218f
  of prefrontal cortex, 313–15, 314f
  of procedural memory system, 238–40,
    239f
  of striatum, 238–40, 239f
  of three memory systems, 200–201, 200f

Animal models
　for amnesia, 105–38. *See also* Amnesia;
　　Monkeys; Rats
　retrograde, 298–302, 300f
　of memory circuit
　　Aplysia, 40–48, 42f
Antidromic activation of long-term
　depression, 64
Antireticularists, 7
AP5. *See* D-2-Amino-5-phosphono-valerate
　(AP5)
Approach and avoidance learning in rats,
　114–16, 115f
Arachidonic acid as retrograde messenger, 63
Arborization, 8, 8f
Artificial grammar test, 95–96, 97f
Association fibers, 218–19, 218f
Associative learning, 46–48, 47f
Associativity and long-term potentiation, 57
Attentional shift protocol, 315
Auditory cortex, 180–82
　classical conditioning of, 184–86, 185f
　fear conditioning and, 272–74
　fear-potentiated startle and, 276
Auditory thalamic nuclei
　in emotional memory pathway, 266
Autonomic nervous system
　in emotional memory pathway, 264
　as part of multiple memory systems,
　　200–201, 200f
Axons
　action potential in, 36–37
　anatomy of, 30–31, 30f
　discovery of, 7–9

Baddeley, Alan, 312
Bartlett, Frederic, 82–83
Basal ganglia, 239
Basolateral nucleus, 289–90
　in emotional memory pathway, 266
　in fear-potentiated startle, 276
Bear, Mark, 65
Behaviorism, 14–15, 15f
　vs. cognitivism, 79–84
　　Packard and McGaugh's experiment of,
　　195–99, 196f
Behaviorist manifesto, 15
Bergson, Henri, 17
Biran, Main de, 197
"Black reaction" stain, 7
Brain
　generic, 6f
　subdivisions of, 6f

Brain stem
　Knowlton's experiment and, 206–8, 207f
　nuclei and striatum, 239–40, 239f
　as part of multiple memory systems,
　　200–201, 200f
Broca, Paul, 19
Brodman, Korbinian, 176, 176f
Brown, Malcolm, 189, 228
Bucy, 264
Burham, William, 23, 283

c-AMP-response element binding protein
　(CREB), 49–50
　fixation of memory and, 286
　in fruit flies, 51
　long-term potentiation and
　　blocking of, 74–75
　　genetic manipulation of, 72–74
　　induction of, 62
c-fos activation, 233
Ca^{2+}. *See* Calcium ions
CA hippocampal area, 54–56, 55f–56f,
　217–19, 218f
　in long-term potentiation
　　anatomic modifications and, 64–65
　　genetic manipulation of, 73–74
Cahill, Larry, 279
　emotional arousal and memory, 288–93,
　　289f, 291f–292f
Cajal, Santiago Ramon y, 7–9, 8f
Calcium/calmodulin-dependent kinase type
　II (CaMKII)
　long-term potentiation and
　　blocking of, 74–75
　　induction of, 62
Calcium ions
　in long-term potentiation, 59–62, 60f–61f
　metabotropic receptors and, 45f, 46
　synaptic transmission and, 38–39, 38f
Calcium/phospholipid-dependent protein
　kinase C (PKC)
　long-term potentiation and, 62
Calmodulin in classical conditioning, 48
CaMKII. *See* Calcium/calmodulin-dependent
　kinase type II (CaMKII)
cAMP. *See* Cyclic adenosine monophosphate
　(cAMP)
Carbon dioxide as retrograde messenger,
　63
Carbon disulfide in olfactory learning, 136
Catalytic subunit, 49
Cathexes, 197
Caudate nucleus, 239

"Cell assemblies" of Hebb, 54, 58, 172–73, 283, 286
Cell body of neuron, 30–31, 30f
"Central executive," 312
Central nucleus
    fear conditioning and, 272
    fear-potentiated startle, 276
Central sulcus and motor processing, 177–78, 177f
Cerebellum
    anatomy of, 238–40, 239f
    motor learning by
        circuitry of, 251–52, 251f
        human experiments for, 255–56
        rat experiments for, 250–55, 251f
Cerebral cortex
    functional organization of, 175–93
        anatomic, 176–78, 177f
        early studies of, 171–73, 172f
    hippocampal memory system and, 214–19, 214f, 218f
    as part of multiple memory systems, 200–201, 200f
    plasticity of
        in adult, 182–83, 183f
        in developing stages, 178–82, 181f
        with learning, 184–87, 185f–186f
        responses to learning, 187–90, 191t
        striatum connections and, 239
"Chaining" of reflexes, 11–12
Chang, 335
Chloride channels and synaptic transmission, 39
Cingulate cortex
    in emotional memory pathway, 262–64, 263f
    hippocampal memory system and, 216
Classical conditioning, 46–48, 47f
    in amnesia, 96–97
    behavioral long-term potentiation and, 67–69, 68f–69f
    Damasio's experiment and, 208–10, 209f
    in procedural memory in humans, 255–56
    tone-cued, 184–85, 185f
Cleft, synaptic, 30–31, 30f
Cleparede, 270
Climbing fibers, 251f, 252
Cochlea and sensory input, 180–82
Cognition theme, 13–17
    behaviorism and, 14–15, 15f
    cognitivism and, 15–17
    described, 3–4
    summarized, 25–26

"Cognitive map" of Tolman, 80–82, 81f
    O'Keefe and Nadel studies and, 117–18
    hippocampal firing pattern studies and, 151–54, 152f
Cognitivism, 15–17
    vs. behaviorism, 79–84
        Packard and McGaugh's experiment of, 195–99, 196f
Cohen, Jonathan, 333–34, 335f
Cohen, Neal, 86–87, 126
Compartmentalization theme, 17–21
    case studies of cortical damage and, 19–20
    described, 4
    experimental neurology and neurophysiology and, 20–21
    organology and, 17–19, 18f
    summarized, 26
Competition of input activities, 178–82, 179f, 181f
Completion condition, 94–95, 94f
Computational models of hippocampal memory organization, 303–6, 304f–305f
Concentration gradient, 34
Conditioned place preference and amygdala, 277–78
Conditioned reflex, 12–13
Conduction
    action potential in, 36–37
    described, 31–33, 32f
    electrotonic, 30f, 32f, 35
    integration of synaptic potentials and, 39–40
    resting potential and, 33–35, 33f
    synaptic transmission in, 38–39, 38f
Confocal fluorescence microscopy, 61
Connection theme, 6–13
    conditioned reflex and, 12–13
    described, 2–3
    neuron doctrine and, 7–9, 8f
    reflex arc and, 9–12, 10f
    summarized, 25
Consciousness and relational memory theory, 125
Consolidation theme, 21–23
    computational models of memory organization and, 303–6, 304f–305f
    described, 4–5
    stages of, 285–309. See also Fixation of memory
    summarized, 26
    types of, 285
    working with memory, 311–37

"Contextual" fear conditioning, 273
Contrast orientation in visual cortex, 179, 179f
Contrasting and relational memory theory, 126
Courtney, S., 334–35
CREB. *See* c-AMP-response element binding protein (CREB)
Cue conjunctions in memory space scheme, 166–68, 167f
Cyclic adenosine monophosphate (cAMP)
    in classical conditioning, 48
    metabotropic receptors and, 45–46, 45f

Damasio, Antonio, 208–10, 209f, 270
Davis, Michael, 274–76, 275f
Deadwyler, Sam, 157
Decerebration studies, 11
Declarative memory, 87
    animal models for, 105–38
        monkeys, 106–13, 107f, 110f. *See also* Monkeys
        properties of, 106
        rats, 106, 113–24. *See also* Rats
    characterizing properties of, 98–99, 125
    emotional memory and, 208–10, 209f
        Cahill's experiments, 291–93, 292f
    expression of, 125
    functional neuroimaging of, 143
    hippocampal memory system and, 214–19, 214f, 218f. *See also* Hippocampus
    hippocampal representation scheme for, 148–50, 149f
    memory space and, 163–69, 166f–167f
    as part of multiple memory systems, 200–201, 200f
    procedural learning and, 206–8, 207f
    relational memory theory and, 124–37. *See* Relational memory
    vs. emotional memory, 270
Decremental conduction, 32f, 33, 35
Deep nuclei in cerebellar circuitry, 251–52, 251f
"Delay cells" in prefrontal cortex, 324–26, 325f
Delay conditioning, 97
    eyeblink conditioning and, 252–54
Delayed nonmatch to sample task (DNMS), 109–12, 110f
    for hippocampal firing patterns, 158–60, 159f
    for inferotemporal cortex study, 188–89
    for parahippocampal cortex experiments, 221–25, 223f, 225f

"Delayed spatial response" task, 107f, 108
Dementia
    and Alzheimer's disease, 23
    and striatal damage, 246
Dendrites
    anatomy of, 30–31, 30f
        alterations with LTP, 64–65
    discovery of, 7
Dentate granule cells, 218, 218f
Dentate gyrus, 217–19, 218f
Depolarization, described, 35
Dermatomes, discovery of, 10
Desimone, Robert, 228
Digestion, Pavlov's studies of, 12–13
DNMS. *See* Delayed nonmatch to sample task (DNMS)
Donoghue, John, 69–70, 70f
Dopamine and striatal activity, 248
Dorsal accessory inferior olive, 253
Dostrovsky, John, 151–54, 152f
Dot patterns test, 95, 96f
"Double dissociation" experiments
    described, 199
    in humans, 205–8, 207f
    in rats, 201–5, 203f
Drugs and fixation of memory, 287–91, 289f, 291f
Dudai, Yadin, 76
Dunce flies, 51

Ebbinghaus, Herman, 13–14
    vs. Bartlett's theory, 82–83
Efficacy, synaptic, 58
"Egocentric" localization, 244
Electroconvulsive shock therapy and amnesia, 286
Electrostatic gradient, described, 34–35
Electrotonic conduction, 30f, 32f, 35
    described, 31–33, 32f
Emotional memory
    brain system for, 261–84
        fear conditioning circuit and, 270–76, 271f, 275f
        first theories about, 262–65, 263f
        learning *vs.* performance distinction, 279–80
        as part of multiple memory systems, 200–201, 200f
        fixation of memory and, 293–94
        pathways for, 265–67, 265f
Endocrine system in emotional memory pathway, 267
Ensemble activity of hippocampal neurons, 157

Entorhinal cortex
  in emotional memory pathway, 266
  firing properties of, 229
  hippocampal memory system and,
    214–19, 214f, 218f
  retrograde amnesia studies and, 300f, 302
Environment and synaptic efficacy, 66–70,
  68f–70f
Epinephrine and memory, 287–91, 289f,
  291f
Episodic memory
  hippocampal processing of, 221
  hippocampal representation scheme for,
    148–50, 149f, 163, 164f
    spatial and nonspatial firing properties
      of, 163–69, 166f–167f
  interleaving in hippocampus of, 127
  relational memory theory and, 125
  vs. semantic memory, 100–102
  vs. working memory, 121
Event memory. See Episodic memory
Everitt, Barry, 278
Excitatory postsynaptic potentials (EPSPs)
  behavioral long-term potentiation and,
    67–69, 68f–70f
  long-term potentiation and, 56f
  molecular bases and, 59
Excitatory stimulus, discovery of, 11
Expectancy, Tolman's cognitive map and,
  82
Experience and cerebral cortex
  organization, 179–82, 179f, 181f
Explicit memory
  relational memory theory and, 125
  vs. implicit memory, 99–100
Eyeblink conditioning, 251f, 252–54
  hippocampus and, 254–55
Eyeblink reflexes in classical conditioning,
  96–97

Face recognition
  amygdala lesions and, 269
  and inferotemporal cortex, 188
  in temporally-graded retrograde amnesia
    studies, 297–98
Fact memory. See Semantic memory
Fanselow, M.S., 300–301, 300f
Fear conditioning
  behavioral long-term potentiation and,
    67–69, 68f–69f
  circuit for, 270–76, 271f, 275f
  fixation of memory and, 286–87
  retrograde amnesia studies and, 300–301,
    300f

Ferrier, David, 20
"Fight or flight" response, 264
Firing patterns of hippocampus. See
  Hippocampus
Fixation of memory, 5
  at brain systems level, 294–95
  cellular events mediating, 285–87
  computational models of memory
    organization and, 303–6, 304f–305f
  drug effects on, 287–91, 289f, 291f
  emotional arousal and, 287–91, 289f,
    291f
  as part of multiple memory systems,
    293–94
  modulation of, 287
  nature of hippocampal–cortical interaction
    and, 306–8
  protein synthesis and, 49, 286
Flexibility
  representational, 126–27
  Tolman's cognitive map and, 82
Flourens, 20
Food preference tests in rats, 134–37, 136f
Forager rats, 134–37, 136f
Fornix, 217–19, 218f
  relational memory testing and, 128–30,
    130f
Fried, Itzak, 158
Fritsch, Gustav, 20
Fruit flies and simple memory circuits,
  50–51
Functional neuroimaging
  of cerebellum, 255–56
  in face recognition, 269
  of medial temporal lobe. See Medial
    temporal lobe, functional
    neuroimaging of
  of motor cortex, 256–57
  of prefrontal cortex, 329–33, 331f
    parcellation of functions and, 333–35,
      334f
  of striatum, 247
Fuster, Joaquin, 188–89

Gabrieli, John, 233–34
Gaffan, David, 278
Gall, Franz Joseph, 17–19, 18f, 175
Galvani, 5
Galvanic skin response and amygdala
  lesions, 267–68
Genes and memory fixation, 49–50
  amnesia studies and, 286
  deficiencies of, 72–74
Geographic recollection, 146–47

Gill withdrawal reflex, 40–43, 42f
Global amnesia, 86
Global information processing and the
    medial temporal lobe, 141–42
Glucocorticoids and memory, 287–91, 289f,
    291f
Glutamate
    in classical conditioning, 48
    long-term potentiation and, 59–62,
        60f–61f
Golden Era, 5, 6f. *See also* specific themes
    cognition theme in, 13–17
    compartmentalization theme in, 17–21
    connection theme in, 6–13
    consolidation theme in, 21–23
Goldman-Rakic, Patricia, 317–18
    delay cell studies of, 324–26, 325f
Golgi, Camillo, 7
Gollins partial pictures task, 90–91, 92f
Granule cells in cerebellar circuitry, 251f,
    252
Graybiel, Ann, 248
Greenough, William, 255
Gustatory cortex and taste aversion
    learning, 76

Habit and memory, 15–17, 201. *See also*
    Procedural memory
Habituation and simple memory circuits,
    41–43, 42f
Hampton Court maze, 14, 15f
Hebb, Donald, "cell assemblies" of, 54, 58,
    172–73, 283, 286
Henke, K., 144
Herpes simplex encephalitis, 208
Heterosynaptic mechanism, 43
Hippocampal-independent memories, 127
Hippocampal memory system, 214–19,
    214f, 218f
Hippocampus
    anatomical characterization of, 214–19,
        214f, 218f
    animal models of amnesia and, 106,
        113–24, 298–302, 300f. *See also*
        Amnesia
    cerebellar activation and, 256
    cognitive map in. *See* "Cognitive map" of
        Tolman
    differential activation of, 233–34
    episodic memory and, 101
        representation scheme for, 148–50,
            149f, 163, 164f
    eyeblink conditioning and, 254–55
    fear conditioning and, 273

firing patterns in
    actions in places, 154–56
    in declarative memory system, 227–28
    early studies of, 150–51
    memory space network, 160–63, 161f
    nonspatial stimuli and events, 156–60,
        159f
    place field studies, 151–54, 152f, 154f
    recording of, 140
    spatial and nonspatial, 163–69,
        166f–167f
in H.M.'s surgery, 88, 88f
learning independent of, 116–17
long-term depression and, 63–64
long-term potentiation and, 54–58, 55f–
    56f. *See also* Long-term potentiation
    (LTP)
    blocking of, 74–75
memory organization and, 220–21, 294–95
    computational models of, 303–6,
        304f–305f
    nature of, 306–8
Olton's view of memory in, 120–24, 122f
Packard and McGaugh's experiment,
    196f, 198–99
as part of multiple memory systems,
    200–201, 200f
protein synthesis in, 62
in relational memory
    role of, 229–33, 231f
    theory of, 124–27
slice preparation of, 54, 55f
White's triple dissociation test and, 202,
    203f
Hitzig, Eduard, 20
H.M. (patient)
    childhood memories in, 91
    exceptions to new learning in, 91–92,
        92f–93f
    features of amnesia in, 102
    history of, 87–90, 88f
    importance of studies about, 85–87
    intact functions of, 90–91
    selectivity of memory in, 90
    semantic knowledge and, 101
    temporally-graded retrograde amnesia
        studies and, 295–96
    vs. monkeys as amnesia model, 108
Hodgkin, Alan, 36
Homosynaptic mechanism, 43
Hormonal activation
    in emotional memory pathway, 264
    fixation of memory and, 287–91, 289f,
        291f

Hubel, David, 179–80
Hunger and amygdala lesions, 268
Huntington's disease and rotary pursuit
    experiment, 246–47
Huxley, Andrew, 36
"Hypercolumn" of visual cortex, 179
Hyperpolarization, 39, 40
"Hyperspecificity" of memory, 102
Hypothalamic-pituitary axis as part of
    multiple memory systems, 200–201,
    200f
Hypothalamus in emotional memory
    pathway, 262–64, 263f

Implicit memory
    relational memory theory and, 125
    vs. explicit memory, 99–100
Inference
    cue conjunctions in memory space scheme
      and, 166–68, 167f
    in relational memory, 126–27
      hippocampal and parahippocampal
        roles in, 229–33, 231f
Inferior olivary nucleus of the medulla,
    251f, 252–53
Inferotemporal cortex (IT), 187–90, 191t
Inhibitory stimulus, discovery of, 11
Inhibitory synapses, 39, 40
Initiation zone, 36
Insight and Tolman's cognitive map, 82
Intelligence in H.M., 90
Interleaving
    memory space and, 127
      nature of hippocampal-cortical
        interactions and, 306–8
    relational memory theory and, 128–30,
      130f
Intermediate-term memory
    parahippocampal cortex and, 220–21
      experiments demonstrating, 221–25,
        223f, 225f
Interneurons
    described, 31
    in habituation circuit, 42, 42f
    in sensitization circuit, 44, 44f
Interpositus nucleus, 253
Ionotropic receptors, 44–45, 45f
    in classical conditioning, 48

Jacobsen, 315
James, William, 15–17
    concious recollection and memory theory
      of, 79
Jonides, John, 329

K+. See Potassium ions
Kandel, Eric, 40
K.C. (patient), 101
Kesner, Raymond, 244–45, 245f, 279, 321
Kinase(s). See Mitogen-activated protein
    kinase (MAPK); Protein kinase (PKA)
Kluver, 264
Knee jerk reflex, 10
Knowlton, Barbara, 206–8, 207f
Kolb, Bryan, 320
Korsakoff, Sergei, 22

Lashley, Karl, 172, 172f
Lateral amygdaloid nucleus
    behavioral long-term potentiation and,
      67–69, 68f–69f
    fear conditioning and, 272–74
Lateral geniculate nucleus, 180
Lateral nucleus in emotional memory
    pathway, 266
Laterality of memory, 141–42
Law of effect, 14
Law of regression, 21
LeDoux, Joseph, 67–69, 68f, 266
    fear conditioning circuit and, 270–74, 271f
Limbic system in emotional memory
    pathway, 262–64, 263f
Lomo, Terje, 55
Long-term depression (LTD), 63–64
    of mossy fiber synapse, 252
Long-term memory. See also Permanent
    memory
    according to James, 16
    hippocampus and, 137
    medial temporal lobe function and, 221
    transition to, 285
Long-term potentiation (LTP)
    anatomical modifications after, 64–65
    "behavioral," 66–70, 68f–70f
    blocking of, 70–72, 73f
      hippocampal plasticity and, 74–75
      outside hippocampus, 75–76
    cerebellar, 257
    genetic manipulations of, 72–74
    hippocampal, 54–58, 55f–56f
    induction of
      cellular basis for, 58–59
      molecular basis for, 59–62, 60f–61f
    maintenance of, 61–62, 61f
    memory and, 66–74
    nonhippocampal, 65–66, 65f
    properties of, 57
    protein synthesis and, 286
    quantal analysis of, 63

MacLean, Paul, 263f, 264
Magnesium ions
  in classical conditioning, 48
  in long-term potentiation, 59–62, 60f–61f
Magnetic resonance imaging, functional
    (fMRI), 139–40. *See also* Functional
    neuroimaging
  hippocampal and parahippocampal
    differentiation and, 233–34
  of prefrontal cortex, 329, 333–35, 335f
Maguire, 144f, 145
MAP kinase. *See* Mitogen-activated protein
    kinase (MAPK)
Maps
  cognitive. *See* "Cognitive map" of
    Tolman
  sensory, 180
Maze studies, 14, 15f
  approach and avoidance learning,
    114–16, 115f
  episodic memory representation and, 163,
    164f
    in memory space scheme, 163–69,
      166f–167f
  Lashley's experiments with, 172, 172f
  O'Keefe and Nadel studies and, 117–18
  vs. water maze task, 124
  Packard and McGaugh's experiment,
    195–99, 196f
  radial-arm, 121–24, 122f
    for striatal habit subsystem, 244–45,
      245f
    triple dissociation test of White and,
      201–5, 203f
  Tolman's cognitive map and, 71–72, 73f
  water, 118–20, 119f
    blocking of long-term potentiation and,
      71–72, 73f
    fixation of memory and, 290, 291f
    Kolb's experiments in, 320
    as reference memory, 124
    relational memory theory and, 128–30,
      130f
    for striatal habit subsystem, 240–44,
      242f–243f
McClelland, Jay, 304–6, 305f
McGaugh, James, 195–99, 196f
  fixation of memory experiments, 287–89,
    289f
Medial geniculate nucleus, 180–82
  behavioral long-term potentiation and,
    67–69, 68f–69f
  fear conditioning and, 272–74

Medial temporal lobe (MTL). *See also*
    Hippocampus
  amnesia and. *See* Amnesia
  computational models of memory
    organization and, 303–6, 304f–305f
  functional distinctions between
    components of, 220–21
  functional neuroimaging of, 139–40
    conscious recollection, 145–47
    early studies, 140–41
    laterality of memory in, 141–42
    stimulus associations and, 143–45, 144f
  hippocampal memory system and,
    214–19, 214f, 218f
  relational memory theory and, 124–25.
    See also Relational memory
Membranes of neurons, 8
Memory. *See also under* various types
  declarative, 87
  emotional, 200–201, 200f
  episodic, 100–102
  explicit, 99–100
  fixation of. *See* Fixation of memory
  implicit, 99–100
  long-term, 16
  nondeclarative, 99–102
  primary, 16
  procedural, 87
  reference, 121
  semantic, 100–102
  short-term, 16
  source, 298, 316
  working, 120
Memory circuits
  complex, 53–78
    hippocampal long-term depression and,
      63–64
    hippocampal long-term potentiation
      and, 54–58, 55f–56f. *See also* Long-
      term potentiation (LTP)
  simple, 40–52
    classical conditioning and, 46–48, 47f
    gill withdrawal reflex and, 40–43, 42f
    habituation and, 41–43, 42f
    sensitization and, 43–46, 44f–45f
Memory space, 126–27
  guiding principles of, 168
  hippocampal network and, 160–63, 161f
  spatial and nonspatial firing properties
    of, 163–69, 166f–167f
  nature of hippocampal-cortical
    interaction and, 306–8
  schematic model of, 148–50, 149f

Memory systems
  anatomy of, 200–201, 200f
  multiple, 173, 195–211
"Mere exposure" effect, 270
"Meta-memory" assessments, 316
Metabotropic receptors, 44–46, 45f
Mg²⁺. *See* Magnesium ions
Miller, Earl, 189, 228, 326–29, 328f, 335
Milner, 295–98
Mirror drawing, 91, 92f
Mirror-reversed words, 86
Mishkin, Mortimer, 222–24, 223f
Mitogen-activated protein kinase (MAPK)
  long-term potentiation and, 74
  in memory fixation, 50
  taste aversion learning and, 76
Miyashita, Y., 190, 191, 335
"Mnemonic scotoma," 326
Monkeys
  as amnesia model, 106–13, 107f, 110f
    delayed nonmatch to sample task and,
      109–12, 110f
    graded retrograde memory loss in,
      111–12
    manual skill tests for, 112–13
    matching-to-sample tests in, 107–8,
      107f
    object discrimination task for, 112
    prospective studies of, 298–99, 300f
    "trial-unique stimulus" test, 109
    visual discrimination tests in, 107–8,
      107f
  with amygdala lesions, 267–68
  in parahippocampal cortex experiments,
    222–24, 223f
  electrophysiological studies of, 228–29
  prefrontal cortex role in, 315–17, 318f
Morris, Richard, 57, 118–20, 119f. *See also*
    Maze studies, water
  blocking of long-term potentiation and,
    71–72, 73f
Moscovitch, Morris, 99, 101
Mossy fibers, 218, 218f
  in cerebellar circuitry, 251f, 252
Motor cortex
  primary, 238, 239f
  processing of, 177–78, 177f
Motor neurons, 31. *See also* Neuron(s)
Muller, Georg, 22–23, 283
Mummery, 144f, 145
Murray, Elizabeth, 222–24, 223f
Muscimol in eyeblink conditioning, 251f, 253
Myelin, anatomy of, 7

N-methyl-D-aspartate (NMDA)
  blocking long-term potentiation and,
    74–75
  in classical conditioning, 48
  fear-potentiated startle and, 276
  in long-term potentiation, 59–62, 60f–61f
    blocking of, 71–72, 73f
    genetic manipulation of, 73–74
  taste aversion learning and, 76
Na⁺. *See* Sodium ions
Nadel, Lynn, 117–18
  hippocampal firing pattern studies of,
    151–54, 152f, 154f
  vs. Olton's theory, 123–24
Nader, K., 286
Naturalistic learning, 134–37, 136f
Nauta, Walle, 265
Navigation
  cognitive maps and, 118–20, 119f
  cue conjunctions in memory space scheme
    and, 166–68, 167f
Nerve cells. *See also* Neuron(s)
  elements of, 7–9, 8f
Networks
  computational models of memory
    organization and, 303–6, 304f–305f
  knowledge and relational memory theory,
    128
  representation of experience and, 147–48
Neuron doctrine, 7–9, 8f
Neuron(s), 20–40
  action potential in, 36–37
  anatomy of, 30–31, 30f
  electrotonic conduction of, 30f, 32f, 35
  integration of synaptic potentials and,
    39–40
  physiology of, 31–33, 32f
  resting potential and, 33–35, 33f
  synaptic transmission in, 38–39, 38f
  types of, 31
Neurotransmitters
  fixation of memory and, 290
  production of, 30–31, 30f
  synaptic transmission and, 38–39, 38f
Neurotrophins and long-term potentiation,
    62
Nitrous oxide as retrograde messenger,
    63
NMDA. *See* N-methyl-D-aspartate (NMDA)
Nodal hippocampal cells, 149
  nature of hippocampal-cortical interaction
    and, 306–8
Nondeclarative memory, 99–102

Nonsense syllable, 14
  in perseveration studies, 23
Nonspatial learning and relational memory
    theory, 131–34, 133f
Nonverbal memory performance, 141–42
Novel information processing, 142–43, 144f
Nucleus of the solitary tract, 289
Nucleus reticularis pontis oralis, 276

Object recognition and inferotemporal
    cortex, 187–88
Ocular dominance property, 179, 179f
Oculomotor delayed-response task, 324–26,
    325f
  Miller's experiments, 326–29, 328f
Odor stimuli for testing rats, 131–34, 133f
  for hippocampal firing patterns, 158–60,
    159f
    memory space and, 160–63, 161f
  naturalistic learning and, 134–37, 136f
  in parahippocampal cortex experiments,
    224–25, 225f
    electrophysiological studies of, 226–28,
    226f
  in prefrontal cortex deficits, 321–23, 322f
O'Keefe, John, 117–18
  hippocampal firing pattern studies,
    151–54, 152f, 154f
  vs. Olton's theory, 123–24
Olfactory bulb in emotional memory
    pathway, 266
Olfactory cortex and parahippocampal
    cortex, 216–19
Olton, David, 120–24, 122f, 320
Opioids and fixation of memory, 290
Optic tectum in frogs, 180, 181f
Organology, 17–19, 18f
Orientation strategy, 123
"Orienting responses" and amygdala
    lesions, 267–68
Overlap in memory space scheme, 165–69,
    166f–167f
Owen, Adrian, 332–33

Packard, Mark, 195–99, 196f
Pain and amygdala lesions, 268
Pain withdrawal reflex arc, 10f
"Pair-coding" neurons, 190, 191
"Pair-recall" neurons, 190, 191
Paired associate test, 131–34, 133f
  cue conjunctions in memory space scheme
    and, 166–68, 167f
  for inferotemporal cortex study, 190, 191
Papez, James, 262–64, 263f

Parahippocampal region
  anatomy of, 214–19, 214f, 218f
  differential activation of, 233–34
  hippocampal memory system and,
    214–19, 214f, 218f
    nature of interactions with, 306–8
  intermediate-term memory and, 220–21
    experiments demonstrating, 221–25,
    223f, 225f
  as part of multiple memory systems,
    200–201, 200f
  role in relational memory, 229–33, 231f
Parallel fibers
  in "acrobatic" training, 255
  in cerebellar circuitry, 251f, 252
Parcellations of working memory, 327
  according to Petrides, 332
Parietal lobe and hippocampal memory
    system, 216
Parkinson's disease
  procedural learning experiment and,
    206–8, 207f
  rotary pursuit experiment, 246–47
"Passive avoidance" test, 114
Pavlov, Ivan, 12–13
  classical conditioning and, 46–48, 47f
Perceptual constancy, 187
Perceptual encoding recollection, 146
Perceptual processing in cortex, 177–78,
    177f
Perceptual skill learning in amnesia, 92–98
  classic (Pavlovian) conditioning in, 96–97
  priming, 93–95, 94f, 96f
  sequence learning, 97–98
  skill learning, 95–96, 97f
Perirhinal cortex
  in emotional memory pathway, 266
  fear-potentiated startle and, 276
  firing properties of, 228
  hippocampal memory system and,
    214–19, 214f, 218f
Perseveration, 23
  prefrontal lobe lesions and, 316, 322
Petrides, Michael, 319, 330–32
"Phonological loop," 312
Picrotoxin and fixation of memory, 287
Pilzecker, Alfons, 22–23, 283
Piriform cortex, 219
  in emotional memory pathway, 266
Pituitary-adrenal axis and memory, 287–91,
    289f, 291f
Place cells. See also Hippocampus
  blocking long-term potentiation and,
    74–75

in cognitive maps of environment, 118
  hippocampal firing pattern studies and,
    151–54, 152f, 154f
  encoding action, 152f, 154–56
  in memory space network, 160–63, 161f,
    165–69, 166f–167t
Place learning. See Spatial learning
Place strategy, 123
Place vs. response learning, 195–99, 196f
Plasticity
  cortical
    adult, 182–83, 183f
    developing, 178–82, 181f
  hippocampal, 74–75
  neuronal, 9
Polyneuritis and amnesia, 22
Pontine nuclei, 251f, 253
Positron emission tomography (PET),
    139–40. See also Functional
    neuroimaging
  fixation of memory and, 293
  of prefrontal cortex, 329
Postrhinal cortex and hippocampal memory
    system, 214–19, 214f, 218f
Postsynaptic element
  anatomy of, 30–31, 30f
  in classical conditioning, 48
  in sensitization, 46
Potassium ions
  action potential and, 37
  in long-term potentiation, 59–62, 60f–61f
  metabotropic receptors and, 45f, 46
  resting potential and, 33f, 34–35
Prefrontal cortex
  anatomy of, 313–15, 314f
  in emotional memory pathway, 266
  hippocampal memory system and, 216
  role of
    in humans, 315–17
    in monkeys, 317–19, 318f
    in rodents, 320–24, 322f
  striatum and, 239, 239f
  temporally graded amnesia studies and, 298
  working memory and, 311–37
    coding mechanisms of, 324–29, 325f,
      328f
Premise pairs, 230–33, 231f
Premotor cortex, 238, 239f
  in conditional motor learning, 257
Presynaptic element
  anatomy of, 30–31, 30f
  in classical conditioning, 48
  in sensitization, 46
  synaptic transmission and, 38–39, 38f

Primary memory of James, 16
Primary visual cortex. See Visual cortex
Priming, 93–95, 94f, 96f
Principal neuron, 31
Principles of Psychology, The, 15, 79
Prism glasses experiment, 255
Probablistic learning, 206–8, 207f
  striatal damage in, 246
Problem solving and prefrontal cortex,
    315–17
Procedural memory, 87
  anatomy of system for, 238–40, 239f
  brain system for, 237–59
  cerebellar involvement in, 255
  characterizing properties of, 98–99
  expression of, 125
  in humans, 255–56
  motor cortex role in, 256–57
  as part of multiple memory systems,
    200–201, 200f
Protein kinase (PKA)
  in long-term potentiation
    genetic manipulation of, 74
    metabotropic receptors and, 45–46, 45f
    taste aversion learning and, 76
Protein synthesis
  eyeblink conditioning and, 253
  fixation of memory and, 49, 286
"Psychic secretion," 12
Purkinje cells
  in "acrobatic" training, 255
  in cerebellar circuitry, 251–52, 251f
Putamen, 239
Pyramidal cells, 218–19, 218f

Rabbits in amnesia studies, 300f, 301
Radial-arm maze studies. See Maze studies
Ranck, Jr., James, 150–51
Rats. See also Maze studies
  "acrobatic" training in, 255
  as amnesia model, 113–24
    "passive avoidance" test for, 114
    prospective studies of, 298–302, 300f
    radial-arm maze for, 120–24, 122f
    relational memory tests in, 128–37,
      130f, 133f, 136f
    "shuttle-box avoidance" test for, 114
    water maze studies for, 117–20, 119f
  fear conditioning in, 270–74, 271f,
    286–87
  fear-potentiated startle conditioning in,
    274–76, 275f
  in parahippocampal cortex experiments,
    224–25, 225f

Rats (*Continued*)
  electrophysiological studies of, 226–28, 226f
  prefrontal cortex role in, 320–24, 322f
  striatal habit subsystem experiments on, 240–45, 242f–243f, 245f
  transitive inference test of, 229–33, 231f
  visual discrimination test for, 115–16, 115f
Receptive fields of cerebral cortex, 177–78, 177f
Receptors for neurotransmitters
  anatomy of, 31
  metabotropic, 44–46, 45f
  synaptic transmission and, 38–39, 38f
Reciprocal innervation, 11
"Reconsolidation" of memory, 287
Reference memory, 121
Reflex arc, 9–12, 10f
Refractory period, 37
Relational memory, 124–37
  formulation of theory, 125–27
  hippocampal and parahippocampal roles in, 229–33, 231f
  hippocampal memory space scheme and, 163–69, 166f–167f
  medial temporal lobe components and, 220–21
  testing of theory, 128–37, 130f, 133f, 136f
    naturalistic learning, 134–37, 136f
    nonspatial learning, 131–34, 133f
    spatial learning, 128–31, 130f
"Relational representation," 126–27
Reorganization of memory, 5
  at brain systems level, 294–95
Repetitive stimulus procedure, 109
"Representational flexibility," 126–27
Resting potential, 33–35, 33f
Reticularists, 7
Retina, sensory input from, 180–82
Retroactive interference, 23
Retrograde messenger for long-term potentiation, 63
Reverberation in cell assemblies, 172–73, 283
Reversal learning and Olton's hypothesis, 123
Ribot, Theodore, 21–22
Robbins, Trevor, 278
Roberts, Angela, 318–19, 318f
Rosen, J., 280
Rotary pursuit experiment, 246–47
Rutabaga flies, 51

"Saccade," 324
Savings scores, 14
Schacter, Daniel, 99–100, 102
Schaffer collaterals, 218f, 219
"Schema" theory of Bartlett, 82–83
Schultz, Wolfram, 248
Scoville, William, 85–87
  temporally-graded retrograde amnesia studies and, 295–98
Scratch reflex, 11
Second messenger, 45
"Second-order conditioning," 278
Secondary memory of James, 16
Semantic encoding recollection, 146
Semantic memory
  relational memory theory and, 125
  vs. episodic memory, 100–102
  vs. reference memory, 121
Sensitization and simple memory circuits, 43–46, 44f–45f
Sensory neurons. *See also* Neuron(s)
  described, 31
Sequence learning
  in amnesia, 97–98
  in striatum, 248–50, 249f
Serial reaction time test, 97, 247, 255
Serotonin
  in classical conditioning, 48
  metabotropic receptors and, 45, 45f
Sherrington, Charles, 9–12
Short-term memory
  according to James, 16
  hippocampus and, 137
  medial temporal lobe function and, 221
  transition from, 285
  working memory and, 312
"Shuttle-box avoidance" test, 114
Silva, Alcino, 72
Simple memory circuits, 40–48
Single cell recording of action potentials, 140. *See also* Firing patterns
Siphon and simple memory circuits, 40–43, 42f
Sixth sense, 10
Skill learning
  in amnesia, 95–96, 97f
  cerebellum and, 256
Skill memory, 201. *See also* Procedural memory
Skinner, B.F., 14
"Slice preparation," 54, 55f
S.M. (patient), 269
Small's maze, 14, 15f

Smith, Edward, 329
Social olfactory learning in rats, 134–37, 136f
Sodium ions
  action potential and, 36–37
  in classical conditioning, 48
  in long-term potentiation, 59–62, 60f–61f
  resting potential and, 33f, 34–35
Sodium pump, 33f, 35
Source memory, 298, 316
Spatial learning. *See also* "Cognitive map" of Tolman; Place cells
  blocking long-term potentiation and, 74–75
  hippocampal memory space and, 163–69, 166f–167f
  Olton's hypothesis and, 123–24
  Packard and McGaugh's experiment and, 195–99, 196f
  relational memory theory and, 128–30, 130f
  striatal habit subsystem and, 240–45, 242f–243f, 245f
Spatial memory. *See also* Spatial learning
  in temporally-graded retrograde amnesia studies, 297–98
Spatial perceptual ability in H.M., 90
Specificity
  hippocampal firing patterns and, 141–42
  long-term potentiation and, 57
Speed reading tests in amnesia, 98
Spinal cord, 9–12, 10f
Squire, Larry, 86–87, 303–4, 304f
Staining method of Golgi, 7
Steinmetz, Joseph, 253
Step-through inhibitory avoidance task, 288
Stimulus response/reinforcer associations, 3
Stimulus-response sequences
  striatum and, 248–50, 249f
Stimulus-reward *vs.* stimulus-response
  amygdala and, 277–78
Stress activation and memory, 287–91, 289f, 291f
Striatum
  anatomy of, 238–40, 239f
  in conditional motor learning, 257
  in emotional memory pathway, 266
  habit subsystem of
    human experiments, 246–47
    rat experiments, 240–45, 242f–243f, 245f
  Knowlton's experiment and, 206–8, 207f

Packard and McGaugh's experiment, 196f, 198–99
  as part of multiple memory systems, 200–201, 200f
  role in habit learning summarized, 250
  White's triple dissociation test and, 203f, 204
Subiculum, 217–19, 218f
  in emotional memory pathway, 266
  fear conditioning and, 273
  in Gabrieli's experiments, 233–34
Substantia nigra
  in emotional memory pathway, 266
  striatal activity and, 248
Summation
  of nerve inputs, 8, 11
  of synaptic potentials, 39–40
Superior colliculus, 180
Suzuki, Wendy, 229
Symmetry test, 134
Sympathetic nervous system and fixation of memory, 287–91, 289f, 291f
Synapse(es)
  anatomy of, 30–31, 30f
  discovery of, 10
  growth of, 50
  long-term potentiation and. *See also* Long-term potentiation (LTP)
  plasticity of, 54
  transmission through, 38–39, 38f
Synaptic potentials, integration of, 39–40
Synaptic "tag," 58
Synaptic weights and memory reorganization, 303, 306

Tactile discrimination learning, 186–87, 186f
Taste aversion learning, 76
Temporal ordering deficits, 316, 319–21
Tetanus-induced synaptic changes, 55–57, 56f
Thalamus
  in conditional motor learning, 257
  in emotional memory pathway, 262–64, 263f
  fear conditioning and, 273
  striatum connections and, 239–40, 239f
Themes in memory research, 1–27
  cognition
    amnesia and, 85–108
    in animal models, 109–38
    described, 3–4, 79–84, 81f

Themes in memory research (*Continued*)
  neuroimaging and cell recording and,
    139–70
  compartmentalization
    cerebral cortex and memory and,
      175–93
    described, 4, 171–74, 172f
  connection
    complex memory circuits and, 53–78
    described, 2–3, 27–28
    neurons and, 20–40
    simple memory circuits and, 40–52
  consolidation
    described, 4–5
    stages of, 285–309
    working with memory, 311–37
  descriptions of, 2–5
Thompson, Richard, 253
Thorndike, Edward, 14–15
"Three-back" task, 330–31, 331f
"Time traveling," 100
Tolman, Edward, 80–82, 81f. *See also*
    "Cognitive map" of Tolman
  on multiple memory systems, 197
Tonegawa, Susumu, 73
Trace-conditioning, 97, 254–55, 300f, 301
"Transfer test," 120
Transitive inference test, 134
  hippocampal and parahippocampal
    functions and, 229–33, 231f
Transmission of signals, described, 31–33,
    32f
"Trial-unique stimulus" test, 109
Trigeminal nucleus, 253
Triple dissociation experiment, 201–5, 203f
Trisynaptic circuit, 217–19, 218f
Tulving, Endel, 100–101
"Two-back" task, 312

Ubiquitin hydrolase, 50
Unconditioned reflex, 12
Ungerleider, L., 334–35
Urbach-Wiethe disease, 208, 269, 293

Vagus nerve
  in emotional memory pathway, 267
  and fixation of memory, 289
Ventral nucleus, 273

Verb generation and cerebellum, 256
Verbal memory performance, 141–42
Vesicles, synaptic, 38–39, 38f
  in *Aplysia* habituation, 40–43, 42f
"Visceral brain," 264
Visual agnosia, 187
Visual cortex
  functional organization in, 178–82, 179f,
    181f
  learning-related reoganization of, 184
  long-term potentiation and, 65–66, 65f
Visual discrimination test
  in monkeys as amnesia model, 107–8, 107f
  in rats, 115–16, 115f
"Visuospatial sketch pade," 312
Voltage-gated channels, 36

Wallace, K., 280
Water maze studies. *See* Maze studies
Watson, John, 14–15
"Weather prediction" game, 206–8, 207f
  striatal damage and, 246
Weinberger, Norman, 184–85, 185f
Weiskrantz, Lawrence, 277
Wernike, Carl, 19–20
"What" and "where" task, 327–29, 328f
Whishaw, Ian, 323–24
White, Normal, 201–5, 203f
Wiesel, Torsten, 179–80
Willis, 5
Win-shift rule, 202, 203f
Win-stay rule, 203f, 204
Winocur, G., 298–99, 300f, 323
Wisconsin Card Sorting task, 315
Witter, Menno, 215
Woody, Charles, 257
Word stem completion tests, 94–95, 94f
  conscious recollection and, 145–46
Working memory, 120–21
  vs. working with memory, 311. *See also*
    Prefrontal cortex
Working with memory, 311–37. *See also*
    Prefrontal cortex

Yerkes studies on apes, 79–80

Zajonc, Robert, 270
Zola-Morgan, S., 298–99, 300f

Taking TRAUMA out of Teen Transitions

Larry Anderson

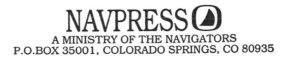

NAVPRESS
A MINISTRY OF THE NAVIGATORS
P.O.BOX 35001, COLORADO SPRINGS, CO 80935

The Navigators is an international Christian organization. Jesus Christ gave His followers the Great Commission to go and make disciples (Matthew 28:19). The aim of The Navigators is to help fulfill that commission by multiplying laborers for Christ in every nation.

NavPress is the publishing ministry of The Navigators. NavPress publications are tools to help Christians grow. Although publications alone cannot make disciples or change lives, they can help believers learn biblical discipleship, and apply what they learn to their lives and ministries.

© 1991 by Larry Anderson
All rights reserved. No part of this publication may be reproduced in any form without written permission from NavPress, P.O. Box 35001, Colorado Springs, CO 80935.
Library of Congress Catalog Card Number: 91-61421
ISBN 08910-96353

Second printing, 1992

Cover illustration: Dan Pegoda

Some of the anecodotal illustrations in this book are true to life and are included with the permission of the persons involved. All other illustrations are composites of real situations, and any resemblance to people living or dead is coincidental.

All Scripture in this publication is from the *Holy Bible: New International Version* (NIV). Copyright © 1973, 1978, 1984, International Bible Society. Used by permission of Zondervan Bible Publishers.

Printed in the United States of America

FOR A FREE CATALOG OF
NAVPRESS BOOKS & BIBLE STUDIES,
CALL TOLL FREE 1-800-366-7788 (USA)
or 1-416-499-4615 (CANADA)

Contents

Foreword   5
Acknowledgments   7

1   The Trauma of Transition   9
2   Teen Passages   17
3   Managing Expectations   33
4   Making Transition Your Ally   45
5   Team Member 1: Knowing God   55
6   Team Member 2: Realistic Goals
    for Traumatized Parents and Teens   67
7   Team Member 3: Maximizing Resources   81
8   Team Member 4: Maintaining Intimacy
    in the Midst of Transition   93
9   Team Member 5: Prayer — Healing Strength
    for the Stressed   105
10 Team Member 6: Managing Time Factors   117
11 Team Member 7: Laughter and Fun as Shelters
    from the Storm   127
12 Release in Transition   137
13 Closing the Book on Transition   147

Notes   155
Bibliography   159

To my wife, Gina,
who brings such grace and hope
to each of life's transitions.
And to my three sons,
Caleb, Joshua, and Aaron,
who have given me the privilege
of walking through life with them.

Foreword

Even the strongest of us tends to get weak-kneed when it comes to certain transitions . . . from carefree student to full-time work responsibilities, from no kids to twins, from a sprawling home in the country to a squashed apartment in the city, from great health to hearing the doctor diagnose a serious condition.

None of us can avoid transitions in our lives, but during the teenage years, young men and women are often terrorized by them.

Almost without exception, we all go through more personal, relational, and societal transitions during the teen years than at any other time in our lives. From childhood to being young adults, from throwing rocks at girls to thinking about marrying them, from majoring in playground to picking a major in college. During these years most of us will make the decision of who our Master is, what our mission in life is, and what methods will get us there.

These are huge transitions! Many of which can set the course of a person's life. Without exception, before our children reach their twenties, they will either be enriched or defeated by how they face these twists and turns in their personal road map.

The task of preparing children to face transitions is one of the most important things any parent can do, but most of us need help in dealing with these turning points ourselves!

That's why I'm glad you picked up this book. When we drive into a large, unfamiliar city, it's great to have a road map. But it's even better to have a personal guide take us by the hand—past all the road construction, one-way streets, and detours—bringing us and our children safely to our destination.

When it comes to the subject of this book, Larry Anderson is just such a guide. He is a nationally respected expert on youth issues, having helped hundreds of teenagers *and adults* take the word *trauma* out of transitions. And he can do that for you in this book.

The Marines teach you to dig your fighting hole big enough for two people. That's because, when the battle comes, it's better to face that trial with a buddy next to you. In even the best of homes, times of transitions can often create a battle-zone atmosphere between parent and child. In all my exposure to youth workers across the country over the years, I can't think of a better, more qualified person to help you and your child win the day than Larry Anderson.

I hope you'll pause and linger over the words and stories in this book. The wise counsel you'll find here will not only help you face the changes your child is going through, but better prepare you to honor God through the transitions you'll face as well.

I'm honored to write this foreword and endorsement for this book, and trust you'll find it to be as helpful and valuable a resource as my wife and I have.

—JOHN TRENT, PH.D.

Acknowledgments

When one of my oldest and dearest friends, Dan Peddie, introduced me to Steve Webb, of NavPress, I had just about given up the idea of writing this book. From there Steve not only became a great editor but a good friend as well. As this book is prepared to be released I want to acknowledge a number of people who have influenced its production. First, I would like to thank Steve for his enthusiasm and support throughout the process of writing this book. He has lent great professional support and skill to a nervous, first-time author.

I would like to express my appreciation to John Trent, who initially challenged me to write a book like this. Without John's support and wisdom, this book would not have gotten off the ground. After John convinced me to go forward on this, he, Tim Kimmel, and Steve Lyon storyboarded the original book concept with me.

I am appreciative of the support of the Young Life family

for their collective support and wisdom over the last sixteen years. Many of the concepts proposed in this book are a result of some great mentors throughout Young Life. I want to especially acknowledge my appreciation to Bob Krulish, my "boss," for allowing me to pursue the completion of this book.

I really thought my first book would be in collaboration with my mother. I had decided that the title should be *Kitchen Table Psychology* for all the wisdom that both my mother, Billie Anderson, and my father, the Rev. Tommy Anderson, supplied me with as parents and continue to supply as parents and grandparents.

I am indebted to the wisdom and the work done by Brennan Manning and Tim Hansel, among others, who are quoted throughout the book. Their winsome style of writing and their personal encouragement has been both helpful and inspirational to me.

Next, a special thanks to Renee McKenzie, who runs the regional office out of our home. Her extra administrative support and computer expertise has been valuable.

Finally, to my wife, Gina, who is an untiring supporter and fan, and to my three sons, Caleb, Joshua, and Aaron, who make life so fun and provide great tests for Dad's theories, thanks, I love you.

• • • • • • • • • • •

CHAPTER ONE

The Trauma of Transition

It was May, and the Arizona sun was typically hot as I wheeled my little Nissan toward the church. But even the sun's piercing heat could not thaw the chill I felt in my heart. As I drove, my thoughts were clouded by doubt and a feeling of failure. Another young person had made the tragic decision that life was not worth living.

Kit came to Young Life all through high school. He went to camp with us and regularly attended our Bible studies. We were good friends. He was such a likable guy. He breezed through high school appearing to enjoy every minute. Somehow, though, after graduation he was unable to make a successful transition to early adulthood and dropped out of college without telling his parents. On the day he should have been graduating he took his life. Without the courage to face his family he chose a harsh and permanent way out of his trauma.

Now I was driving to Kit's funeral feeling pain over his

death and guilt that maybe I could have done more. I knew he was attending a good church and seemed to have some Christian friends there. I continued to play the tape of our relationship over and over in my mind, always searching for a clue to Kit's actions that I was not so sure I wanted to find.

Young people like Kit are not unusual today. Many are unable to contend with the various directions life takes as they grow up. Without the tools to make good decisions they turn to harmful alternatives like drug and alcohol abuse, partying, and sex. They often lash out at their parents or society, looking for someone to blame, or they withdraw because they are afraid to face perceived failure.

My eyes began to glisten and my sight blurred as I caught sight of the book the pastor was holding as he led the service. It was the Bible I had given Kit early in our friendship. As he opened the Bible he began to comment on verses that Kit had underlined. Verses of hope and direction, words of life and joy.

My tears were flowing freely as I fought for understanding in the midst of tragic circumstances. I knew that committing my life to youthwork would mean days like this. I have counseled with many young people from junior high to beyond college who were confused by the changes they were experiencing in their young lives. I have sat with brokenhearted parents lamenting the choices their children had made. Many of these were good and conscientious moms and dads who dearly loved their kids.

As boys and girls approach middle school or junior high, a mysterious metamorphosis begins. Their hormones go into high gear and as their bodies experience enormous change a search begins for two things: *identity* and *independence*.

Mostly, we see the struggle for identity in the way young teens dress and try to "fit in." They can be moody and belligerent. They are children growing up in a culture moving so fast it threatens any sense of stability in their lives. Teenagers' need for acceptance is a natural drive and one that everyone must face. They have been loved by their parents; now they feel the need to be accepted by the world.

In the midst of this, just when many parents would love to shelter and protect them, teenagers begin to pull away. They need some space from their parents. They need to experiment with being on their own. This independence often surprises parents and can leave them somewhere between bewildered and hurt.

As the young person approaches high school, the search for identity and independence becomes more social. I once heard a sociologist claim that high school created a mini-society where a small percentage succeeded and everyone else spent the rest of their lives making up for it. If you doubt how powerful these years are in the life of your child, take a moment to reflect on your own high school experience. Were those years wonderful—full of achievement and popularity—or are your memories a painful and grim reminder of what you dreamed of being but were not?

Perhaps this exercise of memory seems to oversimplify things, but such reflection is intended to provide clues to the transitions your own young people must face during the teen years.

College is a good example. The college years represent the final transition from childhood to adulthood. Unfortunately, this transition is too often only symbolic. In many ways college students, or young people of college age, are the most hard pressed. They know they are approaching a time when they must take on adult responsibilities. The wild parties and recklessness often associated with these years represent either a last fling at childhood with its lack of responsibility, or rebellion at the notion that as young adults they are being forced to grow up. Today, this is often carried over into adulthood in the fast-paced, get-rich-quick attitude of so many young folks just starting out.

I couldn't fathom the tunnel Kit had stumbled into or comprehend how he had gotten so lost. I had served as a compass for a part of his journey. But, in the end, he chose his own route. When Kit had realized he had taken a wrong turn so soon on his life journey, he was afraid to stop and ask for directions. Unable to face the consequences of his decision, he got out.

Perhaps I was too consumed with my own sense of failure. As I sat on the smooth, varnished pew I felt rough and tarnished. My thoughts strayed to how others more capable, or more spiritual, might have changed the course of Kit's life. This is always the game we play. Someone else could have done it better. He or she would have prayed more, had the right words to say, appeared at just the right moments. I wondered how many more Kits I would come in contact with in days and years to come. I wondered how many parents would feel the same sense of failure.

I was startled out of my reflections when the pastor began to speak. At that point in the funeral service he gave me a great gift. He spoke with fondness of the change and impact that Young Life had on Kit and read from the Bible I had given Kit—words of hope Kit had marked during our studies together. Then he said, "The only problem was that Kit didn't wait for God to fulfill His promises." Waiting isn't easy for young people. Yet waiting is part of learning to deal with life's inevitable transitions. And none of us deals effectively with change all of the time.

I realized then that the pastor and I were a team. We had not made an official agreement, but nevertheless we were on the same team, with the same hopes and goals and prayers for young folks like Kit. Now he was supporting me in the same way both of us had sought to support Kit. Sometimes it is crucial to know that we do not battle alone.

TOOLS FOR TEEN TRANSITIONS ARE AVAILABLE

As a parent I have a strong desire to give my children the tools they need to face the transitions of adolescence and early adult life. But as someone who has been in youth ministry all of my adult life, I also have a strong desire to see parents and their kids develop a strong *team* to support and guide them through the tricky and often perilous times in their teenagers' lives.

Too many young people race through their early years unaware and tragically unprepared to deal in healthy ways with the *inevitable* changes they must face. Suddenly, they find themselves in previously uncharted waters with no navigational system and no anchor. They are adrift in a sea of change with no land or hope in sight. These are not necessarily young people from bad homes with difficult lives. Even for successful children from the best of families, the current of transition can carry them to perilous waters. Many will not stay afloat.

Life is never static. It is always changing, moving forward, dynamic. How many times have we as adults felt like screaming, "Stop the world and let me off!"? But time will not stop. No matter how we attempt to alter it or simply slow it down, it marches on. We cannot shield our children from change, therefore we must prepare them for it.

We really have only two options. We either prepare ourselves and our kids for the inevitabilities of transition and the march of time, or we watch as we and our children are pushed, jostled, and occasionally trampled as life surges ahead.

Transitions are points in our journey where we pass from one phase to another. In a novel, transitions can make the story easy to read and enjoyable; poorly done, they render the book choppy and hard to follow. The same is true in our lives and in the lives of young people. The passage of each phase of adolescence can have a lot to do with whether they experience success or failure handling change as adults.

As a high schooler, Kit hadn't anticipated the need to know how to face transition. He had never considered the impact time and change would have on him. When the reality of his choices finally caught up to him, he lost all hope and in his own way he struck back. He wasn't prepared for failure and couldn't bring himself to ask for help.

This is not a book of pat answers and easy antidotes. Nor is it a scientific experiment. I really hope to accomplish two major tasks. First, I want to share what I have observed and learned through years of walking the passages of adolescence and young adult life with hundreds of kids and their parents. And second, I'd like to help draw you closer to the One who desires to reveal Himself in the midst of the storms and changing tides of our lives. He is the One who gives comfort and hope. For He enables us to navigate the perilous waters of transition.

Deeply imbedded in the lines of this book is the conviction that the closer we walk to the heart of Christ, the more we experience His love and mercy—and the more we are able to dispense such love during the tides of change in our families.

To hear of the birth of Christ and then learn of His resurrection is a wonderful thing. Those two events changed the course of human history. Yet, without the stories of His life from childhood through the cross, the account is woefully incomplete. We see something of Jesus' passage from childhood to adulthood when we read of Him as a boy in the Temple courts asking the rabbis questions (Luke 2:41-49). We are filled with wonder when we think of what this event must have meant to Mary and Joseph as they began to glimpse the change that was about to hit their lives.

Another critical transition comes in John 2. A wedding celebration Jesus and His mother were attending was about to come to an abrupt end because of an exhausted wine supply, and Mary began to sense in her heart that maybe this was the moment Jesus would be catapulted into public ministry. Up to this point He had quietly begun to gather disciples and teach in the synagogue. But, if He now did what His mother asked Him to do, His life would never be the same. He would become a miracle worker, a hero, a religious celebrity.

One must wonder if Jesus paused a moment there. This miracle would start in motion a chain of events that would eventually lead Him to the cross. One must also wonder how Mary had perceived that this indeed was the time of a significant transition for her Son.

What a moment!

It is one thing to read the words describing the miracle Jesus performed that day. It is altogether different to try to grasp the significance of this transition in the life of our Savior and the role Mary played in recognizing the necessary turn of events. When He was a child she had protected Him from perceived dangers, now she could not protect Him from the inevitable—the Father's plan.

In a similar sense, we must realize there is no way to protect our children from change. They must eventually face the realities of their growing up, as must we. But we all desire to walk through the phases of our lives with less surprise, less fear, and less sense of failure.

This is a book about growth, about the realization that growing pains are as much a part of maturing as are lost love or lost security. It is about dealing with the trauma of these inevitable teenage transitions.

THE TRANSITION TEAM

In an election year the first place the president-elect turns his focus is to his transition team. The team's job is to make sure the new president has as smooth a transition as possible. They scout ahead for potential disaster, help him choose his administrative team, make sure he shakes the right hands and speaks to the right people, and in general, assure the public they made the right choice. How well the team members do their job will have great impact on how well the president makes the transition to his new role and responsibility.

Perhaps a team like this is exactly what Kit, or his parents, needed. In the following chapters we will be assembling your team. It is my prayer that these tools will provide help and confidence for you parents as you sail the often-troubled sea of transition with your children on their voyage to adulthood.

• • • • • • • • • • •

CHAPTER TWO

Teen Passages

*"There is no reason for you to be embarrassed
about S-E-X," I told my daughter. "Sit down and
I will tell you all I know about it. First, Lassie is
a girl. Second, I lied. Sensuous lips do not mean
fever blisters. Third, I did not conceive you by
drinking the blood of an owl and spitting three
times at a full moon. Here is the bra and girdle
section from the Sears catalogue. If you have any
questions, keep them to yourself."*

ERMA BOMBECK

I n this chapter we explore the various stages of adolescent development. This will give you a framework by which you can view the transitions your son or daughter will face.

Each of us has had to deal with the changes between childhood and adulthood. We challenged the ideas of our childhood and stretched the patience and wisdom of our parents. To say that adolescence is a complex time for parents and children often seems like an understatement. The period of adolescence is not static. It will begin earlier for some children than others. It will be more painful for some than others. But, it is a pivotal time in children's lives, and how they handle it is directly linked to whether their adult development is healthy or not.

THE TWO PHASES OF ADOLESCENCE

For our examination of the adolescent experience we will break the broader period of adolescence into two primary categories. The first is *early adolescence*, those years generally associated with junior high school and running from age ten through age fifteen. The second phase we will call *late adolescence*, which approximately corresponds to the senior high and college years, or ages sixteen to twenty-two. Because the time and intensity of adolescence will vary with every child, it is difficult to be more specific. But these two divisions of adolescence are widely adhered to by experts in sociology, psychology, and education.

EARLY ADOLESCENCE

"Adolescence" comes from the Latin verb *adolescere*, which means "to grow," or "to grow to maturity." While we may be most conscious of the physical changes in our children during early adolescence, this transition in their young lives is far more radical than mere physical change. To aid us in our discussion of this period, we will look at the two most dramatic types of change of the *early adolescent* period: *physical* and *emotional.*

Physical: The Great Awakening. Generally, the first thing that comes to mind when parents think of early adolescence is puberty. That is when we brace ourselves for everything in our family to come unglued. Puberty may be a prelude to confusion and disarray in your home, but that is not always the case.

It is difficult to predict the beginning or the end of the pubertal process. There is about a *six-to-seven-year* range in both boys and girls for both pubescence and puberty. *Pubescence* is the stage of physical growth marked by the maturation of reproductive functions and the primary sex organs and by the appearance of secondary sex characteristics (breasts, pubic hair, changes in voice and skin, and so on). Pubescence lasts about two years and ends in *puberty*, the point at which a person is sexually able to reproduce—and the time of life when the greatest sexual differentiation since the prenatal stage takes place.[1]

Judith suddenly seems glued to a mirror. She is always looking at herself with a critical yet curious eye. For the first time she is recognizing the new contours of her body, and while she is entranced by her body in private, she is very nervous and self-conscious in public.

Many young girls who mature quickly experience a time of insecurity. They may feel conspicuous and out of place among their peers. Parents and teachers may treat them differently, even appear as if they disapprove of the way they look. This can be a very trying, but productive experience for young women as they learn to face differences and challenges for later life.

The same is true for young boys. While sometimes it is fun for them to "look older" than their peers, often they are not mature enough to handle the expectations resulting from their mature appearance. It has been my experience that the "late bloomer" often develops better coping skills as an adult because of the challenges of early adolescence.

Emotional: A Roller Coaster Ride. Adolescence is a period of tremendous emotional upheaval. Transition and change are challenging for any of us, but for a young teenager experiencing the emotional challenges of adolescence, they can be even more difficult.

Here is a list of some of the most prominent causes of emotional tension in teens:

- Coping with physical change
- Setting aside childhood habits
- Lack of social (adult) skills
- Dealing with the opposite sex
- Family stability (or lack of)
- Environmental changes (moving, new schools, new church)
- Failure in school
- Parental conflict (stretching old boundaries)
- Moving from dependence to independence

Any or all of these emotional challenges are bound to bring behavioral consequences with them. Often this is a result of teens' feelings of insecurity and fear.

Here are some of the typical behavioral side effects:

- Aggressiveness
- Self-consciousness and ego-centeredness
- Withdrawal from others
- Aloofness
- False courage (macho)
- Moodiness
- Daydreaming
- Sudden outbursts
- Irritability
- Demandingness
- Materialistic

In *early adolescence* each child experiences these emotions differently and at various times. There is a great deal of moving back and forth. One moment your teen will seem grown-up and you have a feeling of a job well done, then the next moment you will be wondering if that teen will ever grow up. But as we will see, the challenge continues into *late adolescence.*

LATE ADOLESCENCE
While physical maturity and emotional stability are still issues among older teens, two other transitional developments often rush to the forefront: *intellectual development* and *identity.*

Intellectual Development. When a young child is told that his father is no longer going to live with the family, many times he will assume it was because he was bad. This is because children are *concrete thinkers.* They take everything at face value. Teenagers going through *late adolescence* have developed the ability to think *abstractly* to the point where they can weigh various bits of information and draw an independent conclusion regarding the situation.

Developing this skill allows teenagers to take information gathered in the past and apply it to current situations. Young people are therefore capable of hypothetical-deductive reasoning.

Egocentrism. Experts believe that this new ability to reason in adolescence brings with it a unique sort of egocentrism. The teenager begins to act as if others are as preoccupied with her behavior as she herself is.[2]

Although teens are rarely aware of this egocentrism, they act out their need for being "center stage" in numerous ways. Romantic interests, conformity to peers, and even peer relationships can be part of this new attention-getting style. Part of this transition for teens relates to the discovery of *ideals*. This new thinking can inspire and repulse adults. It is a mode of thinking that often forsakes the practical for the adventurous and romantic.

David Elkind describes some adolescent behaviors behind this new thinking:

- Finding fault with authority figures
- Argumentativeness
- Self-consciousness
- Self-centeredness
- Indecisiveness
- Apparent hypocrisy[3]

Parents must view these behaviors as natural and consistent with all adolescent development. This does not mean unacceptable behavior should simply be tolerated in the home, but knowing that these behaviors are generally part of the growth process will help parents take a more objective view of their teen.

Identity. As teenagers begin to view themselves from this new vantage point, a search for identity begins. Ideals often begin to emerge. Teens begin to wonder how their lives can really count in the world. By now they have established some personal views of success and fulfillment.

The entire adolescent period is one of great influence. We often call them "wet cement" years because adolescents are formulating so many views about life. The battle to mold these young minds and hearts is a fierce one. The competition is tough.

One way kids discover who they are is by what Elkind calls *markers*.

> Markers are external signs of where we stand, in Kierkegaard's lovely phrase, in "the stages on life's way." Markers can be as simple as the pencil lines on the kitchen wall that mark a child's progress in height from birthday to birthday, or as complex as a well-deserved promotion after years of hard work and dedication. Markers are signs of progress to others as well as to ourselves.
>
> We all have a "sense of becoming," of growing and changing as individuals. Markers confirm us in our sense of growing and changing.
>
> Giving up old markers also helps the young person become aware of his or her progress toward maturity. There is a direct parallel between the child of six or seven who says, "I don't believe in Santa Claus anymore," and the car-driving sixteen-year-old who says, "I don't ride bikes anymore." In both cases there is a pride in a new accomplishment and in a certain disdain for an earlier skill marker that is now seen as part of a period one has left behind.[4]

If as parents we work hard to recognize the markers in our children's lives, and allow them the privilege to move from one to another, we will help our kids stay on target and give them a better chance to make good decisions.

It is easy for parents, especially fathers, to become emotionally distant or separated from their teenagers. Busy with careers and adult activities, moms and dads often continue to think of their children as just that—children. Sometimes this means thinking of them as still six instead of sixteen; at other times it means comparing them when they hit age eighteen to themselves at that age.

But times have changed and so have kids. They have been exposed to more of the world than we were at the same age. They have more choices to make in school than we did. Sex is an open topic, and drugs and alcohol influence every campus.

While they seem less ready to accept responsibility overall, they are more aware of what adult life is like socially. They have been tutored by the media on all the vices available to the adult, and each lesson is pushed by handsome men and beautiful women eager to get them to try these vices out.

If parents are not able to communicate with their children during this time, it can be a crushing blow for both. For parents it generates a great sense of failure, for kids, a sense of frustration and alienation.

Complicating late adolescence is a strong sense of idealism in young people. Whether they live it out or not, they have a strong sense of justice and right and wrong. This idealism comes from a new view of the hurt and injustice in the world. They become aware that half the world goes to bed hungry every night. While it may not slow down their junk-food habits, it may cause them to criticize their parents for tossing those leftovers when so many are starving.

Often they are very judgmental. This can hurt parents and at times make us angry. Yet of all the generations of parents, we should be the most sympathetic to this phase of growing up. All of us are at least aware of the upheaval of the sixties. The riots and student protests of that era were led by some of you reading this book. Materialism was *out* and all adults, especially parents, were not to be trusted. The lesson we learned in the eighties is that idealism without truth never leads to lasting change. The famous protesters of the sixties became the ravenous consumers of the eighties. If the music of the sixties was protest songs, the sound of the eighties carried a beat that could be exercised to by all those graying hippies seeking youthful bodies again.

Young adults want answers—now! Patience is not very high on their list of virtues. They spurn the well-worn solutions offered by their parents and seek the truth for themselves.

To make matters worse, the questions and struggles of our kids during late adolescence sometimes bring to the surface unresolved issues of our past. We are imperfect people. Recognizing and accepting the gaps in our own lives will make us more tolerant toward our children.

Yet, one of the great gifts of adolescent idealism is that adolescents will not be comfortable with our "brand" of religion if they sense it is not real in us or impacting the world. They will push us to examine our own relationship to Christ. I have seen many families renewed in Christ because of their teenager's witness.

ONE TEEN'S WITNESS

In the desert, surrounded by the affluence and luxury of Scottsdale, Arizona, two lonely people lived in a rented shack. Some college-age volunteer leaders for Young Life noticed Fritz's loneliness. They could not articulate his needs scientifically or academically; they simply saw a young person in need. As Fritz slowly got involved in the Young Life program he began to discover a place of acceptance and nurture. He loved the meetings and the leaders who showed such kindness toward him. He responded to virtually every opportunity for camps and outings, always learning afresh that this was a place he belonged. Acceptance wasn't an issue with these friends, it was a given. Soon Fritz had given his life to Christ and was committed to weekly Bible studies.

As the leaders talked one evening, the subject of Fritz came up. They were all encouraged by the growth they saw in his life, yet there was a nagging feeling that something more was needed. Their sense of justice and their energy for doing it was still in high gear. They discussed numerous possibilities and finally came to a conviction that Fritz now needed a dentist to complete the metamorphosis occurring in his life.

They approached a sympathetic orthodontist, who agreed to greatly discount the cost of the dental work. Some parents, hearing what these young people had in mind, chipped in on the bill. The next time I saw Fritz he gave me a wide smile showing off his new braces. He was proud of the hardware in his mouth. It represented a significant step in his life. Those braces would be a marker he would always look back to.

On a Sunday morning a few months later, our pastor asked if anyone there would like someone to pray with him or her to find Christ. I noticed two hands in the front row go up. To my surprise one hand belonged to Fritz and the other to a gray-haired gentleman next to him. It didn't take me long to figure out who the man was. He was Fritz's dad.

As I made my way toward the front of the church to stand with them, I couldn't help but consider the events that had led to this moment. Fritz had experienced the love of Christ through a group of young volunteers. He had discovered the identity and acceptance that had long eluded him. Now that he had some clear markers to guide his way he had found another important one. He had moved from follower to leader. His father, overwhelmed and intrigued by the changes in his son, had agreed to visit church with him The Spirit of God did the rest.

CONFLICT

Conflict is an inevitable part of adolescence. As teenagers begin to develop their reasoning skills, they will look for opportunities to make decisions on their own. They will challenge our values and take an idealistic approach to our practical advice. While conflict generally escalates during *early adolescence*, it is often not until later that parents suddenly think the disagreeing will never end.

Most arguments between parents and their adolescents focus on normal, everyday goings-on, such as schoolwork, social life, peers, home chores, disobedience, sibling fights, and personal hygiene.[5] Within some normal range, then, conflict with parents may be psychologically healthy for the adolescent's development. A virtually conflict-free relationship may indicate that an adolescent has a fear of separation, exploration, and independence.[6]

It is important to remember the impact of youthful idealism on the world. Much is done because of adolescents' convictions and zeal. They challenge old ideas and force us to defend or discard our positions. In that way, they are good for us, and we must allow reasonable room for them to grow and think for themselves. Listen to General Douglas MacArthur's thought on this.

> Youth is not a period of time. It is a state of mind,
> a result of the will, a quality of the imagination, a
> victory of courage over timidity, of the taste of adven-
> ture over the love of comfort. A man doesn't grow old
> when he deserts his ideal. The years may wrinkle
> his skin, but deserting his ideal wrinkles his soul.
> Preoccupations, fears, doubts, and despair are the
> dust before death. You will remain young as long as
> you are open to what is beautiful, good, and great;
> receptive to the messages of other men and women,
> of nature and of God. If one day you should become

bitter, pessimistic, and gnawed by despair, may God have mercy on your old man's soul.[7]

HIGH SCHOOL

One parenting expert says this about high school: "High School is the central organizing experience in most adolescents' intellectual lives. It offers basic day-to-day learning, a preview of career choices, and opportunities to participate in sports and get together with friends."[8]

This prime social and academic environment is where many of the adolescent transitions blend together. In high school, puberty, abstract thinking, independence, and identity all merge in the teenager. You may well see many of the behaviors associated with adolescence in your child at this point. At the same time, there are some important decisions being made. As most young people begin to think about college and careers, they are forced to ask, "Who am I going to be?" and "What am I going to do?"

I think today we have allowed too much focus to land on "Who will I *look* like I am?" There has been so much emphasis on having money, cars, nice homes, and spectacular vacations that teens are often more concerned about finding a job that will net them a desired lifestyle than they are about living a productive and fulfilling life. While it is obviously true that both fulfillment and financial reward can be attained together, the wrong focus can keep teens from taking a realistic view of what they should get out of life.

My son Josh is in elementary school. He wants to be a pro football player someday. There is very little doubt in his mind about his chances. The elementary school years are generally the fantasy period. My son Caleb is in his junior high school years. He often rebukes Josh for his optimism about a future in football. Caleb would love to play pro basketball someday, but he has begun to admit it may not happen. He is in his tentative period. Before they graduate from college they should move into the realistic period and begin to look seriously and realistically at what they want to do with their lives. In my opinion, the media blitz on young consumers, increased foreign competition that impacts jobs and services, and the frantic rush for financial success in the 1980s has caused many young people to avoid this realistic period. For many the "appearance" of success has blurred their view of fulfillment, the establishment of realistic goals, and the notion of God's call—the most important element in anyone's vocational outlook.

WORK—AN OPTIONAL TEEN TRANSITION

More young people are working today than ever before. While there are a number of positive aspects to this, there is a down side as well.

On the positive side, working can influence your teen's self-image. It can help the teen develop some independence, time management, and a positive attitude about work and authority. If the manager or employer is willing to give thorough training and be sensitive to a teen's other responsibilities (such as family time), working can be a rewarding experience.

In a survey of high school seniors, three out of four had some kind of job income. But on a negative note, the same survey showed that tenth graders who worked more than fourteen hours per week suffered a drop in grades. A similar drop was found among eleventh graders who worked more than twenty hours per week.[9]

DEVELOPMENTAL TASKS

Every culture makes certain expectations of those who are to be considered adults. Certain tasks should be learned if a person is to function adequately in our society. During the adolescent years, the following skills should be developed:

1. Achieving new and more mature relations with age-mates of both sexes;
2. Achieving a masculine or feminine social role;
3. Accepting one's own physique and using the body effectively;
4. Achieving emotional independence of parents and other adults;
5. Achieving assurance of economic independence;
6. Selecting and preparing for an occupation;
7. Preparing for marriage and family life;
8. Developing intellectual skills and concepts necessary for civic obedience;
9. Desiring and achieving socially responsible behavior; and
10. Acquiring a set of values and an ethical system as a guide to behavior.[10]

Helping your teen acquire these skills is a big job. You'll need every member of your *transition team* to help you and your child through this important passage. It is also critical to keep in mind that the adolescent period will go to at least age twenty-two and sometimes later. If your eighteen-year-old has not mastered all of these skills yet, don't start worrying that he or she will never grow up. As we learn to understand the various stages of adolescent development and discover how to make our transition team work, we will find the whole process less intimidating and more enjoyable.

SPIRITUAL DEVELOPMENT

Often as we raise our teenagers the most frightening thought is that they might not choose to follow Christ. The idea of them rejecting something we hold so dearly is a painful thought. But the fact is, teens must "choose" whom they will follow. It is not a decision we can make for them. I am encouraged by Kevin Huggins when he says,

I believe God is at work in kids' hearts. And I believe He is summoning them to nothing less than a life of servanthood for Him. My goal is to provide the kind of environment in the relationship and responses I offer kids that makes them both aware of and accountable for why they do the things they do. When my strategy majors on getting them to just change their behavior to get out of trouble, or just change their circumstances to get out of pain, then I am actually making it easier for them to enter adulthood without grappling with the main issue of life: *Who are they* intending to serve through their actions?[11]

Most people in youth ministry agree that the adolescent years are when kids are most open to committing their lives to Christ. They may challenge the "religion" of their parents and even complain about our "old-fashioned" values, but they are still looking for truth and their hearts are hungry for a sense of wholeness and love. We must give our teens the freedom to choose, while we provide an environment that encourages them toward Christ.

The adolescent period is complex and challenging. There are many points along the way where things can go wrong. But if we can begin to prepare ourselves for what is ahead, we can help our kids set a course for a productive and useful adult life.

From Brennan Manning's book *The Ragamuffin Gospel* come these words from the Indian poet Tagore:

No, it is not yours to open buds into blossom.
Shake the bud, strike,
      it is beyond your power to make it blossom.
Your touch soils it.
You tear its petal to pieces
      and strew them in the dust,
But no colors appear and no perfume.

Oh, it is not for you to open the bud into blossom.
He who can open the bud does it so simply.
He gives it a glance and the life sap stirs
    through its veins.
At his breath the flower spreads its wings
    and flutters in the wind.
Colors flash out like heart longing,
    the perfume betrays a sweet secret.
He who can open the bud does it so simply.[12]

● ● ● ● ● ● ● ● ● ●

CHAPTER THREE

Managing Expectations

Will was one of the finest basketball players ever to grace the courts of our city. He had superb physical tools and the mental tenacity to be a winner. He could score, rebound, block shots, and play defense. In short, he was a coach's dream. He was also a parent's dream.

When our basketball team took the court, invariably most eyes were on Will. He had become a near legend. Most people overlooked the fact that he wasn't a great student. And hardly anyone knew how sensitive he was. Here was a great big kid with unbelievable talent who basically wanted to please everyone.

It was no surprise to any of us when dozens of colleges began vying for Will's basketball talents. Some schools wanted him so badly they were willing to offer some of his less talented teammates scholarships just to get Will to attend their school.

Those were heady days for such a sensitive young guy.

As the time approached for choosing a college, Will asked me for advice. Knowing that he wasn't an outstanding student and just how vulnerable he was by nature, I encouraged him to stay close to home. Several good schools close by could offer him everything he needed, including the support of good friends. The weight and pressure of the decision was beginning to slump his shoulders and slow his step. He could no longer enjoy the simple pleasures of his peers; his was a life of notoriety and constant attention. All eyes seemed to be on him and everyone was guessing which school would be the recipient of his considerable talent. I hoped and prayed he could relax after the decision was made.

Finally, one major event changed the course of his life. He talked to his parents. They had been so proud of his accomplishments and so sure of his future that they actually told him that if he didn't go to a big-time basketball school they would never speak to him again.

I couldn't help feeling it wasn't Will's future they were most concerned about. Will obediently chose the school they recommended.

Everything seemed to go well at first. On the surface, Will was adjusting to college life and contributing to the team. He had grown even taller after he arrived at the university and his potential now seemed limitless. That is, until a series of injuries cost Will his athletic career. No one had noticed along the way that he was barely able to stay in school academically. The average upperclassman playing football or basketball spends thirty hours per week in practice and preparation for games and only twenty-five hours per week in the classroom and studying.[1]

Will was unable to finish his degree. This failure, coupled with the loss of his athletic career, caused his self-esteem to plummet. As a result, he couldn't bring himself to come home for a visit because he couldn't face the family and friends he felt he had disappointed. Can you imagine a young man thinking that a whole community had pinned their hopes on his success? The wave of adulation and the soaring expectations he felt from almost everyone he knew made it impossible for him to face the folks in his hometown.

When I flew out to spend some time with him, Will was smoking one cigarette after another and taking an anti-depression drug prescribed by his psychiatrist.

The addiction to applause had become too great a habit for Will to kick. The disappointment was too heavy a burden to bear. In his adolescent heart he wanted to please. He had developed a chronic need for the praise and respect that had come so early in his life. Nothing had prepared him for this sudden fall from grace.

His parents had an equally hard time adjusting to the change. They grew tired of answering questions and found it impossible to hide their disappointment in Will. When disappointment gave way to resentment, the entire family structure collapsed. Will's mom and dad, now divorced and living in separate cities, rarely see their son and barely know his wife and children. Parental expectations and peer pressure had infected and destroyed a family.

BALANCING OUR EXPECTATIONS FOR OUR KIDS

As parents we all run the risk of expecting too much from our kids. But this does not have to be the case. Often the problem stems from *what* we are expecting. Athletics are not an important enough gauge of a person's worth to shape a life over it. Neither is academic achievement. These are simply convenient measuring sticks to see how our kids stack up against the "competition." We hope our kids can excel in something, and when they do we reward them for their performance. But to major in "outdoing the competition" reveals values that are not rooted in the Scriptures.

Young people want to be valued. Yet one of the greatest frustrations I have heard from kids over the years is that they don't measure up to the expectations of their parents. They seldom hear a "way to go" or "I'm proud of you" from Mom and Dad. Too often, it's, "Why did you get a B in that class instead of an A?"

While we want our children to succeed and develop a work ethic that always strives for excellence, none of us wants to set them up for depression and anxiety down the road. We know the world is rough, and we want them prepared for the hard knocks they must face. So we must be very careful to choose what to focus our expectations on. Somewhere there is a balance. As parents we must be committed to discovering what that is for each of our children.

FOCUSING ON VALUES AND CHARACTER
Tim Kimmel in his book *The Legacy of Love* highlights some important character traits for us to pass on to our children.[2] I appreciate the fact that he didn't give us guidelines for successful-looking children or something like that. He points out rather clearly that our children are in need of the right character, not the right style.

Faith, integrity, poise, discipline, endurance, and courage are the values Tim recommends.[3] If we keep these building blocks in mind, we won't need to worry what *our* peers are thinking. If we want our kids to remember it, we must remember that reputation is a byproduct, not a goal. If you want a good reputation in business, start by planning well, working hard, and showing integrity in your dealings with others. You will find little need for a public relations firm if you start out the right way. When parents focus on helping their children develop character, their reputation will reflect that character.

I have often quoted a little poem penned by an unknown author regarding character.

> Sow a thought
> Reap an act

> Sow an act
>> Reap a habit
> Sow a habit
>> Reap a character
> Sow a character
>> Reap a destiny.

Kids today are conspicuously conscious of what others think, especially their peers. But they often have a difficult time thinking through the consequences of their thoughts and actions. Part of the growing-up transition is learning to think. As parents we will give enormous aid to our sons and daughters if we affirm them as people while asking caring questions about their thoughts and feelings. At the same time, we must be careful to manage our own expectations of them. Our expectations, after all, reveal our own true values.

One of the toughest experiences I have had to face came from an extreme end of the spectrum of parental expectations.

By the seventh grade Mike had already experienced a tough life. His father was convinced that he would grow up to be a good-for-nothing and told him so frequently. If something came up missing at home, Mike got the blame. He rarely received any praise from his folks.

Mike was one of those kids who wasn't really a trouble-maker; he just hung out with some of the wrong kids and seemed to be the one who always got caught. I would look at him with his straight brown hair nearly covering his eyes and he would shrug his shoulders and tell me he really didn't mean whatever it was they were accusing him of this time. Mike was never belligerent. I never saw or heard of him hurting anyone, but he was living out an expectation that he would never amount to anything.

I am convinced Mike committed his heart to Christ, yet he struggled with the wrong set of expectations. At the age of sixteen Mike turned in front of a car while riding his motorcycle and was killed instantly.

He had fulfilled a tragic and unnecessary prophecy. Ultimately he lived up to the expectations that had been programmed in him. I guess I had hoped he could have lived long enough to prove them wrong. When he was killed on the motorcycle, his parents treated the tragedy like it was "one more dumb mistake by Mike."

We can be sure that whatever our expectations are, our kids will probably live up to them.

Because this is so true, parents of adolescents caught in the trauma of transition must be committed to building the character of their children and not simply their personalities. The question should not revolve around how popular, or accepted by your friends, or even by their friends, they are. The key issue is, do they reflect the kind of character that is consistent with their faith?

In today's culture kids have become part of parents' résumés. The success of the child is too often seen as a reflection of the success of the parent. Therefore, teenagers are not allowed to make choices that might change the perception held by their parents' friends and associates. Will had been an important part of how his parents viewed themselves. They loved the attention they received as a result of their son's success. It proved to be as much an addiction for them as it had become for him. Later, when he needed their unconditional acceptance, all he found was disappointment. In their eyes he had squandered a wonderful opportunity. He would never rise to his real potential. As an adult Will is still working through the pain of that ordeal.

THE ART OF ENCOURAGING TEENS

Encouragement is an art. We must work at it constantly.

Young people facing the transitions of adolescence need encouragement. They also need recognition, but we must carefully keep these two separate. By encouragement I am referring to *building up our children for who they are and not for what they do*. As parents we want to reinforce our love and commitment in ways that have nothing to do with their performance. Recognition means acknowledging their accomplishments and hard work.

To really excel at encouragement, we need to move beyond worrying about what our peers may think. If your son or daughter is not the "best" at something, that does not mean he or she will never achieve great things as an adult. In the long run, if your child reaches adulthood with faith intact and a clear sense of right and wrong, I'd say you have a very successful child. The world judges people by the cars, houses, and toys they can purchase. As Christians, we have a much better gauge for our lives. It is to be conformed to the image of Christ.

Telling your children things like "I love you," "You are a great person," and "I am proud to be your parent" for no apparent reason will create a mountain of confidence and security for kids trudging through the valley of adolescence.

Be spontaneous in your praise of the teenager in your home. If you wait for the "right" moment, you will lose a lifetime of opportunity. When your teens succeed at something, be quick to congratulate them, but don't tie "I love you" to those events. Children feel enough pressure to perform without the added suspicion that our love for them is wrapped in a package of performance. Instead, tell them how proud you are that they chose to work so hard to accomplish what they did and that the end results were great.

THE PRODIGAL PARENT: A MODEL FOR MANAGING PARENTAL PEER PRESSURE

The story of the lost son in Luke 15:11-24 is one of the best-remembered parables in Scripture. The father's unsurpassed love and acceptance is a lasting reminder of our heavenly Father's commitment to us. Here a young man had squandered his inheritance and had forsaken the morals and teachings of his youth, put his father through incredible agony and grief, and then was accepted back by his dad without a second's hesitation. It's more than we can fathom.

If this father had been more concerned about his reputation, he would never have allowed his son back so easily. Proper penitence and reparation would have been required. But this father didn't base his action on how he would be perceived by the religious in the community. He was responding to his son who was lost and now was found. Had this father been in a modern church, he may have had to deal with losing a position of leadership in the church because he was not managing his household in a manner "suitable" for someone in his position. He would have had to endure the humiliation of public acknowledgment of his failure as a parent.

We often decry the impact of peer pressure on our children and deny its impact in our own lives. Many times in the Christian community we feel the pressure to raise successful and trouble-free kids. We don't know what to do with those creative free spirits in our home who challenge every rule and thought. We want them to represent the family in a positive way. But we don't want to kill their spirit, either.

We need more parents like the prodigal's father—unashamed of their love for their children and unafraid of the perception of others. As parents we must become more and more confident in our relationship with our Father and less dependent on the approval of others. Our sons and daughters need the freedom to fail in the context of a loving home so they will not become addicted to the drug of pleasing people to gain acceptance.

TEEN PEER PRESSURE

Peer pressure may be the biggest challenge your teenager will face. Never minimize the strain of peer pressure. It is one of the constant forces of the adolescent life. Peer pressure tests the strength of young people. With the onset of adolescence, acceptance by one's peers becomes a need of titanic proportions.

As we learned earlier, most teenagers lack a sense of identity in one way or another. During adolescence they discover a new social order. They begin moving into adult activities and situations. They date, drive, make decisions about what kind of friends to have, and begin to compete for a place on the social ladder. During this pivotal time they are often somewhat closed to the comments and advice of their parents. This is a discovery time and a time to test the turbulent waters of the adult world.

In 1968 only 7 percent of driving-age teens owned cars. Now the figure is 35 percent.[4] A 1988 survey of twelve- to nineteen-year-olds conducted by an advertising firm revealed that 69 percent considered themselves to be adults. Independence was the greatest desire of 69 percent of the sample.[5]

As concern for status and acceptance escalates among our kids, so do other pressures. Playing on these needs, corporate America bombards them with the latest gimmicks for achieving the attention and acceptance they strive for. Teens now spend $55.9 billion annually on their day-to-day needs. This figure is up from $25.3 billion in 1975, even though the teenage population has dropped 15.5 percent since 1980.[6]

As parents we must recognize the needs of acceptance and identity within our teens. We cannot battle nature, but we can create a framework for help in the midst of this chaos. We know that the timing of these transitions and when they peak will be different for every young person. We also know each will respond to the challenges differently.

PREPARING FOR PEER PRESSURE CHANGES

So how do we face the dark clouds on our child's horizon? How will we prepare for the changes ahead?

First, remember that every child does not experience a grave crisis at each intersection of adolescence. Many will integrate most of the changes gracefully and without a great deal of drama. So let's not create a crisis if one is not there. At the same time, let's have our transition team in place and ready in case the need arises.

Pray for your kids. Each day give yourself anew to your heavenly Father, then leave the burdens of parenthood in His protective embrace.

If your household has both mom and dad, work hard together. Discuss the issues ahead of time and try to reach a consensus on the direction you want to take.

Everyone needs to think through the available resources. Ask, who can I call for help? Which institutions and organizations can I network with? Parents who are raising kids without considering every reasonable resource will feel like they are baking a cake with only half the ingredients. No matter how much sugar you add, if you don't add the flour and the rest of the ingredients, you won't have a cake.

If we are making decisions based on the long view of who we are and who we believe our child can be, our emotions and perspective can be healthier. The father of the prodigal son was able to look beyond the filth, both inwardly and outwardly, and embrace his son. He did not do it out of appreciation or even acceptance of the young man's lifestyle, nor was he responding out of fear that he might lose him again. His reaction was one of love and hope. Love for a son who though once lost had now been found and hope that the future would find them in relationship together.

Love is not a matter of public opinion. It is an attitude that recognizes the needs of acceptance and identity and provides the necessary room and the right resources for a son or daughter to find acceptance as a person and identity in Christ.

Let's strive to make the priorities John Baillie sets down in the following prayer our own.

O Lord—let me put right before interest: let me put others before self: let me put things of the Spirit before things of the body: let me put the attainment of noble ends before the enjoyment of present pleasures: let me put principle above reputation: let me put you before all else. Amen.[7]

• • • • • • • • • • •
Making Transition Your Ally

In many ways growing up has never been more difficult. Kids are faced with more choices and are required to make more decisions at a younger age than ever before. It is no wonder that stress and burnout are now observable in the lives of many young people.

Our kids are a product of a high-tech world, and the name of the game in technology is change. By the time they get the latest CD player it is out of date. On top of that, marketing strategists have discovered that kids are a highly profitable consumer group. So young people are being bombarded with ads to buy more and more.

A recently published survey provided this insight:

Teens have money to spend—girls go for make-up, boys spend more on entertainment. Girls' weekly average: clothing, $10.65; food and snacks, $6.50; entertainment, $3.45; cosmetics, $3.35; records and tapes, $1.80. Boys: food and snacks, $10.10; clothing, $6.19; entertainment, $4.35; records and tapes, $1.55; grooming, $1.10.[1]

But these are not just statistics. These are our children. Stacy, a senior who has been involved in Young Life all through high school, juggles school, dating, and Young Life and holds down two jobs to pay for her car and clothes.

Never before have junior high and especially high school students looked and dressed older than they do today. And with the clothes, cars, and money come other things. Surveys taken in 1988 show that 52 percent of seventeen-year-old girls had sex, up from 47 percent in 1979; for boys, it was 66 percent in 1988, up from 56 percent in 1979. Although AIDS cases among teenagers account for only 1 percent of the nation's total, the number of cases doubles every fourteen months, and many AIDS victims who are now developing the disease in their twenties got it during sexual activity in their teen years. The syphilis rate for teens aged fifteen to nineteen has jumped 67 percent since 1985, and condom use among teenagers doubled between 1979 and 1988. About one million teenagers have become pregnant every year since 1973—that's one out of ten fifteen-to-nineteen-year-old girls getting pregnant every year.[2]

We are aware that such activities are reinforced by media influences. Teens watch an average of twenty-two hours a week or about three hours a day of television.[3] And that includes MTV. They're also going to movies, listening to the radio, and reading magazines that are *explicit* and *influential*.

How does all this affect our college students?

A 1989 poll of first-year Harvard students revealed their three highest goals and values in life:

1. Money
2. Power
3. Reputation[4]

BUT THERE ARE STILL "GOOD KIDS" AROUND!

Now you may be thinking, "Things are not as bleak as all of that. There are still plenty of good kids around. After all, somebody's making it!" But the point is that the number of challenges today for those "good" kids has escalated dramatically. If you add to that the children living in single family homes or dealing with the breakup of their parents' marriages, the latchkey kids and young people facing the typical debilitating factors of their age, it paints a very challenging picture for all of us.

Jeff was an early bloomer. From age six until the ninth grade he was one of the best athletes in the city. During his junior high years he became a Pop Warner football legend. The high school coaches couldn't wait for him to arrive. Jeff didn't disappoint them. He was big and strong and had a great attitude. Through the season he rarely got a rest during a game.

By Jeff's sophomore season things had changed considerably. Jeff was still hardworking and aggressive, but other boys had caught up with him physically. He could no longer dominate a game, and it looked like the glory days were over.

I watched Jeff closely. He continued to work as hard as ever, yet by his senior year he barely made the team. I waited for the deep disappointment and rebellion to set in. It is difficult enough for adults to come to grips with their physical changes, but in a kid like Jeff it had to be impossible.

I was wrong.

Like almost everyone, I had underestimated Jeff. Athletics had never been his whole life. By graduation he was one of the top students academically in the school. It wasn't until his athletic career began to wind down that people noticed his other qualities. He made a very difficult transition with remarkable ease because he was prepared. I didn't know his parents well, but I had great respect for their encouragement of Jeff's growth in various areas. It would have been very easy for them to begin in junior high to push Jeff toward a college football scholarship.

I have had the father of an eight-year-old boy tell me that he was gearing his son for a college scholarship in one particular sport. That kind of pressure rarely works.

TEENS CAN OVERCOME PERCEIVED SHORTCOMINGS

Acceptance and identity are too important to teenagers for parents to set them up for failure in these areas. Teens can accomplish so much if we will let them pursue their areas of giftedness and interest.

One of my favorite characters in Scripture is Zacchaeus. His story can be found in Luke 19:1-9. One day Jesus was passing through Jericho, that ancient city rich with the history of God's miraculous power. The city around which Joshua marched the triumphant nation of Israel several hundred years earlier was now filled with disciples and gawkers as Jesus moved along her dusty streets.

One of the spectators that day was Zacchaeus. We are given only two brief but very revealing insights into this man. First, he was a wealthy tax collector (19:2). In the next verse we discover that he was short (19:3).

Let me tell you a secret about Zacchaeus. He was short before he was rich.

Perhaps it was his physical stature that drove him to achieve political and economic success. He certainly had clout. He could charge whatever tax he wanted, and the Roman army helped him collect. He could line his pockets with the hard-earned money of his oppressed and impoverished countrymen and there was nothing they could do.

I have seen hundreds and hundreds of kids in my years of youth work who are driven to make up for perceived shortcomings in their lives. Whether it is physical, social, or economic deficiency—real or perceived—they are working as hard as they can to develop some kind of acceptable stature among their peers. They must find a place in their lives where they measure up.

Like so many of our kids today, Zacchaeus thought he had found his place. He had attained the wealth and power he craved. But somewhere along the way toward recognition and stature, he lost himself.

Loneliness and isolation will sometimes make us do desperate things. Zacchaeus was desperate to see Jesus. Because he was unable to see Jesus over the crowd, he risked his stature and certainly whatever dignity he had in the community and climbed a tree. Above the heads of that throng of people he had his chance not only to see, but to be seen by the Savior.

I have a theory. I believe that Zacchaeus wanted to be found. Not only did he want to see Jesus, but his heart was bursting to be known, to be loved, to be understood. Today's kids want to be found as well. Part of our job as parents, ministers, educators, and youthworkers is to help them be found.

We can imagine how the scene played out. As Zacchaeus crouched among the leaves and branches the crowd was stunned to silence when Jesus approached. The amused chuckles of the followers suddenly became sighs of wonder as Jesus stopped the whole procession to call Zacchaeus by name and start a life-changing relationship with him.

For Zacchaeus the transition was swift and dramatic. The results of being found aren't always that spectacular, but they can be just as miraculous and just as real.

There are obstacles between Jesus and young people today. Their vision is blocked by the towering challenges of adolescence. It is more difficult to see Him than ever before. Money, sex, and fame loom high over our adolescents' heads. The pain of their own deficiencies or those around them keeps them bowed too low to see their Hope. They simply lack the view that comes from experience to see Jesus on their own. Consequently, they are unable to see the only Source of life.

Somehow we must find ways to help these young people

up the tree. Make it possible for them to see over the crowd. Give them a chance to be found.

DEPEND ON YOUR TEAM RESOURCES

This is not a job we can do alone. We must utilize every resource at our disposal. Fortunately, we have an abundance of resources—though we may not have taken the time to assemble those resources.

Let me introduce you to your team.

TEAM MEMBER 1—KNOWING GOD
Nothing in your life as a parent quite matches the experience of losing control over your children. For the first twelve years you have the dominant say in what they think and do. You work hard to set the patterns you believe are necessary to carry them through life. But while you are a flurry of activity for your kids, who is preparing *you* for the changes ahead?

The first step in our journey is to find ourselves in the Lord. Knowing God is the foundation of our team.

When Jim committed his life to Christ as a fifty-year-old, it was largely due to change he had seen in his kids. Several times he talked to me with tears in his eyes about the pain of watching his college-age son rebel and then drop out of several universities. As God began to work in his son's life, Jim was forced to take a hard look at his own. Today Jim is leading a household whose center is Jesus Christ. The family is facing the challenges of transition with new perspective and new hope.

In the next chapter we will discuss how to make your family journey a spiritual one. How we feel about ourselves as people and parents begins with how we view ourselves in Christ.

It has been said that the Bible is as necessary to our safe passage through this lifetime as oxygen is to sustain life. Yet, it often seems that the spiritual disciplines are first to go when transition brings rapid change and panic. I have often said in our Young Life ministry that it is very difficult for people to claim God's promises in their lives when they don't know what those promises are! We must learn to plant God's Word in our hearts and let Scripture change our perspectives.

TEAM MEMBER 2—REALISTIC GOALS

Most people learn early to set goals. They want to get good grades, to excel in a sport, to learn the piano, etc. Then somehow later in life they either set the wrong goals or they allow their goals to be set for them by their jobs or by others. We need to know how to chart a course. We all want certain things in our lives and for our children, yet we are not sure how to start and we become lost in making midcourse corrections in our families. Consequently, we live in a state of panic, or simply survive.

We not only need goals in regard to planning toward our future, but also for the spiritual health of our families and who *we* want to be in the years ahead. Goals are a reflection of our values. They are where we begin to put "legs" to our convictions.

There's a well-worn story of a man who approached a laborer who was laying bricks and asked him, "What are you doing?" The laborer replied, "Can't you see I'm laying bricks?" The man then walked over to another bricklayer and asked, "What are you doing?" And the workman answered with pride, "I am building a cathedral."

Physically, both were doing the same thing. But the first laborer was occupied with the present task, while the other had in mind the ultimate goal. Setting clear and measurable goals will help get you beyond the pain or confusion of the present transition and back on track.

TEAM MEMBER 3—MAXIMIZING RESOURCES

Another invaluable team member is your ability to muster your resources. Who do you call for help during specific times of need in your life? Do you have the right compass and map to help you navigate the unknown terrain of transition?

None of us can make it alone. We must learn to gather around us those people and instruments necessary for our journey. It is inevitable that at some point you will need another adult to come alongside your young person. So often someone else can offer advice and direction that would not be heard coming from you.

TEAM MEMBER 4—INTIMACY THROUGH COMMUNICATION

Far too many men and women today struggle to communicate their feelings during critical times in their lives. Some communicate well because they have always felt the need to maintain an image of strength for others, yet far too many simply have never learned the proper skills to share stress, burdens, fear, or happiness and fulfillment. These skills are a critical part of your team. These communication skills help you draw closer to young people during times of transition and help provide a framework for you to understand more fully what others are going through.

Communication is not a team member that simply helps you talk. It is the tool to help you *get through to those* you want to communicate with.

TEAM MEMBER 5—PRAYER

One of the old hymns I remember singing often as a child ended with the warm refrain, "Take your burdens to the Lord and leave them there." The gift of prayer during times of change in our lives is an enormous one. Prayer can be the difference between being totally overwhelmed by our circumstances or seeing the hand of God in every situation. If we lose the ability to pray, or never develop that part of our relationship with Christ, we are woefully incomplete.

It is true that the first thing that changes through prayer is the one who prays.

TEAM MEMBER 6—MANAGING TIME FACTORS

Time is like a bank account that does not carry a balance from day to day. What you don't use is lost. Each of us has been given the same amount of time in our day. The challenge is to use it efficiently and wisely. There are many time management tools on the market today. But, as a member of your transition team, time management is not just a tool but a perspective bringing peace, hope, and energy. If you feel stressed by the lack of time in your life or your inability to manage all your time commitments, you need a team member that aids you in balancing priorities and commitments and helps you live each day to the fullest.

At the same time you need to be able to get a feel for how long these changes may take. If for example, you have a son or daughter going through junior high and all the changes that period brings, how do you plan for the next stage?

TEAM MEMBER 7—LAUGHTER AND FUN

Laughter is the music of hope. For the Christian it rings of faith that is not bound by circumstances. The ability to laugh says I will choose joy today because I know my God still lives. A family's transition team would be sorely incomplete without laughter. This is not a mirth that is unrealistic about problems and blind to pain. This is a gift to look at life with hope and to experience healing by allowing ourselves to see humor in the passages of our lives.

None of us wants to laugh at hurt. Yet, we need to learn to laugh in spite of hurt.

Not all of your transition team members will apply to each change in your life, or the life of your child. Nor is this an exhaustive list. But if you choose to use this team, you will find great help and hope for your teenager and yourself as you navigate through the various passages of family life with adolescents. Best of all, you will discover you are not alone.

•   •   •   •   •   •   •   •   •   •

CHAPTER FIVE

Team Member 1: Knowing God

Anyone who knew Sarah would confirm that she was both charming and intelligent. Always fun and entertaining to be around, she quickly became one of my favorite people. Sarah could run a PTA meeting and then lead the youth group at church with equal grace and skill. She was one of those ladies that many kids wished they had for a mom.

That is, except for one of her own.

Sarah called me in despair. Her oldest child, sixteen-year-old Heidi, had run away, and Sarah believed she was staying with a man of twenty-one who had questionable values.

For the next two years I walked a painful road with Sarah and her husband, Ed. They applied tough love and tender love; they took Heidi back and asked her to leave. It was a nightmare for this successful and high-profile Christian couple.

Sometime during her eighteenth year Heidi settled down
and began that long process of making peace with her parents and herself. Each time Sarah and I discuss those painful days, she always mentions the moment her faith began
to rise above her torment.

Before Heidi's very open rebellion Sarah had been the
queen of Christian moms. She was loved and admired and
emulated by many. But at times during the family turmoil
Sarah felt worse than a failure. More like a leper, she would
say. She no longer felt fit to lead the PTA or try to teach other
parents' kids right from wrong.

TWO GREAT TRUTHS

Yet, sometime during her grief two great truths emerged.
First, Sarah recognized that her hope was in Christ and
not in her success as a mother, or as a Christian leader
for that matter. When all else failed, the Lord was truly all
she needed. Sarah realized that her experience with Heidi
spurred growth in her own life that she probably would
have otherwise missed. In the midst of sorrow and pain she
learned to enjoy the presence of Christ and discovered a joy
that was not related to circumstance or environment.

We live in a world starving for that kind of joy. It is a joy
that the world can neither give nor take away. It is the joy
that comes from knowing God.

The second important truth that Sarah discovered was
that Heidi, with all her anger and rebelliousness, was still
more important to her than all the committees and boards
and ministries she could think of. Her new discovery of God
in the face of lost prestige had begun to remold her thoughts.
She no longer aspired to be supermom and super Christian.
Her heart now simply longed for Jesus, and she was eter-
nally grateful to rest in the arms of her heavenly Father.

Sarah is living proof of a hard reality: Being a parent is
tough. No question about it. In the midst of coping with life

and all that confronts us as people, we are forceu ir raise another generation and prepare them for the road ahe,

It is no wonder that many people live with the stress and guilt of not being the parents that they perceive their children need. If you have ever experienced the fear of not being the perfect parent, I have great news!

You can't be one.

No one can meet all of the needs of his or her children, or even of a spouse for that matter. At best, we commit ourselves to hard work and growth. We must recognize that perfection is not for this world and our hope must lie in another place.

For this reason, we commit ourselves to One who is capable of meeting our needs. We have a heavenly Father who loves us. We are His children. He desires to see us whole and happy.

STEPS AND MISSTEPS IN SUCCESSFUL PARENTING

The first step to being a successful parent is *not* to become a "successful person." Many parents today are living under this tragic assumption. They equate worldly success with all its whistles and bells to their potential to parent successfully. In the end they achieve, at best, an attractive family, but not necessarily a healthy one.

When a scribe asked Jesus what the greatest commandment was, the Lord answered, "Love the Lord your God with all your heart and with all your soul and with all your mind" (Matthew 22:37). That is the call to men and women everywhere. The greatest commandment is not to accumulate things, or to acquire prestige and power. It does not relate to any of our abilities. It is an act of the will: Will you love God above all else?

If educators are correct, 70 percent of learning is modeling. We can talk about values and morals all day, but unless our young people are seeing them lived out in vital fashion, they are merely words, void of any real meaning in their lives.

We have discovered that most kids believe in God. They just can't seem to figure out why it matters. For years in Young Life we have said, "You gotta walk your talk." We have said something else as well, "You can take a kid only as far as you are in the Lord." As parents we must make our own growth in Christ our first goal. We can only lead and model what we hope our children will embrace from a posture of submission and love for Christ. George Bernard Shaw once commented that the only tragic thing about the Christian faith was that it has never been tried.

WHY WE DESIRE TO KNOW GOD

There are really two reasons to desire to know God. First, it is commanded. God has called us to Himself and He has prepared the way for us to have fellowship with Him through Jesus Christ. We do not come to Christ to be better parents. We do not yearn after God in order to change our kids, or our spouse. We follow Christ because He calls us to Himself and that is enough. Change, we discover painfully, usually begins with ourselves. As we draw nearer to Christ, our parenting will improve naturally. Why? Because God turns our attention from the faults and foibles of others (especially our teenagers) to our own need for Him. We are struck by the great forgiveness we have received and experience a new capacity to dispense forgiveness to others. The more we seek and yearn after Him, the sharper our focus on who *we* are as parents.

My pastor recently said, "God does not react to the *pressure* of faith, but to the *presence* of faith." In other words, we cannot manipulate Him to action. He is not a machine, He is the King.

Second, we all were created with a longing for God. We were made for that relationship, and we are destined to live aimless and unfulfilled without it. You may have heard the old illustration from Pascal that within each person is a God-shaped vacuum. Nothing else will fit, try as we might to find a substitute. Every attempt is akin to forcing a square peg in a round hole. Substitutes just won't do. It may strike you as illogical, but when our eyes are focused on Christ we will see our teenagers more clearly.

FIVE PRINCIPLES TO GUIDE YOU IN KNOWING GOD

If Sarah could discover God in a new way through the turmoil in her life and family, you can too. In the next several pages we will discuss the following five basic principles. These will guide you as you seek to know God.

- You are a product of God's grace.
- God is near.
- You can do all things through Christ.
- The Spirit—your source of power.
- Being heavenly minded.

YOU ARE A PRODUCT OF GOD'S GRACE

"Amazing Grace, how sweet the sound"—familiar words, but often for us an unfamiliar experience. As a high school student I was given a definition of grace that has stayed with me through the years.

God's
Righteousness
At
Christ's
Expense

We experience the grace of God through His unmerited favor toward us. This paints a graphic picture of God's sacrificial and unconditional love. We have such difficulty accepting that love at times. We have grown up in a number of competitive love situations. We competed with our siblings for love, and we competed with various demands on our parents' time. Then we competed at school for the attention and acceptance of our peers. We need to feel loved and accepted in various environments, and that means learning how to act and respond correctly. Finally, when we come to Christ we are struck by the fact that He isn't interested in our acceptance games. He won't force us to prove our worthiness time and time again. We don't perform for Him in order to earn His favor. This is hard to get used to!

As we grow, we discover that by working to earn God's love we are really working against ourselves. The real key is humility and contrition, as King David, the writer of the following psalm, knew so well.

> You do not delight in sacrifice, or I would bring it;
>   you do not take pleasure in burnt offerings.
> The sacrifices of God are a broken spirit;
>   a broken and contrite heart,
>   O God, you will not despise. (Psalm 51:16-17)

Youthworkers will often tell a child that if he or she were the only person on earth, Christ would still die for him or her. His love and commitment to us cannot be earned. His forgiveness is complete and permanent. I have struggled many times with this concept. As much as I recognize my need for God, I often strive to meet Him on my terms. I find that just as I competed for the attention of others as a child, I now compete to prove myself a spiritually sufficient person as an adult. I act out my Christianity for my peers and charges rather than simply loving Christ for what He has done for me. Unfortunately, when troubles come, this self-sufficient lifestyle is woefully insufficient. The apostle Paul summed it up beautifully in 2 Corinthians 12:9: "My grace is sufficient for you, for my power is made perfect in weakness."

The Lord's grace is the key to sustain us. Our transition

team will provide resources, but we experience peace in our heart because we know God's love is unconditional. He is not waiting to see how well we handle transition or struggles before He affirms us. It is often only in weakness and distress that we see His hand in our lives. Most of the time we are simply too busy to notice.

The secret to experiencing God's grace and peace is to daily, moment by moment, give your thoughts and dreams to Christ. It is not an ethereal or mystical concept, but as simple as saying, "Lord, please carry this burden."

Listen to the words of Isaiah.

> But now, this is what the LORD says—
> he who created you, O Jacob,
> he who formed you, O Israel:
> "Fear not, for I have redeemed you;
> I have summoned you by name; you are mine."
> (Isaiah 43:1)

The next time you find the swelling tide of teen transitions threatening to wash you away, first affirm to yourself that you are saved by grace. You are loved and accepted regardless of your circumstances. When within your heart you have a rock-solid conviction of who you are in Christ, you will not be swept away, regardless of the circumstances you face.

GOD IS NEAR

> Rejoice in the Lord always. I will say it again: Rejoice!
> Let your gentleness be evident to all. The Lord is near.
> (Philippians 4:4-5)

When was the last time you felt the Lord was far away and unconcerned about the hurt and trouble in your life? Yesterday, right?

The apostle Paul has good news for you—"Rejoice." He

is *not* talking about being glad for calamity and stress. He is saying that *in the midst of the battle the Lord is near.* The Lord has not left you. *You* may have turned from Him. The obstacles you are confronting may be crowding out your view of Him, but He is there.

Look at the next two verses in Philippians 4: "Do not be anxious about anything, but in everything, by prayer and petition, with thanksgiving, present your requests to God. And the peace of God, which transcends all understanding, will guard your hearts and your minds in Christ Jesus" (verses 6-7).

The peace of God can be ours. He is near.

From his beautiful book *God Came Near*, Max Lucado gives us this challenge: "Would you like to see Jesus? Do you dare be an eyewitness of His Majesty? Then rediscover amazement. The next time you hear a baby laugh or see an ocean wave, take note. Pause and listen as His Majesty whispers ever so gently, 'I'm here.'"[1]

Can you see Jesus in your teenager? The next time your son or daughter laughs, the next time you touch him, or watch her lounge around the house—see His majesty there, in your child, His creation.

You Can Do All Things Through Christ

We're all familiar with stories of men and women who have overcome enormous odds to achieve great things. These heartwarming tales of courage fill us with warmth and encouragement. But then we walk back into our ordinary world where the challenges aren't so clear and obvious.

That is why the apostle Paul left us some very valuable and practical advice in 1 Corinthians 9:24: "Do you not know that in a race all the runners run, but only one gets the prize? Run in such a way as to get the prize."

The last part of this verse is an admonition to run the race with the goal in mind. Most people run the race with the obstacles and challenges foremost in their minds. Paul says run to win. Our goal is usually just to finish the race.

My two brothers both ran the hurdles. I would watch them practice, and in so doing, learned an important lesson. Just as important as speed in running the hurdles is getting your steps down. There are a certain number of steps you need to take to make the transition between hurdles smooth and fast.

To run a strong race the worst thing you can do is watch the hurdles as you run. It always throws off your timing and gets you out of step. The best way to run the hurdles is with your eyes fixed on the finish line.

When we are focused on the hurdles in our lives, our view of the race isn't clear and we are sure to get out of step. Yet if we can keep our eyes focused on Christ during the race, we will see more clearly and the obstacles will not loom so large in our minds.

In Philippians 4:13, Paul says, "I can do everything through him who gives me strength." There is no obstacle too great for those who get their strength from Christ. Such focus requires discipline and commitment. It means every day renewing your pledge to keep your eyes on Him. Then quickly asking forgiveness, not allowing sin to get a permanent foothold in your life, and refocusing when you become aware of taking your eyes off Him.

With each change in our teenager's life we will face a new hurdle in parenting. Keeping a clear focus in our lives doesn't mean we know what to do in each situation. In the midst of unpredictable days we aren't consumed by the hurdles we must go over; rather, we keep our eyes focused on Christ and we run the race to win.

THE SPIRIT—YOUR SOURCE OF POWER

> Jesus said to her, "I am the resurrection and the life.
> He who believes in me will live, even though he dies."
> (John 11:25)

The Resurrection. Not since Creation had the world seen such a display of power. That Jesus Christ would conquer death and usurp its authority in the world represents a power of proportions we cannot comprehend.

But God does not stop there. He makes that power available to us through the Spirit of God who inhabits us. It is His desire to provide the strength we need to wage the battles of our lives. Paul says it well in Ephesians 3:16: "I pray that out of his glorious riches he may strengthen you with power through his Spirit in your inner being."

We will be talking about appropriating this more in a later chapter, but the primary point here is: *Power is gained by waiting on the Lord.* There is no shortcut and no substitute. If we desire to be strengthened by the Spirit of God, we must wait before Him. Remember, it is not by pressure that we experience the Spirit; it is by presence.

Waiting will not always mean being still. If, as we walk through the transitions of adolescence with our kids, we have waited before the Lord, we are prepared and empowered to wait *on* Him. We live with the peace and knowledge that God is at work even during the busiest times of our lives.

BEING HEAVENLY MINDED

A great part of my spiritual tradition lies in the teaching that Heaven is our home and this earth is merely a stop along the way. I can remember as a child singing about Heaven. Those songs gave me two great truths about life.

First, they said, "Don't take this life too seriously." That doesn't mean to be flippant or irresponsible but simply that we are not to be consumed by the cares of this world.

I have heard it said that the life of a Christian in the hands of God is like a bow and arrow in the hands of an archer. God is aiming at something the Christian cannot see.

Being heavenly minded simply helps us leave the shooting to God. He sees things from a vantage point simply not available to us. He knows exactly where to aim.

Second, being heavenly minded means we are focusing on an eternal God and not the temporal things of humankind. Our values are based on eternal commitments and not the fleeting things of this world.

A few years ago, I heard James Dobson share a touching story of a little boy who was dying. One day when his mother arrived at the hospital, the nurses attempted to prepare her for the worst. "He has been hallucinating," they told the mother. "He has been muttering something about the bells."

"Oh," she said as she gently lifted her little one. "I told him that when the pain got too difficult to stand and he didn't think he could take any more to look up in the corner of the room and he would see Jesus. Then to listen very carefully and he would hear the bells of Heaven."

Most of us are too busy to distinguish the bells of Heaven from the noises and sounds that assault our hectic lives. Knowing God means to look for Him. As often as we can we need to be quiet. Quiet enough to hear the bells of Heaven.

There may be no greater gift we could give our children than the picture of us waiting and listening to the Lord. At the same time, as adults we need to be more heavenly minded. Our home is not of this world, therefore we are not overwhelmed by apparent failures or successes. With our focus on Christ we draw on the power God bestows on those who wait on Him. We do this knowing we are here to serve Him until He calls us to be with Him.

I have learned much from watching parents like Sarah live through the trauma of parenting a troubled adolescent. If her despair could turn to peace, so can yours. If her faith can rise above her torment, that strength is available to you and me as well. To know God is to experience His peace and strength. It involves daily taking your cares and fears to your loving heavenly Father. Then in the midst of struggle and challenge you can learn to enjoy the presence of Christ and discover a joy only He can give.

● ● ● ● ● ● ● ● ● ● ●

CHAPTER SIX

Team Member 2: Realistic Goals for Traumatized Parents and Teens

*What lies behind us and what lies before us
are tiny matters compared to what lies within us.*
OLIVER WENDELL HOLMES

J ack sat in my office an angry and confused dad. His son, Mike, had just wrecked his new Trans Am during a high-speed frolic with some friends. "I suppose I should be grateful that no one was killed," he said, as he slumped in the chair. Suddenly, he threw up his hands in a sign of surrender and in a broken voice asked, "Where did I go wrong?"

It would be impossible to count how many times I have heard those words spoken by confused, angry, or frustrated parents. They love their children and have attempted to do everything they can to provide for them. Yet, in the middle of the adolescent storm there is an overwhelming sense of fear and even failure.

My first reaction to Jack's question was to encourage and not let him blame himself. But, I also felt that it was necessary to ask a few questions. "Jack," I asked, "what is your major goal as Mike's father?"

"Well, I guess I just want him to be happy," was his reply.

As I continued to ask Jack questions, it became apparent to me that he had never really considered his goals for raising his son. He knew how to set aggressive goals for his company, and he was well covered for his future retirement. Still, he could not provide a clear blueprint for raising his son.

Finally, I shared with him one thought I had heard from James Dobson a number of years ago: Most people try to pave the way of success for their children rather than preparing them for the bumpy road of life.

Jack was ecstatic. He had been thinking about the process all wrong. He wanted Mike's life to be successful and he worked hard to ensure that. But when Mike failed to live up to his expectations or didn't seem to appreciate his efforts, Jack was often angry and hurt.

I encouraged him to develop a different pattern, one that focused more on character and less on "success." He recognized this trial as a great opportunity to understand the deeper meaning of goals. At the same time it was a great opportunity to guide Mike through a traumatic experience and show a Christlike attitude. Mike, as a person, and especially as his son, was far more valuable than the Trans Am.

GOALS THAT REFLECT DEEPER VALUES

Goals reflect our values. They tell us what our priorities are and help us put "legs" to our beliefs.

There are really two functions of this chapter on goals. One is to make sure you have clearly thought through your own goals. At this stage in life, you may not be able to establish goals for your son or daughter, but you can set personal goals regarding who you want to be and how you will respond to your family. The other is to recognize that "doing" the right things is not as important as charting a course to "be" the right person. You may not be able to "control" the actions or attitudes of the adolescent in your home, but you can respond according to some carefully laid out principles that guide you during difficult times.

There is no greater nor more tender example of clear goals than the story of Jesus healing the sick woman in Luke 8:40-48. Jesus was on His way to the home of Jairus, an influential and powerful religious leader. The notoriety from a miracle on behalf of this man would be significant. Jairus was beside himself. His little girl was dying. The crowd, sensing something special was about to happen, poured into the streets and made it almost impossible for the Lord and His disciples to move.

Jesus stopped. His brow furrowed in concentration, and scanning the vast crowd of people, He asked, "Who touched me?" Only one person really knew what He was asking. For a sick and destitute woman had just touched the hem of His garment and had suddenly been freed from her years of torment.

Now perhaps the most remarkable thing of all happened. She fell down before Jesus and shared why she had touched Him and how she had been healed. With Jairus wringing his hands, and the disciples fretting over the schedule, Jesus stood and listened intently while this little woman who had suffered so much told her story. Then before she got away, and before the crowd could separate them and force Jesus on His way, He blessed her.

He said to her, "Daughter, your faith has healed you. Go in peace."

Nowhere else in the recorded words of Jesus do we find Him calling someone daughter. She must have trembled at those words. The overwhelming joy at the words and warmth of Jesus would have surely burst her heart had not deep and abiding peace filled her soul at that moment. It was a moment when peace and joy were partners.

Jack didn't see instant results in Mike's behavior and attitude. What he did experience was a revolutionary change in how he viewed life and in particular, Mike. Good behavior was no longer Jack's number one goal for Mike. In fact, Jack realized that before he could entertain any thoughts about goals for Mike, he had to make some clear decisions regarding how he would live his life and respond, regardless of the circumstances. He knew that his first goal must be to know Christ personally and to become more like Him. Jack began to find a new peace and joy inside himself. I believed it would only be a matter of time until Mike would begin to experience Christ, too.

GOAL-DRIVEN PARENTING

As we learn to set goals for ourselves and attempt to guide our children in theirs, we must bear in mind the example of Jesus.

First, He is not only our hope, He is our model. He showed us how to love and how to care during those awkward intrusions in our lives that seem so unnecessary and out of place. He knew His goal was not to get to the next meeting as fast as possible. It was to touch people, lost and forsaken men and women, and to touch them one at a time. He valued the individual and, because He knew His ultimate goal, He didn't see the woman as a distraction, but as an important stop on His journey to the Cross.

Second, we can never be too busy to stop for our child. Jesus didn't see the woman as an intrusion, He saw her as a "daughter." His goal was not merely to use His time efficiently but to use it effectively. Too often we attempt to make our household efficient at the expense of effective relationships. While a certain amount of efficiency is helpful, whether it involves household chores or a specific dinner time, these activities must not become the goals. Rather, *our activities must be driven by our goals.* For example, if your goal is to have quality time as a family, you may have to adjust if a common dinner doesn't work.

The most powerful result in setting a goal is that it tells

you what *you* think is significant and puts you in a proactive position to follow your convictions. Instead of waiting around for life to "happen" to you, being proactive means to chart a course for your future.

Jack set a goal for his life that people would see Christ in him in every situation. He began to take some steps in his devotional life, and in his relationship to his son, to see that goal begin to take root in his life. If Jack's goal had remained to change Mike's behavior, he probably would have faced a long and frustrating battle.

GOAL-DRIVEN TEENS

In challenging young people to carefully consider the direction of their lives, we youthworkers often ask them to write their own eulogy. The idea is that they think about how they want to be remembered when they are gone. What will their children say about them? What will their coworkers believe they lived for?

In his very helpful book *The Seven Habits of Highly Effective People*, Stephen Covey does a beautiful job challenging adults with the idea of writing their own eulogy. He calls it "beginning with the end in mind." Covey says that if you carefully consider what you want said of you at your funeral, you will "find your definition of success."

I ask kids to put their thoughts into one phrase that they can memorize and apply to any situation in their lives. For example, "She was a woman after God's own heart." That little phrase says volumes about how you want to be remembered and what your values and goals are.

After we have talked about how they want to be remembered and they have decided on their "life phrase," we can begin to work backward to set some goals for achieving the desired end. We talk about what they need to be doing right now to set the course of their lives.

It is not my intention to tell you what goals you should

set for yourself or your children. People are different, and the best goal is the one you think of and apply to your particular situation and life. Ownership is the key here. Please don't hand your young people a set of goals for their lives. Give them most of the ownership. As children make the transition from junior high to high school, they are beginning to make decisions on their own and won't simply adopt your goals, no matter how valid they appear to you. And if they were to adopt your goals, you must ask yourself if you've helped them achieve even the basic level of independence necessary to survive in high school or college.

Help them ask the right questions. Ask them how they want to be remembered. Sometimes you may feel that they're incapable of thinking that far ahead. Ask how they want to be remembered by their classmates when they come back for their ten-year reunion. I have asked my boys how they want to be remembered after soccer season. I try to avoid letting them get away with cliches like "He was the best player on the team" or even "He was a real example for Christ." Instead I continue to ask what their statement means until we get to *values* like teamwork, working hard, and listening carefully. Then I ask them how they think they will work toward that end. Now the question isn't, "How good are you?" or "How did you play?" Rather, the question is, "Did you see some growth in the areas you established as priorities?" That is almost always a goal they can achieve. And it puts the emphasis on *who they are* and not on *what they do*. It allows them to set goals based on their own values and doesn't limit it to performance.

I am not trying to take away the value of healthy competition or to reward mediocrity. But when you work the hardest, listen the closest, and give the necessary respect to coaches, teammates, and opponents, there is bound to be an impact on your performance.

With this in mind, I would like to point you toward five values you may want to discuss with your son or daughter when setting goals. You can also use these values to guide your own goal-setting and thus provide a model for your adolescent and give you more patience as they pursue their own.

VALUE 1: LOVE GOD

"Love the Lord your God with all your heart and with all your soul and with all your mind and with all your strength" (Mark 12:30).

"Too easy," you say? Then obviously you haven't tried it. But try it you must if it is to be a goal for your child. Remember, your goals are an expression of your values. You will communicate those first by your lifestyle.

We are not talking about going to church here. We are talking about a devotion to Christ that commands the attention of your whole life (and your kid's!).

This is the foundation for the rest of the goal-setting process. Encourage your young people to give it some thought. Ask them what they want their children to say someday about their dad or mom's relationship to God. Ask them how they would verbalize that conviction.

Be content to set small goals. Make promises to yourself that you can keep. For example, one objective in reaching a goal in this category might be to commit to five minutes a day alone with the Lord. Now that may not seem very spiritual, but it is a promise you are able to keep. After ninety days you may want to increase the time.

So, while loving God with all our heart, soul, mind, and strength is no small goal itself, to live with such a high value requires that we start small and set achievable objectives to demonstrate our commitment to it.

VALUE 2: LOVE PEOPLE

"Love your neighbor as yourself" (Mark 12:31).

From his popular book *All I Ever Really Need to Know I Learned in Kindergarten*, Robert Fulghum shares the following thoughts:

ALL I REALLY NEEDED TO KNOW about how to live, and
what to do, and how to be, I learned in kindergar-
ten. . . . These are the things I learned:
- Share everything. Play fair. Don't hit people.
- Put things back where you found them.
- Clean up your mess.
- Don't take things that aren't yours.
- Say you're sorry when you hurt somebody. . . .
- When you go out into the world, watch for traffic,
  hold hands and stick together.[1]

Fulghum gives us a clever description of our attitude
to those around us. Our children are growing up in an
increasingly violent world. That world desperately needs love
modeled in tangible ways. The very first place we demonstrate this attitude is in the home. And it begins with love
for our spouse. Our children's values will be established by
what they see lived out in the home. If love is lived out in a
home, whether or not both mom and dad are living there, the
impact will be far greater than all the sermons and lectures
in the world. As a teenager I would always notice when an
"older" couple held hands. I told myself I wanted to still be in
love like that after years of marriage. If you begin with your
"neighbor" at home, you are well on your way to reflecting
this value in your goals and behavior.

As junior high- and high school-aged kids make the transition from dependence on you to independence, you may
not get the response to your suggestions that you think you
deserve. But the key issue cannot be their response. If your
goal is to love, success is not dependent on their response.
Nor can you demand a response. The issue is who you are,
not how your children respond.

Psychologists tell us that most anger is related to unfulfilled expectations. If you are expecting a certain response
from your son or daughter, you will undoubtedly get angry
over his or her failure to respond. In truth, as boys and

girls pass through adolescence they often *don't know* how to respond. They are searching for a socially acceptable way to relate to others. Their world is changing so fast they may be incapable of responding in a manner acceptable to us.

This is not to say we overlook rudeness, but simply that we can't afford to view no response as necessarily a bad response at the time.

We must learn to share and play fair. And then we must certainly learn to stick together.

Here is one way to express the value to love our neighbor as ourselves. Stepping back, we encourage kids to define who their neighbor is. Then we ask them how they want to live out loving their neighbor, and finally where or with whom they will start. If they have seen a model of that happening in their family, they may start there. But they may choose to start with their peers. That is okay. They will own an objective; that goal will guide them. Don't panic if they don't respond the way you anticipated.

Finally, learn to serve. Demonstrate for your children what the Lord meant when He said, "Whatever you did for one of the least of these brothers of mine, you did for me" (Matthew 25:40). Sometimes our children need to see us serving outside the home in places they wouldn't expect. They need to be exposed to the world around them, which doesn't live the way they do.

VALUE 3: DEVELOP INTEGRITY
In his book *Legacy of Love*, Tim Kimmel has this to say about integrity:

> When I think of a legacy of love, I picture parents who carefully develop a child's integrity. All other skills and talents, regardless of how carefully defined, must submit to the demands of integrity.
>
> That's because integrity protects us. We never have to keep lies straight or catalog the deceptions. There's

never a worry about what we said or what we did. Integrity shines out of our life like an inner light, and people find it easy to place their trust in us.[2]

These are important words about integrity for all of us. Unfortunately, at about the junior high level integrity gets mixed up with another important word: *reputation*. This is a mistake that is too often carried over into adult life. Reputation, whether good or bad, is a by-product of our lifestyle and integrity. Typical junior high students will most often define their reputation in two ways. How they believe they are perceived by their peers is one definition. This used to begin in high school, but is now a junior high or middle school issue. Second, they are influenced by what they see in the media. Much of their view of beauty, masculinity, or success is a product of advertising and the media. A $170.00 pair of basketball shoes may never be on a basketball court, but it can be a symbol for many kids that they are "in."

In reality, we cannot control our reputation any more than Jesus could control His. He was often maligned as a friend of sinners. But many people cultivate a reputation. They strive to look "just right" to those around them. And often this is at the expense of their own personal integrity and spiritual health.

If we have a life goal that places Christ in the center of life, we must allow obedience to Him to supersede our obsession with reputation. By establishing personal goals we can teach ourselves and our children to draw approval from God and not others. That's *real* integrity!

VALUE 4: WORK HARD

E. M. Gray once said, "The successful person has the habit of doing things failures don't like to do." Hard work is easily one of the most difficult values to communicate. The concept of hard work is very confused today. Most people think hard work and long hours away from home are one and the same. That is an unfortunate view of hard work. I have often wondered what kind of values in regard to work I am communicating to my sons if they never see me do any. If most of our work is done outside the home, their view will come from hearsay, or even worse, television and the media.

How do your teenagers think you earn money? Do they have an idea of how hard you work and how long it took you to get where you are today? Most of the time they don't really understand what you go through to provide for them.

I want to encourage you to do a couple of things. First, if at all possible, take them to work with you. Show them around and let them see you in action. Let them see the kind of accountability you face at the job. You could give them a great gift by letting them see some of your life. If it wouldn't be appropriate to visit your job, call on someone who can help you. Maybe a friend has a career that your teen has shown some interest in.

Second, share with them your thoughts about your career. Are you happy with it? Do you wish you had done something different? What are some of your major fears about your future? While you are at it you can let them see some or all of your budget. Let them see where the money goes. When they see the link between a full-time job and family financial commitments they will have a more balanced view of work and money.

Finally, as you model and share about work don't forget to let them know when you stop working. This is extremely difficult in my life and for most of us in the ministry. Too often, I am not able to distinguish between what is work and what is personal time. There are so many needs and so many relationships that seem to overlap. My sons are very aware of not having my full attention even when from their perspective I am not "on the job." To combat this I have always coached one of them in soccer and tried very hard to do things they like on a regular basis. Making time for this is an ongoing challenge.

VALUE 5: PLAY HARD

Do you know the art of leisure? Much of my early understanding on this subject came from Tim Hansel's book *When
I Relax I Feel Guilty.* There is something very central to our
health as individuals and families in learning how to play.

Tim expresses our dilemma with leisure like this:

> Part of our confusion about leisure is the result of
> using as synonyms a number of overlapping and
> ill-defined terms such as *play, game,* and *recreation.*
> Another difficulty lies in the fact that some define lei-
> sure as a certain type of *activity,* while others define it
> as a *state of mind.* One tradition conceives of leisure as
> free time not devoted to paid occupations. The other,
> much older, classical tradition conceives of leisure as
> cultivation of the self and a preoccupation with the
> higher values of life.
>
> If you will excuse me a moment for not speaking
> English, I think you will find it helpful to know the
> background of the word leisure. It comes from the
> Latin word licere, which means "to be permitted." More
> today than ever, we need to learn how to give ourselves
> permission to relax, to play, to enjoy God for who
> he is.[3]

Of course, defining leisure in a way that the whole family
can agree on can be a challenge. Leisure is different from
"kicking back," although that may be a part of it. Watching
television can provide a piece of your family playtime, but it
can have the detrimental effect when it is done in excess.

Young people like variety. They will do simple things if
the setting is right. Too many of us have an expensive view
of play. We buy expensive toys, go on exotic vacations, and
in general see play as something extraordinary that happens
on holidays. But play can be almost a daily occurrence. It is
part of what brings joy into life.

AFFIRMATION AND GOALS

After Jack had finished establishing goals for himself and had begun to talk to Mike about his goals in life, we discussed one final detail. Jack was going to need to learn to affirm Mike and any new goals he might come up with.

This isn't to say Jack could not ask questions and even challenge Mike's position, but he needed to affirm Mike's values, not his performance. He had to look at whom Mike was becoming and not just what he was doing. This would take lots of work and require patience. He would need to genuinely affirm Mike's goals and specifically point out things he appreciated. It would also be very important for Jack not to use these goals in moments of anger to embarrass or humiliate Mike.

Jack was energized and encouraged. He had a game plan now and not only hope for Mike but convictions about his own life as well. If your goals are an expression of what you value, what are they telling you right now?

I pray you will establish goals that will guide you through life and provide a proper model for those who follow.

• • • • • • • • • • •

CHAPTER SEVEN

Team Member 3: Maximizing Resources

O ur society loves celebrities. Folks watch their every move and dream of living their life. With the close attention famous people get from the media, we often get more information than we ever wanted. Most of our would-be heroes are tarnished and brought down by their own actions. Few can pass the test required by a public who likes its heroes bigger than life. As a parent I am constantly paying attention to successful athletes and other celebrities to discern if there is one my sons can latch onto as a role model. Certainly, I am always grateful for the ones who hold high standards and take their role in society seriously.

Parents know that successful role models are not all our kids need in developing a view of who they want to be and in making good decisions about life. The most important role models are right at home. Yet the influence other adults can have on our kids can be critical to their development.

Too many young people are facing the world today without enough resources to guide and support them. They are facing an increasingly hostile and competitive world with only a narrow view of life to guide them. It is in adolescence that these young folks need our help in mustering the resources necessary to aid their passage through these trying years.

Our children need to know that they are not passing through this life alone and that there are resources and helps they can turn to.

When you as a parent think about caring for your son or daughter during the transitions from junior high through young adulthood, you need to know where your resources are as well. You must know whom to call and where to go for help.

SIZING UP THE SITUATION

The first thing you will want to do is take a hard and honest look at what you are facing. No matter what phase your child is going through, there are five basic questions you can ask yourself to begin your assessment.

1. How do my kids view themselves?
2. What is the state of my teenagers' faith?
3. Do my kids have the social and mental skills to handle life on their own?
4. Are my kids surrounded by healthy people inside and outside the family?
5. Are they capable of making healthy independent decisions?

I would encourage you at this point to recruit someone who knows your children and has your trust to help you answer these questions.

Too many people in the United States still hold the view

that they must be self-sufficient. They believe that to accept help is a sign of weakness. They confuse fortitude with solitude. Nothing could be further from the truth. We were created by God to work together. The Body of Christ functions *best* when we are all pulling together. To refuse help is to cripple the plan of God in creation. Even the business world today is coming to grips with the need to work together. The business community expresses it in terms like networking and team building, but the point is, *we need each other.*

One strong resource can offset many deficits or setbacks in the life of a young person. A close family or a strong role model outside the family can carry someone through trials that might otherwise be debilitating. At the same time let me caution that resources need to change and adjust as kids grow up and circumstances change. We must always be ready to seek new resources when necessary.

We can say with a great deal of certainty that our teenagers are going to experience setbacks and failure. These may come in the form of some deficiency or finding they cannot compete and succeed in a certain area. It may be as common as being a jilted suitor, or as painful as missing the prom.

These setbacks are going to occur. The challenge is to have the resources in place to aid your teens through trying times.

TAKING INVENTORY OF YOUR RESOURCES

The second step in maximizing your resources is evaluating what you already have available. Make a list of who you can turn to for support and help. Write down other assets and tools at your disposal, including outside agencies, books and periodicals, and financial resources. And don't forget the all-important asset of *time.*

Let's look at some available resources.

PERSONAL FAITH

This is critical for both you and your son or daughter. Do you have confidence in the Lord? Are you committed to the work that God is doing in your life as well as in your child's?

Personal faith is our number one resource. We may not be able to force our convictions on our children, but we can remain true to these convictions ourselves in spite of all adversity.

FAMILY

Is your family in a position to be a resource? If so, use it. You can't *demand* that your teenager or young adult stay close to the family, but you can work at making the home a warm and comfortable place for your child.

I have often told my mom that she should write a book. I even thought of a title for her, *Kitchen Table Psychology*. I can remember our home vividly from my childhood. When we came home from school, Mom would always have something in the kitchen to eat—cookies, brownies, cake, etc., with an unending supply of milk. When one of us (I had one sister and two brothers) would wander in, she always managed to be around. Then while we were enjoying the treats, she would gently ask us questions about our day and how we were viewing life at the time. Our kitchen table was a secure place and many seeds of maturity were planted right there.

OTHER ADULTS

Significant others are some of the most crucial parts of your transition team. These are adults who have some kind of special relationship with your son or daughter. They may or may not be related, but they hold a place of love and trust in the family. As young people grow up, they reach certain points along the way where they experience some need to be on their own. This may not be a physical separation, but simply an opportunity to make independent decisions. This newfound independence is often frightening and painful for parents. You have made all the major decisions for years and now your teenager either isn't listening or is pressing you constantly for more autonomy.

In your heart you may doubt your teen's ability to make good decisions, but you recognize his or her need to do so. The adolescent environment may not be conducive to healthy choices, so we become concerned about the teen's choice in friends.

At this point you may want to call on another adult who has a strong relationship with your child and who holds to your values and commitments about life. As a Young Life leader, it has often been my job to fill that gap for parents. It is not any youthworker's goal or desire to replace parents or families; instead we prefer to come alongside families in times of transition and need. More important might be an uncle or aunt who has watched your child grow up. Extended family can be an invaluable resource.

The important thing is to be prepared. *Take a minute right now and list the resource people in your life.* Who would be in position to step in if your son or daughter needed an outside voice in his or her life?

A number of folks already know that I may call on them at any time, and they would be ready to spend some time with one of my sons or even have the boys over for a weekend or longer if necessary. One of the most difficult aspects of moving our family a few years ago was separating from the people who had surrounded our boys. If we hadn't been moving closer to a grandma and grandpa, plus uncles and aunts, we might not have moved.

If you don't have much of a list, I would encourage you to talk to your youth pastor. If that is not possible, look for another Christian organization such as Young Life, Youth for Christ, Student Ventures and others, and don't forget Christian coaches or teachers who might take a special interest in your child.

One warning. These people are resources and as such are to *supplement* and *support* you as the parent. Make sure you keep your expectations realistic as to their potential role. Never blame them if things don't work out the way you hope. They are resources and may be part of the team. They cannot be your whole team.

I think the first time I met Doug he was in trouble. I think the last time I saw Doug he was in trouble. In fact, he showed up at my apartment with two friends, all of whom were going to camp under duress. They had gotten in trouble with drugs at school, and I had convinced the vice principal that part of their sentence should include a Young Life camp. I had known the other two guys for a couple of years and they were dragging Doug along.

That week at camp forged a strong relationship between the four of us. Doug made a commitment to Christ and began to make some real progress in his life. Needless to say, his parents were encouraged by what they saw happening.

That is why I was so stunned one day when his dad called me and started to chew me out. In his mind I was the sole key to Doug's health and future. He was seeing a few slips in Doug's life and concluded that I wasn't right on top of the situation. I tried to explain to him the role I felt I played in his son's life, but he had a very different view. I suddenly found myself needing resources to deal with an unexpected problem.

I got together with Doug as fast as I could. We spent a good deal of time together and his attitude started to improve. A couple of weeks later his father called and apologized for his anger. He said some nice things, but the truth of his earlier call still bothered me. I had given all I could to Doug and I knew I couldn't keep it up. Already my relationship with him was costing me more than I had anticipated. As I thought through my options I realized there weren't many. From the day Doug walked into my apartment, I had worked hard to build our relationship. Now that I needed some help there was no place to turn. His father did not want the responsibility for his son's attitude and behavior back, and I had not developed any other resource people. Doug drifted away from the Lord in college and over the years we have lost touch, but I will never forget the lesson I learned early in my ministry. None of us can meet the needs of an adolescent by ourselves. We must develop a network of caring people to come alongside us.

Many friends and relatives out there would probably love to be a resource to you and your family. They have a great desire to see your family succeed. But they cannot replace you. One of the hard lessons we are learning as a nation is how to use our resources wisely. We have squandered so many of the beautiful gifts that God gave us. Our air is polluted, we are short of water, and many animals are living with the threat of extinction. By the same token we must be good stewards of the resources God has placed around our family. They are part of our team.

PEERS
This resource is a very tough one to orchestrate, but easy to encourage. If your child has good friends, be grateful. Conversely, if you are concerned about those friends, you may want to talk to a youth leader about getting some ideas and even some help.

Peers are extremely important during adolescence. They provide much of the social network for kids. One way to influence your child in a healthy way is to make your home a place where kids can hang out. Offer some incentive like food and take advantage of the opportunity to get to know your child's friends. For example, my mom got my friends to hang out at our house for two reasons. First, there was always good food around. Many of my buddies preferred eating dinner at my house to eating at home. Second, she was warm and a good listener. Most of my good friends saw her as a second mom. They would talk to her about things I didn't even know they were worried about. They knew she cared and would listen.

It would have been fun if we owned a pool table or had our own weight room, but you don't have to spend money to make your home a place where kids will hang out. Things like those can be very attractive, but they aren't the most important thing.

One of my favorite people is Jeff. He was a good kid from a good home. It has surprised no one that Jeff has grown up to be a highly respected young man and entered the ministry. But I have seen a number of good kids from good homes who did not turn out like Jeff. After weighing the evidence, I have reached the conclusion that Jeff's success stemmed from a group of buddies he surrounded himself with at Coronado High School in Scottsdale, Arizona. These young guys held each other accountable and hung together. Almost every one of them has done well. It is my opinion that one of the major reasons for the maturity and integrity of this group of young men is the commitment they shared as high schoolers to follow Christ together.

The younger your children, the more influence you can have here. I am not encouraging you to try to pick your children's friends, but make sure you encourage them, especially when they find a friend who is obviously a good influence.

SCHOOL

For some, this is a great source of encouragement and success. If you sense that school is a positive reinforcer, you don't necessarily need to do more than tuck that information away for future reference. On the other hand, if you can see that your teenager is not finding any healthy niche at school, start working with teachers, counselors, and others at the school to build a more positive environment. I know failure is often a better teacher than constant achievement, but an adolescent who doesn't discover any reason to stay in school may become difficult to deal with.

JOB

Again, a job may give a young person a sense of pride, responsibility, and accomplishment. If your son or daughter has a job or is pursuing one, make sure you get to know who he or she is working for. Not every place that hires younger folks worries about the environment they are creating. A new job can provide a very good opportunity to discuss goals and to learn responsibility. Ask questions like "What influence do you think this will have on school?" or "How do you think you will spend your money?" This may be a great time to show your child your family budget.

Having a job doesn't guarantee teens will learn responsibility. Yet, if you have thought it through, a job can be an integral part of your transition team.

BOOKS AND PERIODICALS

A great deal of resource information is available today in books and magazines for kids, young adults, and parents. Do your homework. Many resources deal with specific issues relating to parenting. If you have a daughter going into middle school or junior high, I would recommend you learn something about eating disorders. It may never be an issue in your family, but a little information early on could save you a lot of grief down the road.

You don't need to read everything, but you should regularly be seeking resources to help you grow as a Christian and a parent. A visit to your Christian bookstore or a call to your church or simply to another parent could yield a wealth of information about what is out there. I have placed a short bibliography at the end of the book. While it doesn't contain all of the helpful resources available in print, I trust it will get you started.

PROFESSIONAL COUNSEL

Another important resource is the Christian counselor. There are times when we simply need extra help. You may reach a particular point in your own life where your resource team has dwindled to a dangerous level. At these times I would encourage you to seek the help of a professional. It is important to pick someone who shares your values and has some experience in the situations you are facing.

PROVIDING A SAFE HARBOR IN THE STORM

You are your child's greatest resource.

No one can replace the role a parent has in the life of a child. And none of us should ever minimize our importance as a parent. Here are five things you can do to serve as a resource to your kids.

PRAY
You have no greater tool at your disposal. As we will discuss later, the first thing prayer does is change the one who prays. Be faithful in your prayers for your children.

ENCOURAGE
There are a great many things in the world that will discourage and break young people. We need to learn the art of encouragement. Not praise for what they do, but appreciation for who they are. This is not applause without accountability. Rather, this is a building up and a recognition of the valuable inner person.

TRUST
When possible, demonstrate to your children that you trust them. Give them opportunities to earn more trust. Whenever possible, treat them as adults.

SHARE OPENLY
One of the most effective ways to demonstrate trust and build your friendship with your children is to share how you feel about them and about life. They need to see how

adults work out difficult issues in their lives and feel how adults cope with pain and disappointment. This is not to say that you should burden your kids with every detail of your life, but begin to let them in a little more. This is not simply sharing about how they make you feel. It must include more of your life than that.

LISTEN

They may rarely be in the mood to talk, but when they are, be prepared to listen. Ask good questions and maintain eye contact. Most kids are spontaneous emoters. They will talk when they are in the mood. At that point you will want to be ready to listen. They may not be looking for an answer from you. So be prepared to listen hard for the message *behind* the words. Most of all, show by your body language and your thoughtful questions that *what they are sharing with you is vitally important.* If you do, they will come back again and again.

The average American family moves every four years. It is common for kids to attend six or more schools while growing up.

Americans are taught to be individuals. Our society is hungrily consumed with grabbing for a piece of the American pie. Consequently, young people find themselves isolated and without clear guidance. They are trying to survive through the storms of transition without the necessary resources to keep their young lives on a steady course. Teenagers desire some independence, but there is often a need to find a safe harbor in the storm.

One of those lost in the storm of adolescence was Dottie. Her father was an alcoholic and her mom simply survived. There was virtually no resource team at her disposal.

I met her when she was a sophomore in high school. She faithfully attended our meetings and even went to camps. But she always seemed to be on a collision course with trouble. There were simply not enough people or resources around her to make up for the deficits she was experiencing.

Dottie and I have been friends now for fourteen years. Nothing much has changed. When we are together I can sense a real desire in her to be different. She continually renews her determination to make life work and to follow Christ. But she has never had a resource team in place. Try as I might to pull other resources together for her, she fears failure and won't risk a radical change. Dottie is now an adult who may never have the strength to follow her convictions.

A lot of people are like that. But we can muster resources for our children and give them the opportunity Dottie didn't have. It is going to take some work, but it is worth it.

Finally, one writer had this to say about our ultimate resource:

> The Lord works from the inside out. The world works
> from the outside in. The world would take people out
> of the slums. Christ takes the slums out of people,
> and then they take themselves out of the slums. The
> world would mold men by changing their environment.
> Christ changes men, who then change their environ-
> ment. The world would shape human behavior, but
> Christ can change human nature.[1]

In the trauma of transition our teenagers face, we mustn't try to meet their needs alone. We will find great help and encouragement by gathering resources to aid us. Trusted adult friends, peers, school, a job, books and periodicals, and most importantly prayer are some of the resources at our disposal. We can be certain transitions are ahead. How they affect our children and our lives could be significantly improved with some well-planned help.

• • • • • • • • • •

CHAPTER EIGHT

Team Member 4:
Maintaining Intimacy
in the Midst of Transition

One of the great cries of teens today is for intimacy—the joy and security of closeness and trust with another human being. Too many have been robbed of the potential of real intimacy because of stress, busyness, pride, fear, and more. The lack of intimacy young people feel often causes a panic that forces them into misguided and even tragic relationships.

Marriages and families face great danger from the loss of intimacy or closeness. So much of our children's identity and sense of worth comes from relationships in the family.

What makes intimacy so difficult as kids go through their adolescent years comes from parents' lack of time and energy and teens' lack of response. For many parents, careers are peaking and there are more demands on our time. We are working more and beginning to discover we have less energy than in years past. At this point, we are often as insecure about what is going on as our kids are. We may have felt in control when they were younger, but now we don't know how to read them. Boys' responses are usually monosyllabic and girls' responses can range from chatter bordering on the frenetic, to sullenness with sudden bursts of tears.

When we parents expect the warm and expressive dialogue associated with preadolescence or mature adult conversation (which teens are sometimes capable of), we are generally let down and often feel disappointment, failure, or even anger. We may want to demand an adequate response and use negative reinforcement to accomplish it.

In this chapter we are going to offer some guidelines on maintaining intimacy during these trying times. Our goal is not to control the behavior of our teens, but to determine our response based on our security in Christ, and to develop some additional communications tools.

REMEMBER YOUR GOAL

If your goal is to achieve some preconceived "proper" response from your teen, then you have set the stage for ongoing tension between you and your child. If your goal is intimacy with your son or daughter, then you will look at the situation from a very different perspective.

The first objective is to remember who you are. You are a person who has set your eyes on Christ. Your identity and sense of worth come from your relationship with Him and don't depend on anyone's response.

If we can stay committed to this view of ourselves, the battle will not focus on our children's response. We will operate from a position of strength in Christ. Our own relationship with Christ becomes the foundation for our relationship with our teenagers. The peace and confidence we get from Christ will guide our emotions and responses to the teens in our family. This gives us the power to be proactive.

We can listen to the words being said, and we can listen with our hearts to our teens' silence, moods, or body language.

Gary Smalley and John Trent, in their very helpful book *The Language of Love*, quote current research about the communication of children.

> Researchers have found that from the earliest years little girls talk more than little boys. One study showed that even in the hospital nursery, girls had more lip movement than boys! That propensity keeps right on increasing through the years, giving them an edge at meaningful communication![1]

They go on to report that researchers found that 100 percent of the sounds coming from girls' mouths while on the playground were audible, recognizable words. The girls spent a great deal of time talking to other children, and nearly as much talking to themselves! Yet for little boys, only 68 percent of their sounds were understandable words. The remaining 32 percent were either one-syllable sounds like "uh" and "mmm," or sound effects like "Varooom!" "Yaaaaah!" and "Zooooom!"

This information should give you comfort. Now you know that the grunts that have been frustrating you are genetic and not simply a plot by your son to drive you crazy.

From a position of security and focus in Christ, you don't have to view the grunts and groans of adolescence as a threat. You can begin to develop the perspective that inside the heart of that young person there is a deep need to be loved and understood. God is doing a work in your teen's life just as He is doing a work in yours.

LEARN TO BE AN EMPATHETIC LISTENER

In the movie *Star Wars*, Obi Wan Kenobi tells Luke Skywalker to use his laser sword with his eyes closed. "Trust the force," he admonishes Luke. Luke didn't trust something he couldn't see until he experienced some success in wielding his sword with his eyes closed.

Parents generally put too much stock in what they see with their eyes and hear with their ears. They may even base their success as a parent solely on this criterion. This often creates conflict when they don't see or hear what they perceive as acceptable from their kids. Young persons on the other hand get frustrated because they sense conditions on their parents' love. They think they are loved only if they look and speak a certain way. These kids usually turn to a peer group for acceptance.

As parents we must be skillful listeners. We must constantly ask ourselves questions like, "Do I really understand what my son is saying?" "Am I forming my answer in my mind rather than carefully listening to the question?" "Have I just given my daughter another standard parental cliché?" "Do I present my ideas in ways that my kids can understand?" and "Am I communicating to convince or to understand?" These and other questions help us reflect on our communication style.

When Shawn came by my house one night I could tell things weren't going right. "My dad just blew up at me again," he explained. "He just won't listen when I try to explain how I feel!"

We'd had this conversation before. Shawn was a typical kid in many ways. He wasn't always very communicative, but he had a good heart. His father had great hopes for him and yet found it very difficult to listen to Shawn's hopes and fears.

There are always two sides to every conflict, and I worked hard with Shawn to help him own up to his responsibility in the relationship. But I could never get his dad to engage in a discussion about his own communication style.

"Kids are just spoiled," he would reply. Often he pleaded that what Shawn needed was another camp experience. It had made him so easy to live with for a while afterward.

Shawn's dad based his judgement of Shawn on a certain behavior. Consequently, he often missed what was really going on *inside* his son.

To be an empathetic listener we must step outside ourselves and attempt to view what our adolescent is saying from his or her point of view. The critical need for kids today is not our sympathy; it is our empathy, our understanding.

CLUES TO WHAT'S INSIDE A TEENAGER

The world of young people is one of constant change. Even when it's not apparent in their words or swaggering style, a lot of insecurity is creeping in. Often their words attempt to disguise their feelings. It is a difficult thing for them to admit they are insecure and unsure of themselves. At the same time, these young folks may not have the capacity to clearly express what is going on inside. To really understand them we must look for clues.

Boredom—This is one of the common stereotypes particularly seen in young males. They have a look about them that says the earth could be collapsing all around them and they really wouldn't care. We want to call them zombies, and we fret that they will never amount to anything.

Physical change—The truth is that many times these kids are in a growth phase or physical maturation phase during which their energy is used up from the inside. They may be walking around looking the way they look because it is how they feel. This phase also uses up much of their emotional energy.

Confusion—On the other hand, these teens may be at a point where they really don't know what to do or how they are supposed to feel. So at the moment at least, it may seem best not to worry about it.

A doctor would never prescribe a remedy for a patient without carefully considering the illness. Parents should not prescribe a remedy for their child without doing everything possible to discover where the teen's problems really lie.

Obviously, this involves some risk and a major effort at intimate communication. First, when we work hard to understand another person, we open ourselves up to being influenced by that other person. Our ideas and thought patterns are challenged. But, if our image of ourselves is centered on Christ and not our opinion of ourselves, we will always be open to change. We will see the communication risk as a way of being conformed to the image of Christ.

Second, we risk being wrong. What if after all this effort we misjudge what is actually going on? In response to that concern, I simply want to ask you this question: Wouldn't you rather someone work hard to really understand who you are and what you are feeling, and then with the best intentions be wrong, than to never have had another person risk that kind of love? But these risks must be taken to clear up teenage confusion. Only intimate communication can help teens face their doubts and fears.

Here are four other steps in empathetic listening for you to keep in mind.

1. *Choose a good setting.* If you are ready to listen carefully to your son or daughter, choose a setting that will facilitate communication. Make sure you are not likely to be interrupted. If possible, ask your child where he or she would like to meet.

At the risk of contradicting myself, I must say that even in the best setting communication doesn't always happen. We need to be ready to talk (or just listen) when our kids are ready. That may be in the car, while watching a movie, or just before bed.

2. *Keep your eyes on your teen*—and I don't mean spying. Often you may wonder who your teenager is talking to because of the way he or she looks down or around during a conversation. But your teen is aware if you are not totally with him or her. Work hard to stay focused on your teen. Eye contact is the key to this.

3. *Repeat back to them what you are hearing* in ways that acknowledge and express the content and feelings they are sharing. This will require you to set aside your own judgments on the matter long enough to really hear what they are saying.

When your college student says, "Mom, I hate school!" a typical response might be, "Well, everyone hates things they have to do sometimes. You'll grow to appreciate this opportunity." A more appropriate response might be, "You are really frustrated, aren't you?"

By a simple statement that acknowledges your teen's problem, you are not judging the outburst, and it allows your teen to clarify if "frustration" is an accurate description of how he or she feels.

4. *Respond from their vantage point.* When the opportunity presents itself to share your insight or wisdom, do it from your understanding of *their world*, not from the perspective of how the adult world functions. Show them that you have listened carefully to them and you understand the situation from their point of view.

When your seventh-grade daughter comes home crying and asks why no one likes her, don't say, "Nonsense, you are very popular." Instead, you may want to respond with, "Do you think it's your problem or their problem?"

Her response may tell you how she feels about her looks or how someone hurt her feelings. From here you may let her know that if she feels that way about her appearance there might be some possible solutions the two of you can explore.

To summarize, we must remember to demonstrate that we value our teenager's feelings and perceptions. We do this most effectively when we feel valuable in our own hearts because of what Christ has done for us. Then we work hard at listening and avoid forming our response while our son or daughter is sharing a feeling or trying to make a point. It takes a lot of energy to be an empathetic listener. We may often feel unappreciated by our teen for the effort we are making. But his or her response is not the key. Our commitment and faithfulness will pay off in time.

BEGIN TO MOVE FROM PARENT TO FRIEND

Grandparents will tell you that you never stop being a parent. Yet, in the course of raising children there comes that difficult point when we realize that we must begin to see our child as an adult. Even earlier than that, we must recognize when to begin to communicate more like a friend than an authority figure.

This is a very difficult transition to recognize. Also, we must remember that as our kids go through some periods in the teen years they may need the security of that authority. Beginning to share as a friend can be very intimidating because it may reveal some weak communication habits that we have not been aware of. Following are some tips to make the transition as smooth as possible.

BE HONEST
All of us struggle with communication. Tell your teens how you feel and ask for *their* advice. Make sure they know how much you want to be an available friend as well as a parent. Be clear that you are not giving up your parental role and leadership, but you want to recognize their maturity and growth.

SAY YOU'RE SORRY
If you recognize that you have not communicated in a helpful manner, apologize and make adjustments. By doing this you demonstrate your respect for teens' feelings and perceptions.

GIVE THEM SPACE
Adolescents need room to grow. They need privacy. Becoming their friend does not mean acting like another adolescent.

It means demonstrating an attitude of respect. This means giving them some privacy and independence.

DEVELOP FRIENDS YOUR OWN AGE
Have you ever learned how to be a friend? Have you worked at it? All of us need to learn the art of developing strong peer relationships. Many times parents need the friendship of their young adults more for the parents' sake than the kids'. This can often lead to disappointment and frustration.

DON'T BE AFRAID TO TOUCH
You need to discover appropriate ways to touch your children. This is very important. It may mean a firm handshake instead of tousling their hair. Or a quick hug may be more apropos than plopping the kid into your lap. If you stay committed and observant, you will find out what works and you will discover that, even though kids need change, their need for touch will grow. A standoffish junior high boy can easily become an affectionate collegian.

DON'T TRY TO BUY INTIMACY
You cannot spend enough money to create intimacy. It must come from time, commitment, warmth, and love. It will come from kids who know you both care about them and also provide accountability and parameters. It will come when they discover that you have been on your knees on their behalf.

STAY CLOSE TO YOUR SPOUSE

The trauma of teen transition in a family often exacts its biggest toll on the parents' marriage. Unfulfilled expectations, disagreements about direction, and a preoccupation with the kids can leave wives and husbands feeling left out and jealous. The stress created by children can leave moms and dads bankrupt emotionally and unable to address each other's needs.

We have talked about finding our focus and center in Christ. Next we must guard and nurture our relationship with our spouse. Marriage is hard enough work without the added stress of adolescents, but it can become a great source of strength and encouragement when facing tough times.

Intimacy with our spouse gives us the experience and some of the framework for intimacy with our children.

Shawn and I are still good friends. His father left the family a few years ago and has been remarried for some time. Shawn's mom fought to hold the family together and make life as "normal" as possible for the kids. Shawn has slowly forged a relationship with his dad and has been a great help to his mom. He will never know the kind of intimacy with his dad that he wishes, but they have found some common ground to share interests and opinions.

Shawn remains very close to his mom, and she will tell you he has been her closest friend through everything. Intimacy is often the result of pain and struggle. Many times it is born out of desperation and failure. When we don't have all the answers, we become more human, more approachable. We are forced to admit that the best relationships aren't perfect. The deepest relationships aren't always the ones that are the most trouble free. Intimacy comes from dependence when we recognize our need for each other. It comes from commitment, that willingness to roll up our sleeves and to keep working on our relationship until we see some change (usually in ourselves). And it comes from endurance, our commitment not to give up on each other, but to stay committed through the hard and painful times.

Intimacy is much more a discovery than a feeling. It comes from a journey with many twists and turns along its path. But, if we can stay faithful to the direction set before us, we may discover intimacy along the way. As we move ahead with our transition team, the emphasis from this chapter will be continually underscored. The peace and confidence you have in Christ will empower you to make good choices. This will be important to using each team member well. Also, each additional member of your team is offered to help you respond to your children and not to manipulate a response from them. Then in the midst of your journey through adolescent transitions, you will discover the joy of intimacy with Christ and with your teen.

• • • • • • • • • • •

CHAPTER NINE

Team Member 5:
Prayer—Healing Strength
for the Stressed

To say that prayer should be the first rule of parenting can be frustrating and convicting. We are a society raised on the premise that we need to be self-sufficient and independent. Therefore to reduce our parenting to prayer takes too much power out of our hands. We are unaccustomed to that position.

Far too many Christian parents simply trot down to the nearest bookstore for the latest guide to "successful" parenting. While these books are helpful and encouraging, they were never intended to replace the activity of prayer.

Whether we are aware of it or not, prayer impacts our lives. It may be the *lack of prayer* that results in stress and uncertainty, or it may be the *evidence of prayer* resulting in peace and confidence. There are few things in life more demanding and at the same time more necessary than prayer. It is our greatest resource in the battles we face, yet the most difficult one to master. It is the transition team member we should most often turn to, yet the one we usually find the most troublesome to face.

Throughout history when God's children have faced disaster, insurmountable odds, or tragedy, the common thread of their survival has been prayer. In Exodus 3:7, God told Moses, "I have indeed seen the misery of my people in Egypt. I have heard them crying out."

No one could express the sentiments of a broken and contrite heart like King David:

Have mercy on me, O God, have mercy on me,
for in you my soul takes refuge. (Psalm 57:1)

TRANSITION AND TRANSFORMATION
FOR THE ONE WHO PRAYS

It has been said that the first thing prayer changes is the one who prays. When parents come before the Lord on behalf of their children, they may often walk away with peace in their own hearts. When we ask the Father to change the behavior of one of His children, we are generally confronted with our need for grace and change.

Such was the case with Herb. We had talked often about the rebellion of his oldest son. Herb was a successful businessman and was very embarrassed and hurt by his son's actions. His wife, Marilyn, was a woman devoted to Christ and with a clear understanding of the need for prayer in this situation. As Herb resisted her invitations to prayer, tension grew in their relationship as well as in their family. Their son was being swept away in an angry current of rebellion while they drifted apart from each other in their own sea of confusion and hurt.

Finally, during one of our talks together I worked up the courage to ask Herb to pray with me. We were at a restaurant and with a furtive glance at the surrounding tables he agreed to let me offer a prayer. Bolstered by this response,

I asked Herb if he would be willing to meet regularly just to pray. I let him decide where and when. That was the beginning of an extraordinary journey.

Herb and I met weekly for a number of months. At first our get-togethers didn't look much like prayer meetings, but the Lord was slowly beginning to work in the life of a man who had always prided himself in being independent and strong. Prayer had never been a resource or team member for him. He was discovering a whole new dimension as a parent and person.

In the beginning I kept a log of our meetings. It was simply a piece of paper with a line drawn down the middle. On the left side I would write down what Herb thought we should pray for. I never tried to change his mind in those requests. This was to be part of his growth. Too often I have been guilty of trying to manipulate the lessons the Lord should teach others. This time I wanted to allow God's Spirit to lead and change Herb where necessary. In the process He would also change me, I was quite certain.

I told Herb that on the right side of the page we would record God's answers to our prayers. I think at that point he was willing to humor me. But it wasn't too long before that right side began to fill up.

Sometimes we must look hard for those answers. We expect one response, and when we don't see it we can miss what God is doing. As prayer changes us, we gain a new perspective. We begin to see more from God's perspective and less from ours.

Herb's son, Kevin, did not become a scholar after the first prayer meeting, but he didn't get kicked out of school either. Herb needed to see God's provision in what God was doing, not in what Herb wanted Him to do.

After about eight months of meeting for prayer Herb and I evaluated our time. We had seen tremendous changes in Kevin. Sometimes Herb would come to our meetings with statements like, "I can't believe it; he's like a new kid!" He

began to ask me if there were other things we could be praying for, and started praying for my family as much as his. *In
the midst of all of the concern over Kevin, the most profound
change was in Herb.*

God can change your kids. He will use prayer to ease
the transitions of adolescence. But, if you are not willing
to be changed in the process, you will have a difficult time
sustaining your prayer life.

Adolescents will often disdain our advice simply because
it is ours. If you are a parent of a teenager, you have probably been frustrated many times by the lack of response your
suggestions get. But, let *them* come up with an idea, or worse
yet, *one of their friends*, and it's golden. Let good old mom or
dad offer an idea and it's, "Yea, *right*, Mom" (with the inflec-
tion making it negative).

At such times our most faithful team member, the one
we keep coming back to, is prayer. Here we find strength and
assurance. We are enlisting God's help—the most powerful
force in the universe—to intercede on our behalf. Even in the
midst of the storms of transition, when we are at a loss as to
what to pray for, the Holy Spirit intercedes:

> In the same way, the Spirit helps us in our weak-
> ness. We do not know what we ought to pray for, but
> the Spirit himself intercedes for us with groans that
> words cannot express. And he who searches our hearts
> knows the mind of the Spirit, because the Spirit inter-
> cedes for the saints in accordance with God's will.
> (Romans 8:26-27)

THE KEY TO PRAYER IS SHOWING UP

I will never forget the words of Stephen Winward in his book
How to Talk to God. "The whole of life should be a walk with
God, and all times and all places should be sacred to Him."[1]
Here we are given the admonition to pray our way through

life. There is no magic place or circumstance for prayer. At any place and under any set of circumstances, we can and should bring our needs to the Father.

At the same time, we learn to live in communion with Christ by setting aside specific blocks of time for Him. A specific place or a special chair might help us, but prayer is interior. We must cultivate a quiet heart sensitive to the whispers of the Spirit.

The important point here is to do it. Prayer is something we must give ourselves to. We must open our hearts to the Lord and allow Him to speak back to us. Prayer must become a habit.

The habit of prayer doesn't happen by itself. It is in private moments of focus on Christ that we discover how to open our hearts and minds to Him. The skill of praying will be mastered by practice.

Paderewski, the famous Polish pianist, once said, "If I stop practicing the piano for a day, I notice the difference; if I stop for two days, my family notices the difference; if I stop for three days my friends notice the difference; and if I stop for a week the public notices the difference."[2] Certainly in our lives the lack of prayer is usually more obvious than we care to admit. During the turbulence caused by teenage transitions, we cannot afford to get "rusty" in our prayers. A consistent life of prayer keeps us focused and in touch with the Lord.

When I first asked Herb to pray, he was concerned about saying things right. He was under the impression that effective prayers should be offered in King James language with a lot of "Thees" and "Thous." He had been confused about *how* to approach God. Prayer to him was a formal ceremony done by serious and pious people, not by driven, rebellious folks as he had pictured himself.

I have often felt the same emotions Herb expressed. It was not hard for me to relate to his concerns. Often when I pray, my own fears and sense of failure inhibit my approach to God. I feel guilty asking Him for the same thing again or confessing the same misconduct I confessed the day before. At such times it is crucial that I remind myself that it is my problem and not God's. He is ready and anxious to hear my prayer. He is not shaking His finger at me like a stern school-master. He is holding out His arms, a loving Father longing to embrace His child.

Our Lord told us about prayer in Matthew 7:7-8: "Ask and it will be given to you; seek and you will find; knock and the door will be opened to you. For everyone who asks receives; he who seeks finds; and to him who knocks, the door will be opened."

That is not the wishful thinking of some well-meaning person. It is a promise from Jesus Christ. If we seek Him we will find Him. He listens to our prayers and knows the longings of our heart.

He does not require us to address Him formally any more than we would require that of our own children.

When Herb discovered he could address the Lord with words from his heart, prayer became less formal and awk-ward. Prayer was still hard work, but Herb was beginning a journey that would lead him down a path of discovery and growth.

Brennan Manning recently shared with a group of our staff one of the most remarkable examples of this I have ever heard. Not too long ago he responded to a knock at his door. The woman standing in the doorway asked if he would please come and pray with her ailing father. Soon Brennan was sitting on the edge of a bed talking to a frail, elderly man about life, love, and eternity. The man shared that for years he was intimidated and confused about how to pray. He had asked others for help until someone finally told him he could talk to the Lord just like he would a friend standing right beside him. This had revolutionized his life.

He pointed an aged finger at an empty chair beside his bed and whispered to Brennan that now he simply pretended

Jesus was sitting in the chair, and they would talk. It was a secret he had been afraid to tell anyone else.

Brennan prayed with this dear saint and went home deeply touched and greatly encouraged.

Sometime later he heard from the woman again. This time it was to share the news of her father's passing. "The odd thing," she said to Brennan, "was that he had pulled himself over to the edge of his bed, and when I found him he had died with his head resting on the chair."

We may talk to the Lord as though He were right next to us, but in truth He is even closer than that.

As a parent you know that kids are always asking for something. It can be that constant need for more cash or the keys to the car. Requests for leniency and more freedom are frequent, too. But a relationship solely made up of asking is a tedious one. It has no depth and allows for only shallow perceptions of another's value.

Certainly we would not want to approach God the same way. Prayer that is exclusively asking becomes self-centered. When we ask from a posture of adoration, confession, and thanksgiving, our requests take on more of what God's will might be rather than ours.

Scripture tells us to ask in the name of Jesus: "Until now you have not asked for anything in my name. Ask and you will receive, and your joy will be complete" (John 16:24).

We are given that privilege in Christ to offer our cares and needs to the Father in His name because He has chosen to be our Advocate. Winward offers this further insight: "In the Bible 'the name' means nature; it stands for the person revealed in his character. To pray in Christ's name is to pray in accordance with His nature and character, in harmony with His revealed will and purpose."[3]

There is nothing so small that God is not interested in it or bigger than He is able to do it.

Too often we are tempted to give up. We just can't seem to get our message through. Don't give up. God has given you permission in Scripture to be persistent. You may have heard someone say that God's timing is not our timing. Rarely does God work within the time frame we create for Him. But He always works.

For over fifty years my grandmother faithfully prayed for my grandfather. I am sure that many times during those years she must have wondered if the Lord was listening. My grandfather was a wonderful man who, like so many others, shared a lifetime battle with alcohol. So for more than half a century Grandma prayed for him. And in the waning years of Grandad's life he opened his heart to Christ and went Home in peace.

I hope you are gaining a better understanding of the life of prayer. You see, if we will give ourselves consistently to adoration, confession, and thanksgiving, by the time we begin making our requests we will be changed. And when our hearts are united with Christ, we can approach the Father with confidence and joy.

COMMON BARRIERS TO PRAYER

I have often wondered why prayer is so difficult. If it is such a key transition team member, why do we hesitate to appropriate its power? Of the many possible reasons, I would like you to consider four.

GUILT

When I first began to pray with Herb, he wrestled with a familiar enemy: guilt. "I feel like I'm cheating," he would say. "I have never really prayed before, and to start now when things are such a mess doesn't seem right."

Many of us struggle with guilt because we recognize that we only pray when all else has failed. We resent being treated that way ourselves, and we know it must really irk God when we do it. The truth could not be more different. We have created a God in our image that says we must perform a certain way to have access to Him. That is not the God of my experience and certainly not the God of Scripture, who says,

> And call upon me in the day of trouble;
> I will deliver you, and you will honor me.
> (Psalm 50:15)

We have permission to call upon the Lord in times of trouble and distress. He will not hold our previous prayerlessness against us during those times. He loves us too much. If you have put off praying because you hadn't prayed in the good times, start now! Take your burdens of guilt and failure and lay them at the feet of your loving Father and watch Him take them away. Being a parent is a heavy burden. At times the transition periods in our kids' lives feel like they will crush us. Don't add an unnecessary burden to one already so heavy. Christ bids us in Matthew 11:28, "Come to me, all you who are weary and burdened, and I will give you rest."

FEAR OF THE COST
Another common block to prayer is fear. We fear what it might cost us to enter into a relationship of prayer with the Lord. Let's face it, we twentieth-century adults want a painless solution to our problems. We baby boomers want a quick and easy fix. We hesitate at the thought that something might infringe on our interests and lifestyle. We are afraid if we begin to pray we might be confronted with issues in our lives we are unprepared to deal with.

We have been amazed and at times shocked in our ministry to find a growing number of kids being checked into psychiatric hospitals because they are discipline problems and their parents want someone else to deal with them. Granted, there are times when the situation may warrant such action, but we are seeing a growing number simply put into these institutions because it's quicker and easier.

All of us have some fear of change. It is always difficult to be confronted with areas in our lives that require growth or correction.

We must gather the courage to risk such a confrontation. I don't know if Herb would have had I not pursued him. Perhaps it would be good to find a prayer partner to help you and hold you accountable.

DOUBT

Another reason some balk at prayer is doubt. What if I go to all this trouble, get my hopes up, and God doesn't come through? This is a desperate fear. Often our pain is so real, and on the surface there appears so little reason for hope, that we are not sure if even God can fix it.

The fact is, God may not "fix" our problem or problem child in the way we desire, but He has promised to hear our cries and meet us at our point of need. He has commanded us to "come to Me." Even in our moments of greatest doubt we can approach the Lord in obedience and He will meet us there.

Francois Fenelon, in her *Little Book of Prayers*, wrote, "Lord, I don't know what to ask of You; only You know what I need. I simply present myself to You; I open my heart to You. I have no other desire than to accomplish Your will. Teach me to pray. Amen."[4]

ADDICTION TO BUSYNESS

Lastly, a prayerless life may also result from an addiction to busyness. I find it deeply disturbing when people tell me they don't have time to pray. We have time to worry, we have time to complain, but we cannot seem to find the minutes in our day to go to our Lord in prayer.

Many of us are caught in the *need to produce*. Generally speaking, the busier we are, the better we feel. If we are living a hectic life, at least we appear successful and vital. To be still is to be alone with our thoughts and that may seem threatening. So we maintain the blur we call a life and look forward to the day we can retire and forget all of this.

But King David had a different idea. He wrote, "Be still before the Lord and wait patiently for him" (Psalm 37:7).

If your life is ruled by busyness, you need prayer on your team. When your teenager doesn't seem to respond to anything you do or say, prayer is the team member that offers quiet and peace. It has the potential to bring God's perspective to every situation. As you rally your transition team you will discover that prayer empowers every member.

The *heart* that seeks the Lord is always rewarded. We cannot substitute anything in its place, and a life of prayer will eventually leave its mark.

A *prayerful spirit* is a spirit to which God can speak. The more sensitive and responsive our hearts become to the voice of the Father, the more confident we are that He hears us.

Learning the *discipline of prayer* radically changed the direction of Herb's life. I want to encourage you to sit down and read Psalm 27 today. Make the words of the psalm your prayer. The last verse beautifully sums up this chapter.

> Wait for the LORD;
>> be strong and take heart
>> and wait for the LORD. (Psalm 27:14)

In conclusion, we join with John Baillie as he prays for vision, faith, and love. "Eternal God, you have been the hope and joy of many generations, and who in all ages has given men the power to seek you and in seeking you find you, grant me, I pray you, a clearer vision of your truth, a greater faith in your power, and a more confident assurance of your love. Amen."[5]

● ● ● ● ● ● ● ● ● ● ●

CHAPTER TEN

Team Member 6:
Managing Time Factors

I went out Lord,
*   men were coming and going,*
*   walking and running.*
In spite of all their grand efforts,
*   they were still short of time.*
*   Lord, you must have made a mistake in your*
*   calculation.*
Lord, I have time.
*   I have plenty of time, all the time you give me,*
*   the years of my life,*
*   the days of my years,*
*   the hours of my days.*
Mine to fill quietly, calmly,
Up to the brim.

AUTHOR UNKNOWN

I first met Bill Piel when I was in eighth grade and he was in seventh. I certainly had no idea that our lives would be linked together from then on.

Bill and I played on our elementary school flag football team. None of us on the team understood the changes swirling through Bill's life. His mother was remarried that year and he suddenly became Bill Hamilton. Since becoming adults, Bill has shared with me the amazing events surrounding that experience. It became one of the turning points in his life. Up until then his reputation was less than desirable. His mother was overwhelmed with the task of raising five kids on her own. Bill and his older brother often found themselves without any supervision. Even though he was not a "bad kid," he had some minor brushes with the law and was on the verge of heading the wrong way for life.

For some reason, this change of name encouraged Bill to seek a change in his life. He thought with a new name a be he could become a new person. The marriage had put Bill in a different school where he was not known. He had a chance to be different.

Now Bill is a husband, father, and full-time minister. He is highly respected in his community and very effective in his work. We have been partners in reaching kids all our adult lives. But, he would be the first to tell you that it wasn't changing his name that rerouted his life. Bill's life-direction was still up for grabs until our Young Life leaders, Dr. Bob and Rillie Lee, got hold of him. It was through this remarkable couple that Bill found Christ. Still, all through high school Bill struggled with allowing the faith he held in his heart to manifest itself in his life. That's the part that took time. As a youngster he had experienced a name change, yet he still had to rely on the Lord to change and build his character.

Each of us "changed our name" when we came into the family of God. We call ourselves Christians and serve a new Master. Still, each day we face transitions as we allow our Father to change and mold us to the image of Christ.

I find there is a great deal of interest in shortcuts today. Too often we are consumed by a desire to move quickly past the challenges and changes in our lives. Many folks today want instant spirituality. They want to win the race without experiencing the agony of training for the event. If we push this on the adolescents in our home, we keep them from a healthy growth process.

In the next two chapters we will be looking at transitions from the vantage points of crisis, transformation, and change. To understand the scope of the transition your son or daughter is experiencing, you will want to view him or her from one of these vantage points.

When Bill changed his name and determined to change his lifestyle, he underwent a transition of transformation. He gained a feeling of newness and hope for the future. In this he reminds us of a valuable fact: transitions do not have to result in crisis. In fact, most transition is very normal and healthy.

A transition from crisis may be the result of the loss of a family member, a close friend's death or suicide, your own brush with death, or a divorce. Yet for teenagers without a support team and the correct coping tools, a serious crisis may emerge from what would be merely a simple transition for someone else.

TRANSITIONS OF GROWTH

As we discussed earlier, adolescence can be viewed in two broad time periods—early adolescence and late adolescence. We know that from approximately ages ten through fifteen kids go through tremendous physical and emotional change. Then from sixteen through about age twenty-two they go through late adolescence. During this time, you can expect greater intellectual development and need for independence.

Every child will face the basic transitions of growth and maturity differently. Some children reach puberty earlier than others. We can't do much about *when* puberty will strike, but there is a lot we can do when we see it approaching. Puberty is a major transition and the physical changes are very obvious, yet the greatest challenges are often not so visible. Many young people are plagued with feelings of insecurity and inferiority during this transition. They wiggle out of the warm cocoon of childhood and face competition and comparisons they have never felt before. Tall, gangly boys often look awkward and clumsy. Their voices are changing and nothing seems to fit anymore. Suddenly they become aware of how people see them. Many times they lack the social skills and confidence to relate to girls. They stumble through their first bout with love and panic at the potential for disaster.

As puberty approaches for your son or daughter, you can anticipate these challenges and provide coping resources.

For example, I have known parents who took their teen on a date. One dad took his daughter out to dinner and then to a movie. He opened the car door for her and made polite conversation all evening. He tried his hardest to help her relax and have fun, and he succeeded. Then at the end of the evening he asked her how she felt about the way he had treated her. "Daddy," she quietly replied, "now I think I know what I want dating to be for me. Thank you." When he received a positive response he left her with this challenge: "Never settle for less in your relationship with a boy." His daughter never forgot that invaluable lesson.

It may be helpful to call on one of your resource people to take your son or daughter on a date. Sometimes we need an outside voice in our child's life. A younger adult makes the date more comfortable for the teen. If you have thought through your team, you will likely know just who to call.

Physical attractiveness is one of the great threats to a young person's self-image today. We live in a society that places far too much emphasis on our body's appearance. We can point out all their good attributes, but most kids are simply going to go through a stage in early adolescence where they hate something about their physical appearance. They are too tall, too short, too heavy, too thin; they have pimples, or freckles, or "uncool hair."

Parents can have a positive influence on their adolescent kids in a variety of ways. If you are comfortable with the way you look, it will help. Also, be sensitive to styles and fashion. As much as you may hate to give in to the cost of fashion these days, allowing your son or daughter *some* current styles or even a brand name or two may give them some confidence in the face of drastic physical and emotional changes.

Our goal is not to speed up the transition process, but to help our children adapt to the various changes they are experiencing.

As parents we want to look for signs in our kids' ability to cope and integrate changes into their lives. We want to help them develop coping resources to move with as little strain as possible through the inevitable changes they will face.

Remember team member goals? We must remind ourselves to keep the end in mind during these crazy times. We must ask, what are we hoping the long-term results of this short-term discomfort will be? If you are firmly rooted in your goals, who you are, and how you will respond to your son or daughter, you won't panic during transition times. (A little panic is allowed in crisis, however!)

Our culture will continue to tell young people that they need to look a certain way, drive a certain car, and wear certain clothes to really have it together and be happy. We will not help the transition process by ignoring these messages or pretending they aren't there! Nor will we help them by giving in to every passing fancy. But, if we are thoughtful and take every opportunity to build up our children for *who* they are and not how they look or perform, we will give them an invaluable tool for adapting to change.

YOUR RESOURCE OF TIME

Here are three principles for managing time during transitions in an adolescent's life:

- Don't become a crisis manager.
- Make time for your children.
- Give your teenager time to grow up.

DON'T BECOME A CRISIS MANAGER

Most of us spend a good deal of our time managing crises. We are always putting out fires or trying to recover from the last major blaze. Time management means exactly what it says. We are to manage our time. Decide on what is important and then do those things. I remember Gordon McDonald saying that too many of us spend our lives doing good things when we need to focus on what's best.

If we can commit ourselves to pursuing what is "best," it can help us make good decisions.

Remember, choose your battles wisely. If your daughter wants to wear some clothes that you aren't sure about, ask yourself a couple of questions. Is this something that is truly inappropriate, or am I struggling with my own insecurity here? Check out the clothes she normally wears. Is this new outfit a fad or style that will be gone in a few months? Or does it represent some pattern I am concerned about? A "time manager" will carefully consider these and other questions before making a judgment.

Through part of my college career I chose to wear my hair pretty long. My parents were pastors and my shaggy looks must have caused them a fair amount of embarrassment. But they had a commitment to look beyond my hair and work hard to know the young man underneath. They saw me involved in ministry and working my way through college. So, aside from some good-natured kidding, they never made my hair a barrier in our relationship. They showed me a good deal of respect and didn't create an unnecessary need for me to flex my "independent" muscles. By the time I graduated from college my hair was a respectable length and my relationship with my parents as strong as ever.

If you focus on the strengths of your children and refuse to panic when you see something new, it helps create an environment where change can occur without as much trauma.

Make Time for Your Children
If you have browsed through a bookstore lately, you will notice many books for the stressed, busy, and burned out. Life provides plenty of challenge and everyone's schedule feels out of control. When you add the time kids require, it is no wonder parents shake their heads and throw up their hands. But, no matter how busy you may feel there is still

some discretionary time in your schedule. We must choose to give time to our children. As important as once-a-year vacations are for your family, this is not what I have in mind.

All of us have time we cannot control. In the Los Angeles area where I live many people commute hours to and from work. Most of us feel our free time is greatly reduced by travel. Still, we have certain hours we must make choices about. Those need to be wise choices. Let me give you a couple of suggestions. Don't put off your personal relationship with Christ. Often if we don't wake up quite on time in the morning, we put the Lord off to the next day. This can become days, weeks, and years. The guilt and frustration we originally felt can become hardness and apathy. However, when we see such values modeled by our children, we know we have missed the mark. Unfortunately, even if we model a strong spiritual life—even a balanced, nonthreatening one—it's no guarantee our kids will, too. But if we don't, more often than not, our children won't, either.

The next priority is your discretionary time. You need to spend it with your primary relationships—spouse and children. I know many of you are thinking, *What about time for myself?* We often feel we are so busy caring for others that we have no time for ourselves. Please understand that time with Christ is the most powerful, positive, and healthy time you can give to yourself. If you think devotional time is duty and work, something you do "for God," think again. We spend time with Christ because in the hustle and stress of our everyday lives He is the only One who can take our ragged clothes of burden and care and exchange them for a fresh and clean garment of peace and rest.

Likewise, if we are giving time to our other primary relationships, we will have a great sense of freedom and release when we do spend time on ourselves.

And, of course, we must have some personal time. I love to exercise and read. That combination really helps me. The exercise is tough to get in regularly. I drive a lot (I live in L.A.!)

and other priorities often get in the way. I also try to read at least a little every day. I generally have three books going at once and almost always one is a novel or something fun. The point is, if we ignore our own personal time, and time with significant others, it will damage our own emotional life, as well as our children's.

GIVE YOUR KIDS TIME TO GROW UP

Transitions happen for different teens at different times. According to James Dobson, puberty "may occur as early as nine or ten years of age or as late as seventeen or eighteen, but each boy and each girl has his or her own timetable."[1]

Obviously, we can't orchestrate that change. We can, however, be prepared for the results and have our transition team in place. We should be especially aware of the following issues.

Many young people today are growing up too fast. Early dating is a concern in many affluent communities. Boys and girls, from age ten up, are begging their parents to allow them to date. "More affluent families want their children to be more socialized. They feel that social dealings, as well as academic programs, are somehow a race; the earlier you start, the better," says David Elkind, author of *The Hurried Child*. Elkind believes one cause of this trend is television and other "contemporary influences."[2]

On the other end of the spectrum we have the "boomerang" children. The term *boomerang* refers to young adults who have moved back into their parents' home for one reason or another. For many families this can be healthy and happy. But for others, parents *and* children, it can be embarrassing and frustrating.

The high cost of buying or renting a home these days is a key to this trend. Many of these young people are from more affluent communities. Often their income on their own would not allow them to live in the way they desire.

Parents must decide, based on the real needs of their

children, whether moving back in is an option. It is critical, though, to keep a few things in mind.

Family life with adult kids will not be the same as it was when they were children. Make up your mind immediately not to set your expectations at impossible levels. A young man or woman moving home should not be treated the way he or she was at sixteen. Don't become a maid or a butler. Make sure some guidelines are clearly stated and give the arrangement a timetable so you can regularly evaluate how it is going. Finally, if possible, charge them rent. To charge them what they would pay somewhere else may not be appropriate, but some kind of rent is critical for maintaining your peace of mind and their dignity.

The storms accompanying transition come in many sizes and levels of intensity. It is very difficult to judge when they will hit or how long they will last. The key to navigating the typical changes in a teenager's life is in the parents' ability to *adapt and integrate* these changes into the family's lives. A solid support base (your transition team), carefully nurtured values, forgiveness, and patience all help provide the stability necessary to keep the ship on course.

Managing the time trials of adolescent life will test both you and your teenager. Keep in mind the two basic categories of adolescent development—early adolescence and late adolescence. Remind yourself of the common characteristics of each stage. Then you can anticipate certain changes and be better prepared. If your daughter has suddenly become moody, you will be in a much better position to help her if you remember that teens commonly ride an emotional roller coaster when they reach puberty. On the other hand, if you react as though it is simply rebellion, it will likely end up that way. Further, stay committed to doing the "best" with the time you have. There are many "good" things and events that crowd out what we really value.

The challenge of mastering our time in today's culture is a formidable one. I don't think "mastery" is really the issue.

It is simply a matter of deciding what is important in your life and then making time for it.

One night in the course of writing this book, I played Boggle. As anxious as I am to make deadlines and keep everyone happy, I can seldom resist joining the rest of my family in playing a game. I want to make time to play with my three sons. These years of family life are over with so soon. So I reflect and make time for my three boys now, before I miss out on having any memories of them at all! Prayers like this one by Rev. Wilferd A. Peterson make me think:

Slow Me Down, Lord

Slow me down, Lord.

Ease the pounding of my heart by the quieting of my mind.

Steady my hurried pace with a vision of the eternal reach of time.

Give me, amid the confusion of the day, the calmness of the everlasting hills.

Break the tensions of my nerves and muscles with the soothing music of the singing streams that live in my memory.

Teach me the art of taking minute vacations—of slowing down to look at a flower, to chat with a friend, to pat a dog, to smile at a child, to read a few lines from a good book.

Slow me down, Lord, and inspire me to send my roots deep into the soil of life's enduring values, that I may grow toward my greater destiny.

Remind me each day that the race is not always to the swift; that there is more to life than increasing its speed.

Let me look upward to the towering oak and know that it grew great and strong because it grew slowly and well.[3]

• • • • • • • • • •

CHAPTER ELEVEN

Team Member 7:
Laughter and Fun as Shelters
from the Storm

A cheerful heart is good medicine,
but a crushed spirit dries up the bones.

PROVERBS 17:22

There is little in life that produces more good for body
and soul than laughter. Laughing not only releases certain enzymes in your body that promote good health, but
it also just feels good. To regain a healthy perspective on life
we must cultivate our sense of humor. In the middle of the
change and uncertainty of raising teenagers that may seem
like a tall order.

Most of us have a few people in our lives who can make
us laugh. If you stop to think about it, there may be quite a
few. As we muster our resources we may forget to add the
friend who can bring laughter back to our lips. When I was
a child, my younger brother found in me the ideal audience.
I always laughed at his silly antics and one-liners. These
days my wife, Gina, and I laugh more with our kids than
with anyone else. They seem to provide plenty of accidental
and intentional comic relief.

Throughout this chapter I would like to share with you

127

a few stories and people who always make me laugh. I also want to share with you some thoughts on laughter and fun that may provide a framework for you during the otherwise dark hours of transition in your family. We will add laughter and fun to our arsenal for managing the trauma of transition in our lives and family.

High school can be a particularly awkward time. Young people stumble through the challenges of growing up. They are met with new experiences every day and are forced to gauge their success on how they fare among their peers.

While many of these experiences seem tough and humiliating when they're happening, often when we take a closer look we find some memories there to store away for the times we need to laugh.

"THE DATE FROM HELL"

Carl had dreamed of his prom for months. He couldn't wait for the night to actually arrive. Cindy, the girl he had always wanted to date, had said yes. Carl's feet had not touched the ground since. This was going to be the most romantic night on record. *Cindy will be so completely swept off her feet she'll be putty in my strong, manly hands,* thought Carl with a mental swagger. From now through eternity, when young people dreamed of true love and romance, the story of Carl and Cindy would be their example.

As he dressed for the big date, Carl rehearsed each moment of the evening. Every word he would say, each move he would make, were carefully and thoughtfully choreographed. Nothing was going to spoil this evening.

He pulled up in front of Cindy's house in his mom's newly washed and waxed car. As he approached her front door he frantically went over the mental notes he had made on how to react to her new dress and how to win over her parents with his maturity and charm.

Overall, Carl was pleased with how this first stage went

as he led Cindy to the car. He had endured the photo session and had made polite and articulate conversation with Cindy's folks.

He opened the car door for Cindy and his heart leaped to his throat as he thought of driving alone to dinner. As he scooted behind the wheel and turned the key in the ignition, the nightmare began. The car wouldn't start. With Cindy in the car and her entire family watching from the living room window, Carl tried to be nonchalant. He turned the key again. Nothing. Then he got out of the car and raised the hood hoping that this act might create some self-healing magic.

Still nothing.

As he got back into the car his eyes riveted on his mistake. In his excitement to pick up Cindy he had forgotten to put the car in park. He coughed and tried to distract Cindy as he quickly put the console gearshift back to P. When he looked up Cindy was giggling and to his horror so was her entire family.

Carl's heart began to sink as he drove away.

Dinner took forever. The service was slow and the waiter, weary of high schoolers' tips, was not greatly helpful. Carl kept wondering, *Why, when you are paying so much more, does the service get progressively worse?* Conversation was stiff, and Carl began to long for the crowded prom with its noise and familiar faces. He barely had enough money for dinner and for a fleeting second pondered what it would be like to have to ask Cindy for help.

By the time they got to the dance it was just about over. Still, it was an unmatched thrill for Carl to escort Cindy to the dance floor. He felt every eye in the place on them as he used the steps he had rehearsed for hours alone in his bedroom.

After the dance came the party. A good friend of Carl's was hosting the affair, and Carl was anxious to see his buddies there. He picked up a plate of munchies for the two of them and headed back to where Cindy was sitting with some friends.

He forget about the step. There was a step down into the next room and missing that step was disastrous. He went head first toward the floor and landed face down in the plate of food. Some of his friends thought "Crazy Carl" had done it on purpose, and his misstep actually turned out to be the highlight of the party.

All the way home Cindy assured her dejected suitor that she had had a wonderful time. As Carl walked her to the door he had one more chance for true love: a goodnight kiss. He stood shyly at the front door like a first grader meeting an adult for the first time. Just as they were about to embark on that epic kiss Cindy spoke up, "Carl, isn't that your mother's car rolling down the street?"

First in stunned amazement, then in panic, he saw the car rolling down the hill toward a truck. He sprinted into the street and quickly grabbed the door of his runaway vehicle.

It was locked.

The car continued to roll as Carl fished the keys from his pocket, unlocked the door, jumped in, and stopped it about one foot from the truck.

Carl was panting, sweating, and humiliated. He started the car and began to turn, hoping to go home and never be seen again, when he heard a tap on the window. Cindy was standing outside the car. He rolled down the window, red-faced and sweating, and looked into the eyes of the girl of his now-shattered dreams.

Then in an instant his world was turned back around. Cindy looked down at Carl, told him again that she had had a very nice time, leaned through the window, and gave him a kiss on the cheek.

Life *can* be beautiful.

Carl and his buddies have laughed many, many times about that evening. And each time I think of it I smile. Life has many funny moments.

ENJOYING LIFE REQUIRES PERSPECTIVE ON PAIN

For many teenagers and their parents life is full of deep pain, completely lacking in fun and laughter. As a result, it becomes almost impossible for these folks to embrace the idea that our lives need laughter. Yet life must not be completely boiled down to situations or surroundings. Our quality of life is not always determined by our circumstances, and even in the worst of situations joy can be an option.

Tim and Pam Hansel are two of my role models. Tim was an athlete and adventurer until a mountain-climbing accident left him in constant pain. Pam has worked alongside Tim through the darkest hours of his injuries. Through all of this both have maintained a remarkable perspective and sense of humor.

Tim has this to say about pain: "Pain is inevitable, but misery is optional. We cannot avoid pain, but we can avoid joy."[1] Indeed, we often avoid enjoying life because we only deal with pain externally.

In one of his books I found this poem, written by a young Jewish girl from a Nazi concentration camp.

> From tomorrow on
>   I shall be sad
> From tomorrow on—
>   not today.
> Today I will be glad,
>   and every day
> no matter how bitter it may be
>   I shall say
> From tomorrow on I shall be sad
>   not today.[2]

This poem and the status of its author should poignantly and appropriately startle us with the idea that joy is a choice. We don't have to like our surroundings and circumstances, yet in the midst of change and fear we can choose joy.

In Galatians 5:22-23, Paul lists for us the fruit of the Spirit. These products grow in the lives of those who are connected to the Vine that is Christ Jesus. It is not our job to produce this fruit; it is our challenge to stay rooted to the Vine. The fruit of the Spirit is a byproduct of our relationship to the Vine. One of the characteristics of the fruit is joy. It represents a happiness that the world cannot give and cannot take away.

Winning the lottery will not produce joy. It may create a sense of happiness for a time, but true joy cannot be won that way. It will only come as a result of carefully tending our relationship with Christ.

Joy is not a giddy response to tragedy. Nor is it an irresponsible approach to life. It is not to deny the pain and suffering we all experience. The fruit of joy comes from deep inside our souls, constantly assuring us that no matter how bad it gets or how hopeless life seems, there is life and hope and help in Christ alone. We live with the assurance that we are supremely loved and the very God of the Universe is aware of our plight.

The Apostle Paul underlines the fact that God is in control in his letter to the Romans.

> And we know that in all things God works for the good of those who love him, who have been called according to his purpose. . . . What, then, shall we say in response to this? If God is for us, who can be against us? He who did not spare his own Son, but gave him up for us all—how will he not also, along with him, graciously give us all things? (Romans 8:28,31-32)

This is one of the reasons that we begin with adoration when we pray. Circumstances do not change who God is. We can be confident in Him and find joy in remembering His mighty works.

Shout with joy to God, all the earth!
    Sing the glory of his name;
    make his praise glorious!
Say to God, "How awesome are your deeds!
    So great is your power
    that your enemies cringe down before you."
        (Psalm 66:1-3)

You may want to take a few moments right now to give God thanks and to accept the joy He offers.

In the midst of transition in our families we often find ourselves saddled with limited choices. Many times the choices we do have range from bad to worse. If we are dealing with change in our family or tough circumstances that require tough choices, we may still choose joy. Please don't confuse joy with happiness. Happiness can be derived from any number of sources. Joy only comes when we are drawing our strength from the Vine who is Christ.

Young Life staffer Bob Krulish asks the rest of us regularly if we are "enjoying" Christ. By this he means, are we more in love with Christ now than we were six months ago? Do we find ourselves more and more wanting to kneel in His presence and find ourselves in Him? Bob always finishes the conversation by saying, "He is enjoying you."

IDEAS FOR KEEPING TEENAGERS
(AND THEIR PARENTS) LAUGHING

When I was in high school one of our club leaders was Jan Webb. As a fifteen-year-old girl she had contracted polio. A healthy, fun-loving teenager had been struck with a disease that seemed to trap her within her own body. She began a lifelong struggle and challenge both physically and emotionally. But though Jan felt keenly the restrictions of her body, she did not allow her disease to keep her spirit from soaring to new heights and impacting the lives of everyone she met.

I will never forget the many nights we cheered in anticipation as Jan made her way to the front of our Young Life club meetings on crutches. Her sense of humor not only made us laugh, but it amazed us. She was creative and at the same time in touch with what would appeal to kids. She could tease but would never go over the line by putting down or embarrassing anyone. There wasn't a kid in our school who had not heard of Jan. I don't know how many kids were won to Christ through Jan's humor, but many were attracted to the Savior by this winsome servant, and I know all of us grew to count on Jan. Her wit could always lift us no matter how we felt.

Today she has a new generation of fans, and I am deeply grateful that my three sons are among them. Whether it is making bird calls or pulling a dime out of their ear, Jan always creates a lot of laughs and fun. You see, along with her pain, in spite of her own physical challenge, Jan has learned to allow the joy of Christ to infect her own life and everyone around her.

You can't "make" people have fun. They must choose to have fun just as you do. Our responsibility is to find our joy in Christ and then to live that out in our family.

Here are some fun ideas you may want to try:

- *Take your teenager on a date.* Let the teen pick the restaurant; you decide on the activity afterward. Kids almost always enjoy plays and musicals more than they think they will. Try to think of something other than a movie to take them to.
- *Make your teen breakfast in bed.* Do you have a hard time getting your teen up in the morning? At least once, make getting up an event your teen will always remember.
- *Have a "welcome home" party after school.* Place your teen's favorite snack or dessert in some conspicuous place and put a few decorations around. If you

and your spouse both work, leave the treats out and attach a note.
- *Offer a dollar for the joke of the day.* Set certain standards for the kind of joke allowed, then at night or mealtime give everyone in the family a chance to share his or her funniest moment of the day or a joke.

Each family must work to discover fun. For me, as the father of three sons, almost any kind of sports is fun. We play, watch, and discuss sports. I have to work to make sure that sports is not the only way we have fun together, though. For many families, camping is a great way to enjoy each other and have fun. Still others work on cars, or play card or board games. Families must look for opportunities to have fun. But the secret is to let your joy in Christ "infect" everyone around you.

There are a number of resources available with fun things to do as a family. You may have tried them all. But, perhaps the key to adding fun to transition is your own attitude. Your kids may not be at an age where playing games or taking little trips will work, but you can still be a joyful person who is fun to be around.

We know we cannot "make" things fun if our teenager is determined not to participate. I am not always able to feel joyful either. When I experience those moments, it is usually because I have been focusing on my own feelings or circumstances and not on the truths of God's Word.

There is no denying the pain we all experience in life. Sometimes I feel so overwhelmed with my own emotions and pain that it is difficult to even focus on my kids. During those times I must turn to other members of my resource team like Scripture, prayer, and trusted Christian friends to gain the strength and perspective I need. I confront myself with the "facts" of the Christian faith — God loves me (John 3:16), He died for me (Romans 5:8), He is near (Philippians 4:4-5).

In the midst of life's transitions we can choose joy. We can find God's peace for our troubled souls, not in our ability to withstand pain or remedy every problem, but in our willingness to find Jesus each day and rely on Him for our strength and joy.

Finally, for those days when we need a little boost, here are a few one-liners I've gathered over the years from various sources. I hope they bring a smile to your face and lighten your heart.

- Middle age is always fifteen years older than I am.
- There is no safety in numbers, or in anything else.
- A verbal contract isn't worth the paper it's written on.
- Eat a live toad first thing in the morning and nothing worse will happen to you the rest of the day.
- The lion and the calf shall lie down together, but the calf won't get much sleep.
- Being in politics is much like being a football coach. You have to be smart enough to understand the game and dumb enough to think it's important.
- Nobody notices when things go right.
- An ugly carpet will last forever.
- When you're in it up to your nose, keep your mouth shut.
- You can lead a horse to water, but if you can get him to float on his back you've got something.

• • • • • • • • • • •

CHAPTER TWELVE

Release in Transition

Tears. You never know what may cause them.
The sight of the Atlantic Ocean can do it, or a
piece of music, or a face you've never seen before.
A pair of somebody's old shoes can do it. Almost
any movie made before the great sadness that
came over the world after the Second World War,
a horse cantering across a meadow, the high
school basketball team running out onto the gym
floor at the beginning of a game. You can never
be sure. But of this you can be sure. Whenever
you find tears in your eyes, especially unexpected
tears, it is well to pay close attention.

They are not only telling you something
about the secret of who you are, but more often
than not God is speaking to you through them of
the mystery of where you have come from and
is summoning you to where, if your soul is to be
saved, you should go to next.

FROM *WHISTLING IN THE DARK* BY FREDERICK BUECHNER

Sometimes the trauma of adolescent transitions feels like a time bomb just a few seconds from detonation. Parents and teens, their stomachs in knots, become anxious and irritable and find it difficult to stand still. We know if we don't somehow escape this situation for a while, we may explode.

In the midst of such stress, we must know where to turn for support. We must learn how to handle stress and allow the pressure to slowly dissipate, thus avoiding those painful explosions.

UNDERSTANDING STRESS

The word *stress* is often misunderstood. Archibald Hart, author of the book *Adrenalin and Stress*, makes these very helpful comments:

It [stress] is a multifaceted response that includes changes in perception, emotions, behaviors, and physical functioning. Some think of it only as tension, others as anxiety. Some think of it as good, others as bad. The truth is that we all need a certain amount of stress to keep us alive, although too much of it becomes harmful to us. (When most of us use the term, stress, we usually are referring to this harmful aspect—overstress.)[1]

We all have a natural response to any emergency or demand. In these situations a "complex chain of responses is set in motion to prepare us for what has been described as a 'fight or flight' response."[2] When we are under stress our body is preparing itself to either fight or flee the situation.

Here are a few examples of stress:

- You are rushing around getting everyone ready on Monday morning and you notice your teenager is still in bed. You have gone over this a hundred times and he still can't or won't get himself out of bed on time. You can't afford to be late for work again and you begin feeling anxious and angry. You are under stress.
- You have a great deal of responsibility at work, at church, at the PTA, and at home. You love to serve and get very positive strokes for your effort. At the same time, you are gone almost every night and often too tired to really participate when you are at home. You feel guilty about all the time away, and yet you can't decide what to give up in order to be at home more. Something has to give and whether you are willing to face it or not, that something is probably you. You are under stress.
- As you stack the dishes in the dishwasher, you find your eyes brimming with tears. Your teenage daughter has dropped out of school and you can't seem to

control her anymore. Your husband wants to kick her out of the house, and several times your discussions with him have turned into shouting matches. You had so many dreams for your life and for your daughter's life. Now these have crumbled and been blown away by the winds of life. You are under stress.

Stress is an overexcitement of our body that can be caused as much by things we find pleasurable and rewarding as by things unpleasant or painful. The body does not distinguish between types of stress.

CAUSES OF STRESS

A variety of things cause stress. Anything that mobilizes your body for "fight or flight" is stress. It can be a painful experience or a pleasurable activity. The key is, too much stress without release or relief is unhealthy.

Stress can result from anything that:

- annoys you
- threatens you
- prods you
- excites you
- scares you
- worries you
- hurries you
- angers you
- frustrates you
- challenges you
- criticizes you
- reduces your self-esteem.[3]

DISCOVERING RELEASE FOR STRESS

The Apostle Paul offers sound advice about relieving stress. He writes, "Do not be anxious about anything, but in everything, by prayer and petition, with thanksgiving, present your requests to God" (Philippians 4:6).

When we know the God of Peace and have learned to take our burdens to Him, we can experience the peace that only He can give. It is a peace the world can't give—one that comes from deep within, rooted and solid, unshakable and strong.

Okay, we know this works. It is spiritual and mature. Yet, I often find that it is harder than it sounds to experience peace and release from my emotions when I face hard times. I have spent so many years being self-reliant that I don't always follow the prescribed remedy of prayer and focus on Christ immediately. While I certainly hope I am arriving at that place sooner now than in the past, I am still confounded by my own actions. It is during these times that I find I need a bridge from my emotions to my heart.

I don't cry very often. And when I do it is never for long. But tears are truly the rain of the soul. In California, where we now live, I have developed a special appreciation for the rain. After it rains I want to run out and look at everything. The mountains, stark against a clear sky, are always the most beautiful then. To our smog-choked area rain brings a few short hours when the earth and the sky look fresh and clean. There is something fresh and clean about the release from stress that can be produced by tears. Especially when we are baring our soul to our Father in Heaven.

If anyone ever appreciated this truth it was King David. He was one of the all-time great criers. We probably learn more about crying out to the Father from him than anyone except Christ.

> In my distress I called to the LORD;
>   I cried to my God for help.
> From his temple he heard my voice;
>   my cry came before him, into his ears.
>   (Psalm 18:6)

Out of the depths I cry to you, O LORD;
O Lord, hear my voice.
Let your ears be attentive
to my cry for mercy.
(Psalm 130:1-2)

Then David himself gives us the next step to releasing stress.

I wait for the LORD, my soul waits,
and in his word I put my hope.
My soul waits for the Lord
more than watchmen wait for the morning.
(Psalm 130:5-6)

When men and women cry out to the Lord, they should wait for an answer. The discipline of waiting is crucial. For when we have cleared our mind with tears, we must wait for the Lord to fill the void with His peace and assurance. We will not find it if we, embarrassed by our outburst, rush off to find the shelter of busyness and activity to hide us from our feelings.

Wait for the LORD;
be strong and take heart
and wait for the LORD.
(Psalm 27:14)

I waited patiently for the LORD;
he turned to me and heard my cry.
He lifted me out of the slimy pit,
out of the mud and mire;
he set my feet on a rock
and gave me a firm place to stand.
He put a new song in my mouth,
a hymn of praise to our God.

Many will see and fear
and put their trust in the LORD.
(Psalm 40:1-3)

From the mud and mire of our distress, the Lord desires to set our feet on solid rock. When we feel like our lives are stuck in a swamp of pain, our Father hears our cry and rewards our waiting with sure footing and a new song in our hearts.

Sometimes I wait on my knees. But on days when waiting comes hard you may find me walking somewhere. It may just be around the block or even around the house. When possible, I walk on the beach or along a path in the hills. Walking helps me clear my mind. It allows me to be more receptive to the voice of the Lord. I know others who find jogging accomplishes the same thing for them. Exercise can relieve just enough tension in our bodies to get us refocused, or at least calmed down.

CONNIE'S STORY
Connie was a driver. She put a tremendous amount of effort into everything she did. Even though she did not hold down a full-time "paying" job, I have rarely met anyone more busy. When schoolkids were scheduled to go on a field trip, Connie was the first mom called and then she arranged the rest of the transportation. She was always the team mom for soccer or Little League and was an aide in the classroom. On top of this, she was the caretaker for her aging parents and just as involved in church as she was at the kids' school.

Sometimes all the activity and busyness would get her down. Fred, her husband, would put his foot down and they would try calmness for a while. But it simply couldn't last. One of the children would have trouble with a teacher and in she would go. The cycle had begun again.

Connie was obsessed with the need to be a great mom.

As the children grew older life began to change for

Connie. She had a difficult time adjusting to her diminished control in her teenagers' lives and was genuinely hurt by their demands for autonomy and privacy. Before she knew it, Connie had made the transition from obsessed to distressed. She felt rejected by her kids and at a loss for how to find meaning in her life. She began to manipulate her family by constantly letting them know how much she had done for them and how hurt and lonely she was. This only caused more alienation and resentment within the family. Connie's carefully constructed world was beginning to crumble. She thought maybe she was going crazy.

Little did she know that a group of women who met weekly had begun to pray for her. They had seen her distress and began taking their friend before the Father. Then they invited Connie to join them and she jumped at the chance.

During the early weeks of Connie's involvement, she dominated the time. She would bring the group up to date on the hurt in her life from an unappreciative family. The other women would listen and then pray with her. Slowly a change began to take place in Connie. A transition team began to emerge. She discovered resources she hadn't known before. Friends and confidantes to share with. Through these loving sisters she learned that venting her hurt was not enough. She must give it over to God. Gradually she embraced the peace that comes from waiting on the Lord. Her feet landed on solid rock and the changes in her family couldn't shake her. Most important, Connie got the log out of her own eye.

As Connie rediscovered life she met Joy and Laughter. Her children would come home and hear the joyful sounds of praise songs as they came through the door. Home was no longer a prison for them, and each one began to quiz mom about what had transpired in her life. Connie was no longer obsessed about being a great mom. She was one.

Connie found a release from the mire of transition. She discovered grace and truth through some friends, then she appropriated it in her life.

If you have not discovered an outlet for your own stress yet, let me offer some steps.

1. *Find a person or small group to share with.* There are three rules to follow here.

  a. If you cannot choose your spouse or a couples group, then choose a person or persons of the same sex.
  b. Use this as an opportunity to express feelings and hurts, not to gripe about your family and friends.
  c. Make prayer the central focus of your time together.

2. *Learn to wait on the Lord.* Waiting may include walking, crying, or singing hymns, but commit to developing a listening ear to the Father.

3. *Choose joy.* You are a child of the King. His greatest desire is that you experience His joy and peace. The choice is yours.

HELP FOR YOUR TEEN

Teenagers also have the need to release the stress from transitions in their life. They are going through changes so rapidly that their mood swings are often very difficult to read. A stable Christian home is the first line of defense. You create an environment of love for Christ and family, and no matter how much they buck it, at least they will always know that home is a safe harbor in a storm.

You may not be able to choose your kids' friends for them, but you can recruit caring adults who will help you keep in touch with your son or daughter.

I would like to encourage you with six things you *can* do to help your teen learn to release tension during times of change.

1. *Be a careful and thoughtful listener.* When teens express anger or explosively react to transition, listen to understand, not simply to respond. Empathize with your kids. Listen for what is in their heart as well as what is coming from their mouth. Many young people are living with fragile egos. They need to know that someone really cares enough about them to listen.

2. *Don't become the judge.* Too often parents simply want to solve problems and then get on with life. Or, they overreact to what their teenager just said. Take a deep breath before you respond to something said. Make sure the statement requires a response before you speak. Your kids need your acceptance. Often they are simply trying out new ideas and exploring foreign concepts or reacting to stress they're not sure how to articulate.

Isn't it better they do that *with you* than a peer? If we are quick to pass judgment on what they are saying, they will eventually stop talking to us.

3. *Model what you want them to be.* If you want your children to have a vital relationship with Christ, work on yours. If you want them to experience joy, then choose joy in your life. Don't manufacture something you think they need to see, but rejoice because you have taken your burdens to your Father and left them at His feet.

4. *Encourage teens to get exercise.* You would be surprised how many young people today are out of shape. Exercise is a great stress breaker. Set a goal to run a 10K together, or go on a bike trip. There are lots of options. Be creative.

5. *Learn to know when they need "space" and privacy.* Respect their right to some time alone. When, with the best intentions, we don't allow our kids some space, we will force them to find that space outside the home. As we have said before, it is a natural part of adolescent life to need some privacy and space away from mom and dad. We can't let our own transition crisis interfere with their need at that point.

6. *Know when to ask for help.* If you notice behavior in your teen that concerns you, ask a professional for advice and counsel. For example, if your teenager suddenly stops hanging out with his or her friends and just sits in the bedroom listening to music, ask the teen how he or she feels. If you can't get a response, begin looking for other symptoms of stress. Have his or her eating habits changed? Does the teen look well? If you see too many things you don't have answers for, ask for help. Decide right now who you would call first. Keep your resource team handy and up to date.

In the first chapter of this book I shared a painful story about Kit. He did not have the coping resources to manage the transitions in becoming an adult and no one noticed. In retrospect, I believe he was avoiding many of us who knew him well. Then when the hole he had dug for himself was too deep to go unnoticed any longer, he buried himself in it.

Almost every kid in the world thinks about suicide sometime during adolescence. We won't be able to stop that. But we can create an environment of hope in our homes. It begins with us. Our growth in Christ and the coping resources we deploy in the midst of change in our lives will be the first step in creating that "safe place" for our kids.

My friend Tim Hansel is fond of saying, "Until further notice, celebrate life!" And to this my dad would add, "If you have the joy of the Lord in your heart, don't forget to inform your face."

Can the Lord relieve the stress in your life?

Maybe you should wait and see.

••••••••••

Chapter Thirteen

Closing the Book
on Transition

T here is a legend about the Apostle Peter in which it is said he was fleeing Jerusalem after hearing he was being sought for execution. As Peter fled down the dusty highway he saw Jesus walking toward him.

"Where are You going, Master?" Peter is supposed to have asked as he came to a halt in front of the Lord.

"I go to die for you a second time," was the Savior's reply.

With those words Peter is said to have turned on his heels and headed back to Jerusalem and certain death.

As we live through the trauma of transition with our teenagers, the temptation to run is a common one. We feel the changes in life smothering us under the dark quilt of the unknown. We long to escape the pace and pressure of our hectic lives and find a place of peace and rest.

WE HAVE FOUND THE PLACE AND IT IS YOU

We now call upon our team members of prayer and Scripture. Through these two gifts we are able to find a quiet place in our hearts, regardless of the storms raging in our lives. There is help for our distress and it begins and ends with knowing Christ. This is not wishful or unrealistic thinking. These disciplines take our focus off our circumstances and place our attention on the Lord.

Find a quiet place and you will discover a quiet heart.

He who had the power to calm the storm when the disciples feared they would perish is the same God who can still the tempest of our souls. In Mark 6:45-51, Jesus "makes" His disciples get in a boat while He dismissed the crowd that had been with them all day.

I don't know what the disciples were thinking as they began their journey across the lake. Perhaps they spoke in quiet reverence of the miracles they had witnessed that day. Maybe they discussed the unusual and haunting parables that Jesus had spoken in their presence. Whatever the topic, their conversation was suddenly broken by panic.

A great wind came against them and their muscles bulged as they pulled the oars through angry waters.

These men had done nothing in particular to deserve this plight. They were merely obeying orders. In fact, had they time to think, they may have considered their situation unfair.

Many of us won't go so far as to blame God for the storms of transition in our life. But we often harbor notions that somehow the whole thing is unfair. After all, we have been trying our best in a difficult situation we never asked for, and now we find ourselves in the middle of a storm.

Our only hope is to raise our heads and look out into the storm. Somewhere on the horizon we will see Jesus. He walks on the waters of our storms. He is not overwhelmed by our troubles. He has authority over the crashing waves of change.

As we work toward seeing the Lord, other team members begin to emerge. Our perspective on time gains clarity and we understand more of the nature of change among kids. Where we may once have been confused by the seemingly slow march of days and hours, now we look resolutely forward to the adults God is building in our sons and daughters.

When resources are marshaled and key people put in place, we can approach each change in our teen's life with new hope and confidence. We worry less because those who have surrounded our family encourage us and step into the gap when needed.

WHEN WE'RE NOT AFRAID TO PICK UP THE PHONE

Adolescence can be a very difficult time for young people and their parents, but it doesn't need to be impossible. Help is available if we know who to call and aren't afraid to pick up the phone.

Laughter is available to jump start us toward joy. Brennan Manning offers this thought:

> Here is the root of Christian joy and mirth. It is why theologian Robert Hotchkins at the University of Chicago can insist: "Christians ought to be celebrating constantly. We ought to be preoccupied with parties, banquets, feasts, and merriment. We ought to give ourselves over to veritable orgies of joy because we have been liberated from the fear of life and the fear of death. We ought to attract people to the church quite literally by the fun there is in being a Christian."[1]

Joy becomes a byproduct of those who find their life in Christ. It is a happiness the world can't give and the world can't take away. Too many people today work at *creating* joy or happiness. They work and plan and dream about the day when they will have nothing else to do but be "happy." Yet true happiness cannot be manufactured. The kind of joy God offers us grows out of a life that is focused on Him. Like a carefully groomed tree that bears fruit in season, so shall we bear fruit as we are connected to the vine which is Christ and are pruned by the Father (see John 15).

Even in her nineties, my Granny Pierce never lost her joy. A wisp of a woman with an unquenchable fire for Christ in her soul, Granny bubbled with zeal for the Savior. She had the ability to enjoy Him even in old age and declining health. From her bed when she grew too old and frail to get about, we could hear her singing and praying at the top of her lungs, never lamenting her failed health, but with her focus on Christ clear and unwavering. Anyone who came to visit her was struck by her love for the Savior and a joy that seemed to fill the room.

If joy is a byproduct of our walk with Christ, then tears are His gift to clean the room in our heart for joy to fill.

Tears. They may come as a result of the untimely death of one too young and vulnerable. They may spring from the frustration of watching sons and daughters make bad choices and risk their future for insignificant pleasures. Or, they may simply fill the little creases in the corners of our eyes as we watch the relentless march of time.

Whatever the reason, tears will flush out the pain and sorrow and give us the opportunity to fill our hearts with something else. It is our choice.

To choose joy requires one major ingredient: trust. We must believe that God will fill our hearts with His peace. We must believe Him capable of fulfilling His promises to us. Trust begins when we acknowledge that we are accepted by God regardless of our ability as parents. His love is unconditional and never-ending.

As our children begin to emerge from childhood into adolescence and we are faced with separation from them and their quest for independence, we must have the freedom to let them grow. Our perception of ourselves is not dependent on how responsive they are, or if the folks at church applaud us as "Christian Parents of the Year." We are saved by grace;

our joy is not a result of success, but acceptance. We were accepted by our loving Father when we didn't deserve it, and we will always be accepted by Him regardless of our performance or failure.

Brennan Manning puts it this way: "You may be insecure, inadequate, mistaken, or potbellied. Death, panic, depression, and disillusionment may be near you. But you are not that. You are accepted. Never confuse your perception of yourself with the mystery that you are really accepted."[2]

DANIEL'S STORY:
THE FINAL KEY TO MANAGING TRANSITION

I don't exactly remember when Daniel first came to our Young Life club. He was just there and we were glad. Daniel had muscular dystrophy and other complications. He walked awkwardly on his toes and often lost his balance. He had none of the social skills of his peers and as a result had virtually no friends at school.

He loved coming to our group every Monday night to sing and laugh and be one of the gang. He began to feel accepted, and when some of the kids he met at the meetings recognized him at school, he felt like he was in Heaven.

As an outlet his parents let him take voice lessons, and we would often let him help us lead songs. Monday nights were the highlight of his week and a window to a world he had never known.

As an elementary student and even in high school, he had been brutally teased. His tormenters would say cruel things, mark his face with magic markers, or knock his books out of his hands as he walked to class. With no recourse, Daniel would endure the humiliation while a great hate and rage boiled in his heart. At home he would tear up his room at the end of the day.

When we became friends he was on medications for his illness and his anger.

Late in the fall when Daniel expressed a desire to go on a weekend retreat, we were all thrilled. He had never been away from home alone, except for being in the hospital. I still remember vividly heading up to camp early to make preparations and thinking about the responsibility of having Daniel with us for the weekend.

In the mystery of God's providence, all of Daniel's medication was somehow lost on the trip up. I called his dad to share the bad news and asked if Daniel could stay anyway. I promised that at the first sign of trouble I would drive him home myself.

Daniel had the time of his life. And there were two primary reasons. First, two popular, dedicated guys in our cabin decided on their own that the terrain around the camp might be too difficult for Daniel by himself. So they positioned themselves on either side of him and stayed there all weekend, making sure he didn't fall. There is no doubt Daniel walked straighter and taller than ever in his life that weekend, and I can't even write about it without feeling some tears of gratitude for those two young men. Daniel had never really experienced friends outside his family, and suddenly he had two sticking with him.

Second, Daniel heard about the love of Christ while he was seeing it on either side of him. The combination was too powerful, and he committed his heart to Christ.

He knew he had been accepted. For the first time in his life he understood that fitting in and being accepted were activities that had been done for him. He had been accepted by Christ and he belonged to that family.

The impact of that experience pierced my heart when I saw Daniel at a track meet several months later. In his dreams he had scored winning touchdowns and won gold medals, but in his real life he would never know the feeling of competing and wearing a team uniform. Yet Daniel had something infinitely better.

I watched him during a distance race. He had positioned himself in the middle of the infield and was screaming encouragement to one of the runners.

Can you guess which one?

He was cheering for a little guy who was in last place and about to be lapped by the leaders. Daniel yelled for this boy like an Olympic gold medal was at stake. He empathized with anyone running last and wanted to help that runner.

It was a picture I'll remember the rest of my life. This physically challenged young man scooting around in a little circle yelling, "Come on, Ross! You can do it!" While everyone else at the meet was focusing on the strong, the successful, the winners, he was giving all he had to the one who needed him the most.

I watched in utter amazement as Daniel cheered Ross to the very end. Even as others were preparing for the next race, he matched each step with a word of encouragement.

I was very proud of him and walked over to tell him after the race. As we talked he shared with me another event in his day. Just before coming to the meet he had stuck his head in to watch the pom-pom girls' practice session. One of them spotted him and asked him if he wanted to dance with them. They all laughed as Daniel left and made his way onto the track.

As he was telling me this story my blood pressure was reaching dangerous heights. I was thinking about how to punish those girls, I mean, really make them pay, when Daniel recaptured my attention. He looked me in the eyes and, somehow sensing my anger, shrugged his shoulders and said, "It's okay, because I like myself now."

Suddenly my anger was replaced by wonder. Here was someone who with all his physical problems seemed healthier than me. I realized that humiliation was nothing new to him. He had experienced it before. Rejection by a few kids was not going to kill him. He had survived it many times. Two of the things I feared most were almost daily occurrences for this dear young man. And he could say, "I like myself."

He had been accepted for who he was by the One who made him, and he was happy with the results. Daniel's story illustrates for us the key to handling teen transitions: As the changes in our children and our own lives threaten the image we have of ourselves, *we need the courage that comes from knowing we are accepted.* If we have experienced grace, we can dispense grace.

THE GREAT TRANSITION

If the humiliation of looking like a failure as a parent causes us to rush toward hasty solutions, we only need to look at the humiliation Christ experienced on the cross to stop us in our tracks.

As we try to run from the fear of rejection, whether from our teenagers or anyone else, we must hear the voice of Christ say, "I go to die for you a second time." And only when we will turn on our heels and face life's dangers will we know the great transition of becoming like Christ.

Your transition team awaits. Your teen's future is at stake. Sound the alarm and let them join you in the battle.

Notes

CHAPTER TWO – TEEN PASSAGES

1. Diane E. Papalia and Sally Wendkos Olds, *A Child's World*, 4th ed. (New York: McGraw-Hill, 1987), page 466.
2. John W. Santrock, *Life-Span Development*, rev. ed. (Dubuque, IA: William C. Brown Publishers, 1986), page 356.
3. As quoted by Papalia and Wendkos Olds, pages 496-497.
4. David Elkind, *All Grown Up & No Place to Go* (Reading, MA: Addison-Wesley, 1984), pages 93-94.
5. Santrock, page 369.
6. Santrock.
7. General Douglas MacArthur, as quoted in Brennan Manning, *The Ragamuffin Gospel* (Portland, OR: Multnomah, 1990), page 193.
8. Papalia and Wendkos Olds, page 500.

9. Santrock, page 360.
10. Elizabeth B. Hurlock, *Adolescent Development* (New York: McGraw-Hill, 1955), page 5.
11. Kevin Huggins, *Parenting Adolescents* (Colorado Springs, CO: NavPress, 1989), page 237.
12. Manning, pages 205-206.

CHAPTER THREE—MANAGING EXPECTATIONS

1. Bruce Newman, "Classroom Coaches," *Sports Illustrated,* November 19, 1990, page 63.
2. Tim Kimmel, *The Legacy of Love: A Plan for Parenting on Purpose* (Portland, OR: Multnomah, 1989), page 35.
3. Kimmel.
4. *Youthworker Update: The Newsletter for Christian Youth Workers,* vol. 4, no. 7, March 1990, page 1.
5. *Youthworker Update.*
6. *Youthworker Update,* vol. 5, no. 1, September 1990, page 2.
7. John Baillie, *A Diary of Private Prayer* (New York: Charles Scribner's Sons, 1949), page 61.

CHAPTER FOUR—MAKING TRANSITION YOUR ALLY

1. *Youthworker Update: The Newsletter of Christian Youth Workers,* vol. 5, no. 1, September 1990, page 1.
2. *Youthworker Update,* page 1.
3. *Youthworker Update,* page 1.
4. Cited in "Young Adults: the Foundation of Tomorrow's Families," *Implications: Taking Research Beyond Information to Application,* Spring 1990, vol. 3, issue 1, pages 2-3.

CHAPTER FIVE—TEAM MEMBER 1: KNOWING GOD

1. Max Lucado, *God Came Near: The Chronicles of the Christ* (Portland, OR: Multnomah, 1987), page 85.

CHAPTER SIX—TEAM MEMBER 2: REALISTIC GOALS FOR TRAUMATIZED PARENTS AND TEENS

1. Robert Fulghum, *All I Really Need to Know I Learned in Kindergarten* (New York: Ivy Books, 1986), pages 4-5.
2. Tim Kimmel, *Legacy of Love* (Portland, OR: Multnomah, 1989), page 67.
3. Tim Hansel, *When I Relax I Feel Guilty* (Elgin, IL: David C. Cook, 1979), pages 29-30.

CHAPTER SEVEN—TEAM MEMBER 3: MAXIMIZING RESOURCES

1. Ezra Taft Benson, as quoted in Stephen R. Covey, *The Seven Habits of Highly Effective People* (New York: Simon and Schuster, 1989), page 309.

CHAPTER EIGHT—TEAM MEMBER 4: MAINTAINING INTIMACY IN THE MIDST OF TRANSITION

1. Gary Smalley and John Trent, *The Language of Love* (Pomona, CA: Focus on the Family, 1988), page 33.

CHAPTER NINE—TEAM MEMBER 5: PRAYER—HEALING STRENGTH FOR THE STRESSED

1. Stephen Winward, *How to Talk to God: The Dynamics of Prayer* (Wheaton, IL: Harold Shaw Publishers, 1961), page 23.
2. Winward, pages 17-18.
3. Winward, page 78.
4. Francois Fenelon, as quoted by Bob Benson and Michael Benson, *Disciplines for the Inner Life* (Waco, TX: Word Publishers, 1985), page 28.
5. John Baillie, *A Diary of Private Prayer* (New York: Charles Scribner's Sons, 1949), page 115.

CHAPTER TEN – TEAM MEMBER 6: MANAGING
TIME FACTORS

1. James Dobson, *Preparing for Adolescence*, rev. ed. (Ventura, CA: Regal Books, 1989), page 73.
2. David Elkind, as quoted in *Youthworker Update: The Newsletter for Christian Youth Workers*, vol. 4, no. 10, June 1990, page 2.
3. Quoted in Tim Hansel, *When I Relax I Feel Guilty* (Elgin, IL: David C. Cook Publishing Co., 1979), page 9. Used by permission.

CHAPTER ELEVEN – TEAM MEMBER 7: LAUGHTER
AND FUN AS SHELTERS FROM THE STORM

1. Tim Hansel, *Ya Gotta Keep Dancin'* (Elgin, IL: David C. Cook Publishing Co., 1985), page 55.
2. Quoted in Tim Hansel, *When I Relax I Feel Guilty* (Elgin, IL: David C. Cook Publishing Co., 1979), pages 61-62. Used by permission.

CHAPTER TWELVE – RELEASE IN TRANSITION

1. Archibald Hart, *Adrenalin and Stress*, rev. ed. (Waco, TX: Word Books, 1988), page 20.
2. Hart, page 22.
3. Hart, page 30.

CHAPTER THIRTEEN – CLOSING THE BOOK
ON TRANSITION

1. Brennan Manning, *The Ragamuffin Gospel* (Portland, OR: Multnomah, 1990), page 149.
2. Manning, page 25.

Bibliography

A Dad Named Bill [pseud.]. *Daddy, I'm Pregnant.* Portland, OR: Multnomah, 1988.

Arterburn, Stephen, and Jim Burns. *Drug-Proof Your Kids.* Pomona, CA: Focus on the Family, 1989.

Clark, Chap. *Next Time I Fall in Love.* Grand Rapids, MI: Zondervan, 1987.

Dobson, James. *Preparing for Adolescence.* Ventura, CA: Regal Books, 1978.

Huggins, Kevin. *Parenting Adolescents.* Colorado Springs, CO: NavPress, 1989.

Melton, Tom. *Sex From Inside Out.* Englewood, CO: JTM Press, 1989.

Sizemore, Finley H. *Suicide: The Signs and Solutions.* Wheaton, IL: Victor Books, 1988.

Smalley, Gary, and John Trent. *The Language of Love.* Pomona, CA: Focus on the Family, 1988.

Swindoll, Charles. *Growing Wise in Family Life.* Portland, OR: Multnomah, 1988.

Author

Larry Anderson is the Regional Director for Young Life in greater Los Angeles. He has been on the staff of Young Life for more than fifteen years, during which time he has served as Area Director for Phoenix/Scottsdale and Regional Director for Arizona.

Larry holds an M.Div. from Fuller Theological Seminary and is an ordained Assembly of God minister. He has written numerous leadership training materials for Young Life. He is married and has three children.

BOURGEOIS

ELIZABETH AVEDON EDITIONS

VINTAGE CONTEMPORARY ARTISTS

VINTAGE BOOKS

A DIVISION OF RANDOM HOUSE NEW YORK

A Vintage Contemporary Artists Original, November 1988
First Edition

Library of Congress Cataloging-in-Publication Data

Bourgeois, Louise, 1911–

Louise Bourgeois.

(Vintage contemporary artists)
"Elizabeth Avedon editions."
Bibliography: p.
1. Bourgeois, Louise, 1911–   —Interviews.
2. Sculptors—United States—Interviews.
I. Kuspit, Donald B. (Donald Burton), 1935–
II. Avedon, Elizabeth.   III. Title.
NB237.B65A35   1988   730'.92'4   [B]   88-40177
ISBN 0-394-74792-5 (pbk.)

COVER PHOTOGRAPH © 1988 by Richard Avedon

BACK COVER: *Nature Study*, 1984.
Bronze, unique; 30" x 19" x 15". Collection of the
Whitney Museum of American Art, New York.
Courtesy Robert Miller Gallery, New York.
Photo: Allan Finkelman.

Manufactured in the United States of America
10 9 8 7 6 5 4 3 2 1

AN INTERVIEW
WITH
LOUISE BOURGEOIS
BY DONALD KUSPIT

INTRODUCTION

Louise Bourgeois's art conveys an extraordinary sense of the uncanny. Her works, in whatever medium, seem to have generic
unconscious import, as though instantly transporting us to a universal subjective realm. Whatever her art's source in her own
personal history and memory—and she has spoken much about
her childhood and the subtleties of the relationship between her
parents, to which she was attuned as only a brilliant child can be
—its subjective logic is not particular to her. Her work has been
celebrated for its basic emotional power, its way of revitalizing and
freshly objectifying universal symbolic forms, making them seem
to speak urgently in the present. Her art offers us life from the
inside, as it were, by reason of her ability to make her materials
evocative and provocative, as though they had depths that had
never been plumbed until Bourgeois worked with them. At once
full of subliminal innuendo and outspoken meaning, her sculptures
resonate powerfully.

Bourgeois's recognition took a long time coming, partly because she was a loner, partly because her work seemed marginal to
the apparent stylistic mainstream, and partly because the horizon
of expectation on which it could be properly received was a long
time in developing. It was only in the late seventies, when, as has
been said, a pluralistic atmosphere developed in the art world,
along with a dissatisfaction with formalist art—so-called self-
referential art, exemplifying the ideal of purity of medium, of doing
little else but to declare its conventions and material—that the

way was open to an appreciative awareness of Bourgeois's work. Her stylistic innovation in sculpture is inseparable from her use of it to articulate and concentrate meanings not ordinarily available on the everyday surface of life. Also, a new sociopolitical context —feminism—provided an important framework for the understanding of Bourgeois's art.

In general, Bourgeois's art answered the call for a renewed and strong interest in the autobiographical, a new acceptance of stylistic diversity and intricacy, and a new sense of expressive possibilities and complexity. Bourgeois was already the master of seemingly contradictory styles, from symbolic representation to abstraction, which she had anticipated in a manner that came to be recognized as postmodernist. She was in fact a postmodernist pioneer, with her strong sense of self, and her sense of the psychodynamic dimension of art. She was able to effect the kind of complex synthesis of styles—in the very act of acknowledging stylistic diversity—demanded in the postmodernist situation. She is certainly central to what has been called the "new subjectivism" of the eighties. Intuitively in possession of her ideations, she knew every nuance of their existence within her being, every ambiguous move they might make. One might say that she was in full possession of her ambivalence, which she articulates with a rare stylistic complexity and a self-possessed, exploratory, risk-taking restlessness.

As Deborah Wye, the author of the major study of Bourgeois's art, wrote in the fine catalogue essay accompanying the retrospective at the Museum of Modern Art in 1982/83—an exhibition that brought Bourgeois, born in 1911, long overdue recognition—"Encompassing abrupt changes in medium and form, [Bourgeois's work] moves unexpectedly from rigid wood poles to amorphous plaster nests; from pliable fusions to stiff protrusions in rubber and plastic; from bulbous bronze configurations hanging on hooks or cords to their reappearance in solid marble on sturdy bases; from a tiny four-inch [self-portrait] pincushion to a room-size environment."[1] Along with this amazing variety of modes of work is Bourgeois's use of an impressive variety of materials, correlated with an unusually varied and complex iconography. Especially in the sixties—when Bourgeois was already in her fifties—did this extraordinary fertility and brilliant inventiveness declare itself. As Wye says, after making drawings, prints, and sculptures of wood, Bourgeois "experimented with plaster, cement, rubber latex, and plastics, as well as marble and bronze." Her themes, which have a masochistic dimension, include: "woman and self-image; pregnant woman; human body shaped as a weapon; human body in relation to nature; body parts as isolated shapes; weapons, skeins, tapestry shuttles, nests; fecundity, nurturing, food; landscape, earth, topography; growth, seeds, sprouting; the terrain of the unconscious; hiding, protection, inner sanctums; mystery, fear, pain, anger; the human world in relation to the animal world; individuals, groups, families; balance and harmony; formlessness and loss of control."[2] Bourgeois can be alternately humorous and serious, coy and direct, uncompromising and ironic, whimsical and austere—sometimes both extremes at once. She has almost always pursued the elusive unity of opposites, which in part generates the uncanny effect of her works. Her work is like a private encounter with contradiction and self-contradiction, in which each pole wrestles the other, seeking for its blessing as Jacob did when he wrestled the angel, not knowing if it was an angel of death or of life, whether it was merciless or compassionate.

Louise Bourgeois was born in France. Her parents found and restored tapestries in Paris. This idea of finding and restoring in effect became the method of Bourgeois's work. Art was a self-evident part of her environment. It was acceptable to study art. When she was a teenager and in her twenties, Surrealism was the dominant stylistic mode and intellectual orientation in Paris. While her art is far from conventionally Surrealistic, it was inevitable that Bourgeois assimilate Surrealistic ideas. There was always the independence that kept her loyal to herself. Her relationship to Surrealism is complex, as is her relationship to abstract art, the other, more obviously formal, pole of her work. Suffice it to say that it justified her obsession, self-exploration, and self-articulation. Also, it legitimatized her curiosity about materials, and the inherent poetic quality of materials, however late in her life that interest explicitly emerged. Much of her work can be understood—although it is ultimately uncategorizable—under the auspices of the Surrealist conception of the poetic object, based on the notion of the found object. In the interview here, and in interviews elsewhere, Bourgeois has acknowledged her use of found objects. Marcel Jean has said that "the found object is always a rediscovered object. Rediscovered in its symbolic—original or acquired—meaning, which endows it with a fullness that a 'created' object rarely reaches. Bricks, molten glass, root, pipe, star-shaped wafer, tabernacle for who knows what demented games: found objects reveal our multifaceted irrational life."[3] The found object is the basis for many of Bourgeois's creations, and she wants to give us the sense of finding what later artists oriented to Surrealism called "enigmatic objects." Moreover, her great variety of materials —her tendency to search out always new materials, both traditional art materials and materials that only modern technological invention permits the use of—has an affinity with Jean's list of found-object materials. Jean celebrated "the *expectant* air that emanates from surrealist objects,"[4] and it is this expectant air that Bourgeois achieves in her art, to greater effect than many Surrealist poetic objects, in my opinion, because she combines the idea of the found object with the created object, to greater artistic potency. The key difference between Bourgeois and the Surrealists is that she works with raw materials, which she transforms by a deliberate art process, while the Surrealists tended to use already "refined" objects, which were left untransformed, or were minimally transformed, by being juxtaposed with one another.

There are many other relationships that can be made between

the Surrealist orientation and Bourgeois's works. Jean's notion of creating objects that imply "a *potential* motion of a great poetic violence: an expectation, as in the common object waiting to be used for some vital need" seems useful for an understanding of her work.[5] Salvador Dalí's notions of "psycho-atmospheric-anamorphic objects" and of "the 'dialectical process' of the 'surrealist object' " seem tailor-made for many of Bourgeois's sculptures, however unlike Dalí's pictures they are.[6] Bourgeois has extended these concepts into unexpected realms of production. Even the black humor of many of her works can be regarded as Surrealistic in connotation, if hardly Surrealistic in any programmatic sense.

In 1938, Bourgeois married an American professor and moved to the United States, where she has lived ever since. It was in the security of her new life and country that she was able to begin to explore and articulate her feelings about her childhood and life as her parents' daughter. This became her art's basic—but far from ultimate—subject matter. It was as though Bourgeois had deliberately set out to articulate her deepest memories and feelings—those of her formative years (in my opinion in part responsible for the sense of her art as always "in formation," in primordial process, in effect forever unfinished)—in a seemingly systematic way. Out of her extraordinary awareness of her own psychic process and of her emotional "position" in her childhood—her incredible ability to regress in the service of her contemporary artistic ego, to recover the sense and perspective of childhood—she developed a more general, and equally profound, awareness of the psychophysical basis of life, especially of sex and death. She has finally come to articulate both the life force and the death wish with startling directness, sacrificing nothing of her art's formal subtlety. She is clearly the major woman artist working today, her art touching a range of issues in art making and life beyond the reach of much contemporary art.

1 Deborah Wye, "Louise Bourgeois: 'One and Others,' " in *Louise Bourgeois* (New York: The Museum of Modern Art, 1982), p. 13.

2 Ibid., p. 23.

3 Marcel Jean, "The Coming of Beautiful Days," in *The Auto-biography of Surrealism*, edited by Marcel Jean (New York: Viking Press, 1980; Documents of 20th-Century Art), p. 304.

4 Ibid.

5 Ibid.

6 Salvador Dalí, "Psycho-atmospheric-anamorphic Objects," in *The Autobiography of Surrealism*, p. 296.

COLOR PLATES

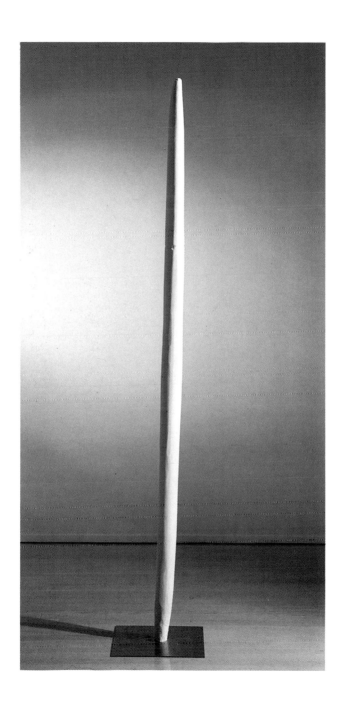

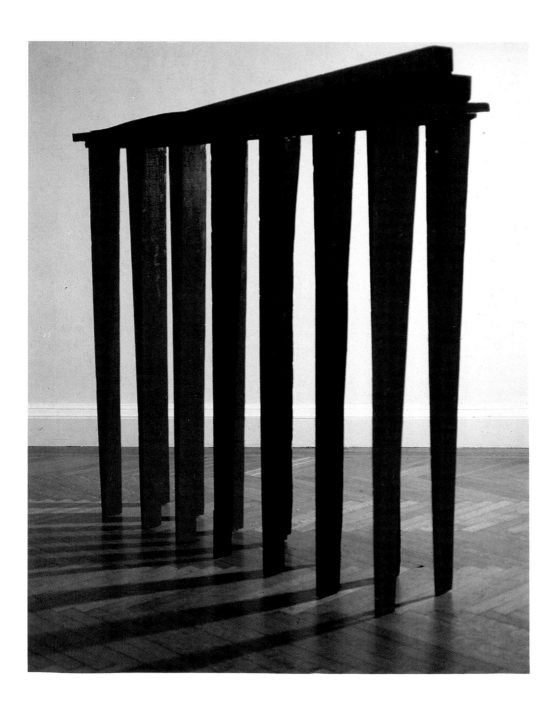

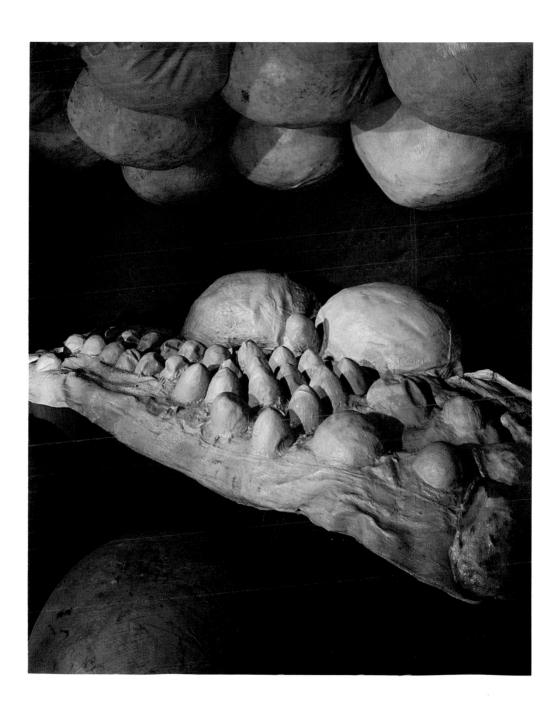

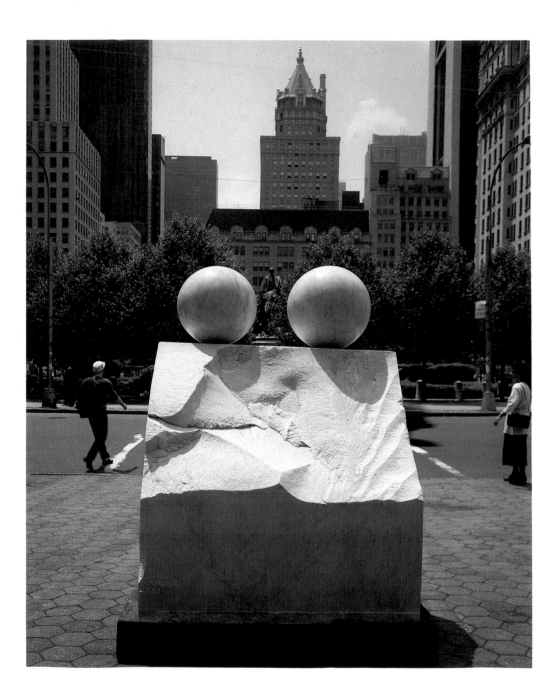

UNTITLED, 1947–49.
Painted wood; 75½″ high.
Collection of the artist.
Courtesy Robert Miller Gallery, New York.
Photo: Allan Finkelman.

THE BLIND LEADING THE BLIND, c. 1947–49.
Painted wood; 67⅛″ x 64⅜″ x 16¼″.
Private collection, London.
Courtesy Robert Miller Gallery, New York.
Photo: Peter Moore.

THE DESTRUCTION OF THE FATHER (detail), 1974.
Latex, plaster and mixed media; c. 108″ x 132″ x 108″.
Collection of the artist.
Courtesy Robert Miller Gallery, New York.
Photo: Peter Moore.

EYES, 1982.
Marble; 73″ x 65″ x 45″.
Collection of the Metropolitan Museum of Art, New York.
Courtesy Robert Miller Gallery, New York.
Photo: Peter Bellamy.

THE INTERVIEW

DK: I know you have told the story of your familial situation, the story of your upbringing, over and over again, and you have told how it was such a great influence in your art—that it is the emotional substance of your art. You have said that your art originated in response to your familial situation. Could you tell the story once again?

LB: You must understand that I am completely at ease with my art and that I like it. I am not afraid of my art at all because at the beginning, when I first became an artist, it was through my family situation. I was introduced to art as a useful thing. You could never understand this here in America. I was about ten or twelve, and completely involved in school. And one Saturday morning, when the whole family was there, when my father was there—one Saturday morning my mother said we would have to deal with this matter having to do with art.

But my mother was repairing a tapestry which was very large. It was maybe twenty feet by ten feet. It was one of those typical allegorical subjects. And she needed a draftsman. Monsieur Genault, the draftsman who worked at Gobelin, was a prima donna, and once in a while he simply did not show up when he was needed. There was no telephone to call him. The whole operation needed him. It could not be done without a draftsman. So my mother turned to me and said, "Louise, since you make drawings all the time, why don't you help me make a drawing on the tapestry so that we can go on. We can proceed if you can help us."

So I did that; I made the drawing. That was very important, because it meant I could draw and be valuable. It was very simple.

My father was not terribly interested in repairing the tapestries; he was interested in finding. He and my mother complemented each other, but they were very, very different. They had different gifts, and they appreciated each other. I was told by my father, "You cannot work for us, you are a pain in the neck, you are a useless mouth"—as Simone de Beauvoir put it, *la bouche inutile*— so I am very much a feminist.

The tapestries were always torn at the bottom. They were originally used as moving walls. The rooms they were used in were not very clean, and the tapestries always got torn at the bottom. Their lower parts were actually lost; the feet on the figures were often missing. I drew one foot for my mother. I became an expert at drawing feet. I still do it; I still do lots of feet. I was very satisfied with them, very satisfied with the feet I drew for my mother. It was a great victory. And it also taught me that art is interesting, and that it can be useful, which is completely unknown today. It can restore. So it gave me great pleasure. Everybody thought my feet were wonderful, the feet I restored. I didn't think so, but they did. That is how my art got started.

DK: That is certainly very interesting. But it is not the usual story you tell, the story you have told in the past. It does explain the family connection to some extent, but I was really asking you about your personal psychological history, the history you have spoken about before, the history of the complexity of your relationship with your mother and father and his mistress. You have told that story before, and I wanted you to tell it again, if it's no trouble for you to do so.

You have many works that have been interpreted as aggressive against the male figure, including the father. You have let such interpretations stand, even seemed to encourage them. One of them is a very famous piece, The Destruction of the Father, *the very important environmental sculpture you made in 1974. In explanation of it, you offered, according to Deborah Wye, "a long and fantastic tale" about your "childhood dinner table." You talked about your "burdensome and*

self-important father holding forth to his captive family night after night."
Finally you fantasized, in response to the situation, the family dismem-
bering and devouring him. As you said, you wanted to make "other
people relive that experience."

From what kind of personal, familial situation did these very intimate
works of art emerge? By your own past testimony, they do not simply
seem to have happened. I remember that in your last interview you said
that all art came from the unconscious, was about the unconscious. You
said this very explicitly.

LB: Definitely. It does, it is.

DK: I would like to know more about your unconscious situation, so to
speak.

LB: Let us take an example. *The Destruction of the Father* deals with
fear—ordinary, garden-variety fear, the actual, physical fear that I
still feel today. What interests me is the conquering of the fear,
the hiding, the running away from it, facing it, exorcising it, being
ashamed of it, and finally, being afraid of being afraid. This is the
subject.

I'm not an expert, but I know what fear is; I know what fear
will make you do. The fear—garden-variety fear—what do you do
about it? Do you run away? There is a long, long list of what you
can do. The way immature people can conquer—they don't conquer it, but they feel that they make the fear disappear—is by
falling in love. Right? You deceive yourself, you pretend to yourself
that you love in order not to feel that pang of the fear. You "fall
in love" with somebody that you are afraid of, and it short-circuits
the fear; you do not feel the fear. If you take a snake and a bird—
the bird is fascinated, right? It's exactly the same. It's mesmerized.
He doesn't suffer, he's not afraid—in fact he's thrilled—and the
snake gobbles him up. That's it! All my thinking is in terms of
images. This is my trouble. But the difference from real love is that
it does not come to sex; there is no real desire. I think that the
test of being in love—real love—is that you want to give.

But you cannot "love" everybody to obscure the fear—it is completely time-consuming and unproductive. You'd never grow up! So you go from puppy love to puppy love, and you don't feel afraid; you feel that you have conquered something. But you have conquered nothing! And the years pass, you have not experienced love—since that kind of love usually does not materialize—and you have wasted your time. And that waste of time is expressed by a great anger, because you feel that you have not lived, that life has passed you by. This is what *The Destruction of the Father* is about.

Obviously there was denial in this fear, and I deny this denial. I am a tease in my art; I tease with the unconscious. I was terribly afraid of them and I could not face it. And I still have that fear today. I am ashamed of my fear.

DK: Are you talking about your fear of your parents, which still continues, after all these years?

LB: Yes. But the important thing is that I am afraid of my fears. If you were not my friend I would never have said that I was afraid of you. I am ashamed of it, but I could say it. In my art, I can say it. It is a terrible thing to say you are afraid, but a necessary thing. There is the constant image that comes from Turenne saying to his horse: "You are a trembling carcass under me but you would tremble much more if you knew where I am leading you."

DK: You speak of yourself as an underling. You have this top-dog, underdog way of thinking.

LB: Yes, right.

DK: Is it a repetition of your family situation? When you were a little girl, were you an underling, so to speak? Were you made to feel like an underling in your family?

LB: They didn't try to make me feel like one.

DK: *They didn't try.*

LB: They didn't try to make me feel that way, they just did.

DK: *And you articulate this situation in your art?*

LB: To date I do.

DK: *Only to date? Can it still change, after all these years?*

LB: Yes.

DK: *How do you do so?*

LB: I do so in my art because I have denied it all my life.

DK: *What exactly do you deny?*

LB: I deny that I was so afraid because I was an underling.

DK: *But in your art you can acknowledge you are afraid.*

LB: Yes, because I am fearless in my art. I am not interested in anybody when I make my art. I am completely independent and fearless.

DK: *But you have also said your art reflects back or in some way relates to the situation of intense childhood fear that made you feel like an underling.*

LB: Yes, definitely. But it is because I am absolutely fearless when I am in my art that I can make the connection with my fear.

Now, the purpose of *The Destruction of the Father* was to exorcise the fear. And after it was shown—there it is—I felt like a different person. Now, I don't want to use the word *thérapeutique*, but an exorcism *is* a therapeutic venture. So the reason for making

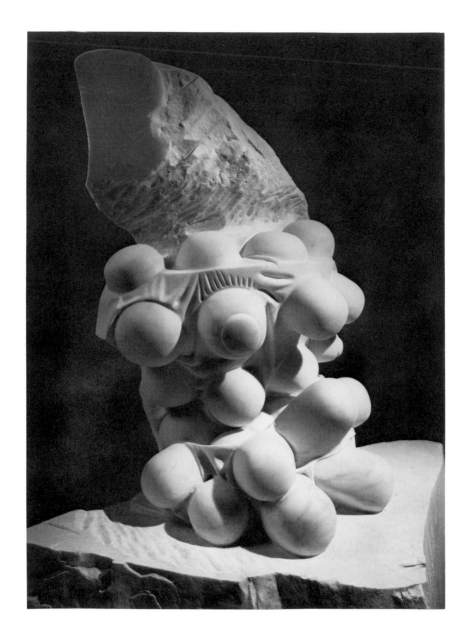

BLIND MAN'S BUFF, 1984.
Marble; 36½″ x 35″ x 25″.
Courtesy Robert Miller Gallery, New York.
Photo: Allan Finkelman.

the piece was catharsis. What frightened me was that at the dinner table, my father would go on and on, showing off, aggrandizing himself. And the more he showed off, the smaller we felt. Suddenly there was a terrific tension, and we grabbed him—my brother, my sister, my mother—the three of us grabbed him and pulled him onto the table and pulled his legs and arms apart—dismembered him, right? And we were so successful in beating him up that we ate him up. Finished. It is a fantasy, but sometimes the fantasy is *lived*. I have seen the sudden onslaught of a victim, when —if you remember—two or three years ago when Khadaffi teased us and pushed us, and suddenly it was enough and he was bombed out of his mind. Never heard about him again! With *The Destruction of the Father*, the recall was so strong, and it was such a lot of work, that I felt like a different person. I felt as if it had existed. It really changed me. That is the reason artists go on—it's not that they get better and better, but they are able to stand more. So when I talk about success it is not a material success that I'm talking about, it is about the successful outcome of the making of a work of art.

(Shows painting.) This is the story of an erotic attraction. It has to do with a man of whose presence I am intensely aware—physically, erotically. And when he is gone, as an exorcism, I visualize —not visualize, I *concretize*—his *columne vertébrale*, his spine. This is the spine of somebody I love. Suppose you—in French one says, *avoir le begat*—you have the hots for someone. Now, for reasons of your own—maybe the guy's married, he has somebody else in mind —you have to forget about him. It's very, very painful. I can do that by actualizing, by visualizing—by rendering concrete the feelings that I have. It works. But this is not to seduce somebody; it's the opposite, to get rid of somebody, to destroy the spell. I render the spine because it's very important, it's the gait, it's the way somebody walks—the main attraction of this guy is his gait. The main attraction—that's why I do so many eyes, and so on—the spell is usually (not with me, since I don't dare to look at anyone) in the eye contact. The spell doesn't go away suddenly, but this exorcism makes it more manageable. I talk in analogy. That used

to drive my husband crazy; it threw him off balance. I never made him out, and he never made me out. He felt that he had found a diamond that he loved—rough, very rough—and I felt that he was really a catch. But we didn't understand each other, so that each of us remained forever, forever, mysterious to the other.

DK: So your art is useful to you in your life, as you have suggested in other interviews. On the basis of what you have said before, it seems possible to say that it helps you live, it helps you endure. We all have our ways of coping with our history and emotions and memories, and you have suggested that your art helps you cope. This is certainly a well-known, even traditional function of art. It helps us deal with our inner life. It has been acknowledged, in one way or another, ever since Aristotle wrote of catharsis, the pity and terror aroused in us by tragedy. Certainly your work has a heroic, tragic dimension, in the classical sense.

In any case, can you tell me how, specifically, in your imagery and form, and perhaps in your techniques, your childhood fears manifest themselves?

LB: For instance, there is a piece called *The Blind Leading the Blind* in the Australian National Gallery. It represents an army of legs, two by two, that holds together. Eight pairs of legs. The reason this blind army of legs does not fall, even though the legs are always afraid of falling, since they come to a point, is that they hold on to each other. This is exactly what I felt when I was a child, when I was hiding under the table. My brother was following me like a shadow; I was blind with fear and so was he. My brother was a little younger than I and I used to protect him—I still feel protective toward men. I feel compelled to take care of them, whether I want to or not. I don't like it too much sometimes. But there we were under the table and we would look. I don't know what we were looking at. But I was watching the feet of my father and mother from under the table, while they were preparing the meal. And I thought to myself, What are they doing? What is their game? What is their purpose? How do I relate to them? And in the end I considered that they were not friendly. I decided that the outside was not friendly. And I was afraid, simply afraid. I couldn't understand their purpose, which was to prepare lunch. I didn't understand why they were walking around the table. Why would one pair of legs interfere with the other visually, physically? There were their legs and the table's legs. It really just made me wonder where I fitted in. Where did I fit in? I couldn't manipulate anybody since I didn't know what the issue was. I remedied the bewilderment by trying to understand how you could manipulate people—the end being how you could manipulate people to have them like you. I had to make an object of, physicalize this problem.

DK: So what is the relationship between manipulating material to make art and manipulating people?

LB: It's training—I get better and better every time. I realize the problem, I solve the problem at this physical level, and it gives me an insight into somebody else.

DK: The idea of the childlike aspect of many works of modern art, the idea that they are informed by a childhood vision, that a child's sense of things is especially compelling in them, is of course a well-known one. It is part of the so-called "return to origins" involved in much modern art, and it correlates with abstract art's return to elementary form. Certainly your art seems involved in this general—perhaps generic--modern idea, which goes back at least to Baudelaire, who writes about the child's point of view in his essay "A Philosophy of Toys." Is it worth acknowledging that there is an affinity between the legs you drew for your mother's tapestry, the missing legs, and the legs in The Blind Leading the Blind? *In the tapestry the feet were missing; in the sculpture you found feet, as it were. You have an interest in legs in general.*

LB: Yes, there is a connection. There are also the recent hanging rubber legs, hanging bronze leg, the imprints of legs in the recent stone pieces. There are many, many legs.

DK: *Then your works with legs come out of the association of the tapestry legs and the legs of your parents that you saw from under the table?*

LB: It is a coincidence, a very big coincidence, that their legs and the legs of the tapestry were the same.

DK: *No doubt it's a coincidence, a very pointed one. Perhaps it articulates your feeling of being little and looking at the legs of the adults, which confirmed your feeling of being little. Perhaps you thought they would kick you, and you kicked them back with your art.*

LB: Absolutely. I was looking up, which confirmed that I was small.

DK: *You were looking up as a little girl, but in your art you don't look up. Is it fair to say that you looked down?*

LB: Certainly in my art it is the opposite situation. I am impudent, manipulative, I do what I want to do. I do not hide under the table. And I succeed, too.

DK: *You certainly succeed. What does it mean to succeed?*

LB: First, you have to conceptualize what you want to do; you have to have an idea. The idea, as I said before, comes from a failure somewhere, a failure of power somewhere. For instance, if you have had a disagreement with the people you work with, if you have a problem to solve—with your children, for instance —you have to deal with it and show no criticism and no tension, and it is a terrific strain. There are many kinds of tension, but the one I am trying to deal with, to alleviate, is a social tension. My trouble is that it is absolutely impossible for me to put them together in a sequence, to organize my material so that it comes to a certain . . . I'm not trying to convince you of anything—and I *couldn't* convince you of anything. All I can do is to have these flashes of intense experience that are represented by this, and this, and this, and this. And all these entities have no connection with each other. This is one of the bases of my repeated work—that I have to make a whole out of all these parts, and it is not possible for me because every time I take a position, it shakes me so much that the thinking process does not take place.

It is by thinking about what is missing there, thinking about it little by little, in the night or when I travel, and so on—"What is wrong? What is wrong?"—that I find a way of repairing the difficulty by making a piece. This is a conception at a certain level; it is a way of thinking. The problem is purely one of organization. It has to do with survival at the everyday level—art is about life. So in order to put through what I have to put through, I have to prove to myself that I can organize and I am going to make the piece. That is at the very beginning. It is not deductive, it is intuitive—you have to read Pascal!

I have to admit something terrible: for breakfast I have tea with sugar, and I am extremely sensitive to sugar. That carries me until around eleven, and at eleven I become worried. At about eight-thirty I go by car to Brooklyn, to my studio. I spend all day there, until five or six. I have to be completely alone.

I do my thinking in the morning; the physical work I do in the afternoon. I think, and I do my sketches, and I do the conceptualizing. But I cannot conceptualize if I am afraid, if I am under stress. It is not possible to conceptualize if you are afraid. That's why some children do not learn—they're petrified. These strange— how would you describe these?—these are what I call my "nests." It is a form of apology, for not thinking completely straight. I am attacked by so many images when I think that I do not think straight. I see images next to each other, or overlapping each other —the whole thing is visual; I think visually. So these nests are an establishment of priorities, priorities in different subjects. There is no sequence here; there is a priority in size—obviously this is more important than that. Here is a list, but it doesn't move me; it doesn't mean anything to me. I'm trying to be a Descartes—it's terribly difficult for me. It is my way of dealing with a problem.

Personal problems—everything I am interested in is a personal problem. And I have to see my problems in physical shape before I can deal with them. So this is a first attempt at physicalizing them, of differentiating values, of putting them in order. The work in the afternoon is to make realizations of them—three-dimensional models of them.

DK: Can every problem be attacked that way?

LB: For me, yes. Every problem. Absolutely.

All afternoon I really work on the pieces. And then I come back on the subway from Brooklyn. This is the most intense social encounter that I have, seeing the people on the subway. For me, that is a fantastic experience. I notice people's faces, and even if they are strange, they are not hostile; I do not feel hostility any-where. I am in admiration of the differences between them. This is what really gets me—how people are separated, and this is expressed in their faces—that people are all alone, that they live in a world of their own is written on their faces. I love that. I am very sensitive to the way people look at me, and I have noticed that the way people look at you is a reflection of the way you look at them. If I have friendly eyes, they're reflected immediately. I want very much for them to like me; I'm very sensitive to that. It is not fifty-fifty; it's seventy-five–seventy-five—you have to give a lot.

So after the trip in the subway I get back here and I have to unwind in two ways. I have to unwind physically, so I start clean-ing, and I have to unwind from the stress. I do that by reading a boring book—not a boring book, but a book that does not present problems, that does not stimulate me, that doesn't make demands on me.

So, when the working time is over for me, I have sometimes managed to make a tangible thing of what I wanted to express. Usually, usually, usually I do succeed. There is a mounting tension, arising from my physical encounter with the physical material. There is always this mounting tension, and out of it grows what I want to say. Suddenly in this mounting tension you get it, you express what you want. Suddenly there is total release; it is like waking up and you are hungry. So this is a sign. When you are hungry you have succeeded.

DK: That's a very interesting account of your sensations when you work. What about the work itself, about the history of your work? Haven't you been associated with the Surrealists?

LB: No—with the people outside, on the fringes of Surrealism.

DK: Do you regard yourself as a Surrealist?

LB: No, even though I knew the Surrealists socially. They were my elders. Marcel Duchamp could have been my father. The Surrealists had a gallery called Gradiva, which was near the building where I lived. I saw them every day after lunch, when I was a student. They were of course famous artists. They were father figures.

DK: Do you feel an affinity with their ideas, with their notion of the work of art as a kind of manufactured dream? Wye, whom I know you admire, writes that Surrealism encouraged you "to tap the complex texture" of your personal life. She says that where the Abstract Expressionists utilized Surrealist automatism, you "moved toward a greater psychological literalness through representational work of a symbolic nature." Can't we say that such symbolic representations are in effect dreams?

LB: I have never mentioned the word *dream* in discussing my art, while they talked about the dream all the time. I don't dream. You might say I work under a spell, I truly value the spell. I have the privilege of being able to enter the spell, to enter this very arid land where you are likely to find your birthright. To express yourself is your birthright. In the spell I can express myself.

31

DK: Isn't being in a spell also a Surrealist idea?

LB: The spell and the dream are not the same. The spell is more friendly than the dream. The "spell" is acted out on a physical level; it's not a passive state, like a dream. The dream blinds you; the spell does not. It is a friendly process.

DK: In this friendly spell, what do you have in mind? When you were making your sculptures, what did you have in mind? What were you trying to achieve stylistically?

LB: Stylistically the background is always the extraordinary tapestries with which I grew up. I lived with them since I was born. It has to do with the stories. I am telling the same stories as the tapestries told, but with different means. For example, the story of Pyramus and Thisbe. This is a favorite story of mine.

DK: Does it have something to do with the relationship of your mother and father?

LB: Yes, to an extent, I suppose, but they were not really like the figures in the tapestry stories. And there were other subjects, antique subjects, and subjects from the Old and New Testaments. They were stories about pleasure and reason. All these were really everyday subjects, which is why they had a great reality. They were part of my education. I am an American artist; I am not even shown in France very much. I am shown much more in Germany and Scandinavia and so on. But I am French way back—all the formation, and the ideas, the values and all—are solid French. La Fontaine was my street education. La Fontaine is simply the *sagesse de nation*—how to defend yourself, how to keep alive. *Le loup et l'agneau* was most important to me—the *loup* comes and pontificates to the *agneau*, in order to eat him—that was my father! And *Le corbeau et le renard*—it's very real—you just have to flatter people; that's where everything starts. I'm still carrying those images, of taming birds. . . . But the French, being very sure of themselves, have a recipe for everything. My father would say, if

32

you want poetry, take the classics; if you want truth—downright horrible truth—you take the Old Testament. And the *sagesse de nation* really comes more from the Old Testament.

But Pyramus and Thisbe is not a *sagesse de nation*. It is a classical theme, from the Greek. It especially interested me because it was a story of love and death. Very early in life I associated lovemaking with death. In the story, the lovers tell each other that if one of them should happen to die first, the other would not wish to survive, as a sign of their love for each other. My parents would say the same thing to each other. They would play Pyramus and Thisbe. This is their story, not my story. They would coo their love to each other. This was a very strange thing, because my father was promiscuous and betrayed my mother every chance he had, and she knew it. This is one of the peculiar things about my father—that this man who was promiscuous and slept with just about everybody had as his ideal Pyramus and Thisbe. He expected his wife to die if he passed away—I'm not so sure it worked the other way around! My mother was not given to foolishness, but he would say things like that—"I love you so much that I would want to die if you passed away!" The day before, he had lipstick on his face—my father always had lipstick on his face. So much for protestations of love. They always lead to death. They conceived of love as distinct from sex.

DK: But your parents kept the act going, the pretense of devoted love. They played Pyramus and Thisbe very well.

LB: Love is eternal; it's sex that leads to death. This is a child's vision. They lived with a kind of elegance that we can no longer live with. They tried to believe their love story. I know my mother believed it, and my father tried to believe it. They believed their roles.

DK: Their marital roles.

LB: Yes. The French have a saying that you love your wife and you simply love everybody else you can and yet you still love your wife. Divorce is never considered, is never the word. My father was given to proverbs—he had proverbs for everything. He had to glorify everyone that he victimized.

DK: *How does this affect your art? You have mentioned classical themes, Old Testament themes, New Testament themes. But now you are talking about your real theme, the betrayal of love, and the taking of revenge for it, the revenge that was never taken in life.*

LB: Maybe. That is too easy. I will explain what my art is about by talking about my first sculpture. Here is a life-size model of it, a work of 1945 or 1946. It is made of milk containers folded and notched together. These are models for plaster and wax molds.

DK: *What does it mean, if you want to talk about that.*

LB: It is a kind of attempt to create order out of chaos. Every artist would say that. It is a cliché. But it is true. In the desolation of human relationships, their chaos, my way of making order is to group them and to see to it that they touch each other and are close together. The same problem exists now, forty years later. The problem is to put everybody in place, to give them a place, and especially to be sure they are together.

DK: *As they are not really in life? It seems to be an abstract fantasy of the way things should be. It seems to be an abstract analogue for an ideal family intimacy and unity that rarely exists. You once said you are always dealing with the problem of the one and the many, the individual and the group, separateness and togetherness.*

You are showing me cylinder-shaped elements, each of a different thickness. All belong to the same family of form. Each is in effect a surrogate for a person. Wye has said that "for Bourgeois a plank of wood can, on some level, be identified as a replacement for a specific person rather than as a symbol of that person." The problem is to bring them harmoniously together, to make them touch in an emotionally good way. Is that correct?

LB: Yes. They do in fact belong together, even though they may not know how to stay together.

DK: *You want them to have a harmonious relationship they do not have in life.*

LB: Yes.

DK: *All the elements are piled up. There is an accumulation of elements which don't quite add up but which you make hang together.*

LB: Right. The whole of them together is more than the sum of the parts.

DK: *They neatly come together, even though they are different in size and shape.*

LB: Yes. I was guilty about making them come together, but they had to. It was a privilege for me to make art; I felt guilty about it.

DK: *Why should you feel guilty about your sculpture?*

LB: It is because of the symbolic quality of the thing. I worked with found objects, and I found a magic overtone in them.

DK: *The breast is the moral background of the milk bottle.*

LB: It is the opposite; the milk bottle is the symbol for the feeding breast. It was once important that the objects I used be found in the house.

DK: *Why is that?*

LB: Because such objects are rejected objects, are lowly objects. They are used daily and are indispensable. This is why the milk container was for me the principal object of that time.

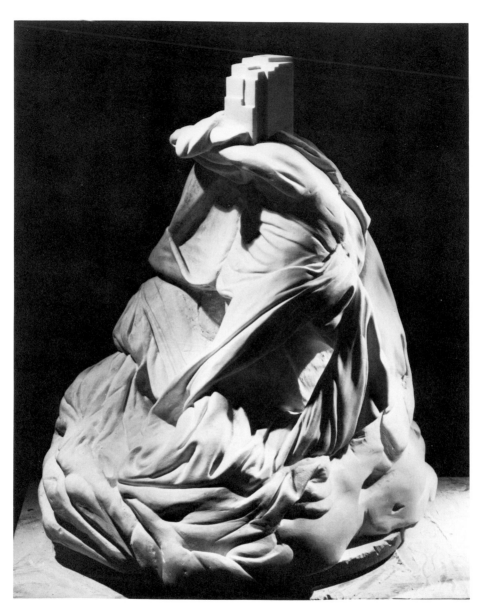

FEMME MAISON, 1983.
Marble; 25″ x 19½″ x 23″.
Courtesy Robert Miller Gallery, New York.
Photo: Allan Finkelman.

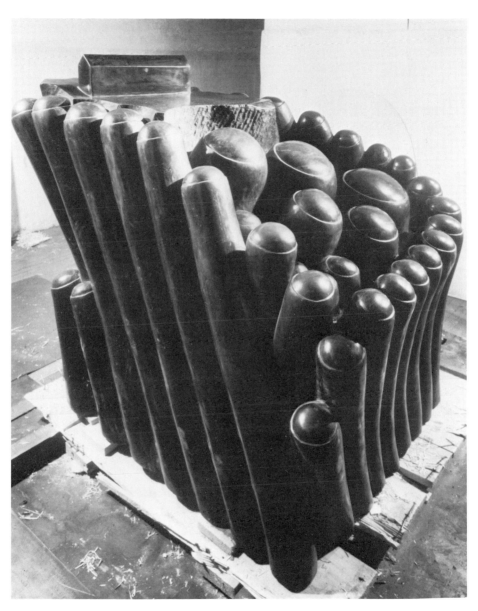

FEMME MAISON, 1981.
Marble; 48⅛″ x 47″ x 49⅞″.
Courtesy Robert Miller Gallery, New York.
Photo: Allan Finkelman.

DK: The milk containers here look old, used.

LB: Yes, it is important that they show their age.

You might mention as a general characteristic, to understand the tenor of my work, that I am a masochist. Whether that is the general attitude of women, I do not know. The masochism expressed itself at the time of the *Femmes Maisons* in the feeling that I didn't have the right to have children, and that I didn't have the right to be an artist. This was a privilege. So if you consider art as a privilege, then, by definition, you feel that you do not deserve it. You are continually denying yourself something—denying your sex, denying yourself the tools that an artist needs—because to be a sculptor costs you money. If you consider art a privilege instead of something that society will use, you have to save and suffer for your art, for what you love; you have to deny yourself in the cause of the art. I felt I had to save my husband's money rather than do sculpture that cost money. So the materials I used in the beginning were discarded objects. This was given a poetic meaning by saying that the discarded object has a value. That's true as well, but certain artists—for instance in black neighborhoods you will see that people will make sculpture with refuse because they don't have the money to buy new wood. The Surrealist object, on the other hand, was in the direction of *preciousness,* of rarity—rarity in time, in that there are very few left, and rarity in space, in that you don't find it so much. Rarity, preciousness, "beauty of material" . . . Joseph Cornell. But this is not me at all.

Here is a discarded object, *Shredder*—but certainly nothing to do with the Surrealists. It is an eight-foot wheel, a spindle for cable. It is typically American; it is a part of the discarded landscape here. And today, they are not made of wood, they are made of metal, so this represents a certain period—maybe twenty years —in American industrial history. Another discarded object was *The Fallen Woman*—but that was not *objet trouvé* at all. *The Fallen Woman* is a discarded object, but it is not made from discarded objects; it had to be made of clay.

Look at this.

DK: It is a photograph of yourself with your two children and with a bottle of milk.

LB: It is a gallon bottle.

DK: And your two children are in front of a chess board. The game is set up. It is a very beautiful photograph. I suppose you know that the big bottle of milk is a symbol of nourishment.

LB: Absolutely. It is important.

DK: So you knew what you were doing all the time? It was not just a blind unconscious expression?

LB: Yes, because it reflected our everyday life. The children lived on milk; we had big containers of milk everywhere.

DK: Is it farfetched to say that some of your work—some of your most important sculptural objects—signifies the good breast, the nurturing breast, both yours and your mother's? Are those big stone sculptures, which you open up, whose hardness you penetrate, surrogate breasts, capable of giving milk, the way it is said water can miraculously come from a stone? Is it silly to say that?

LB: I wouldn't know. I wouldn't know if they are breasts.

DK: The arrangement of the figures in the photograph is interesting. The one boy is holding your hand with both his hands; the other doesn't seem to want to hold your hand.

LB: He is the master of his fate, he has an ego. You can see that; he doesn't want to touch.

DK: So the point is again the intimacy. When was this photograph taken?

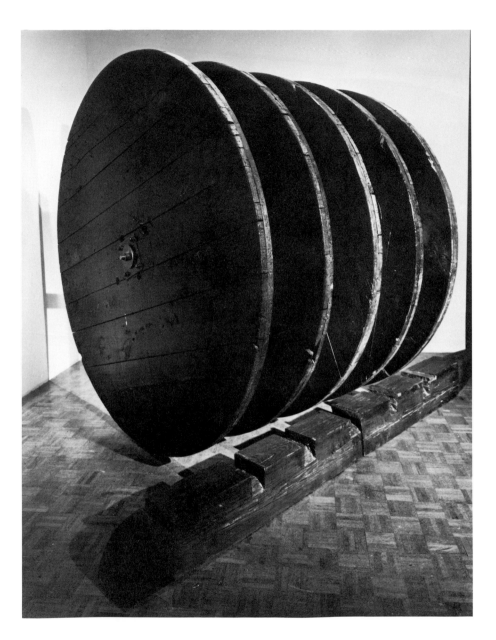

SHREDDER, 1983.
Wood and metal; 83″ x 59″ x 83″.
Private Collection.
Courtesy Robert Miller Gallery, New York.
Photo: Allan Finkelman.

LB: In 1950, the same year as the sculpture.

DK: *So it is the background of the sculpture; it is information about the sculpture. It is about the situation of intimacy you are always dealing with.*

LB: Yes. Here is another photograph, of a sculpture. It is from 1968.

DK: *What is it called?*

LB: *Cumul.* It was exhibited in a show of works that could be understood by the blind. It is a very tactile sculpture. Again there are these elements hanging together. They are emerging from the drapery. The drapery falls away and they come to light. All this around is drapery. This sense of something completely covered and then emerging—that is important to me. There is one element isolated from the others.

DK: *Tell me more about the work. Tell me its story.*

LB: Well, this represents the coastline, and this the open sea, and this element is about to go off alone and be herself.

DK: *So you are picturing the family.*

LB: Right. It is like a family that is too comfortable, too tight.

DK: *Too constrictive.*

LB: Right.

DK: *This continues the problem of the milk-bottle work.*

LB: Well, I don't know. Other people see different things in them.

DK: *What do you see in them?*

LB: I really see things as mother figures.

DK: *All these things in the sculpture?*

LB: Yes. Even these tight, little ones here.

DK: *So it's a kind of personal allegory for you?*

LB: Right. And a kind of personal vortex.

DK: *It's like a landscape.*

LB: Definitely.

DK: *It is a self-contained landscape.*

LB: Right.

DK: *You've made other kinds of works like this one, works with the elements tightly grouped together, in a variety of media. Does the medium make a difference to you?*

LB: A great difference. For instance, this sculpture is supposed to be filled with water.

DK: *Again, there is the implication of a life-giving liquid, as in the case of the milk bottles.*

LB: Yes. You see this flowing drapery underwater. It has all kinds of elements that change shape.

DK: *What kind of stone is this?*

LB: It is marble, like the other ones, but the idea is not the same in it.

DK: *Why is that?*

LB: Because I work in series, especially when I am intensely concerned with a subject. I will start small, in a certain material, and then change material, and the change will change the subject. You get different things from different materials. Eventually, after going through many changes of material, I will get the subject that interests me most, and the most resistant material. The fact of resistance is challenging, perhaps the most challenging fact about sculpture for me. It is overcoming resistance.

DK: *Does that have something to do with subject?*

LB: Right. I go over the material and the subject as something I have to deal with and fight to the finish. What the piece finally is depends of course on the material I work with, but I usually work with hard material. I am attracted to it.

DK: *Is there a psychological reason for this? You spoke in psychological terms of the waves and forms and the way they are grouped together.*

LB: Oh, definitely. The picking of the challenge is altogether psychological. It has to do with my sense of myself. That perhaps sounds ridiculous.

DK: *It doesn't sound ridiculous. Tell me more about it. Wye has remarked that the sense of self is fundamental to your art, inseparable from it. How does your sense of yourself relate to your using what might be described as a stubborn material? Are you deliberately setting yourself a difficult, almost impossible, task? Are you taking yourself to task, as it were, setting yourself a hard task as a kind of penance?*

LB: No. I deserve the privilege of my self-expression. But my self-expression is very aggressive, and this causes me a certain tension. When students come to me, I tell them I don't want to be bothered, or that they know more than I do, anything to push them away, so that they don't experience my aggression. It is very bad.

DK: *Pushing people away?*

LB: Yes.

DK: *Does the hard material represent these people you are pushing away?*

LB: Yes. Right. It is also a way to prove to myself that I am a very strong person.

DK: *Meaning isolated. Meaning that you can be yourself, stand on your own.*

LB: Yes. I can take care of myself. I am not dependent.

DK: *You want to demonstrate that you are not dependent by overcoming the material on which you are dependent?*

LB: Right.

DK: *But you articulate situations of dependence.*

LB: The fear of dependence is crucial for me, and is partly what my art is about. The challenge is to show that I am independent. It is a constant challenge. I have to prove it.

DK: *Yet you show in these forms identifying with a nurturing mother figure, on whom others are dependent.*

LB: Exactly.

DK: But it is also an isolated figure, to show its independence of those dependent on it.

LB: Yes, it also wants to have fun and forget everybody and not nourish anybody. *(Laughs.)*

DK: It wants to remain high on itself, on its own.

LB: Very true.

DK: What about when you work in softer materials? I know you've used wood as well.

LB: First I work on a drawing, then I will translate the concept into cardboard and then into corrugated cardboard. Here, let me show you. I get hooked on a subject and I make sketches and drawings. It means the obsession is going to last for several months. Then it will disappear, and reappear several years later. I am involved in a kind of spiral, a spiral motion of motivation. The material itself, stone or wood, does not interest me as such. It is a means; it is not the end. You do not make sculpture because you like wood. That is absurd. You make sculpture because the wood allows you to express something that another material does not allow you to.

DK: You seem to move from sketch to cardboard model to corrugated cardboard model to wood to stone. And you apparently feel free to stop at any one point in the process and dig into that material, to linger with it and work with it. Is that correct?

LB: Yes.

DK: In other words, sometimes the sculpture ends at the wood stage, and sometimes at the stone stage.

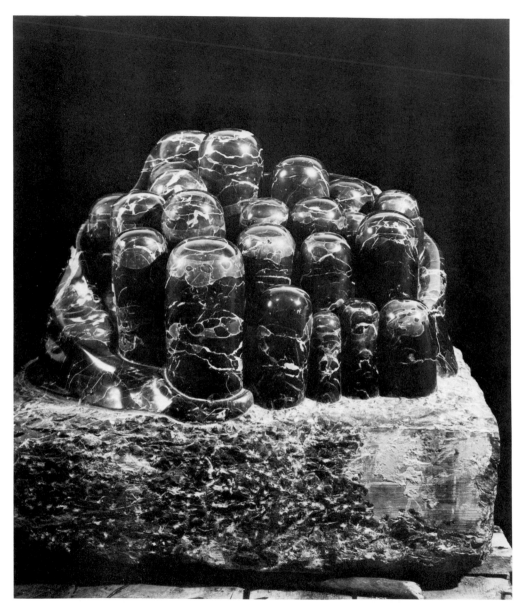

Noir Veine, 1968.
Marble; 23″ x 24″ x 27″.
Courtesy Robert Miller Gallery, New York.
Photo: Peter Moore.

LB: That is true. But at each stage it is sculpture. Every part of the series belongs to it, from the smallest sketch to the marble.

DK: *But you seem to prefer the marble. You seem to prefer the hardest material, the material with the most resistance.*

LB: Yes, I would say that. I think I do express myself best in marble. It permits one to say certain things that cannot obviously be said in other materials.

DK: *What kind of things?*

LB: Persistence, repetition, the things that drive you toward tenacity, that force you to be tenacious. I am a tenacious person.

DK: *I'm aware of that.*

LB: Art comes from life. Art comes from the problem you have in seducing birds, men, snakes—anything you want. It is like a Corneille tragedy, where everybody is pursuing somebody else. You like A, and A likes D, and D likes. . . . Being a daughter of Voltaire and having an education in the eighteenth-century rationalists, I believe that if you work enough, the world is going to get better. If I work like a dog on all these . . . contraptions, I am going to get the bird I want.

DK: *Does that sometimes happen?*

LB: Very little. The end result is rather negative. That's why I keep going. The resolution never appears; it's like a mirage. I do not get the satisfaction—otherwise I would stop and be happy. There is no resolution, but you are very pleased with yourself because you have done everything you could and you have been efficient. You have understood the problem, and the understanding of a problem is a very high objective. Lots of people remain at the level of collecting—collecting objects, or collecting women, if it's a man—which is a lower activity than understanding. Of course, there are lots of artists, and most of them are completely uninteresting, because self-expression is not an end in itself—or rather, self-expression *is* an end in itself, but it is not interesting. Millions of people have breakfast in the morning; it's very difficult to make breakfast interesting, from an objective point of view.

I work very hard and I never—never!—get people to understand what I mean. I want them to understand tenacity as a virtue, an end in itself. More than that, they must understand that I had to equate sex and murder, sex and death. They could never understand the problem of this equation. I should be softer on myself, I should not pursue such a mystery, but it is still a mystery, and I still pursue it.

DK: Are you talking about the relationship between sex and death?

LB: The mystery is why I can't trust sex as a good thing, why I am afraid of it, why this destroys its thrill, why this makes it like death. It reaches a point where you do not know if it is pleasurable or repulsive. You do not know if death is pleasurable or repulsive.

DK: Painful.

LB: Painful. You lose your sense of where the edge is. You lose the thrill of the poor guy who bets on the horses and doesn't know if he is going to win, become rich, or end up dying under a bridge. The fear of death destroys your sense of the edge in sex. It is this same moment, when death and sex are one, that I want to get in my work.

DK: I am reminded, by your talk about the peculiar, paradoxical relationship of those seeming opposites, sex, the life force, and death, its exhaustion, about what Marius Bewley has written about the intentions in the symbolic imagery that appeared in the prints published in He Disappeared into Complete Silence, *which you produced at Atelier 17 in 1947. Bewley wrote: "They are all tiny tragedies of human frustration: at the outset someone is happy in anticipation of an event or in the possession of something pleasing. In the end, his own happiness is destroyed when he seeks to communicate it, or, perversely, seeks to deny the necessity for communication. The protagonists are miserable because they can neither escape the isolation which has become a condition of their own identities, nor yet accept it as wholly natural." This was written some time ago, but it seems to beautifully describe the situation of frustration embodied in the age-old dilemma of the relationship of sex and death that you are so interested in. Can one say that much of your work attempts to articulate the difficult, even impossible, very intimate situation—tinge—of emotional frustration that the association of death with sex implies?*

And would this have something to do with the fact that your father repeatedly betrayed your mother, making sex untrustworthy, a pawn in the game of relationship? Does it have something to do with your unhappiness about the French notion of marriage as a situation in which a man loves his wife but sleeps with as many women as possible? That is a very pure, rarefied betrayal. It is legitimized, institutionalized adultery.

LB: It is true. My father acted as he did because he was not an adult. He remained a child all his life.

DK: An adolescent in attitude?

LB: Right. And my mother was extremely reasonable, very reasonable, reasonable to a fault—foolishly reasonable. She was completely reliable, and my father was unreliable, emotionally. It is only because of her that I am able to build up a little trust.

DK: Is it correct, then, to say that your sculpture is always from the point of view of woman?

LB: Yes. But I *am* a woman.

DK: Yes, you are, but what I mean is that your sculpture is always from the point of view of the reliable woman who has been betrayed, who has tasted death, whose sex with her husband is tainted because he has been with other women, and she thinks that is the way it should be, that is customary, allowed, even though she dislikes it intensely, unconsciously. Your mother was a model for you, as you yourself have suggested. Is your persistence against the stone, your determination in the situation of the hardness of stone, like your mother's reliability? Is your persistence your adult mother's endurance of your infantile father, whom you have destroyed in spirit in several of your works—destroyed him for your mother's sake, to revenge your mother?

LB: I don't know all that for sure. I think what is going on in my sculpture is even more personal than that.

DK: How would it be more personal?

LB: It is about how I am unable to make myself loved. The resistance of the stone is that I am unable to make myself loved.

DK: Are you saying that you feel you are unlovable, and that your art is about your unlovableness?

LB: You said it, I didn't.

DK: I asked it, I didn't say it.

LB: I said that I am presented with a game, a game I don't know how to play, a game of love which looks like a game of death. I don't know if the game is correct, but it exists, it is given, it is the family.

DK: It is the only game in town, the game of family betrayal.

LB: Right. It is easier to feel that people do not love you so that you do not break down when they betray you. So that I am unable to be trusting in love. That's it. Of course it's painful.

DK: So in a sense, the making of your work is an articulation of this difficult, even impossible, very intimate emotional situation.

LB: Right. Only the making of art makes it valuable. Valuable.

DK: Because you can endure the struggle.

LB: Right.

DK: Because you can present the struggle, in whatever elusive, abstract way.

LB: Yes. And the work is valuable in itself, as art.

DK: I wouldn't deny that.

LB: If it is valuable in itself, what enters is the celebrity factor, the way the work is understood and celebrated. I believe in that.

DK: But you said before that you felt people didn't understand your work.

LB: It is not my responsibility whether they understand it or not, only that I express it. Nonetheless, the celebrity factor, the work's reception, gives it a place. I do not care if it has the right place. I do not claim that my work is a communication, because that is like a game also. I do not play the communication game, because one will always be betrayed in communication as in love.

DK: Let's talk more about your life, about your life after you left home, which clearly had its problems. You married the art historian Robert Goldwater and you moved to the United States.

LB: I married, first of all, an intellectual. He was interested in nothing but ideas. That means he was interested in what is true and what is not true. This is a great compliment to him. My father was also a skeptic, a disbeliever. He said you always have to prove something to him.

DK: Did your husband say that also?

LB: No, my father did, and I admired it. He said, "I do not believe in anything unless you prove it to me. It's up to you to prove it to me." Intellectually, basically he had the same idea, the same approach. But Robert Goldwater was a completely rational person; he had the same qualities as my mother had. He did not betray me. He did not betray anyone. I never saw him angry in my life. Ever. And I never heard my mother raise her voice, ever. That is something.

DK: Yes, it is quite unusual.

LB: It is amazing. I could appreciate it, because I threw tantrums. The tantrums that I threw made me feel that I was not lovable. The tantrum never gets you anywhere, certainly not in love. Some people say, "Oh, you're immature, out you go." So even now that I have success with my art I do not feel like a successful person. I do not feel welcome.

DK: But you seem to enjoy your success, your celebrity.

LB: I am selfish, like all artists. But I do not take any nonsense, all this nonsense connected with success.

DK: Did your husband's work influence yours? Were there ideas that you shared?

LB: His Penguin book called *Symbolism* was published in 1971. This is a common interest we shared.
   I am not interested in art history. My husband taught it, so I had my fill at home! I do believe in it as an activity, as a form of

intellectual pursuit, but it did nothing for me—except that it kept me at a certain bracing level of intellectuality.

In general, my work portrays and encompasses the whole tradition of art. It is baroque, for example. I have even called one work *Baroque*, a work made about 1970. My art involves other styles as well. I privilege no one style or material.

DK: Can you tell me how this is shown in your art?

LB: Yes. Look at the "No" poster, which was reproduced in *The New York Times*. It is graphic design in the strictest sense.

DK: Is it that poster on the wall?

LB: Yes. The word *no* is presented in letters of different sizes. That is modern design.

DK: Does this work represent your skepticism, your saying no to everything?

LB: I didn't think of it then, because the work was made for a specific occasion, but yes, I can say it does.

DK: What is the specific event it relates to?

LB: The specific thing is that people say you must think this way or that way. I say "no" to it all. You know, you have many religions in the world, maybe eight or ten, not just one or two or three. And each of them tells you how to express yourself; each of them tells you it is incomparable. I say "no" to all of them: I will express myself. They have nothing to tell me; they can show me nothing. You can express yourself by comparing them, but none of them can express you.

DK: So you are saying "no" to any dogma that claims to speak for you.

LB: They cannot speak for anyone; they have to prove what they say. Everyone must prove what they say. I can say I like you because you are a very nice person, but what do I mean by that? I must prove it. Robert [Goldwater] was saying that all the time: you have to prove it. He would say, "But Louise, how can I prove it? How can you prove it?"

DK: *I want to ask you something about the arrangement of posters and letters you have on the wall where the "No" poster is. I see that you also have a photograph of one of your sculptures, the one with the eyes.*

LB: Right. It is called *Eyes*. The staring, unflinching eyes stand for scrutiny.

DK: *Could you tell me whether this scrutiny is related to your skepticism you mentioned before, the skepticism of Voltaire you once called it?*

LB: Absolutely. It is the skepticism embodied. I have in general been preoccupied with the idea of eyes for many years. I often isolate the eyes. In general, I am interested in body parts, and most come in pairs, because the body is symmetrical. I am interested in this doubleness, just as I am interested in opposites.

DK: *Can you tell me a little more about the meaning of this work, which seems to present another side of you, a more autonomous side, the independent side you mentioned, far from the family situation, with all its emotional complexity? It is as though here, at last, I am looking at the real Louise Bourgeois; her strong identity and powerful self-expression are self-evident. I see her free of her involvement in her parents' relationship, of her unconscious identification with one or the other and her uncertainty and confusion about her own place in the family. Even though this critical, strong self derives from your father's skepticism, it seems more entirely your own, more entirely you, than the works of the mother with whom you identify, the breast works, as it were. In Eyes I see Louise Bourgeois's all-seeing, sharp eyes. In Eyes I see the power of consciousness embodied in a spherical form that is simultaneously organic and abstract, bodily and universal. It is simultaneously a pure form and an impure part of the body that yet engages in pure seeing, pure knowing.*

LB: What counts, our whole purpose, is to try to understand what we are about, to scrutinize ourselves. Art is an aid in this. It involves a quality of scrutiny. I once said, "Every day you have to abandon your past or accept it, and then, if you cannot accept it, you become a sculptor." It is of course a privilege to be able to scrutinize, especially in the mode of art. Scrutiny presupposes tenacity, the tenacity to see, to concentrate. Skepticism clears the way for scrutiny, clears away the blindness of dogma, of easy belief, easy seeing.

DK: I think it is wonderful to think of your sculpture as concentrated scrutiny, as declaring the imperative of scrutiny.

LB: That has always been the quality I have sought in my work. But it depends on my power of scrutiny and concentration, and this has reduced itself to the few hours of the morning.

DK: Do you feel your work has become less concentrated as you have aged?

LB: No, more concentrated. I have become less concentrated in general. But perhaps in those few early hours I have become more concentrated.

DK: You know, we are all aging, we are all growing old, and it seems more evident as the world continues to pretend to be young. But that only makes us more tenacious. It is a way of respecting ourselves, our power of scrutiny. Your work seems to me stronger than ever. You are as tenacious as ever, perhaps more openly tenacious. Your work seems to embody what the psychoanalyst Sandor Ferenczi said is the great gift of old age, the combination of wise vision and youth's sense of freshness.

LB: Yes, that is true. I always feel the last work is the best, the most concentrated, the strongest, the most tenacious.

DK: *What are you working on now? What is your most recent work? Tell me about it.*

LB: I don't think I can do that without the work in front of me.

DK: *You must have some ideas about it that you can talk about now.*

LB: But I am still inside that work; I do not know where I am going, what I can do, exactly what is happening, what I am seeing. I am passionately going somewhere, but I am not sure that I know where, where it is.

DK: *I understand. You're still deeply in process, so you are reluctant to talk about it. You are afraid that its spell might dissipate. But would it be fair to assume that it involves some of the ideas you have already spoken about?*

LB: Yes, definitely.

DK: *Is it a work in stone?*

LB: Yes, it is a work in stone.

DK: *And are you fighting it, struggling against its resistance?*

LB: You can say that. But the stone is not a very hard stone. It is not a very hard stone at all. So, let us say that we have a cube of stone. It has happened many times that I have had such a cube of stone. The cube is a hostile entity, more hostile than the stone. It is more intact than the stone. It resists me more than the stone. I cannot destroy it! It is a problem I have to resolve. How am I going to attack the problem? What is the technique of resolving the problem of the resisting cube? How shall I get at and overcome its truth, the truth of its existence, as hard as the hardness of stone, which is its truth?

DK: *You haven't worked with the cube too often, except in recent years. Why have you turned to it now? Does it symbolize your concentration? Does its perfection make it the perfect object of your scepticism?*

LB: It's true that I haven't used cubes very often, except recently. I have decided to respect the way stone is given, the way it comes to me. It comes from the quarry in the form of a cube. I want to preserve that sense of the quarry.

DK: *Do you know the "Altar of Good Fortune" by Goethe, which involves a cube and a sphere, two contrary forms of perfection, two axiomatic forms, brought into conjunction? Are you interested in the perfection, the completeness symbolized, the perfection that seems to come raw from the quarry? Are you aware of the symbolic meaning of the cube? Are you trying to make a philosophical work, a conceptual sculpture?*

LB: No, I don't know the symbolic meanings. I am not sure that I want to make a philosophical sculpture.

DK: *Goethe's piece was a kind of minimalist work. Are you trying to be minimalist?*

LB: I understand what Goethe was doing. He probably thought he had created a complete harmony, bringing the cube and sphere together. And so it was his good fortune.

DK: *Right.*

LB: It is the opposite for me. I see the cube as a problem, a problem you have to enter. I see it as a physical cube, not as a symbolic cube or as a concept. My problem is to penetrate the physicality of the cube. Modern technology allows you to do that. It allows something that was not possible in the past. If Goethe could have drilled into the stone cube, he might not have thought of it as perfect.

DK: It is an aggressive act to penetrate the cube.

LB: Yes, so that my work could not have been made in the eighteenth century. I take great pride in the solitary cube, and great pride in the fact that I can penetrate it. My work with the cube is very modern. It does not repeat former work.

DK: Are you working only with this one cube?

LB: No, there are three of them.

DK: So where is the solitariness of the cube, and the unique destruction of its hardness and givenness?

LB: With three of them I can get at the truth. Three of them represent an investigation of the truth. The investigation is the driving into the cube. Each time I drive into it in a different, more thorough way.

DK: I remember you once told me that you used workmen to make the initial penetration of the stone, and then you followed on the trail they had blazed.

LB: Yes. They are very special people. They are people who do nothing but drill stone. What is important is that they do not relate to my work, they relate to their machine. They come with this machine and with this very particular drill, which they know very well. They are special kind of men.

DK: You clearly respect and admire them.

LB: I do. They raise for me a very important question, the question of the relationship of the artist to the technician, to the man of skill. It is an important question for me.

DK: *Does it raise the issue of dependence on technique for you, a concern that technique may do the whole work?*

LB: I am interested in technique. I respect the men with technique. I try to help by congratulating them all the time. But they are not interested. They are extremely sensitive, extremely proud. They are proud because of the prowess of their machine. They are not people-related; they are machine-related.

DK: *I take it you tell them where to drill, and what size hole to make. That is already the beginning of the work. What do you do after they have drilled, after they have made their penetration?*

LB: We work for one day at it. It is exhausting.

DK: *What do you do then?*

LB: I contemplate the penetrated cube for a long time. Then I try to express what I have to say, how I am going to translate what I have to say to it. I try to translate my problem into the stone. The drilling begins the process by negating the stone. The problem is how to complete the negation, to take away from the stone, without altogether destroying it, but overcoming it, conquering it. The cube no longer exists as a pure form for contemplation; it becomes an image. I take it over with my fantasy, my life force. I put it to the use of my unconscious.

DK: *Can we say that geometry casts another kind of spell for you, over you? To work on the stone cube still seems to have symbolic significance for you, but the significance now seems more obscure, although it is related to your idea of skeptical scrutiny—the skepticism of your scrutiny.*
In any case, this is a different approach than you used in the past.

LB: Yes, it is.

DK: *In the past you added materials; you accumulated them. You put a lot of different things together.*

LB: Right. And now I attack.

DK: *You attack. You empty the stone. You scoop the cube out.*

LB: Yes. Now I want to know. I want to ask questions. That is to penetrate. I used to be frightened and have to recover when I made work. Now I ask questions, I scrutinize with questions, I am not frightened.

DK: *Now you are aggressive against the stone. You are not frightened of any material.*

LB: Right.

DK: *You enter the material. You want to empty it out.*

LB: I am not aggressive in that fashion. I want to find something out.

DK: *Something inside the cube.*

LB: The cube represents my concern. The cube represents a problem.

DK: *So you are attacking a problem. As you talk about it, it doesn't seem like a personal problem; you speak of the cube in an impersonal way—you regard it impersonally. And yet you don't seem to be talking entirely of a technical problem, of making something out of the cube, of changing the raw stone cube into a refined sculpture. It still seems more than an issue of making an art object. To work on the stone cube still seems to have symbolic significance for you, but the significance now seems more obscure, although it is related to your idea of skeptical scrutiny. I have it: you want to undermine the dogma of the cube, its dogmatically given form, to express skepticism of that form the way Voltaire, whom you once told me your father admired, expressed skepticism of religion. No religion of the perfect cube for you!*

LB: It is true. But I am also going back to basics. Part of skepticism is to go back to basics, to call for a return to basics.

DK: Is that itself the problem you spoke of, to go back to basics?

LB: The problem is always the same.

DK: But this return to basics seems different than the old family problem. The return to basics does not seem to have any personal dimension.

LB: It is the same problem.

DK: How so?

LB: It is always the same problem.

DK: Then you are articulating it in a different way?

LB: Oh yes. I am still ashamed of the problem.

DK: You don't seem ashamed.

LB: I am not as ashamed as I was when I worked with the cube.

DK: Why are you less ashamed? Is it because the problem is transformed in the cube?

LB: Yes. It is now the problem of the voyage.

DK: Voyage?

LB: Right. It is the voyage inside the cube. After the penetration by the technicians, comes the voyage. That is the art. I am now alone; I do not need anyone around any longer. I am just going on with this investigation, this voyage by myself. Inside the cube, I am on my own.

DK: *Is it correct to say that in the 1968 work you showed me before, you are pointing to the problem of the voyage that you have now realized in the isolation of the cube?*

LB: Right. I am totally on my own in the cube. There is no family, no forced togetherness. I accept the challenge. I am not terrified by the challenge. I just accept it.

DK: *You have been quoted as saying, with respect to your study of solid geometry, "I got peace of mind only through study of rules that nobody could change, that were safe."*
    I remember that once you spoke of your work as an exorcism. Is the exorcism complete in the cube works? Is that why you can be on your own inside the cube?

LB: Yes. The process of making is an exorcism. Sometimes it works, sometimes it doesn't. In the cube works it has worked.

DK: *How do you know when it works?*

LB: When it works you know it. You can redo it, reshow it, as in the three cubes, one after another. It works in this piece. (*Holds up a photograph.*)

DK: *What is that called?*

LB: *The Witness.*

DK: *From what year? It looks very early.*

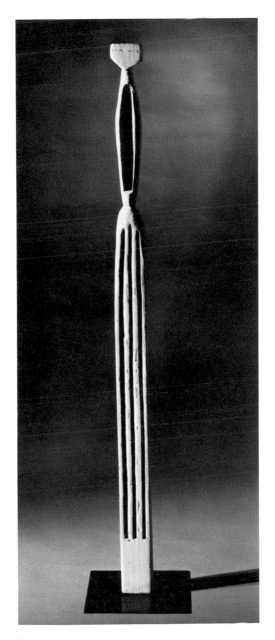

PILLAR, c. 1949.
Painted wood; 64⅜″ high.
Courtesy Robert Miller Gallery, New York.
Photo: Allan Finkelman.

LB: It is a work from 1947.

DK: *Does the exorcism work in it?*

LB: No. The exorcism came later. These figures were very precarious. Their position was precarious. In fact, they couldn't stand by themselves. This one is later; the figure repeats. The witness is still terrified.

DK: *That seems apparent in the hands and arms.*

LB: Yes, the terror is in the stiffness.

DK: *The arms are close to the body.*

LB: And the witness has no feet.

DK: *There you are with your foot problem again, Louise.*

LB: Right, right. The figure tries desperately to be level, but it can't.

DK: *It tries to be on the level, but it's not.*

LB: Right. Once I had a man who wanted to do my taxes—he really wanted to do them. I gave him a carpenter's level as a joke, a long level. And I said, "Are you on the level?" You know, he did not cringe. It did not threaten him. That was how I knew he was honest.

DK: *He did not feel offended by your subtle aggression?*

LB: Not at all. He was delighted. He hung the carpenter's level on his wall. He was not offended.

DK: All these figures you are showing me have the same desire to be on the level, but they cannot stand alone on the level.

LB: Right.

DK: Why are they?

LB: That was what I was blamed for, for not being able to stand up alone. You are not good, you cannot take care of yourself, much less of others, I was told. The exorcism happened when I could. In the cube I can take care of myself. The cube is on the level.

DK: Who said those things to you?

LB: Well, this is very personal. In a closed society, the first child in the family would inherit the wealth, whatever wealth there was. Sometimes there was nothing to inherit, but the first child was expected to have the values, the good judgment. If there was a house, the first child would have it. The second would have the intangibles, or a little money, or something like that. The third child would join the foreign legion. This was a very cruel world, a really cruel world. You had constantly to prove to everybody that you were worthwhile, that your life was worth something. You had to prove to your parents that you were worth having. Your parents had you only because the Church said they should have you. This is the world I was born into. It was a very cruel world.

DK: What order were you born in? Were you the firstborn?

LB: My sister was the firstborn. She was born out of wedlock, because my parents escaped . . . I mean eloped.

DK: When were you born?

LB: My sister was six years older than I was.

DK: Were you the second born?

LB: Just a minute. I must think. My mother lost a child. I don't know if it was the first one or the second one. Anyway, I was the third girl born. Of course, my father wanted a son. So I was an embarrassment when I was born. It is a fact. My mother, who, as I said, was very rational and a very cool person, my mother said to her husband, to my father: "Don't be disappointed with that little girl. You know, she is your spitting image. Don't you think so?" It was not clear that he thought so, but my father said, "Yes, she is pretty nice." And my mother said, "She is your spitting image, and we are going to name her for you." You see, my mother was trying to sell me to him. And she succeeded to an extent. But my father was still disappointed that he did not have a son. My brother finally came, but my mother had problems. She was quite a strong woman, from the mountains in central France. But soon after my brother came she contracted Spanish influenza; it was all over Europe at the time, in 1918. She recovered, but not totally. She contracted emphysema as well. She remained ill the rest of her life. After that, maybe their sex life was not quite the same, not as it had been. It was then that my father looked at other women, looked. His behavior became very, very childish. Immature. Not childish, but immature. After the war, the First World War, he was desperately trying to find peace, and women were his way of doing so.

DK: How old were you when you came to America?

LB: I was twenty-six.

DK: Why did you come?

LB: I came because I was married.

DK: Why did you like Robert?

LB: The fact is that Robert had some attraction to me because he could put my father in his place. Robert was the only person who ever could. My father had this strange humor. He would tell these stories that he thought were funny. But at the end of the story Robert would say, "Is that supposed to be funny?" My father literally fell apart. He didn't know what had happened. Robert was really effective.

DK: You had three sons with Robert.

LB: Right. The marriage did work. Right. But Robert did not want any children. He used to say, "You have me." He was actually bothered. And then as soon as my sons came, I lost interest, and he picked up—he took care of the children. He was a very tender father. Men are strange. I'm supposed to be the one to be tender, but he was the one. You really don't need children. God knows, the world didn't need more children.

DK: But family is so important to your art. How did having children affect your art? Were you making art during the time you were having children?

LB: Oh, definitely. Because I felt that I did not deserve the children, that they were a privilege. And the art was a privilege also. Art is a privilege, a blessing, a relief. Privilege means that you are a favorite, that what you do is not completely to your credit, not completely due to you, but is a favor conferred upon you. Privilege entitles you when you deserve nothing. Privilege is something you have and others don't. Art was a privilege given to me, and I had to pursue it, even more than the privilege of having children. The whole art mechanism is the result of many privileges, and it was a privilege to be part of it.

DK: So you had to keep making art to prove your privilege, to live up to it?

LB: Absolutely. The privilege was the access to the unconscious. It is a fantastic privilege to have access to the unconscious. I had to be worthy of this privilege, and to exercise it. It was a privilege also to be able to sublimate. You have to learn to sublimate. A lot of people cannot sublimate. They have no access to their unconscious. There is something very special in being able to sublimate your unconscious, and something very painful in the access to it. But there is no escape from it, and no escape from access once it is given to you, once you are favored with it, whether you want it or not.

DK: Is your sublimation of your unconscious— of which you seem very conscious— into art an escape?

LB: Absolutely. To escape you have to have a place to go. You have to have the courage to face risk. You have to have independence. All these things are gifts. They are blessings.

Sublimation is a gift; lots of people cannot sublimate. The life of the artist is basically a denial of sex. I really think my power of sublimation, my power of total recall, is due to the education my parents gave me—the discipline, and also the notion of what you can expect. Today I see people who have expectations—you have a poor kid out of engineering school who thinks to himself, "What does Donald Trump have over me? What does he have that I don't have?" This is absolutely ridiculous.

DK: You had three sons. Your mother had three daughters. Do you have any thoughts about that?

LB: Yes, of course. Everything comes back in time, but in a different way. I want to show you a sculpture that is based on that idea. It is called *Clouds and Caverns*. It is a five-sided world, a little world built up of five facets.

DK: *Are you saying that it is your family world, and your parents'* *family world? You and your husband had three sons; your parents and* *their three children.*

LB: Yes. And a pentagon, like married life, is completely uneventful, or at least my married life was. All my work is about the first pentagon, which is also the title of the work. The first pentagon is my family. But children do not like their parents; the wheel goes the other way around—the parents of course love their children, and the wheel, the momentum, goes in that direction only. Again, it's A who is interested in B, who's interested in C.

DK: *Let me change the topic. Let's talk about your current status in the* *New York art world. You must be aware of the fact that you have* *become an important symbol for many New York artists. You are an* *older artist who has finally had serious recognition, after great persis-* *tence. Your tenacity, as you call it, has succeeded. And you are a* *woman artist, which has made your success even more important, even* *more necessary, to feminists. To many people, you are a beacon of hope* *in a dark, difficult, male-chauvinist art world.*

LB: I am totally unaware of that, of any of it.

DK: *Certainly you must be aware of your own struggle for recognition;* *you must have some feelings about it. You must remember the crowds* *of women artists who came to the opening of your retrospective at the* *Museum of Modern Art, who celebrated you. You have become a* *symbol like Georgia O'Keeffe. Your work has been called a "rallying* *point" for feminist artists. Even if you are not aware of this, how do* *you respond to the idea of it? Are you a feminist? What do you think of* *feminism in the art world? How do you respond to the idea of being an* *important woman artist?*

LB: Well, I don't think it is particularly flattering.

DK: *This surprises me. You don't find it flattering to become an important symbol of a breakthrough for women artists?*

LB: Not at all flattering. Since it took me so long to prove my point, my importance, I can hardly be flattered that I am at last recognized. It doesn't matter to me.

DK: *Didn't you feel neglected over the years? Didn't you feel the Museum of Modern Art exhibition was vindication for your long career?*

LB: Not at all. No, no, no. I did not feel neglected. I just worked. I am happy about my success only because it has brought me to the attention of the younger generation. Only the younger generation likes me and understands me. I want to speak to the younger generation. My own generation is indifferent, as I am to it.

DK: *What about your position as a woman artist? Do you have any thoughts about feminism, particularly in the art world?*
The feminist aspects of your work were pointed out long ago. As early as 1947, in response to your second one-person show at Norlyst Gallery, a critic wrote, quite accurately: "Hers is a world of women. Blithely they emerge from chimneys, or, terrified, they watch from beds as curtains fly from a nightmare window. A whole family of females proves their domesticity by having houses for heads."

LB: I don't feel I have suffered more than any other artist. Man is a wolf to man, you know. That is a general truth. It exists in the art world, like everywhere else.
But feminism is important to me. *The Blind Leading the Blind* is a piece that brings me to the feminist cause. Another, which is very close, is C.O.Y.O.T.E., which was the name of the prostitutes' group. All they can do is hold on to each other. Individually, they couldn't even stand on their feet, but holding on to each other, they make it. It's also a comment on failures, on shortcomings, on being disabled. They huddle together, and through their positive attitude toward each other they summon the energy nec-

70

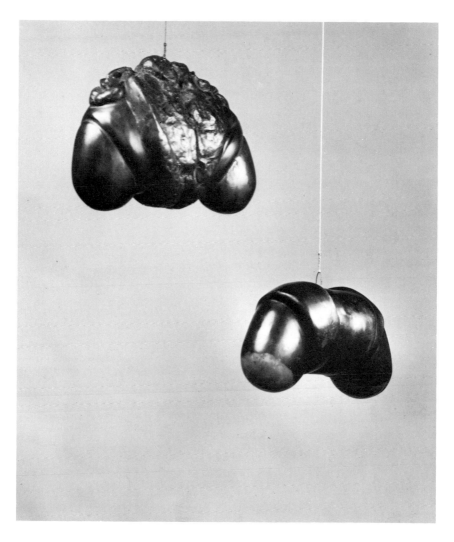

Janus Fleuri, 1968 (left).
Bronze; 10⅛″ x 12½″ x 8⅜″.
Private collection.
Courtesy Robert Miller Gallery, New York.
Photo: Allan Finkelman.

Janus, 1967 (right).
Bronze; 11″ long.
Private collection.
Courtesy Robert Miller Gallery, New York.
Photo: Allan Finkelman.

essary to stand against the world. They conquer their fear enough to finally express themselves and be what they are.

My feminism expresses itself in an intense interest in what women do. But I'm a complete loner. It doesn't help me to associate with people; it really doesn't help me. What helps me is to realize my own disabilities and to expose them. Another very sad statement is that I truly like only the people who help me. It is a very, very sad statement.

DK: But you don't feel there is any special prejudice against women artists?

LB: No. Many artists have been ignored. This is the problem. To be ignored is not the same as to be discriminated against. I don't think many are discriminated against, but many are certainly ignored. It is part of the situation of man being a wolf to man; it is part of the way man is a wolf to man.

DK: So you don't feel you have been discriminated against because you are a woman?

LB: No, I don't. I feel that I have been completely ignored, and that is the fate of many. But it is nobody's fault. It is the condition of the world.

DK: You don't feel it has anything to do with the art system? Why do you feel you were completely ignored, if not because of the art system?

LB: I was ignored because nobody showed me then. It is part of the indifference of the system, but that is true of every system, which favors only the few. But my work is still there.

DK: I want to persist: why do you think nobody showed you then?

LB: It has to do with success. As the saying goes, nothing succeeds like success. Unless you break into what is called success, you simply don't exist. People are not going to hurt you, at least not deliberately; they are going to ignore you unless you have success. What success means is not always clear, but everyone knows when you have it. After you have success, you have wonderful friends, and everything is very nice, but it changes nothing.

DK: *Are you saying that these people who flock to you because you are famous are not your real friends?*

LB: No, of course not. My real friends are the people who helped me to come to success.

DK: *When you started making your work, didn't you have success in mind? Didn't you want success? Didn't you want people to approve of your work, which is one definition of success?*

LB: No. I did not make my work for everybody, perhaps not for anybody. I made my art as a means of survival. It was a basic necessity for me.

DK: *You were really not interested in success?*

LB: No, I was not. That is why I have lasted so long. I have ridden out my success because it was not really the purpose of my work to be successful. My work will outlive its success, be more enduring and stronger than success. I was never disappointed when I never had success, which is why I never destroyed any of my work. Many artists destroy their work not because it is bad, but because it is not successful—because other people aren't interested in it, because other people don't attend to it. When the dealers finally began to look me up, finally came to me, all my work was there. It was on the shelves. I will admit that I now take better care of it than I did. I used to just let it sit, untouched, gathering dust. I have a cannibalistic attitude to my work. I would let it sit until I could use it to make new work. It had to reach a certain state of familiarity. Then I could incorporate it in a new work. I had already worked on it, and this prepared it to be worked on further, once I had assimilated it, digested what I myself had done.

DK: *I was speaking to someone the other day, a well-known artist, who remembered that you had an exhibition in the forties, just after the war. He said it was a stunning exhibition, and everyone said so. He said it was in fact the most marvelous exhibition he had seen at the time, and for some time afterward. That was success, but it seemed to have disappeared until relatively recently. Did that success affect you? Did it encourage you?*

LB: Yes, it was the show at Norlyst Gallery. It was in 1946 or 1947. Some artists noticed it.

DK: *What happened after the show? What was its effect on you?*

LB: What happened is that today those objects are very valuable. But then, after the show, they disappeared. They went underground for many years. Nothing changed. I did not change.

DK: *When was your next show?*

LB: It was in 1948, at Peridot Gallery.

DK: *So you had a certain number of shows in the 1940s. You were not entirely neglected. You were visible, even regularly visible. You were known. You cannot say you were neglected. Perhaps that is why the woman's issue does not interest you. What was the critical reception to your shows?*

LB: It was mild and it was not discouraging. But the work was not taken seriously; it was neutrally accepted. To really be noticed, you have to put out a fantastic amount of time and energy into entertaining and cultivating other people. Maybe I didn't have that energy. Maybe it was not my motivation to be really noticed, to be taken so seriously by the art world. Maybe I did not want to be processed by it.

DK: *The fact remains, you were regularly shown, and it seems to have had nothing to do with your being a woman. Nobody seems to have identified your art as explicitly woman's art. Did you sell any works?*

LB: Alfred Barr bought one work, the *Sleeping Figure*.

DK: *What year was that?*

LB: That was 1951.

DK: *So you have at least one work in the Museum of Modern Art's collection. Did they buy any other work?*

LB: Not in the fifties. It was after the Pompidou in Paris bought work. But I now have about seven works in the Museum of Modern Art collections.

DK: *Were there sales in the years in between? What happened?*

LB: I worked by myself.

DK: *You worked resolutely by yourself.*

LB: Absolutely. It did not matter if I sold or did not.

DK: *But you had exhibitions.*

LB: Yes. I had pieces at Betty Parsons's Gallery. I had exhibitions with the Stable Gallery. At the time, Leo Castelli was supporting the Stable Gallery, was paying the rent. I stayed with the Stable Gallery through the time Warhol started, and Robert Indiana, and Twombly. That was the period, the particular period. The director, Eleanor Wood, showed me. She was a nice person. I do not quarrel with the galleries.

DK: *But all that time, for over twenty years, not a museum purchased your work. You were outside the money system.*

LB: It is generally true. I do not recall the details, but it was generally true. But it did not affect the evolution of my work.

DK: *And you never thought that it had anything to do with your being a woman artist, even with the advantage of your being French?*

LB: No. But I have a strange feeling. I am not sure that I should speak of it here. I think I know why the Museum of Modern Art did not buy my work. The truth is very difficult to speak of. There was a certain style of collecting at the Modern which had to do with . . . I think I should watch my words.

DK: *Why? Don't watch your words. You have lived long enough to tell the truth.*

LB: Well, it had to do with the trustees, with pleasing the trustees. Alfred Barr was not a trustee; he was an employee, like all the rest. The trustees had real buying power. Alfred Barr had special skills, but he was not part of the Board of Trustees. He was on the other side. The artists who succeeded in selling at the time—Calder, Mark Rothko, Ben Shahn, they were the three—pleased the trustees. You had to entertain the Board, and these Three Stooges knew how to do that, knew how to socially entertain these important people, these trustees. I did not mind that, as a woman, but I could not do it.

Women had to work like slaves in the art world, but a lot of men got to the top through their charm. And it hurt them. To be young and pretty didn't help a woman in the art world, because the social scene, and the buying scene, was in the hands of women —women who had money. They wanted to be entertained—they were very lazy and sometimes stupid, and they wanted to be entertained by men of a certain age. So these charmers were what was called in the eighteenth century a *pique-assiette* in French, somebody who picks at your plate, who will come entertain for dinner, like a buffoon—it is a kind of profession that interests me very much. And they are picked from among artists because there is a certain prestige to being an artist, but from a professional point of view they are more entertainers than artists. They relate to the storyteller, which was a profession. The storytellers of the Middle Ages were men who went from place to place, telling their tales, and sometimes reached the top because of their acting and verbal abilities.

Because of the profession and personality of my husband, I lived among these people. It was interesting. And because I was French and kind of discreet, they tolerated me—with my accent I was a little strange, I was not competition—and I was cute, I guess. They took me seriously, on a certain level, but they refused to help me professionally. The trustees of the Museum of Modern Art were not interested in a young woman coming from Paris. They were not flattered by her attention. They were not interested in her three children. I was definitely not socially needed then. They wanted male artists, and they wanted male artists who did not say that they were married. They wanted male artists who would come alone and be their charming guests. Rothko could be very charming. It was a court. And the artist buffoons came to the court to entertain, to charm.

Now it has changed, now the younger men are in—older women and younger men.

DK: These artists, then, played the role of courtiers, which you could not play. That is how they sold their works to the museum. It had nothing to do with the quality of the works even though the works may have had quality.

LB: Absolutely. And you will notice that the buffoons were never women.

DK: *So being a woman had something to do with your difficulties in selling and getting recognition?*

LB: I could write a book about this period. Now, in this respect, I am a little bit of a feminist. But it is subtle. I was still not discriminated against. I would not call it that. I was not openly rejected. I was there, on the scene, but by accident, as it were. I was simply not suitable to these situations, and so in a sense invisible.

DK: *Why do you think the Museum of Modern Art finally gave you a retrospective exhibition?*

LB: It had to do with one person, that wonderful, wonderful woman, Deborah Wye. She worked very, very hard. She convinced them, she got all the information, she cleared up many of the dates of the works, she convinced them that I was important.

DK: *Was this time—if I recall correctly, it was in the early eighties—an appropriate moment for recognition for you? It was certainly an important event in the women's art movement, and in general an important victory for feminism.*

LB: I was very pleased by it personally.

DK: *How old were you at the time?*

LB: I was in my seventies.

DK: *All those years in limbo. Was the Modern's exhibition your first major retrospective? Did you have any before, in France?*

LB: No. But there is a big retrospective being organized now in Germany, Holland, Switzerland and France for 1989.

DK: *Surely it must bother you a little bit, that you had to wait so long for full-fledged recognition, for recognition on that scale, for that matter on any scale. And that your native country was also indifferent.*

LB: Well, you have made me say it, with all your pressure, your persistence. I will say it. But it is true that men could be successful at the Museum of Modern Art, had the chance to be successful, but that I was not, that I was not even in the running, because I was a woman.

DK: *So women were, after all, shut out, in your perception?*

LB: They could not attend the court; they could not be courtiers. Of course, this spared them the fate of becoming buffoons. They did not have the opportunity to make fools of themselves, to be sycophants.

DK: *They had the privilege of being invisible.*

LB: Right. People didn't know they existed. They were ignored. The male artists were charmers. Rothko was a great charmer. Being the daughter of a charmer, I can spot one. I know when I see one.

DK: *Has William Rubin come to your studio?*

LB: Many times.

DK: *Really?*

LB: Yes, he has come many times. But I was not a charmer. John Graham was another charmer. There have always been a number of artist charmers. They always succeed.

DK: *You don't like them, do you?*

LB: I am indifferent. I am not terribly involved. I feel sorry for them. I am interested in the syndrome of the charmer, which is pervasive in the art world, but I am basically not involved. But the syndrome of the charmer has to be exorcised; it interferes with art making, it corrupts the art world and, perhaps inadvertently, it confuses.

DK: *I recall some psychoanalyst once writing that people who are able to maintain their charm in the face of great anxiety are not to be trusted. Are you suggesting the charmers are not to be trusted?*

LB: Many of them are good artists, but they are not to be emotionally trusted. And they are all men. They will betray you sooner or later. I could give you a list of famous artists who were charmers, at least a dozen, much of whose success depended on their charm. Brancusi was one, for example. So was Calder.

DK: *Do you think these artists made a point of being charming in order to succeed in the art world?*

LB: I am not talking about artists. They may call themselves artists, but I am talking about men who made it in the art world. What is important for making it is that they are men and charming, not that they are artists.

DK: *Is that what it finally takes to make it in the art world?*

LB: I am not sure. But I respect their charm, the presence it gives them. I notice their charm more than their work. Nobody in the art world is really interested in a woman's charm. It is the opposite of the larger world, where women must be charming and beautiful. But that is a way of not taking them seriously. Whereas it makes us take men more seriously, because we do not expect them to be really charming. Who can be seriously interested in a beautiful woman, after the first look? It is absurd. But an artist, let's say like a Léger, may be a peasant, but if he has charm, all is forgiven; he has a certain social presence, charisma.

DK: I'd like to ask you a few last questions about your art. You have spoken of it as encompassing the whole history of art, but I wonder if you have any special consciousness of modern art. What do you think about modern art in general, if you want to talk about it generally? How do you see yourself in the history of modern art?

LB: I am not interested in art history, in the academies of styles, a succession of fads. Art is not about art. Art is about life, and that sums it up. This remark is made to the whole academy of artists who have attempted to derive the art of the late eighties, to try to relate it to the study of the history of art, which has nothing to do with art. It has to do with appropriation. It has to do with the attempt to prove that you can do better than the next one, and that a famous art history teacher is better than the common artist. If you are a historian, you have to have the dignity of a historian. You don't have to prove that you are better than the artist.

But I can say this. I studied in Paris in the thirties at a time when artists had ateliers that were open to students. My favorite teachers among many were Fernand Léger, Othon Friesz and Paul Colin. Michèle Leiris and André Breton were also part of my education. Also, I taught for a long time and was given many honorary doctorates. Flattering as it is, it has little to do with my ongoing self-expression. Also, I valued my friendships with Corbusier, Duchamp, and Miró, Arp, Brancusi and Franz Kline and Warhol. Today I value my friendships with Robert Mapplethorpe and Gary Indiana.

DK: Which artists do you like?

LB: I like Francis Bacon best, because Francis Bacon has terrific problems, and he knows that he is not going to solve them, but he knows also that he can escape from day to day and stay alive, and he does that because his work gives him a kick. And also, Bacon is not self-indulgent. Some people will say, "What do you mean by that? He always paints the same picture." That's true—he always paints the same picture, because he is driven. But he is not self-indulgent. Never.

DK: Apart from your history of involvement with modern artists, what does modern art as such mean to you?

LB: What modern art means is that you have to keep finding new ways to express yourself, to express the problems, that there are no settled ways, no fixed approach. This is a painful situation, and modern art is about this painful situation of having no absolutely definite way of expressing yourself. This is why modern art will continue, because this condition remains; it is the modern human condition.

DK: Do you feel modern art has a special relationship to the painful difficulty of self-expression in the modern world?

LB: Definitely. It is about the hurt of not being able to express yourself properly, to express your intimate relations, your unconscious, to trust the world enough to express yourself directly in it. It is about trying to be sane in this situation, of being tentatively and temporarily sane by expressing yourself. All art comes from terrific failures and terrific needs that we have. It is about the difficulty of being a self because one is neglected. Everywhere in the modern world there is neglect, the need to be recognized, which is not satisfied. Art is a way of recognizing oneself, which is why it will always be modern.

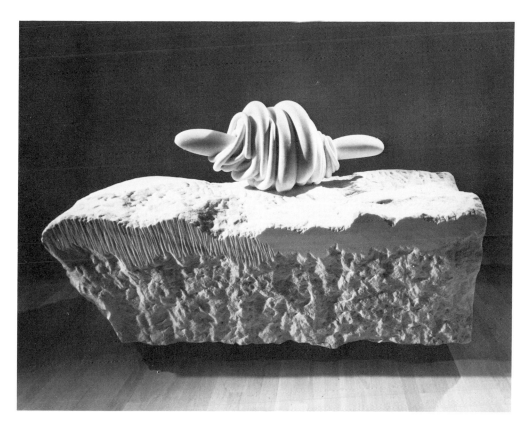

Nᴀᴛᴜʀᴇ Sᴛᴜᴅʏ, 1986.
Marble; 35″ x 61″ x 29″.
Courtesy Robert Miller Gallery, New York.
Photo: Allan Finkelman.

APPENDIX

SOLO EXHIBITIONS

1947   Norlyst Gallery, New York.

1949/50   Peridot Gallery, New York.

1953   Peridot Gallery, New York.
Allan Frumkin Gallery, Chicago.

1959   White Art Museum, Cornell University, Ithaca, New York.

1964   Rose Fried Gallery, New York.
Stable Gallery, New York.

1974   112 Greene Street, New York.

1978   Xavier Fourcade Gallery, New York.
Hamilton Gallery, New York.

1979   Xavier Fourcade Gallery, New York: "Louise Bourgeois Sculpture 1941–1953 plus one new piece."
University of California, Berkeley Art Museum.

1980   Xavier Fourcade Gallery, New York: "Louise Bourgeois Sculpture: The Middle Years 1955–1970."
Max Hutchinson Gallery, New York: "The Iconography of Louise Bourgeois."

1981   Renaissance Society at the University of Chicago: "Louise Bourgeois: Femme Maison."

1982   Robert Miller Gallery, New York.

1982/83   Museum of Modern Art, New York: "Louise Bourgeois: Retrospective"; traveled to Contemporary Arts

Museum, Houston; Museum of Contemporary Art, Chicago; Akron Art Museum, Akron, Ohio.

1984 Daniel Weinberg Gallery, Los Angeles.
Daniel Weinberg Gallery, San Francisco.
Robert Miller Gallery, New York.

1985 Serpentine Gallery, London.
Galerie Maeght Lelong, Zurich.
Galerie Maeght Lelong, Paris: "Louise Bourgeois: Retrospective 1947–1984."

1986 *Eyes,* Doris Freedman Plaza, New York.
Robert Miller Gallery, New York.
Texas Gallery, Houston: "Louise Bourgeois: Sculptures & Drawings."

1987 Robert Miller Gallery, New York: "Paintings from the 1940s."
Yares Gallery, Scottsdale, Arizona.
The Taft Museum, Cincinnati: "Louise Bourgeois"; three-year traveling tour.
The Art Museum of Florida International University, Miami: "The Louise Bourgeois Exhibition."
Gallery Paule Anglim, San Francisco: "Sculpture 1947–1955."
Janet Steinberg Gallery, San Francisco: "Paintings & Drawings."

1988 Robert Miller Gallery, New York: "Louise Bourgeois Drawings 1939–1987."
Museum Overholland, Amsterdam: "Drawings 1939–1987."

GROUP EXHIBITIONS

1943   Metropolitan Museum of Art, New York.
        Museum of Modern Art, New York.

1944   San Francisco Museum of Art, San Francisco.

1945   Whitney Museum of American Art, New York.
        Los Angeles County Museum of Art, Los Angeles.
        Art of This Century Gallery, New York.
        Curt Valentin Gallery, New York.

1946   Whitney Museum of American Art, New York.

1948   Brooklyn Museum, Brooklyn, New York.

1949   Museum of Modern Art, New York.

1951   Museum of Modern Art, New York.

1953   Whitney Museum of American Art, New York.

1954   Walker Art Center, Minneapolis.

1955   Whitney Museum of American Art, New York.

1957   Whitney Museum of American Art, New York.

1958   Allen Memorial Art Museum, Oberlin, Ohio.

1960   Dallas Museum of Art, Dallas.
        Allan Frumkin Gallery, New York.
        Claude Bernard Gallery, Paris.
        Whitney Museum of American Art, New York.

1962   Whitney Museum of American Art, New York.
        Museum of Modern Art, New York.

1963 Whitney Museum of American Art, New York.

1965 Musée Rodin, Paris.

1966 Rhode Island School of Design, Providence.

1968 Whitney Museum of American Art, New York.

1969 La Jeune Sculpture, Paris.
La Biennale di Carrara, Carrara, Italy.

1970 Knoedler Gallery, New York.
Whitney Museum of American Art, New York.

1973 Storm King Art Center, Mountainville, New York.

1974 Sculpture Now, Inc., New York.

1976 New Orleans Museum of Art, New Orleans.
Whitney Museum of American Art, New York.

1977 Rose Art Museum, Brandeis University, Waltham, Massachusetts.

1979 Marion Locks Gallery, Philadelphia: "In Small Scale."
Hamilton Gallery, New York: "Gallery Artists."
112 Gallery, New York: "Artists Against Nuclear Power Plants."

1980 Graham Gallery, New York: "Originals."
Helen Serger, La Boetie, Inc., New York: "Pioneering Women Artists 1900–1940."
Art Expo 180, New York Coliseum: "Sculpture at the Coliseum."
Max Hutchinson Gallery, New York: "10 Abstract Sculptures: American and European 1940–1980."
Neuberger Museum of the State University of New York at Purchase: "Hidden Desires."
Frank Marino Gallery, New York: "Heresies Benefit."
Henry Street Settlement, New York: "Exchanges II."
Grey Art Gallery and Study Center, New York University, New York: "Perceiving Modern Sculpture: Selections for the Sighted and Non-Sighted."
Xavier Fourcade, New York: "One Major New Work Each."

Xavier Fourcade, New York: "Small-Scale Paintings, Drawings, Sculpture."

1981 Westbeth Gallery, New York: "Voices Expressing What Is."

Max Hutchinson Gallery, New York: "Sculptors and Their Drawings."

Grey Art Gallery and Study Center, New York University, New York: "Permanent Collection Installation."

Drawing Center, New York: "Sculptor's Drawings."

Marisa del Re Gallery, New York: "Sculptures and Their Related Drawings."

Whitney Museum of American Art, New York: "Decade of Transition: 1940–1950."

Grey Art Gallery, New York University, New York: "Heresies Benefit Exhibition."

Robert Miller Gallery, New York: "Summer Exhibition 1981."

Xavier Fourcade, Inc., New York: "Sculpture."

Stamford Museum, Stamford, Connecticut: "Classical Americans."

Oscarsson-Hood Gallery, New York: "The New Spiritualism: Transcendent Images in Painting and Sculpture"; traveled to Jorgensen Gallery, University of Connecticut, Storrs; Robert Hull Fleming Museum, University of Vermont, Burlington.

Forum Gallery, New York: "Sculpture in Wood and Stone."

Institute for Art and Urban Resources at P.S. 1, Long Island City, New York: "Figuratively Sculpting."

Zabriskie Gallery, New York: "Art for ERA."

Graham Gallery, New York.

1981/82 Sewall Art Gallery, Rice University, Houston: "Variants: Drawings by Contemporary Sculptors"; traveled to Art Museum of South Texas, Corpus Christi; Newcomb Gallery, Tulane University, New Orleans; the High Museum of Art, Atlanta.

1982   Marisa del Re Gallery, New York: "Selected Works on Paper II."

Montclair State College, College Art Gallery, Upper Montclair, New Jersey: "Visiting Artist Invitational."

Harcus Krakow Gallery, Boston.

Robert Miller Gallery, New York: "Landscapes."

Fuller Goldeen Gallery, San Francisco: "Casting: A Survey of Cast Metal Sculpture in the 80's."

San Francisco Museum of Modern Art, San Francisco: "Twenty American Artists: Sculpture 1982."

Roger Litz Gallery, New York: "The Erotic Impulse."

Contemporary Arts Center, New Orleans: "The Human Figure."

Sculpture Center, New York: "Houses."

1983   Daniel Weinberg Gallery, Los Angeles: "Drawing Conclusions: A Survey of American Drawings: 1958–1983."

Philadelphia College of Art, Philadelphia: "Artists in the Historical Archives of the Women's Interart Center of New York City."

Whitney Museum of American Art, New York: "1983 Whitney Museum Biennial Exhibition."

McIntosh/Drysdale Gallery, Houston: "Small Bronze."

Whitney Museum of American Art at Philip Morris, New York: "Twentieth-Century Sculpture: Process and Presence."

Wave Hill, Bronx, New York: "Bronzes."

American Academy and Institute of Arts and Letters, New York: "Works by Newly Elected Members and Recipients of Honors and Awards."

Renaissance Society, Chicago: "The Sixth Day."

Robert Miller Gallery, New York: "Surreal."

Jersey City Museum, New Jersey: "Selected Drawings."

Bethune Gallery, State University of New York at Buffalo: "Portrait Sculpture: Contemporary Points of View."

Susanne Hilberry Gallery, Birmingham, Michigan: "Drawings."

Fayerweather Gallery, University of Virginia, Charlottesville: "Sensuous Art."

1983/84 International Sculpture Center, New York: "Bronze at Washington Square."

1984 Fayerweather Gallery, University of Virginia, Charlottesville: "Excating Clouds, Dismantling Silence."

Paula Cooper, Inc., New York: "Artists Call, Benefit Exhibition."

Archer M. Huntington Art Gallery, The University of Texas at Austin: "New American Painting: A Tribute to James and Mari Michener."

Tracey Garet Gallery, New York: "Drawings."

University of South Florida Art Galleries, Tampa: "Humanism: An Undercurrent."

Sidney Janis Gallery, New York: "American Women Artists (Part I: 20th-Century Pioneers)."

Hill Gallery, Birmingham, Michigan: "Sculpture."

Parrish Art Museum, Southampton, New York: "Forming."

Rutgers University, New Brunswick, New Jersey: "Women Artists Series."

White Columns, New York: "Bunnies."

Holly Solomon Gallery, New York: "The Innovative Landscape: New Approaches to an Old Tradition."

Ronald Feldman Fine Arts, New York: "Socialites & Satellites."

Weatherspoon Art Gallery, University of North Carolina, Greensboro: "An Other Vision: Selected Works by Women Artists in the Weatherspoon Collection."

Parrish Art Museum, Southampton, New York: "Forming."

Monique Knowlton Gallery, New York: "Ecstasy."

Galerie Maeght Lelong, New York: "Sculpture on a Small Scale."

Laforet Museum, Tokyo: "Correspondences: New York Choice 84."

Blum Helman, New York: "Drawings."

1984/85   Hirshhorn Museum, Washington, D.C.: "Content: A Contemporary Focus, 1974–1984."

Whitney Museum of American Art, New York: "The Third Dimension: Sculpture of the New York School."

The Museum of Modern Art, New York: "Primitivism."

1984/86   Sonoma State University, Rohnert Park, California: "Works in Bronze: A Modern Survey"; traveled to Redding Museum and Art Center, California; Palm Springs Desert Museum, California; Boise Gallery of Art, Idaho; Cheney Cowles Memorial Museum, Spokane, Washington; University Art Gallery, California State University, Stanislaus; University of California, Santa Cruz.

1985   Hill Gallery, Birmingham, Michigan: "Sense and Sensibility."

Philadelphia Art Alliance, Pennsylvania: "Forms in Wood: American Sculpture of the 1950s."

Robert Miller Gallery, New York: "Works on Paper."

Whitney Museum of American Art, Stamford, Connecticut: "Affiliations: Recent Sculpture and Its Antecedents."

Larry Gagosian Gallery, Los Angeles: "Actual Size: "An Exhibition of Small Paintings and Sculptures."

Galerie Maeght Lelong, New York: "20th-Century Master Prints."

Contemporary Arts Center, Cincinnati: "Body and Soul: Aspects of Recent Figurative Sculpture."

University of Pittsburgh Gallery, Pittsburgh: "Sculpture by Women in the Eighties."

Weatherspoon Art Gallery, University of North Carolina, Greensboro: "Art on Paper 1985."

New York Studio School of Drawing, Painting and Sculpture: "Ontogeny: "Sculpture and Painting by 20th-Century American Sculptors."

Fay Gold Gallery, Atlanta: "20th-Century Masters."

1985/86   Museum of Art, Fort Lauderdale: "An American Renaissance: Painting and Sculpture Since 1940."

Stamford Museum and Nature Center, Stamford, Connecticut: "American Art: American Women."

Temple Gallery, Tyler School of Art, Philadelphia: "Small Monuments."

Kunsthaus, Zurich: "Traces: Sculpture and Monuments."

1986   Nohra Haime Gallery, New York: "Drawings by Sculptors."

The Mendik Company, New York: "Universal Images—People and Nature in Sculpture."

Galeries Contemporaines, Centre Georges Pompidou, Paris.

Los Angeles Museum of Contemporary Art, Los Angeles: "Individual: A Selected History of Contemporary Art 1945–1986."

Arnold Herstand Gallery, New York: "American Sculpture—A Selection."

Pictogram Gallery, New York: "Odd and Intense."

Centro Cultural de Arte Contemporáneo, Mexico City.

Cheney Cowles Memorial Museum, Spokane, Washington: "Works in Bronze: A Modern Survey."

Robert Miller Gallery, New York: "Summer Group Show."

Sierra Nevada Museum of Art, Reno, Nevada: "Works in Bronze—A Modern Survey."

Dolan/Maxwell Gallery, Philadelphia: "Avery, Bourgeois, Hayter: Atelier 17 in 1947."

Temple Gallery, Tyler School of Art, Philadelphia: "Body Electric: Four Currents."

Freedman Gallery, Reading, Pennsylvania: "The Freedman Gallery: The First Decade."

1986/87   Carlo Lamagna Gallery, New York: "Traps."

Bernice Steinbaum Gallery, New York: "Elders of the Tribe."

Galerie Maeght Lelong, Zurich: "The Draughtman's Eye."

1987   Art Advisory Service Exhibition, A Project of the Associate Council, The Museum of Modern Art, New York, Loaned to General Electric Company: "Black and White."

Whitney Biennial, New York, Spring 1987.

Ein Ausstellungsprojekt Zeitgenössischer Kunst in der Psychiatrischen Klinik der Universität Mainz (Germany): "Von Chaos und Ordnung der Seele."

Kunstmuseum Lucerne: "L'Etat des Choses I."

Kent Fine Art, New York: "Assemblage."

Galerie Maeght Lelong, New York: "Group Show."

Blum Helman, New York: "Sculptors' Drawings."

Paris–New York–Kent Fine Art, Kent, Connecticut: "22 Artists: The Friends of Louise Tolliver Deutschman."

CIAC Montreal International Centre of Contemporary Art, Montreal: "The 100 Days of Contemporary Art of Montreal 1987: Stations."

M-13 Gallery, New York: "Lust One of the Seven Deadlies."

Siegeltuch Gallery, New York: "Black."

Zabriskie Gallery, New York: "Sculpture from Surrealism."

Iannetti-Lanzone Gallery, San Francisco: "After Pollock: Three Decades of Diversity."

Musée Cantonal des Beaux-Arts, Lausanne: "La Femme et le Surrealisme."

Grossman Gallery, School of the Museum of Fine Arts, Boston: "Undercurrents: Rituals and Translations."

Edith C. Blum Art Institute, The Bard College Center, Annandale-on-Hudson, New York: "Process and Product: The Making of a Contemporary Masterwork."

Kemper Gallery, Kansas City Art Institute, Missouri: "Drawn Out: An Exhibition of Drawings by Contemporary Artists."

Sander Gallery, New York: "Boundaries: Works on Paper."

George Dalsheimer Gallery, Baltimore: "Contemporary Sculpture."

Galerie Maeght Lelong, New York: "Sculpture."

Pat Hearn Gallery, New York: "Sculpture."

Harcus Gallery, Boston: "In Defense of Sacred Lands."

1988 Barbara Mathes Gallery, New York: "Sculptors' Drawings: 1883–1965."

New York Studio School, New York: "The New Sculptor Group—A Look Back: 1957–1962."

Greenville County Museum of Art, North Carolina: "Just Like a Woman."

Whitney Museum of Fairfield County, Connecticut: "Enduring Creativity."

Museum of Modern Art, New York: "Committed to Print."

Whitney Museum of American Art, New York: "Vital Signs."

The Queensborough Community College of the City University of New York: "The Politics of Gender."

COLLECTIONS

Albright-Knox Art Gallery, Buffalo.
Australian National Gallery, Canberra.
Denver Art Museum, Denver.
Detroit Institute of the Arts, Detroit.
Kunstmuseum Luzern, Lucerne.
Metropolitan Museum of Art, New York.
Musée d'Art Moderne, Paris.
Museum of Fine Arts, Houston.
Museum of Modern Art, New York.
New Orleans Museum of Art, New Orleans.
New York University, New York.
Portland Museum of Art, Portland, Maine.
The Rhode Island School of Design, Providence.
Storm King Art Center, Mountainville, New York.
Whitney Museum of American Art, New York.

SELECTED BIBLIOGRAPHY

PERIODICALS

R(eed), J(udith) K. "Exhibition review, Bertha Schaefer Gallery." *Art Digest,* June 1945, p. 31.

"Exhibition review, Bertha Schaefer Gallery." *Art News,* June 1945, p. 30.

Devree, Howard. "Exhibition review, Bertha Schaefer Gallery." *The New York Times,* June 10, 1945, sec. 2, p. 2.

"Exhibition review, Bertha Schaefer Gallery." *New York Herald Tribune,* June 10, 1945.

"Exhibition review, Norlyst Gallery." *New York Sun,* October 31, 1947.

"Exhibition review, Norlyst Gallery." *Art News,* November 1947, p. 42.

"Exhibition review, Norlyst Gallery." *The New York Times,* November 2, 1947.

"Artists." *Magazine of Art* (New York), December 1948, p. 307.

Bewley, Marius. "An Introduction to Louise Bourgeois." *The Tiger's Eye* (New York), March 15, 1949, pp. 88–92.

G., M. "Debut as Sculptor at Peridot." *Art News,* October 1949, p. 46.

Preston, Stuart. "Exhibition review, Peridot Gallery." *The New York Times,* October 9, 1949, sec. 2, p. 9.

"Exhibition review, Peridot Gallery." *The New York Times,* October 9, 1949.

"Exhibition review, Peridot Gallery." *New York Sun,* October 14, 1949.

S(harp), M(arynell). "Telegraphic Constructions." *Art Digest,* October 15, 1949, p. 22.

The Tiger's Eye (New York), October 15, 1949, p. 52 (illus. only).

G., R. "Exhibition review, Peridot Gallery." *Art News,* October 1950, p. 48.

L(evy), P(esella). "Exhibition review, Peridot Gallery." *Art Digest,* October 1, 1950, p. 16.

Preston, Stuart. " 'Primitive' to Abstraction in Current Shows." *The New York Times,* October 8, 1950, sec. 2, p. 9.

Fitzsimmons, James. "Exhibition review, 'Recent Painting and Sculpture,' Peridot Gallery." *Art Digest,* May 1, 1952.

———. "Exhibition review, Peridot Gallery." *Arts and Architecture* (Los Angeles), April 1953, p. 35.

P(orter), F(airfield). "Exhibition review, Peridot Gallery." *Art News*, April 1953.

G(eist), S(idney). "Louise Bourgeois." *Art Digest*, April 1, 1953, p. 17.

Krasne, Belle. "10 Artists in the Margin." *Design Quarterly* (Minneapolis), no. 30, 1954, pp. 9–12.

Munro, Eleanor. "Explorations in Form." *Perspectives USA* (New York), Summer 1956, pp. 160–72.

Goldwater, Robert. "La Sculpture actuelle à New York." *Cimaise* (Paris), November–December 1956, pp. 24–28.

Hess, Thomas B. "Mutt Furioso." *Art News*, December 1956, pp. 22–25, 64–65.

M.J.R. "Whitney Annual." *Arts Magazine*, December 1956, p. 52.

Hess, Thomas B. "Inside Nature." *Art News*, February 1958, p. 63.

"Sculpture 1950–1958." *Oberlin College Bulletin* (Oberlin, Ohio), Winter 1958, p. 66.

Berckelaers, F. L. (Michael Seuphor). "Le Choix d'un critique." *Oeil* (Paris), January 1959, p. 28.

Ragon, Michel. "L'Art actuel aux Étas-Unis: Art Today in the United States." *Cimaise* (Paris), January–March 1959, pp. 6–35.

Pearlstein, Philip. "The Private Myth." *Art News*, September 1961, pp. 42–45, 62.

Oeri, Georgine. "À Propos of 'The Figure.' " *Quadrum: Revue Internationale d'Art Moderne* (Brussels), vol. 13, 1962, pp. 49–60.

E(dgar), N(atalie). "Exhibition review, Stable Gallery." *Art News*, January 1964, p. 10.

"Exhibition review, Stable Gallery." *New York Herald Tribune*, January 11, 1964.

Preston, Stuart. "Exhibition review, Stable Gallery." *The New York Times*, January 19, 1964, p. 23.

"Exhibition review, Stable and Fried Galleries." *New York Post*, January 26, 1964.

R., V. "Exhibition review, Stable Gallery." *Arts Magazine*, March 1964, p. 63.

Robbins, Daniel. "Sculpture by Louise Bourgeois." *Art International* (Lugano), October 20, 1964, pp. 29–31.

Oeri, Georgine. "The Object of Art." *Quadrum: Revue Internationale d'Art Moderne* (Brussels), vol. 16, 1964, pp. 14–15.

"Waldorf Panels 1 and 2 on Sculpture." *It Is* (New York), Autumn 1965, pp. 12–13.

Robbins, Daniel. "Recent Still Life." *Art in America*, January–February 1966, pp. 57–60.

Antin, David. "Another Category: 'Eccentric Abstraction.' " *Artforum*, November 1966, p. 56.

Ashton, Dore. "Marketing Techniques in the Promotion of Art." *Studio International* (London), November 1966, pp. 270–73.

B(ochner), M(el). "Eccentric Abstraction." *Arts Magazine*, November 1966, p. 58.

Lippard, Lucy R. "Eccentric Abstraction." *Art International* (Lugano), November 20, 1966, p. 28.

Andersen, Wayne. "American Sculpture: The Situation in the Fifties." *Artforum*, Summer 1967, pp. 60–67.

Bourgeois, Louise. "Fabric of Construction at MoMA." *Craft Horizons*, March–April 1969, pp. 30–35.

Rubin, William. "Some Reflections Prompted by the Recent Work of Louise Bourgeois." *Art International* (Lugano), April 20, 1969, pp. 17–20.

Bourgeois, Louise. *Art Now* (New York), September 1969.

Elsen, Albert. "Notes on the Partial Figure." *Artforum*, November 1969, pp. 58–63.

Art International (Lugano), February 1970, cover.

Glueck, Grace. "Women Artists Demonstrate at Whitney." *The New York Times*, December 12, 1970, p. A19. (Reprinted in *A Documentary Herstory*, New York: Women Artists in Revolution, 1971.)

Nochlin, Linda. "Why Have There Been No Great Women Artists?" *Art News*, January 1971, p. 37 (illus. only).

Nemser, Cindy. "Forum: Women in Art." *Arts Magazine*, February 1971, p. 18. (Reprinted in *A Documentary Herstory*, New York: Women Artists in Revolution, 1971.)

Marandel, J. Patrice. "Louise Bourgeois." *Art International* (Lugano), December 20, 1971, pp. 46–47.

Bourgeois, Louise. "Letter to the Editor." *Art in America*, January–February 1972, p. 123.

Alloway, Lawrence. "Art." *The Nation*, March 27, 1972, pp. 413–14.

Brumer, Miriam. "Organic Image: Women's Image?" *The Feminist Art Journal* (Brooklyn, New York), Spring 1973, pp. 12–13.

Seiberling, Dorothy. "The Female View of Erotica." *New York*, February 11, 1974, p. 54.

Andre, Michael. "Exhibition review, 112 Greene Street Gallery." *Art News*, February 1975, p. 100.

"Artists Talk on Art." *Women in the Arts Newsletter* (New York), February 1975.

Lippard, Lucy R. "Louise Bourgeois: From the Inside Out." *Artforum*, March 1975, pp. 26–33. (Reprinted in *From the Center: Feminist Essays on Art*, New York: Dutton, 1976.)

Sondheim, Alan. "Exhibition review, 112 Greene Street Gallery." *Arts Magazine,* March 1975, p. 23.

Baldwin, Carl R. "Louise Bourgeois: An Iconography of Abstraction." *Art in America,* March–April 1975, pp. 82–83.

Henry, Gerrit. "Views from the Studio." *Art News,* May 1976, pp. 32–36.

Alloway, Lawrence. "Women's Art in the '70's." *Art in America,* May–June 1976, pp. 64–72.

Robins, Corinne. "Louise Bourgeois: Primordial Environments." *Arts Magazine,* June 1976, pp. 81–82.

Bloch, Susi. "An Interview with Louise Bourgeois." *The Art Journal* (New York), Summer 1976, pp. 370–73.

Ratcliff, Carter. "Exhibition review, Nassau County Museum of Fine Arts." *Artforum,* October 1976, p. 63.

Duncan, Carol. "The Esthetics of Power in Modern Erotic Art." *Heresies* (New York), January 1977, pp. 46–53.

Kuspit, Donald. "New York Today: Some Artists Comment." *Art in America,* September–October 1977, p. 79.

"The Great Goddess Visuals." *Heresies* (New York), Spring 1978, p. 15.

Russell, John. "Exhibition review, Biv Gallery." *The New York Times,* June 9, 1978, p. C18.

"Louise Bourgeois at the Hamilton Gallery of Contemporary Art." *Art Now Gallery Guide* (New York), September 1978, p. 2.

Russell, John. "Exhibition review, Hamilton Gallery." *The New York Daily Metro,* September 22, 1978, p. 20.

Marandel, J. Patrice. "Louise Bourgeois." *Arts Magazine,* October 1978, p. 17.

Frank, Peter. *The Village Voice,* October 2, 1978, p. 121.

Poroner, Palmer. "Is Bourgeois Blossoming?" *Chelsea Clinton News* (New York), October 5, 1978, p. 16.

———. "Bourgeois' Special Chemistry." *Chelsea Clinton News* (New York), October 12, 1978, p. 12.

Ashbery, John. "Art/Anxious Architecture." *New York,* October 16, 1978, pp. 161–63.

Harnett, Lila. "Exhibition review, Hamilton and Fourcade Galleries." *Cue,* October 27, 1978, p. 20.

Zucker, Barbara. "Exhibition review, Xavier Fourcade and Hamilton Galleries." *Art News,* November 1978, pp. 177–79.

Ratcliff, Carter. "Making It in the Art World: A Climber's Guide" and "A Prejudiced Guide to the Art Market," *New York,* November 27, 1978, pp. 61–67, 68–71.

Gibson, Eric. "New York Letter: Louise Bourgeois." *Art International* (Lugano), November–December 1978, p. 67.

Ratcliff, Carter. "Louise Bourgeois." *Art International* (Lugano), November–December 1978, pp. 26–27.

Lippard, Lucy R. "Complexes: Architectural Sculpture in Nature." *Art in America,* January–February 1979, p. 87.

Munro, Eleanor. "The Rise of Louise Bourgeois." *Ms.,* July 1979, p. 65.

Pels, Marsha. "Louise Bourgeois: A Search for Gravity." *Art International* (Lugano), October 1979, pp. 46–54.

Russell, John. "Art: The Sculpture of Louise Bourgeois." *The New York Times,* October 5, 1979, p. C21.

Rickey, Carrie. "Louise Bourgeois, Xavier Fourcade Gallery." *Artforum,* December 1979, p. 72.

Gardner, Paul. "The Discreet Charm of Louise Bourgeois." *Art News,* February 1980, pp. 80–86.

Lorber, Richard. "Women Artists on Women in Art." *Portfolio,* February–March 1980, p. 72.

Ashton, Dore. "Exhibition review, Xavier Fourcade, Inc." *Artscanada* (Toronto), April–May 1980, p. 43.

Tallmer, Jerry. "An Intimate Life Goes on Show." *New York Post,* September 6, 1980, p. 30.

Larson, Kay. "Louise Bourgeois: Body Language Spoken Here." *The Village Voice,* September 24, 1980, p. 83.

———. "For the First Time Women Are Leading Not Following." *Art News,* October 1980, pp. 64–72.

Ratcliff, Carter. "Louise Bourgeois." *Vogue,* October 1980, p. 343.

Kramer, Hilton. "Art: Contrasts in Imagery, 2 Views of Louise Bourgeois." *The New York Times,* October 3, 1980, p. C29.

Tully, Judd. "Bourgeois' Marbles." *Art World* (New York), October 17–November 14, 1980, p. 1.

Cohen, Ronny H. "Louise Bourgeois, Max Hutchinson Gallery." *Artforum,* November 1980, p. 86.

Lawson, Thomas. "Exhibition review, Max Hutchinson Gallery." *Flash Art* (Milan), November 1980, p. 45.

"Exhibition review, Max Hutchinson Gallery and Xavier Fourcade, Inc." *Art News,* December 1980, p. 189.

Gardner, Paul. "Confessions of a Plantain Chip Eater; or, Artists Are Just Like the Rest of Us." *Art News,* January 1981, p. 138.

Ratcliff, Carter. "Louise Bourgeois at Max Hutchinson and Xavier Fourcade." *Art in America,* February 1981, p. 145.

Larson, Kay. "Louise Bourgeois: Her Re-emergence Feels Like a Discovery." *Art News,* May 1981, p. 77.

Kirshner, Judith Russi. "Exhibition review, Renaissance Society at the University of Chicago." *Artforum,* November 1981, p. 88.

"The Art Economist on Building on Solid Foundations." *The Art Economist,*
   November 22, 1981, pp. 2–3.
Lippard, Lucy R. "The Blind Leading the Blind." *Bulletin of the Detroit Institute
   of the Arts,* 1981, pp. 24–29.
"Engravings from 'He Disappeared into Complete Silence.' " *Harvard Advocate*
   (Cambridge, Mass.), Summer 1982, pp. 17–36.
Brenson, Michael. "Sculpture Takes on a Fresh Prominence." *The New York
   Times,* September 12, 1982, sec. 2, p. 33.
Fletcher, Florence. "Museum review." *New York,* September 20, 1982,
   p. 53.
Brenson, Michael. "A Sculptor Comes into Her Own." *The New York Times,*
   October 31, 1982, sec. 2, p. 1.
Glueck, Grace. "Louise Bourgeois, a Life in Sculpture, at Modern Museum."
   The New York Times, November 5, 1982, p. C1.
Brenson, Michael. "Sculpture Louise Bourgeois, A New York Retrospective
   Brings a Loner into Focus." *International Herald Tribune,* November 16,
   1982.
Hughes, Robert. "A Sense of Female Experience." *Time,* November 22, 1982,
   p. 116.
Larson, Kay. "Women by a Woman:. . . Louise Bourgeois Is Finally Where
   She Belongs: Among the Top American Sculptors and at the Apex of
   Feminist Art . . ." *New York,* November 22, 1982, pp. 74–75.
Levin, Kim. "Review." *The Village Voice,* p. 68.
"Building on Solid Foundations." *The Art Economist,* November 22, 1982,
   pp. 2–3.
"A Project by Louise Bourgeois." *Artforum,* December 1982, pp. 40–47.
Art Now/USA: The National Art Museum and Gallery Guide. December 1982,
   p. 13.
Raynor, Vivien. "Art: Louise Bourgeois Closes Her Own Dossier." *The New
   York Times,* December 3, 1982, p. C21.
Smith, Roberta. "Art: Parts and Sums." *The Village Voice,* December 7, 1982,
   p. 83.
Ratcliff, Carter. "New York: Louise Bourgeois at the Museum of Modern Art."
   Flash Art, January 1983, p. 62.
Rose, Barbara. "Two American Sculptors: Louise Bourgeois and Nancy
   Graves." *Vogue,* January 1983, pp. 222–23.
Howe, Katherine. "Landscapes at Robert Miller." *Images & Issues,* January/
   February 1983, p. 65.
Sozanski, Edward J. "The Feminine Aesthetic Is Here in Abundance." *The
   Philadelphia Inquirer,* March 1, 1983, p. 1D.
Johnson, Patricia C. "The Ambivalence That Is Life." *Houston Chronicle,*
   March 20, 1983.

Kalil, Susie. "Art: Louise Bourgeois Retrospective." *The Houston Post,* March 27, 1983, p. 1F.

Storr, Robert. "Louise Bourgeois: Gender & Possession." *Art in America,* April 1983, pp. 128–37.

Russell, John. "Philip Morris Building Plus Whitney Branch Combine Office Space and Art; Art: A Sculpture Court for Midtown." *The New York Times,* April 7, 1983, p. C17.

Larson, Kay. "All-American Energy." *New York,* April 11, 1983, pp. 61–63.

Raynor, Vivien. "Art: Neo-Expressionists or Neo-Surrealists?" *The New York Times,* May 13, 1983, p. C27.

Artner, Alan G. "The Return of the Human Touch: Figurative Sculpture Is Really Back in Vogue." *Chicago Tribune,* May 15, 1983.

Glatt, Cara. "Sculptors Look at Human Form." *The Herald* (Chicago), May 25, 1983, p. 10.

Larson, Kay. "The New Ugliness." *New York,* May 30, 1983, pp. 64–65.

Cameron, Daniel. "Biennial Cycle." *Arts Magazine,* June 1983, pp. 64–68.

Russell, John. "It's Not 'Women's' Art, It's Good Art." *The New York Times,* July 24, 1983, p. C1.

Curtis, Cathy. "Louise Bourgeois: Blending Emotive Dualities." *Artweek,* October 1, 1983.

Whitcher, Ann. "Sculpture Show." *Reporter,* November 10, 1983, p. 13.

Brenson, Michael. "A Living Artists' Show at the Modern Museum." *The New York Times,* April 21, 1984, p. All.

Braff, Phyllis. "From the Studio." *The East Hampton Star* (New York), August 2, 1984.

Russell, John. "American Art Gains New Energies." *The New York Times,* August 19, 1984, sec. 2, p. 1.

"Album: Louise Bourgeois." *Arts Magazine,* September 1984, pp. 48–49.

Hogrefe, Jeffrey. "New York, New York: Call of the Wild." *The Washington Post,* September 18, 1984, p. E7.

Glueck, Grace. "Louise Bourgeois/Robert Miller Gallery." *The New York Times,* September 28, 1984, p. C27.

Larson, Kay. "Bourgeois at Her Best." *New York,* October 1, 1984, pp. 60–61.

Wilson, William. "Louise Bourgeois/Daniel Weinberg Gallery." *Los Angeles Times,* November 16, 1984, part VI.

Gardner, Colin. "Louise Bourgeois: An Outspoken Woman." *Artweek,* November 24, 1984, p. 1.

Silverthorne, Jeanne. "Louise Bourgeois at Robert Miller Gallery." *Artforum,* December 1984, pp. 81–82.

Bellony-Rewald, Alice. "Paris: Louise Bourgeois." *Beaux Arts* (Paris), February 1985, p. 84.

Huser, France. "Papa, je te mangerai." *Le Nouvel Observateur* (Paris), February 8–14, 1985, p. 7.

Dagan, Phillippe. "Louise Bourgeois." *Quotidien de Paris*, February 14, 1985.

Lebovici, Elisabeth. "Louise Bourgeois: Toujours." *L'Événément du jeudi* (Paris), February 14–20, 1985.

"Louise Bourgeois, la vieille dame phalique." *Libération* (Paris), February 16, 1985.

Cabanne, Pierre. "Louise Bourgeois: Sculpteur pour tuer le père." *Le Matin* (Paris), February 18, 1985.

Marangoni, Federica. "Mostre, Parigi: Galerie Maeght-Lelong: Louise Bourgeois." *Grand Bazar* (Italy), February–March 1985.

Larson, Kay. "Women in the Vanguard." *Harper's Bazaar*, March 1985, p. 276.

Genevieve, Breerette. "Les Sculptures autobiographiques de Louise Bourgeois." *Le Monde* (Paris), March 2, 1985, p. 15.

"(Frauen-) Körper Zwischen Fragilitat und Stärke." *Kunst*, April 12, 1985, p. 46.

Boucher, Norman, and Tennen, Laura. "In Search of Fulfillment: Six Meaningful Lives." *New Age Journal*, May 1985, p. 32.

Silverthorne, Jeanne. "The Third Dimension: Sculpture of the New York School." *Artforum*, May 1985, p. 111.

Russell-Taylor, John. "Louise Bourgeois at Serpentine Gallery." *The Times* (London), May 28, 1985.

"America's Lost Generation." *The Times* (London), May 28, 1985.

Holman, Martin. "Louise Bourgeois: Sculpture and Drawings." *The Literary Review* (London), June 1985.

Taylor, Robert. "Unclothed Figures Stripped of Meaning." *Boston Sunday Globe*, January 1986, p. 2.

Stapen, Nancy. " 'Nude, Naked, Stripped' at MIT." *The Boston Herald*, January 1986.

"Louise Bourgeois." *The New York Times*, May 23, 1986, p. C24.

Indiana, Gary. "Insomnia." *The Village Voice*, May 27, 1986.

Brenson, Michael. "A Bountiful Season in Outdoor Sculpture Reveals Glimmers of a New Sensibility." *The New York Times*, July 18, 1986, p. C1.

Gounaris, Demetri. "Bourgeois Sculpture Transforms B-Way." *Columbia Daily Spectator* (New York), September 29, 1986.

Morgan, Stuart. "Louise Bourgeois at Robert Miller." *Artscribe*, September/October 1986.

Revol, Jean. "La Sculpture: État des Lieux: Hommage à Louise Bourgeois." November 1986, pp. 83–91.

Burkhart, Dorothy. "The New Sculpture—Take That, Minimalism." January 11, 1987, pp. 16–17.

Russell, John. "Early Paintings by Louise Bourgeois." *The New York Times*, January 16, 1987, p. C28.

Kuspit, Donald. "Louise Bourgeois—Where Angels Fear to Tread." *Artforum*, March 1987, pp. 115–20.

Wolff, Theodore F. "Fun, Flashy, and Fashionable." *The Christian Science Monitor*, April 16, 1987, pp. 22–23.

Flam, Jack. "Apples to Videos: Retro at the Whitney." *The Wall Street Journal*, April 29, 1987, p. 28.

Golany, Amy; Harris, Ann Sutherland; and King, Elaine A. "Sculpture by Women in the Eighties." *Dialogue*, May/June 1987.

Findsen, Owen. "Bourgeois Exhibit Like a Fine Dessert." *The Cincinnati Enquirer*, May 7, 1987, p. C1.

Gardner, Paul. "Sculpture's Grandes Dames." *Signature*, June 1987.

Russell, John. "Art: Met Favorites, Outdoors and In." *The New York Times*, July 31, 1987, p. C27.

Read, Mimi. "Louise Bourgeois' Machine for Living." *New York Newsday*, August 27, 1987, p. 3.

Fremon, Jean. "Louise Bourgeois." *New Observations*, September 1987, p. 8.

Rose, Barbara. "Sex, Rage & Louise Bourgeois." *Vogue*, September 1987, p. 765.

Smith, Roberta. "Art: 'Sculpture,' The Works of Five Women." *The New York Times*, October 2, 1987, p. C26.

Morgan, Stuart. "Taking Cover: Louise Bourgeois Interviewed by Stuart Morgan." *Artscribe International*, January/February 1988, pp. 30–34.

Smith, Roberta. "Louise Bourgeois." *The New York Times*, January 22, 1988, p. C25.

Larson, Kay. "In the Abstract." *New York*, January 25, 1988, pp. 61–62.

Gardner, Paul. "Working Habits: Louise Bourgeois Makes a Sculpture." *Art News*, Summer, 1988, pp. 61–64.

D O N A L D K U S P I T

A 1983 winner of the prestigious Frank Jewett Mather Award for Distinction in Art Criticism given by the College Art Association, Donald Kuspit is a contributing editor at *Art in America* and a regular contributor to *Artforum*. He is also the editor of *Art Criticism* and writes for *Artscribe* (London), *Contemporanea* (New York), *C Magazine* (Toronto) and *Wolkenkratzer* (Frankfurt), among other magazines. He holds doctorates in philosophy from the University of Frankfurt and in art history from the University of Michigan and is a professor of art history and philosophy at the State University of New York at Stony Brook. He has written over five hundred articles, exhibition reviews and catalogue essays. His most recent book is *The New Subjectivism: Art of the 1980's*. He has also written *Leon Golub: Existentialist/Activist/Painter; Clement Greenberg, Art Critic* and *The Critic Is Artist: The Intentionality of Art*. He is a consultant for UMI Research Press, for which he has edited a series on contemporary American art critics, art theory and contemporary art.

Other books in

ELIZABETH AVEDON EDITIONS

VINTAGE CONTEMPORARY ARTISTS SERIES

FRANCESCO CLEMENTE

---

interviewed by Rainer Crone
and Georgia Marsh

ERIC FISCHL

---

interviewed by Donald Kuspit

ROBERT RAUSCHENBERG

---

interviewed by Barbara Rose

DAVID SALLE

---

interviewed by Peter Schjeldahl

DONALD SULTAN

---

interviewed by Barbara Rose

Best Friends at the Bar

The *New Balance* for Today's Woman Lawyer

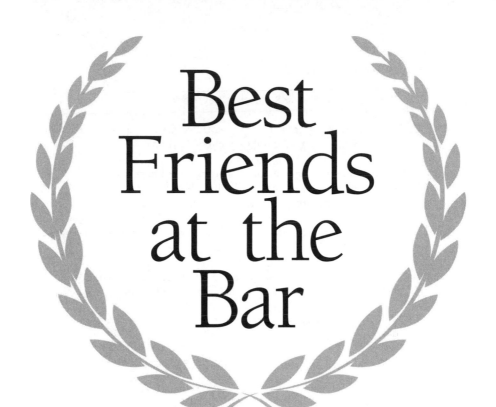

Best Friends at the Bar

The *New Balance* for Today's Woman Lawyer

Susan Smith Blakely, Esquire

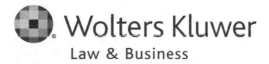

Wolters Kluwer
Law & Business

Printed in the United States of America.

1 2 3 4 5 6 7 8 9 0

ISBN 978-1-4548-2249-3

Library of Congress Cataloging-in-Publication Data

Blakely, Susan Smith, 1946-
   Best friends at the bar : the new balance for today's woman lawyer / Susan Smith Blakely.— 1st ed.
      p. cm.
   ISBN 978-1-4548-2249-3   1. Women lawyers United States.   2. Law—Vocational guidance—United States.   3. Women—Vocational guidance—United States.   I. Title.

   KF299.W6B588 2012
   340.082'0973—dc23

                                                            2012020084

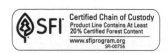

About Wolters Kluwer Law & Business

Wolters Kluwer Law & Business is a leading global provider of intelligent information and digital solutions for legal and business professionals in key specialty areas, and respected educational resources for professors and law students. Wolters Kluwer Law & Business connects legal and business professionals as well as those in the education market with timely, specialized authoritative content and information-enabled solutions to support success through productivity, accuracy and mobility.

Serving customers worldwide, Wolters Kluwer Law & Business products include those under the Aspen Publishers, CCH, Kluwer Law International, Loislaw, Best Case, ftwilliam.com and MediRegs family of products.

CCH products have been a trusted resource since 1913, and are highly regarded resources for legal, securities, antitrust and trade regulation, government contracting, banking, pension, payroll, employment and labor, and healthcare reimbursement and compliance professionals.

Aspen Publishers products provide essential information to attorneys, business professionals and law students. Written by preeminent authorities, the product line offers analytical and practical information in a range of specialty practice areas from securities law and intellectual property to mergers and acquisitions and pension/benefits. Aspen's trusted legal education resources provide professors and students with high-quality, up-to-date and effective resources for successful instruction and study in all areas of the law.

Kluwer Law International products provide the global business community with reliable international legal information in English. Legal practitioners, corporate counsel and business executives around the world rely on Kluwer Law journals, looseleafs, books, and electronic products for comprehensive information in many areas of international legal practice.

Loislaw is a comprehensive online legal research product providing legal content to law firm practitioners of various specializations. Loislaw provides attorneys with the ability to quickly and efficiently find the necessary legal information they need, when and where they need it, by facilitating access to primary law as well as state-specific law, records, forms and treatises.

Best Case Solutions is the leading bankruptcy software product to the bankruptcy industry. It provides software and workflow tools to flawlessly streamline petition preparation and the electronic filing process, while timely incorporating ever-changing court requirements.

ftwilliam.com offers employee benefits professionals the highest quality plan documents (retirement, welfare and non-qualified) and government forms (5500/PBGC, 1099 and IRS) software at highly competitive prices.

MediRegs products provide integrated health care compliance content and software solutions for professionals in healthcare, higher education and life sciences, including professionals in accounting, law and consulting.

Wolters Kluwer Law & Business, a division of Wolters Kluwer, is headquartered in New York. Wolters Kluwer is a market-leading global information services company focused on professionals.

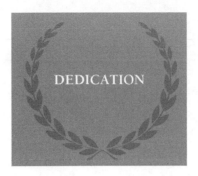

DEDICATION

I dedicate this book to my family and to all of the young women lawyers who distinguish themselves every day in our profession in spite of the special challenges and barriers that still exist for women in the law. They have my complete admiration, and it is my hope that a book like this will help them to persevere and reach their goals. As one of the women profiled in this book states so well, "Reach for the stars, and you will be happy if you land on the moon."

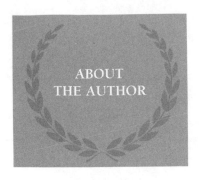

ABOUT
THE AUTHOR

Susan Smith Blakely is an attorney and former teacher whose experiences include practicing law, with a specialty in construction contract litigation and land use, serving as chief of staff to an elected official, and teaching in public school systems throughout the United States. She holds a Bachelor of Science degree from the University of Wisconsin and a Juris Doctorate from Georgetown University Law Center, where she was a teaching fellow for legal research and writing. This is Ms. Blakely's second book in the *Best Friends at the Bar* series. The first book, *Best Friends at the Bar: What Women Need to Know about a Career in the Law*, was published by Wolters Kluwer/ Aspen Publishers in 2009. Ms. Blakely speaks at law schools, law firms and law organizations throughout the country about her books and the *Best Friends at the Bar* project. For more information on the project and her services, please consult her web site at www.bestfriendsatthebar.com, where you also will be able to access her daily blogs and her monthly newsletters.

Ms. Blakely lives in Great Falls, Virginia, with her husband Bill, also an attorney. They have two children: Elizabeth, a graduate of the University of Virginia and Seton Hall University School of Law, and Derick, also a graduate of the University of Virginia, who works as a consultant in the defense industry. Ms. Blakely enjoys reading, playing the piano, gardening, architecture and design, traveling, and being with family and friends when she is not writing and speaking.

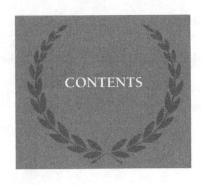

CONTENTS

Foreword .... *xiii*

Acknowledgments .... *xvii*

Prologue 1

1   You *Really* Need to Love What You Do 19

2   You *Really* Need to Get Serious 25

3   You *Really* Need to Be Who You Are 33

4   You *Really* Need to Put Yourself First—At Least
    Part of the Time 49

5   You *Really* Need to Gain Perspective 61

6   You *Really* Need TIME—And All the
    Help You Can Get! 67

7   You *Really* Need Your Friends 91

8   You *Really* Need to Live Within Your Means to Keep
    Your Options Open 105

9   You *Really* Need to Take Credit for What You Do 111

10 You *Really* Need True Grit 121

11 You *Really* Need to Be the Best Lawyer You Can Be 129

12 You *Really* Need to Think About Career Transitions 135

Where We Are and How We Got Here 144
The Starting Point 148
Typical Transitions 149
   The Law Firm Practice Model 149
   From Law Firm to In-House Corporate Practice 157
      Profile of Sally Blackmun 164
      Profile of Amy Yeung 168
   From Law Firm to Public Interest/Non-Profit Lawyer 173
      Profile of Bonnie Brier 175
   From Law Firm to Government Lawyer 181
      Profile of Kathleen Tighe 188
   From Law Firm to Solo Practice 191
      Profile of Laura Oberbroeckling 196
   From Traditional Law Firm to Non-Traditional
   Law Firm 201
      Women-Owned Law Firm 201
      Profile of Kathryn Smith Spencer 202
      Virtual Law Firm 205
      Profile of Stephanie Kimbro 206
   From Law Firm to Law Firm Consultant 209
      Profile of Karen Kaplowitz 210
   From Law Firm to Academia 213
      Profile of Deborah Burand 215
      Profile of Markeisha Miner 220
   From Law Firm to the Judiciary 224
      Profile of Honorable Marianne Short 226
   From Law Firm to Alternative Dispute Resolution 230
      Profile of Victoria Pynchon 231

Epilogue: From a Queen of Reinvention 237

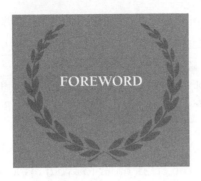

FOREWORD

Susan Blakely's *Best Friends at the Bar* project is an important new approach to success in both law and life for women in the legal profession. Reaching beyond the traditional analysis of entitlement and equal opportunity, Ms. Blakely takes a practical view of the state of women in the law and provides strategies for avoiding disappointment and failure. She encourages women law students and women lawyers to have realistic expectations about their career options that are grounded in their personal circumstances. She also underscores the importance of being *part* of the system in order to *change* the system. Following her lead can make the difference between a satisfying and successful career in the law and the disappointment associated with abandoning a profession because of challenges that were not anticipated or effectively addressed.

Susan Blakely wants to make success easier for today's women lawyers. She understands work-life struggles and the challenge of being part of a male-dominated profession, and she refuses to accept the inevitability of very low retention rates for women lawyers. She has taken on the challenge in an impressive way. This is her second book in three years, and she readily admits that she is on a mission.

I can relate to that mission. Like Ms. Blakely, I have personally experienced some of these challenges in both the private and public sectors. After becoming one of only a dozen female law school deans in 1989, I watched too many young women graduate from law school with impressive records only to find disillusionment and disappointment in the workplace. I salute Susan Blakely for working for better futures for the current generation of women lawyers and those who follow them.

There is still a lot of work to be done, and Susan Blakely wants us all to become part of solving the problem. Her first book, *Best Friends at the Bar: What Women Need to Know about a Career in the Law*, was her way of throwing out lifelines to help women lawyers to make good decisions and good choices early in their careers in order to avoid dissatisfaction, disappointment and unfortunate departures later.

This book continues where the first one left off and digs deeper into the work-life struggle and the quest for balance that women lawyers with family and home responsibilities inevitably will face. It introduces a "new balance for today's woman lawyer," including the important consideration of "self" in arriving at a satisfactory balance. The author provides sound advice to women lawyers including the importance of being true to themselves and valuing and maintaining friendships that are essential to achieving the happiness and balance that will lead to successful careers and lives. She understands the time demands and the near impossibility of being all things to all people, but she does not let her readers surrender to those limitations and pressures. She offers extensive lists of helpmates and service providers, and she also throws in generous amounts of encouragement, tough love, and practical options for those times when particular career paths don't work out. She concludes the book with profiles of twelve women lawyers who have transitioned from large law firm practice to other practice settings and who present excellent role models for her readers.

Best Friends at the Bar: The New Balance *for Today's Woman Lawyer* comes at exactly the right time. Today, women in our country are realizing that things they took for granted are again under attack. Women must fight hard, both in the workplace and at the ballot box, to preserve their rights and privileges. It is widely recognized that women will make up the most important voting block in the 2012 national election, and women are finding that they must stick together to make their collective voices heard. That is what makes the "Women Helping Women" theme of Susan Blakely's books both timely and important.

Susan and I share the vision that women's success in the workplace depends on how much and how effectively women help each other. Gone are the days when women believed that they would get ahead simply because it was "the right thing for employers to do." We know better today. It will take hard work, dedication, effective mentoring, and solidarity, but it is possible. Susan Blakely and her *Best Friends at the Bar* project will help women lawyers get where they want to *go* and where they need to *be* to enrich our profession and to make it better for the next generation of women lawyers.

As a woman, as a lawyer, and as a law school professor and dean, I applaud the *Best Friends at the Bar* project. I thank Susan Blakely for bringing this project to all of us, and know that you are in for a "good read." I wish you all great success and happiness in your law careers.

Judith Areen
Paul Regis Dean Professor of Law and
Dean Emeritus of Georgetown University Law Center
June 2012

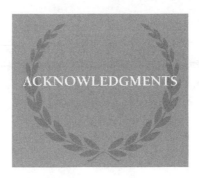

ACKNOWLEDGMENTS

I am very grateful to many people who have contributed to this book and made it possible, especially Wolters Kluwer Law & Business and its editors for, once again, having faith in the *Best Friends at the Bar* project. They continue to recognize the special challenges for women in the law and the need for books like these.

Thank you also to Judith Areen, the former dean of my law school, for writing the *Foreword* to the book. Her participation provides great affirmation for my project.

I also am grateful to the twelve women who are profiled in the book. They all are women of substance, and their time is very valuable. Yet, they took time out from busy schedules that include law firm management, presidential appointments, and university administration to provide me with interesting and relevant information to assist my readers in finding their own best places in law practice. Writing the profiles of these impressive women was pure pleasure for me, and I will always be grateful to them for sharing their stories.

I also want to thank my daughter, Elizabeth Blakely, who recently graduated from Seton Hall University School of Law, for contributing to the Profiles. She also took time out of her challenging routine of working, going to class, and being an editor on the law journal to participate in this project. It is my hope that she will become an even greater contributor to the *Best Friends at the Bar* project in the future.

I also want to thank my research assistant, Dede Potts, a rising 3L at George Mason University Law School.

Both Elizabeth and Dede are featured in the Spotlight! on my web site, www.bestfriendsatthebar.com, and you can read more about them there.

Prologue

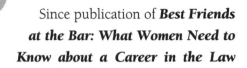

Since publication of **Best Friends at the Bar: What Women Need to Know about a Career in the Law** ("Book One"), I have traveled around the country speaking at law schools, law organizations and law firms to spread the messages of the book and reach as many young women lawyers and law students as possible. The goal of these activities is to inform young women lawyers and law students about critical practice information that they do not receive in college pre-law programs, law schools and, often, in their first years of practice. It is my hope that, with this information, young women will go into the profession with their eyes wide open, develop realistic approaches to their careers, and find ways to stay in their chosen profession. This is particularly important because of the work-life struggles that uniquely affect women professionals and the alarmingly low retention rates for women lawyers.

This has been a very rewarding experience. The young women in law school today are a confident and impressive group, and I enjoy meeting them and speaking with them. They are eager for information, and they understand that there are great challenges ahead of them. They do not understand the depth of those challenges, but that is my job and the job of other experienced women lawyers—to educate them and to help them to accept those challenges and to rise above them.

Book One has been very popular, and I have received many endorsements and acknowledgments from my readers and my audiences. It has been reprinted twice, and it has found its way into the hands of many

1

young women lawyers and law students. These young women have bene-fitted from what *Best Friends at the Bar* has to say, and I am continually asked whether a second book is on the way. My answer always has been "Yes" because I understand the critical need for more of this kind of infor-mation, and I want young women law students and lawyers all over America—if not the world—to have it.

To bring my readers the most useful content in a follow-up book, I ask the young women I meet what further kinds of information they need the most. I am impressed that they are so practical in their responses, and, although answers differ in form, most are concentrated on the same theme: How do I REALLY overcome the challenges of the work-life struggle and have a successful legal career *all by myself*?

So, this book was born, and, as you suspected, the truth is that you don't make it happen *all by yourself*. In most cases, you cannot do it all alone. You must be able to rely not only on yourself but on mentors and others in your life who have stakes in your future.

In my interactions with readers and audiences, I have found a great deal of enthusiasm from young women law students and also an equal amount of disenchantment from women practicing attorneys. I had expected the latter responses, but they were more profound and disturbing than I had anticipated.

As time went on, I began to understand that success for women in the law is about more than just the good planning and good choices and personal definitions of success that we explored in Book One. It is about a philosophy of living, and, in that respect, it is much more gender neutral than I had expected. It is a discussion that goes to the heart of how we approach professional life in America and the value that we put on personal time. It is all about *balance*.

The fact is that we don't do the profession of law very well in America—at least not in terms of the lifestyle and well-being of practi-tioners. Too often, we operate under rules that encourage workaholic be-haviors and lead to stress-related illnesses and dependencies. Researchers at Johns Hopkins University found that lawyers suffer from alcoholism and illegal drug use at rates far higher than non-lawyers. The divorce rate among lawyers, especially women, also appears to be higher than the divorce rate among other professionals. Lawyers are the best-paid professionals, but they are disproportionately unhappy and unhealthy. ("Why Are Lawyers So Unhappy," www.businessinsider.com, December 5, 2011) We end up with a workforce of professionals at the end of their careers, consisting of burned out and resentful lawyers. This is very unfortunate because the law profession is an honorable pursuit and deserves more.

It is sometimes hard for lawyers to consider other styles of practice because they do not like to admit that they are not as important to making the world go around as they might like to think they are. After all, convincing yourself that the firm cannot run without you there 24-7 is a strong statement about how important you are, even if you are the only one who believes it!

Often it helps to bring in more objective observers. In an August 11, 2010 article on work-life balance in the *ABA Journal* on line (www.aba-journal.com) titled "Why Lawyers Should Work No More than 40 Hours a Week," Debra Cassens Weiss relies heavily on the observations and writings of Margaret Heffernan, media entrepreneur and CEO of multiple businesses.

According to Cassens Weiss, lawyers, doctors and others in the service industry can be more productive and creative if they put away their Blackberries and iPhones and stopped working so much. She gets support for this hypothesis from Heffernan, who argues that multitasking causes distraction, and Blackberry/iPhone addicts lose focus and concentration.

The article goes on to quote Heffernan's assertions that manufacturing executives already understand "asset integrity"—preserving plants and machinery from damage due to wear and tear so that they will last longer. In analogizing that concept to professional service industries, Heffernan states,

"The professional service industry should do the same by preserving their greatest assets: the minds of their workers. . . . For the last 100 years, every productivity study in every industry has come to the same

3

conclusion: After about 40 hours in a week, the quality of your work starts to degrade. You make mistakes. That's why working 60 hours may not save you time or money. You'll spend too much of that time fixing the mistakes you shouldn't have made. . . . That's why software companies that limit work to 35 hours a week need to employ fewer QA (Quality Assurance) engineers: There isn't as much mess to clean up. Leaders need to take seriously a century's evidence that 1) overwork doesn't make us productive, it makes us stupid, 2) looking away from a problem is often the best way to solve it, and 3) burnout is what happens when people are asked to work in ways that obliterate all other parts of their lives.'

There is a lot to think about in that article, including some good stuff to use in trying to improve your working habits and your workplace. However, in making the case to your managing partner, I recommend that you leave out the "stupid" part!

Even though we recognize the problems with overwork and burnout and there is a lot written about discontentment among law practitioners, we as a profession have myriad excuses for why we cannot change this pattern and practice. However, change we must, and we may get a push in that direction from clients and from Generation X (those born between roughly 1965 and 1980) and Generation Y (those born between roughly 1977 and 2002) lawyers.

Many of the changes on the horizon in law firms today are being forced by clients, who want more value for less money, who want more diversity in their representation and who are disenchanted with the billable hour and insisting on alternative fee arrangements. Although it may take an entire realignment of our economic and business systems to bring about that kind of change, it already is beginning to have an effect on the way law is practiced in America. The alternative to change, of course, is that we may be stuck with much of the "same old same old" for years to come. The definition of insanity comes to mind here: Continuing to do the same thing over and over and expecting a different result. Insane, indeed.

The change issue also is being nudged along these days by concerns for law firm succession that are confronting law firms in recognition that the Baby Boomers must move on and that the Generation X (Gen X) and Generation Y (Gen Y) lawyers who will remain may not see things quite the same as their predecessors. Many Gen X and Gen Y lawyers, especially, do not favor the workaholic lifestyles they have seen in their parents and predecessors, and, yet, these are the lawyers who presumably will lead law firms into the next generation.

To assure a talented and competitive work force, firms are beginning to look at alternative practice models to assist in retaining talent and creating the critical mass of competent practitioners that will be necessary to lead the firm successfully into the future. We are seeing an attempt to restructure firms away from the lockstep method of promotion, which is based predominately on billable hours, to more of a lattice structure, which includes many different practice models and considerations for promotion. These new law firm models may end up benefitting women attorneys who typically are efficient multi-taskers and for whom billable hours are a poor measure of competency. The new models also may include more opportunities for women lawyers in terms of flexible work schedules in attempts to retain talent.

So, it is an opportune time for us as individual professionals to examine the way that we do business and the effect it has on our personal lives. It is a time when we can adjust ourselves in ways that are likely to improve our happiness and satisfaction in all aspects of our lives, including our lives as practicing lawyers. Not only is it possible to do this, I believe that it is imperative to do it. To ignore the low retention rates for women lawyers and the discontent of lawyers as a whole is to ignore the value of human talent and to squander natural resources.

After contemplating this dilemma time and time again, I kept coming back to the same conclusion: If we are going to improve the retention figures for women lawyers, we need to address the *underlying problems* affecting lawyers as professionals. We need to start with a fundamental analysis of what it takes to be happy in both our professional and personal lives so that we can give professional success the best chance possible. We must examine the issues of balance and figure out what it really takes to make us happy. If we can identify some basic tenets of successful living and combine those with the personal definitions of success that I stressed in Book One, we will have a much better chance for advancing satisfied and successful young women lawyers.

In addressing these issues, I recognize that my readers are a whole new breed of women lawyers. They will not practice as their mothers did or, for that matter, as their fathers did. They have different values, different goals and different approaches to their lives, and I applaud that. It is progress, and we must embrace it because it is our future. As with all progress, there also will be change, and one of those changes will affect the traditional attitude about work-life "balance." In lieu of the traditional concept of work/home and family, I believe that a new balance is necessary and needs to be explored. That new balance is work/*self*/home and family. Without putting the element of "self" front and center in your lives as professionals, I doubt that many of you will succeed in the professional growth and satisfaction that you are seeking.

So, that is my purpose in writing a second book. I have seen these themes played out over and over again, and I believe that the issues identified and discussed in this book will help young lawyers hold true to their new attitudes within the confines of an old profession. At least I hope so.

What other positive prospect do we have for the future generation of lawyers? Gen Y already is disenchanted and is rejecting what is identified as the flawed work ethic of the prior generation. That part is clear. What is unclear is what Gen Ys intend to do about it. In too many circumstances, I think that these young people simply will refuse to go into professions like the law because they are afraid of the traditional lifestyle. Or, they will leave the practice prematurely and perpetuate the dismal retention figures. That, of course, is unfortunate because many of them would make excellent lawyers, and the profession would be enhanced by their presence.

Instead, regrettably, some of the best and the brightest of this new generation will choose other walks of life because we have done such a miserable job of demonstrating alternatives to the dysfunctional model. That surely is our loss.

For more on the way Gen Ys (aka "Millenials") will affect the future, I recommend an article in USA Today entitled "Graduates, You Can Have It All" by Laura Vanderkam, author of *168 Hours: You Have More Time Than You Think* (May 27, 2010). The theme of the article is that as Millennials increasingly demand a work-life balance, they might just teach the other generations a thing or two. It is thought provoking and worthy of your time.

The book you are reading is different from those that have come before it. Other books take the 30,000-foot view and tell you how women fit into the global picture, in both today's world and historically. I did that with Book One, at least partially, and I think it was appropriate there. However, in this book I choose YOU over the statistics and metrics. In this book, I try to get at the HEART of it, and the heart of most everything discussed here is the feeling of happiness that we get from being successful and satisfied in our personal and professional endeavors. To achieve that happiness, we must find the right balance.

My goal is to communicate to you as effectively as possible. Believe me, that sounds a whole lot easier than it is. Inherent in this communication is the fact that most of you do not know what you do not know. You are aware of the generational divide between you and the senior women lawyers, but you cannot relate to the difficulties and hardships of the past. That is understandable, but you must also be aware that, in certain respects, the glass ceiling is so much higher today than it was for women like me. There are so many more of you today and, with that increased talent pool, there are fewer opportunities to stand out from the crowd. There is increased competition for relatively few prizes.

Although there were so many fewer women lawyers back "in the day," we had the common elements of minority and suffering that united us and were incredibly effective motivators. Your generation does not have that in equal measure, and what you do have is the expectation that everyone gets a trophy just for showing up. Quite honestly, the women of my generation worry that you will not wake up to the challenges and the realities and the possibilities of a legal career until too late.

Unfortunately, as a result of our concern, we senior members of the profession can become preachy and that is not effective. We must find appropriate and effective voices to help you and prepare you for the realities, and that is our challenge. We must be authentic without being judgmental, caring without being condescending, and helpful without being patronizing.

You know us, we are your mothers, and this will not be easy! However, it is completely doable if we all focus on the end game and everything that you have to gain from our help. Simply put, our mission is not to *scare* but to make you *aware* so that you have the courage to *dare*.

I am neither a psychologist nor a sociologist. I am only a woman lawyer who has lived the struggle to find the happiness and the balance, and I have access to many other women who have been on that same journey and succeeded. I think that I understand you, and I am confident that I can frame the issues and put you on the springboard to face them in your own life. As women lawyers, we are at that point, and we cannot be mired down in the impersonal world any more. What we have to deal with is VERY personal, and we have to explore those personal issues to come up with solutions.

So, I chose this format, a professional self-help book, to move the marker forward. Enough of the statistics and metrics. Let's talk about what you REALLY NEED to find the balance and to be happy. The conversation must begin or there will be little audience left,—and those in the audience will see only the burdens of the profession and not the possibilities. Let's start the useful dialogue and gain the communications skills that will be necessary when you go to management with your proposals—which most of you will one day. At that point you will need not only the metrics and the statistics but also a language that you feel comfortable with—one where you can conjugate the verbs easily. Men in management positions understand the impersonal stats and the metrics, and you must help them understand the rest. It is important that you know what to say and how to say it.

As you know from my work, women lawyers continue to be my focus. However, I do not disregard the issues addressed in this book as they affect male practitioners, and often I am asked by young male law students and lawyers: *What about us? We have work-life issues as well, and the profession is equally as hard for us.* I tell them that I feel their pain but that currently I have my hands full trying to help you young women lawyers. Maybe I will get to them later or maybe one of their enlightened male colleagues will jump into the abyss.

Until that time, young male law students and lawyers can learn a lot from this book, and I hope that you will help them get comfortable with the concepts. Practically speaking, it may be difficult to get the young men to read a book focused on women, so you young women may have to read it and explain it to the men in your lives. It won't be the first time you have to do this . . . or the last.

It is important that we draw the men into the discussion. Those young men will have wives who are lawyers, one day they will have daughters who are lawyers, and they will be managing women lawyers throughout their careers. This is stuff they all will need to know.

You also will notice that most of the themes addressed in this book are equally as applicable to life outside the legal profession and will be lessons for all women in business and in other professions. That should not be surprising. After all, law is a business—the business of law—as I discussed at length in Book One. My women doctor friends and friends in the financial world tell me that the issues they face are parallel to, if not the same as, the ones discussed here, and I hope that you will share this book with some of your friends outside the profession of law.

This book is about getting what you need to survive in one of the most challenging professions in the world regardless of how you choose to approach that career. This book goes beyond Book One and helps you to understand that all of the work-life struggle is not about raising children and caring for families. It also is about safe-guarding your personal life and your relationships so that *you are happy*. You will find that being happy in your personal life opens up many greater possibilities for happiness in your professional life.

Whether you are single, married without children or married with children or some other variation on those themes, this book is about what you need for success *because you are a woman*. It is a topic that is not often explored when it comes to strong, independent women, and maybe that is part of the problem. Strong and independent does not mean that you do not have needs. If you get that straight right off the bat, we will make some real progress between the covers of this book.

Similarly, identifying what we really need from others is not always easy for women, who have a tendency to think that we can do everything ourselves. This is no place to try out that flawed theory. You *do* have needs, and unless you address them, you are much less likely to be happy and to find satisfaction and success in your professional and personal lives.

Let's look at those specific needs and get you started on the road to finding the help that you deserve—from yourself and from others. Just as you learned in Book One, it is a "Pay It Forward" process. By learning to get the help you need, you will learn to *give* the help that someone else needs. Women helping women. You know how passionate I am about that.

Let's learn how to be happy lawyers. We are intelligent, competent professionals, and we need to apply those skills to the subject of happiness. That may sound trite to you, but that reaction is the result of years of negative conditioning. After all, we are supposed to be cerebral and intellectual to the exclusion of all else, right? NOT! We are supposed to be *happy* so that we can bring the best of everything that we have to offer to both our professional and personal lives. Being happy is not trite. Far from it!

In exploring what the book has to offer, you will need strong practice models. However, the practice models that we will explore in this book are different than the 60-plus Contributors you "met" as role models in Book One. The practice models here will help you address the question, "What if I choose wrong?" or "What if I need something different?" You will find that nothing is forever, and you will be presented with information about transitions that may change your life and save your career. We are taught that change is good and that we should embrace change. That does not make it easy, but I will try to make it *easier* for you.

Much of what I have to tell you, at least in the first part of the book, has less to do with law practice than it has to do with being a happy and successful professional. Unfortunately, that is the part that is too often overlooked in law school, and, yet, it is so important to your future. In law school, you are taught about constitutional law, about contracts, about temporary restraining orders and about the danger from a banana peel left on the floor of the supermarket, but you are not taught how to pace yourself and care for yourself so that you will have years of successful practice to try out all of those intriguing legal theories you learned in school.

Unfortunately, many of our best legal institutions do not think that teaching practical skills is important enough to include in the law school curriculum. They even are reluctant to make changes to the curriculum to produce practice-ready graduates, as pointed out in a very provocative law review article titled "The Changing Cultures and Economics of Large Law Firm Practice and Their Impact on Legal Education" by Neil Dilloff, a partner at DLA Piper, published in the *Maryland Law Review*, Volume 70, March 2011. As you can imagine, law schools are even more reluctant to introduce courses and clinics on practical issues of balance and its effect on professional happiness and survival skills for women in a male-dominated profession.

I have had many discussions with law educators about this problem and the necessity for putting more "practicum" into the law curriculum. If you agree with me, have those same conversations at your law schools and alma maters. At some point our voices will be heard, and we already are seeing some signs of hope. In the last few years, schools like the University of Michigan Law School, Northwestern University Law School, the University of Maryland Law School, the University of Detroit Mercy Law School, the University of Texas Law School, and Washington and Lee School of Law have taken important first steps toward adding more practicum to their curriculums, including some programs tailored to issues facing women lawyers. I am particularly proud of the recent efforts at my alma mater, Georgetown University Law Center (GULC). The clinical programs and practicum courses at GULC are very impressive and have become models for law schools across the country. These programs were highlighted at the Women's Forum held at GULC in the Spring of 2012, particularly as they relate to preparing women law students for practice. All of these schools are to be congratulated, and I hope that they have started a trend among their competitor schools.

Perhaps law school administration and faculty need to be reminded that the longer their graduates practice and the happier they are in the law, the more likely they will be to give generously to their law alma maters for years to come. Perhaps they also need to be reminded that the opportunities to place graduating lawyers are directly related to the number of alumni in practice. Feel free to pass those thoughts on when you have those discussions with your law schools.

For more information on this issue, I suggest that you read anything you can get your hands on from Professor William Henderson at Indiana University Mauer School of Law. I find his remarks and writing on the subject of practice-ready lawyers "spot on" and hope that you, too, will enjoy what he has to say. Here is one of my blog entries about his work.

Feb 24, 2011

Law Schools Need More Practical Curricula to Prepare Young Lawyers for Law Practice

Last week I gave you information about Professor Bill Henderson at Indiana University Law School and his comments on the value of LSAT scores and the downside to law firms in relying too heavily on them. Hope you found it interesting.

12

Even more important from my perspective are Professor Henderson's thoughts on the future of law school education. He is a proponent of more practical course work in the curriculum and more team work and cooperative ventures among students in problem solving settings. Although he acknowledges the value of competition and he recognizes that it brings out the best in students in some settings, he believes that the cut throat nature of law school needs less emphasis than it gets. Check out his thoughts in this radio interview on http://shillingmesoftly.blogspot.com/2011/01/sms-hall-of-famer-prof-william.html.

This issue of the need for more "practicum" in law school curricula was addressed at a conference I attended at American University Washington College of Law last week. Professor Jim Moliterno of Washington & Lee Law School (http://law.wlu.edu/faculty/profiledetail.asp?id=298) and Dean Dana Morris of the University of Maryland Law School (http://www.law.umaryland.edu/faculty/profiles/faculty.html?facultynum=084) reported very innovative programs at their schools, including devoting the third year of law school to practicum at W & L Law. Professor Moliterno pointed out that medical schools adopted the practical approach to professional education years ago and that law schools should use that as a model. He pointed out that "medical schools have been preparing doctors and law schools have been preparing law professors—not lawyers." That got my attention!

I long have been a fan of this approach, and I am so pleased to see these developments. I hope more schools follow the lead and put more emphasis on practical skills in their curricula. Graduating law students and the firms that hire them would benefit mutually from this approach as law graduates would have enhanced skills in drafting agreements, negotiating agreements, preparing motions, arguing motions, the business of law and assorted other disciplines that would make graduating law students think and act more like lawyers and actually feel more like lawyers. Feeling more like lawyers is important. It is disappointing for graduate lawyers to go to law firms and feel "light" on the fundamentals of practice. I know because I hear it repeatedly from the young associates.

I am very happy to see these new developments, and I will be interested in finding out more about the programs at the University of Maryland Law when I am at the law school in March to participate on a panel devoted to issues of young women in the law. More on that later!

In the meantime, while law schools figure this out, I am trying to do all that I can through the *Best Friends at the Bar* books and speaking opportunities to prepare you for the practical aspects of law practice. You know my goal: To see young women lawyers as happy and satisfied as possible so that they continue in the profession to help make it a better place for all women lawyers and for the profession itself.

It is as simple as that. I hope together we will succeed.

I cannot emphasize too much that NOW is the time for you to get real and to focus on your own well-being—long before your situation reaches crisis dimensions and you look like a deer in headlights with no good place to run.

Having said that, I realize that very often you do not have the time you need to focus on your career and your happiness. Rest assured, I get that, I have heard you, and it is why I wrote a second book.

I know you. You are the law student who is working during the day to defray at least some student loan debt and going to class at night. Or you are the law student who is on a law journal or participating in a clinic to get valuable experience that will lead to a good job—all while trying to maintain a modicum of relationships with your friends and family . . . and the beat goes on.

Or, you are the young lawyer who is working at the law firm from early morning until late at night—or into the wee hours of the next morning—trying to keep up with the demands of your supervising attorney, trying to attend professional programs to network and build clientele, trying to carve out something of a personal life . . . and your beat goes on. I have lived it, and it is no walk in the park. My daughter is living it now, and I am grateful for each day that goes by when she stays healthy and does not buckle under the stress of it all.

I see it clearly. Time is your enemy. You do not have enough of it. That is why I have devoted a chapter of the book to the subject of time.

Even though I "get it," I urge you to make a commitment to yourself that you will refrain from the "I do not have time for that" response as you read this book. I know that you will be tempted by that response because you feel that you do not have the capability to put the advice into action. If you do that, you simply will be perpetuating the habits of all of those discontented lawyers who have gone before you.

All of those lawyers who did not have *time* for their spouses, who did not have *time* for their children, who did not have *time* for their friends, who did not have *time* for exercise, who did not have *time* to eat right, who did not have *time* to sleep well, who did not have *time* to see the doctor . . . all because work came first *all of the time*. Well, I think you know that many of those personal lives ended up on the junk heap of history, and I do not think that is where you want yours to go.

You have a choice. You either can go blissfully on without taking precautions to protect your life and your future, or you can take *time* out to avoid these kinds of disastrous results. The retention rates will not change until we change them. We are pretty much doomed in that pursuit if we carry on business as usual.

Instead, vow to make an investment in your future. You will find it *time* well spent. And, if taking out such a relatively small amount of time for yourself and your personal life interferes with the requirements of your practice, then you may be in the wrong practice or practice setting. You may have to choose a transition where you can continue to use your legal education AND have a satisfying personal life. For some that will mean an alternative work schedule, and for some that will mean a transition to a different type of practice altogether.

What you do not want is to become another statistic. You do not want to fall by the wayside as another dropout because you did not take the *time* to figure out who you are and what you need. Wouldn't that be a waste? As my mother so often says woefully about people who do not live up to their potential, "All that education . . ." If she was from my generation or yours, she also would be saying, "All that money . . ." It is hardly imaginable to people of her generation that law educations cost $150,000 plus today, and my mother would tell you that you should want to get your money's worth.

In the interest of your *time*, I will try to simplify your personal introspection by suggesting what you REALLY NEED. We will cut to the chase and focus on what you need the most and how you can get it. We will establish a pecking order of priorities and try to stick to them to get you where you want to go. We will use the lessons of Book One to go further in discovering what women really need to become satisfied and successful lawyers.

A Brief Review

To give you the best chance of success in understanding this book, let's briefly review the major themes of Book One. *Best Friends at the Bar* is a continuum, and these themes are important because they are the foundation upon which we will apply the lessons of this book. Although this book will go further in suggesting specific approaches for a successful and satisfying legal career, the foundation of Book One is important and cannot be overlooked.

Best Friends at the Bar: What Women Need to Know about a Career in the Law started with a recognition of the alarmingly low retention rates for women in the law today. We faced the stark realization that as many as 42% of women abandon their professions mid-career (UC Hastings Center for Work-Life Policy 2009 Report) and 76% of female law school graduates who choose Big Law after law school leave that employer within the first five years (*Working Mother* on line, "Focus on Best Law Firms—Part-Time Practice," November 16, 2008). Although some of those women transition to other practices, the statistics show that two to three times as many women leave law careers as men. We also addressed the unfortunate circumstances that have resulted in fewer than 20% women equity partners in law firms across the country (National Association of Women Lawyers (NAWL) 2011 Report).

We explored the reasons for these dismal figures. Those reasons include the difficult work-life struggle experienced by many women lawyers and the hard and sometimes complicated choices women lawyers must make if they want personal lives that include family and childcare responsibilities.

When you view these statistics within the context of other statistics about women in the law, they are particularly bothersome. As most of you know, women make up almost 50% of all students entering law school today, and, correspondingly, women make up almost 50% of all graduating law students (www.catalyst.org, "Women in Law in the U.S.", January 2012). Women are very often at the top of their graduating classes in terms of GPA and honors, and many of those women go on to top jobs in top firms making top salaries. Yet, fewer than 20% of the equity partners in law firms today are women, and that percentage is not increasing at a pace that was once predicted.

This is a serious dilemma for our profession, and there are no clear solutions. However, there has to be a better approach than watching talented young women lawyers set themselves up for disappointment and failure. Choosing well and addressing the correct career path early on was the topic of my first book, and I hope that you have paid close attention to that better approach.

In Book One, we explored the value of good plans that lead to good choices and of having realistic expectations for your careers, personal definitions of success, setting achievable goals and celebrating when you achieve your goals and experience success. The emphasis was on preparedness, identifying priorities and avoiding impetuous decision-making.

Book One also addressed the lessons that my Contributors and I identified as important to help young women lawyers avoid the pitfalls that had plagued some of our careers and had been evident in the professional lives of some of our colleagues. My Contributors and I shared anecdotes to keep the readers from tripping over themselves on the way to their success in what is still a male-dominated profession.

These are important lessons, and I hope that you all took them to heart. They can often be the difference between success and failure—or, at least, lack of meaningful success.

There were no value judgments in Book One, and there are none here. Book One particularly emphasized that the work-life struggle will not impact all of you the same way. The women who choose to have a significant role in family lives that include children will be impacted the most. For other women who do not have these responsibilities or responsibilities for ill, disabled or aging family members, there may be no greater impact on them from work-life struggle than for the men who occupy the offices next to theirs.

So, that was Book One, and now let's get on with Book Two. There is so much more to explore.

And, I know you have the *time!*

1

You *Really* Need to Love What You Do

I guess I have been lucky. I always have loved being a lawyer. Yes, it is a hard job, and I have had my share of transitions to deal with lifestyle issues, but I have never been sorry that I chose the law. For me, being a lawyer is challenging, it provides opportunity to do good, it allows me to use my brain to its maximum, and it brings me in contact with people from all walks of life, who I learn from and who help me gain important perspectives that enrich my life. Being a lawyer, and practicing as I have chosen to practice, has given me the additional opportunity to show my children the value of hard work and the reward of a job well done. There are many ways that I could have been a good role model for my children, and this is only one of them. But, it was a good one and has served us all well.

Being a lawyer also pays the bills and provides me with the opportunity to have a comfortable lifestyle, but that is last on my list—*really*. The other things are so much more important to who and what I am.

19

This is why an article in a recent edition of the *ABA Journal* had such a profound impact on me. It was written as a sort of love letter to the law profession, a valentine in the February 2011 issue, titled "Why I Love Being a Lawyer (Seriously)." Just the title itself resonated with me, but the content was very interesting. Before I share some of the practice nuggets with you, let me share the introduction.

> "We've all seen the downbeat headlines—surveys show as many as half of all lawyers wouldn't enter the profession if they had it to do over, wouldn't recommend their children become lawyers, would rather be digging ditches or breaking rocks. As the profession struggles to recover from the Great Recession, it's certainly not easy being an attorney.
>
> But what about the other half of the profession—the half that doesn't grab the headlines, that finds satisfaction in their jobs? There's still much to recommend the practice of law, starting with serving clients and the public good."

The article goes on to share some thoughtful words from practicing lawyers on why being a lawyer can be an extraordinary calling. Some of those quotes follow so that you understand the possibilities and what you are fighting for.

Yes, you will have challenges similar to mine. Yes, there will be days when you might rather pound rocks into powder for a living. Yes, you will feel overextended and just plain exhausted at times. And yes, you will reach frustration levels that you did not know even existed.

But, what else will you feel? What are the possibilities for good feelings that come with the territory when you are a lawyer in a practice that you enjoy? Let's hear from some of the contributors to the *ABA Journal* story to answer those questions.

> "I love being a lawyer because when I stand up before a jury and thank my clients for the privilege of representing them (and I usually feel

pretty emotional whenever I say that, with chills) I realize I am being trusted to present them, what they feel, what they believe. And I take that very seriously."

"[Being a lawyer] is the best job in the world: I get paid to read, write, think, talk and argue—all things I would do anyway."

"Why do I love being a lawyer? Because, once in awhile, you get the opportunity to help someone who desperately needs your help. It feels good to be that person."

Here is a benefit of the practice that you may not have thought about. After failing to convince the jury of the guilt of the defendant in a rape case, the lawyers representing the rape victim were feeling defeated. However, it ended up providing one of those lawyers with an "ah-ha" moment:

"I turned to the victim with our sincerest apologies. But she wasn't upset. She hugged us both and thanked us profusely for believing in her and for fighting as hard as we had. I knew then that I loved being a lawyer. I loved protecting people in a court of law. I loved the feeling of accomplishment I get from helping others fight—win or lose."

This next contributor goes to the Gospel for his inspiration:

"One thing I love about being a lawyer is beating up on bad guys. And I take the biblical injunction to 'protect widows and orphans' seriously. . . . I've had several cases where elderly people were duped into signing over deeds to their houses to relatives. One involved a recent widower who was blind.

Another contributor loves the flexibility of the law:

"What I love the most about being a lawyer is freedom. In 25 years, I have had three different careers in law, and even within those careers, I have been free to pursue my own professional desires."

Sometimes it takes only one case to give you the satisfaction of an entire career. One contributor was involved in filing a *pro bono* brief on behalf of Amnesty International and more than 50 other human rights organizations in a case where the Inter-American Court of Human Rights sanctioned the nation of Mexico for the torture and killing of women in Ciudad Juarez in what has become known as the "cotton field case." In reaching its decision, the court referred to that *pro bono* brief. The contributor wrote:

"I remember thinking that I could retire after this decision and still have had a completely satisfying legal career."

And don't make the mistake of thinking that you have to be bored as a lawyer. Here is how one contributor put it:

"What I love most about being a lawyer is that it never has to be boring. As a lawyer, you always have the opportunity to redesign your practice to accomplish different goals. In 30 years of practice I have seen the way in which law practices change radically and rapidly. I hope it keeps on changing."

One contributor was hooked from the very beginning:

"When I opened my first-year property law casebook and read the first case, I knew right then that I had made the right decision to become a lawyer. I still have that same feeling of excitement whenever I sit down to read a brief or an opinion of the Supreme Court. . . . I often have to pinch myself to convince me it is real."

Here is one that is likely to surprise you:

"I love that the law never sleeps and doesn't require that all be done 9 to 5. I could spend the morning as an attorney *guardian ad litem* representing kids who were in foster care, the afternoon as a mom with my kids and then the evening into the wee hours of the morning tackling esoteric legal issues arising from complex litigation."

Well, I think you get the point. There are many ways to enjoy practicing law, and they are not all within the hallowed halls of Big Law. Clearly, however, at least one of these contributors appears to be from Big Law, and he seems to be having a pretty good time fighting the bad guys from high up on that perch as well.

I hope that you all love what you do enough to fight for it. After all, you must have liked it enough to last three or four years in law school—even if you were one of those default students who chose law school because you could not think of anything else to do and someone let you in the door. Liking it enough and having interest in what you were learning must be what kept you there after the first semester.

You will need to remember these things as you navigate law practice to find the best practice for you. Remembering these things will go a long way when you get discouraged and are thinking of "throwing the baby out with the bathwater." Just remembering the professor who used that hackneyed cliché in your constitutional law class may remind you of some of the other reasons to love the law—like human rights and civil rights and scores of other higher callings—to help you keep the faith and use your talents to make a better place for yourself in the profession.

So, keep an open mind and pay attention to your options. If one type of practice does not suit you, another may, as you will find out from the profiles in transition at the end of this book. The most important thing is to find a place where you can be happy so that you will be on the side of half the lawyers in our country who appear to enjoy practice. And, if you are lucky, like me, you will be able to say, "I love being a lawyer."

I do not take that for granted, and neither should you.

For a follow-up article on what lawyers like about their jobs, see the May 2, 2012 *ABA Journal* on-line article, "What Continues to Inspire You About the Practice of Law" at http://www.abajournal.com/weekly/article/what_continues_to_i . . .

2

You *Really* Need to Get Serious

So, now you know that I love the law and that I am very serious about being a lawyer and working in the law. If not, I would have followed advice from some of my friends by now and be on a tropical beach somewhere sipping Mai Tais. But, I am not. I choose the law, and that is why I started the *Best Friends at the Bar* project. It is why I continue to write books, give speeches and work on behalf of women lawyers even when it gets a little discouraging. In other words, I choose *you*.

But, what about you? What do you choose? How serious are you about this law career stuff? Did you go to law school for the right reasons or because you were a good student, a good standardized test-taker and you had the opportunity to go AND you could not think of anything else to do after undergraduate school? Are you a victim of this classic default situation?

If you went for any of those wrong reasons, you are likely to see that decision catch up with you at some time early in your career. Or maybe you will get lucky and begin to love the law in the process. That would not be such a bad thing.

The practice of law is demanding, and if you are not serious about your reasons for being in the profession, you likely will not have "what it takes" to survive. If you are just casually committed to a law career, you will not be able to withstand the struggles and the challenges that are surely to come your way, particularly if you choose large law firm practice. If that is the case, you may as well hang it up right now and save yourself and the people who employ you some time and agony.

I know this sounds harsh, but I hear this all the time from seasoned lawyers, and, believe me, I do not like hearing it. They tell me that they think that too many young women lawyers today lack commitment and that they are not willing to work hard enough to make valuable contributions to employers. Admittedly, I hear this most about law firm practitioners, but I also think that it might be applicable more broadly—but it does not show up as much in the non-billable arenas. And, I hear it from both male and female practitioners. After all, lawyers who are truly committed to the well-being of their business ventures cease to see things as male or female after a while. They just want the business to prosper.

Now is the time to do your gut-check seriousness analysis. I am pretty sure that you are somewhat serious about your profession because you are taking the time to read this book. But there are different levels of commitment that are necessary in different types of jobs. At the top of the commitment scale, along with some kinds of criminal prosecution work, is large law firm practice. That practice setting has a real draw for many young women, but let's take a look at what it takes to succeed in Big Law. Once we have done that, you can scale back the commitment requirements and apply them to other practice settings.

You can start by asking yourself how willing you are to put in long hours, network at legal and business events early in the morning or late at night, and participate in client development activities when you are off the clock. All of these things take time—time away from your personal life—but they are all necessary for your professional growth and for the contribution that is expected of you in large firm practice.

If you are serious about your place in large firm practice, it is not enough to meet the minimum billable hour requirement of your law firm. You must go well beyond that to fulfill the responsibilities mentioned above and to take advantage of the face time with decision-makers and power brokers in your firm. You will not be able to hide in your cubicle, drum out 2200 billable hours, and have that be the end of your commitment. That will not put you in a position to be regarded as a valuable asset to the law firm. Even if you have no aspirations of being a partner in the firm, you still must be regarded as valuable to have a secure place in law firms where the business bottom line is EVERYTHING.

I hope by now you are beginning to see the conflict. You want time to enjoy your personal life, and work gets in the way. If that is your thought process, you are probably in the wrong work setting and you may also be in the wrong line of work altogether. If personal time *always* takes priority for you, that can be a problem—a BIG problem. This does not mean that you should not value your personal time, but it does mean that you have to learn *when* to value it. That is what true balance in this profession is all about.

Being serious about your profession and committed to being the best lawyer you can be (which is explored in a later chapter) essentially means knowing *when* to walk away—when to leave work behind in favor of the personal side of your life. Here are some examples.

It is not the right time to choose your personal life over your professional life when you do not have confirmation that the motion that you are responsible for was successfully filed with the court on time. It is not the right time to walk away when you are expected to be at the client dinner, and it is not the right time to walk away when your legal team is convening on Saturday morning to caucus on the big client meeting the following week. It is not the right time to walk away when there is one last proofread left on the brief—even if *you* think that it is in final form. Others may not share that opinion.

Your colleagues and your clients need to be able to count on you for the best legal services you can produce. Walking away in situations like those described above does not give them the warm fuzzy feelings that you are there for them when they need you.

So, what does this mean? Does it mean that you must devote yourself completely to your job?

No, that is not what it means, but you have to know when to stay totally committed and focused on the job and when that is not required. The law is like any other job, there are peaks and valleys in terms of work-load, and there will be valleys when you can put more emphasis on the personal side of your life. You must remain flexible enough to take advantage of the work valleys when they come along, and that is when you will experience real balance.

As further discussed in Chapter 5, balance is probably a myth in the context of work-life in the legal profession. What you really have to do is know *when* to take time for work and *when* to take time for the rest of your life. Unfortunately, in a business like the law, the "when" is very often dictated by others like your supervisor, your client, opposing counsel, and the judge. Unfortunately, too many times you are last in line for making that determination.

I can hear some of you now saying that this is just too much to expect. This is no life, and you will not do it. Well, that is certainly your choice. If you know that you cannot live up to that kind of commitment, then be honest with yourself and either find a law practice setting that better fits your lifestyle goals or leave the profession altogether.

I know that you may be shocked to hear me say that—me the one who wants all of you to stay in the profession and succeed as lawyers. Well, it is true that I want you all to succeed, but I also want women lawyers to retain a strong reputation in the profession. All of us suffer when law firm managers experience too many examples of lack of commitment, and soon we start to hear women lawyers referred to in "fluffy" and negative terms—the kind of terms that really annoy those of us who have fought so hard for you to be able to be lawyers at all.

Unless young women lawyers are committed to their careers, there is little chance that we will get to the point, some time in the future, when women will be represented at management levels in acceptable numbers and when women will be able to make policy that will address the work-life struggle in positive terms. It just ain't going to happen.

Simply stated, if you are not serious, you will not be taken seriously, and that is a big problem for the future of women in the profession. Those of us who take great pride in women lawyers sometimes would prefer that you did not enter the arena at all if you are not prepared to be serious about being a lawyer.

What I am talking about here is a level of commitment that is not dictated by external factors. It is the level of commitment that you feel for the law and the practice of law, and if you do not have that level of commitment from the get-go, there is little likelihood that you are going to be able to figure out any way of dealing effectively with that real work-life struggle when it comes along—the work-life struggle that includes two kids under five years of age and other family responsibilities. That is the real struggle. If yours is a casual commitment that results from a default choice about your future (as in "I do not know what else I want to do, so I think I will go to law school"), that will probably become obvious under those circumstances, and you will end up as one of the loss statistics at your law firm.

However, if you care enough about helping people solve legal problems, making the world a better place for those who cannot advocate for themselves, and righting all sorts of wrongs, you may be a survivor. Even if you are not a survivor in the law firm setting, you will find a way to be a survivor in another setting. If you truly care, it will show. If you do not, that will show also.

So, think about your level of commitment. It is not about how much money you will make, how cool a car you can drive or how expensive a house you can buy. It is not about affording designer suits or having a decorator's dream office. It is about being the best lawyer you can be—quite apart from any of those other things.

Why does this matter so much? It matters because you are one of a group of lawyers. You belong to the "women lawyers" group, and you have been raised up on the shoulders of women who fought hard for your right to have the choice to be a lawyer. You do well, and we all do well. You screw up, and, unfortunately, we all screw up to a degree. That's what it is like for minorities, whether we like it or not. Guilt by association—not pretty but often true.

Does this mean that you cannot practice law without being committed to the Big Law lifestyle of private practice? No, not at all. But if it is the Big Law lifestyle that you choose—and so many of you will—do not kid yourself about the kind of commitment required for that practice setting. You will not be cut any slack, and do not expect it. Yes, there are flexible schedules available at most law firms today, but they are not always satisfactory. For instance, if you transition your practice to part-time, you probably will work just as many hours as full-time attorneys but for less money. Or, at least, it will feel like that most of the time.

Do not expect any one to feel sorry for you or change the rules for you. Law is a business, as I stressed in Book One, and businesses have bottom lines. The law is just as much about making money as any business. You are either profitable for the law firm or you are not. Even as a part-time lawyer, you are still expected to promote work, attend social events and seek out opportunities to help the firm. If you are not prepared to do that, you may be in the wrong practice setting.

Many of you may not be able to continue in private practice under the pressures of the true work-life struggle that I have described. And, that is OK—*really*. It is your choice, it is your personal definition of success that matters, as you discovered in Book One, and no one should judge what is best for you. And you should not be so hard on yourself about it either.

However, to avoid being really disappointed when private practice does not work out and blaming others for the outcome, you must be honest with yourself about the commitment issues both early on and when the going gets tough. If you simply cannot meet the commitment requirements of the job any longer, admit it and move on to a practice setting where that is not as much of a problem. There are many talented and serious women lawyers who find the need to do just that, and it is OK. It often leads to the kind of success and satisfaction that they would not have found in Big Law.

The alternative is disastrous. Not being able to meet the commitment requirements of the job and staying in the job in spite of the limitations is a recipe for disaster. And that is what I—and so many others like me—want you to avoid. We want you to avoid the pain and stigma of having people think you are letting them down. We want you to avoid feeding the perception that women just do not have what it takes to do the job. We want to spare you the experience of seeing your stock as a lawyer erode over time to the point that you do not even recognize your professional self any more.

In other words, we want to save you from yourself, and we also want you to spare all of the women in our profession from being imputed with the results of what will surely be perceived as your lack of commitment. Unfortunately, it is unreasonable to expect a male-dominated profession to attribute the failings to anything else.

So, here are a few things to think about in demonstrating a serious attitude about your career and your place in the large firm setting.

- Are you prepared to stretch yourself professionally and seek out opportunities to improve yourself as a lawyer and benefit your firm?
- Are you prepared to seek out and embrace leadership opportunities and positions?
- Are you prepared to make it a priority to gain and retain new clients for the firm and take advantage of promotional activities?
- Are you prepared to put in the long hours when necessary to assure that you and your firm are delivering the best legal services?
- Do you have the courage to speak up for yourself and take credit for the work you do?

These are not easy things for me to say to you. It is the kind of tough love that I do not always feel comfortable with. However, I would rather have you face the issues early and decide the level of commitment that is realistic for you and apply that to the decision about where you fit on the legal landscape. There are no right or wrong answers, just the answers that are right for you. Ignoring the realities and putting off the decision can lead to a great deal of dissatisfaction and disappointment in the profession, which then leads to the low retention that we all should want to reverse.

Choose early and choose well, just like you learned to do in Book One. Deciding how serious you are about your profession and what level of commitment fits your lifestyle best is important in making those decisions and avoiding disappointment.

Good luck with it! The next chapter may help you in the important soul searching about who and what you are and where you fit.

3

You *Really* Need to Be Who You Are

This sounds simplistic, but it is so often overlooked in our profession. Being yourself is critically important in anything you do. It is important for men just as it is important for women, and failing to pay attention to this need can lead to real discontent in your life and in your law practice.

You have to be true to who you are because bad stuff can happen if you are not. For instance, in your law practice, trying to be someone you are not will usually lead to disappointing results. As one of my colleagues once said to me, you cannot be a fiery litigator if "fiery" is not your nature. It just does not work. You are better off being an exacting trial attorney and win your cases with a precise demonstration of proof than to try to win the day with a poor Clarence Darrow imitation. And, you most likely will make a fool of yourself in the process. At that point, when your confidence is on the wane, practicing law can lose its appeal. "Be authentic in all things" should be your mantra.

This is good advice, and it can be applied to many other aspects of law practice. Figure out who you are and what you do best, and play to your strengths. Let the other guy wax prolific in front of the jury throwing hands in the air in great demonstrative gestures. It just may not be who you are, and you need to have a different approach. There is no one winning strategy to being a successful lawyer, and you must figure out what approach is the most comfortable for you. We will explore this more in Chapter 11, where we explore Being the Best Lawyer You Can Be.

You also must be true to who you are in your personal life. The law is a very demanding profession, and you need to have pleasures to look forward to in your personal life in order to have the balance that you need and to maintain the professional effort that will be required in your job. Most of you will find that this is true no matter how much you enjoy being a lawyer.

This is very important because being authentic will help to keep you happy, and being happy with yourself is critically important to being satisfied in your work and in all aspects of your life. Trying to be someone and something that you are not usually will result in falling short of the mark and may lead to depression and lack of self esteem. These are not characteristics that will serve you well in reaching your goals as a lawyer.

It is all about working hard and playing hard—and by that I am not talking about hedonistic life styles. I am using "playing" to represent the purely pleasurable parts of your life that provide so much joy and can help you survive and prosper at the more difficult and demanding parts. It is what weekends were designed for, I think, until the law profession mucked it all up in the last fifty years. Weekends were for recharging your batteries with pleasurable pursuits, whether they took the form of golfing, fishing, taking the kids on hikes, going to the theater or myriad other pleasurable pastimes. That, however, may as well be ancient history for most lawyers.

We need to get back to this balance to avoid professional burnout and to continue to find pleasure in our work lives. It is so much easier to deal with the challenges and demands of practice if you have weekend pleasures to look forward to and weekend memories to ponder when the going gets tough the following week.

You work hard in order to be able to afford to do some of the things that you love, and that perspective is important to keeping you on an even keel. Without that, you are very likely to find that you no longer enjoy the law and either drop out or take a "drudge" approach to your professional life. Either result is disappointing, and you want to prepare yourself for something different.

Of course, I am not naïve enough to think that you will be a nine-to-five, five-day-a week lawyer. That is not a reasonable expectation. But you do not have to be a 365-day-a-year lawyer either. You must find a compromise between those two extremes by identifying what makes you happy and pursuing it as often as possible.

There always are exceptions. We all know lawyers who live exclusively for work. They will tell you that they do not need anything but work to make them happy, and we must take them at their word. After all, happiness is the goal, and their needs appear to be met. However, I think that you will find that these particular practitioners have very little else in their lives and are being less than honest with themselves.

Being yourself arguably can be more difficult for women than for men in a male-dominated profession. Although it has never been *easy* for women in our profession, the reasons for the discomfort are different today than they were in the past. In the past, it was particularly difficult for women because there were so few of them and positive role models were scarce. Today half of the students in law school and half of the attorneys starting out in practice each year are women, and finding successful women role models is not the problem that it once was.

However, today's women lawyers, however, are of much more diverse descriptions than in the past and that can lead to a different kind of discomfort. Only the "brainy" girls went to law school out of my college graduation class—and, incidentally, I was *not* one of them! Typically, they were very serious students without a lot of other interests. Of course, there were exceptions—and I am pleased to count some of the exceptions as my good friends—but those situations were rare. By contrast, today's young women lawyers include not only the "brainy" one-dimensional types but also the smart, competent young women who also enjoy being girls and indulging in "girlish" behavior—and lots of other types in between.

We need to pay close attention to this uniquely girlish group of young women lawyers. They are growing in numbers, and, although it may be a delicate discussion, this book would not be complete without exploring this new constituency among women lawyers. If you know anything about my work, you know that I do not ignore the elephant in the room. So, here goes.

I will refer to the young women in this group as the "Girly Girl Lawyers." It is not a derogatory term, and it is very descriptive of them. "Girly Girl" is well-established in today's vernacular by recognized publications like the *Huffington Post* and popular on-line sources like *Wikiipedia* and *Urban Dictionary*, and there are no negative judgments or references in the definitions. These sources are reflections of our times, and we need to call it what it is.

First, we need to put a little meat on those bones—so to speak. "Girly Girl" women are defined as those who are very feminine. They wholeheartedly embrace their femininity and make no excuses for it. They work hard at it. They include the girlish professionals, who are prevalent today in not only the law but in many other professional settings. I understand that most of you are girlish in some respects, but the young women in this group are probably the *ultra-girlish* types.

You know who they are. They are very smart, very talented and very competent like most of the young women in law school today, but they also enjoy all of the typically feminine pursuits. They like fashion, shopping, interior design, having cosmopolitans with their girlfriends—or is it mojitos these days?—and even watching *The Housewives of Wherever* on TV and howling at the escapades. Quite honestly, these are some of the things that make them *really* happy, and tuning into the Bravo channel can relax them after a hard day at the office. If these young women gave up the things that generate this kind of pleasure and enjoyment in their lives, they would change as individuals and they likely would fail to be as happy. This ultimately would affect their job performance and how they view their lives as lawyers.

Examining this group is important because these young women may find themselves under particular pressure to sacrifice what makes them happiest in their personal lives for the sake of a male-dominated profession like the law, and, in that sense, they may be more at risk than others. Conveniently, this group provides an excellent model for the purposes of our discussion about being "who and what you are" to achieve the work-life balance that works for you. The needs of the young women in this group can be articulated and understood easily, and it is this simplicity that will make my point in the most effective way.

This is not to say that you fit into this group or that you do not. It is just to say, "Follow the Lead" and apply the principles to your own life and your own circumstances. If you are on your high horse about the description of Girly Girl Lawyers, now is the time to get off that bucking bronco. Your anti-Carrie Bradshaw predispositions have no place here. Keep your mind open, and you may learn something valuable. You are all different, and you all deserve acknowledgment. My job is to help *all* of you.

So, the Girly Girl Lawyers will be our guides.

Today, I see a lot of Girly Girl Lawyers when I visit law schools, law organizations and law firms across the country. As a result, I suspect that I may be talking to a lot of you through the pages of this book. These young women are not difficult to spot, and I enjoy meeting them because I admire their versatility. I love that they are smart and dedicated and accomplished and comfortable with their femininity, and I know that they are going to make great lawyers. And I do not want them to change who and what they are and put their bright futures in jeopardy just as I do not want *any* of you to go down that path.

I think there also is a recognition today that girls want to be girls in this profession as well as in other walks of life, and the young women in serious professions are not hiding their femininity as much as young women professionals have done in the past. A recent Neiman Marcus catalogue included this quote from a designer at the Valentino couture design house, "We believe that women now are more feminine but in a new way, more rock 'n' roll, not so classic." If the fashion industry is spending time on it, you know it has to be BIG!

Maybe it also has something to do with the popularity of the TV show and movies *Sex and the City* and Miranda's character that made the female viewers believe they could be fashion mavens, devoted to their girlfriends and scary-smart lawyers to boot. However, I am more inclined to think that Miranda and her crew fulfilled a prophecy that was already being driven by the advent of many more ultra feminine women in business and in positions of power. Eventually it was sure to make its way to the profession of law, and, at some point, we saw the Girly Girl Lawyers come out of hiding in law schools and law firms around the country.

The problem is that protecting their authenticity may be more of a challenge for these young women than for young women lawyers of other descriptions. Women continue to have problems competing in our male-dominated profession, and there is a tendency—by both men and women alike—to treat women who demonstrate uniquely feminine characteristics as less cerebral and less professional.

I wish that I could tell you that this is not the case and that our profession has reached the ultimate in enlightenment when it comes to women. However, I cannot. It is very appropriate to ask, "Is a male attorney perceived to be less cerebral and less professional because he is obsessed with athletic pursuits? Is reading *Sports Illustrated* any different for a male lawyer than reading *InStyle* is for a female lawyer?" Of course, the answer to each of those questions is "no," but somehow the comparable scenarios continue to be received a little differently in the workplace. Women who demonstrate uniquely feminine attributes are still at risk of being perceived as lightweights instead of the competent, talented and multidimensional young women they are.

You don't have to be a Girly Girl Lawyer to care about this. If you are not a girlish type, maybe your friend is. Or maybe your sister or your niece is. You will want them to have all the same chances at satisfying and fulfilling careers that you have, and that is why you need to be aware of the particular challenges they may face.

If you are not a Girly Girl Lawyer, this is where you should be substituting some other characteristics about yourself in the model—things that are important to *your* personal life and make *you* who you are. Just as it is important that some women lawyers safeguard their girlishness, it is likely that you have something to safeguard, too. Maybe you are a committed jock or someone who enjoys working with animals, gardening, cooking, mountain climbing, learning ancient Arabic languages, mastering the intricacies of Japanese origami or playing a musical instrument. This is what makes you happy, and you want to hang onto that to protect the joy and the balance that it brings to your life.

Recall the biography of Sandra Day O'Connor that I cited to on several occasions in Book One. Talk about multidimensional! SDO is about as multidimensional as they come, and she never hid behind it. She did not disguise her attractiveness, and she worked hard at sports like golf and tennis to keep fit. She was a pretty good dresser, a compassionate mother and grandmother, and the most devoted and loving wife you can imagine. In fact, she gave up her seat on the United States Supreme Court to care for her ailing husband. AND she was one of the most talented constitutional lawyers and judges in the land. She alone should have put this issue of femininity and professionalism to rest, but I am afraid it has not worked exactly that way. Some of the inequity and bias, both express and implicit, lingers on, and you will have to deal with it.

For the most part, women are not to blame for this unfortunate perception, and you should not have to sacrifice your pursuits as an ultra feminine type on the altar of male dominance. But, you will have to work hard to change the negative perception that persists, and one way to change that perception is to remember that there is positive "girlish stuff" and negative "girlish stuff." You should know the difference—especially if you read Book One. If you didn't—and shame on you!—here is one of my web site blog entries to make it clear for you.

May 31, 2011

Dressing for Success Is Challenging in Hot, Steamy Weather

If you live anywhere on the East Coast, you know that the weather is just darned hot these days. I had a lunch meeting today and nearly collapsed of heat stroke walking between the parking lot and the restaurant. It got me thinking about all of you and the challenge to dressing professionally for young women lawyers—especially in this hot, steamy weather.

If you read my book, *Best Friends at the Bar: What Women Need to Know about a Career in the Law,* you know that this is a serious subject. Too many young women professionals are compromising their dress to their desires for comfort or their desires to play up the "sexy" side. There is a difference between feminine and sexy, and I am quite sure that you know where that line gets drawn. If you passed Federal Income Tax and Secured Transactions, this should not be too difficult to figure out. In case it is not obvious, take advice from the Seventh Circuit judges at a judicial conference in 2009 where they "groused" on the inappropriateness of thigh length skirts and plunging necklines in the courtroom.

This type of dress is not appropriate in the office and sends the wrong signals. You want your colleagues and your clients to treat you like a professional, and you must dress like one and act like one. Off-color jokes are not appropriate in the office, so why would clothing that is reminiscent of nightclub attire?

The Seventh Circuit judges also commented about attire that is too casual for the courtroom. Should anyone have to be told that sweatsuits are not on the appropriate list???? Apparently so. Flipflops also are not on the list, but we still hear of summer associates showing up at Big Law in shorts and flipflops on casual Friday. Casual does not mean beach attire, and it is a really good idea to check the rule book for what casual means in your firm before experimenting. It could be a real career changer to get called to a client meeting at the last minute without backup appropriate attire. And, who wants to carry a suitcase to the office with various clothing choices to cover all odds? Not worth it. Just dress appropriately from the get-go, and you will have no problems. To paraphrase the judges of the Seventh Circuit, dress as a serious person who takes her profession seriously.

Back to the weather and its influence on your clothing choices. Yes, it may be 95% outside, but no, you are not expected to wear stockings—aka panty hose. Even First Lady Michelle Obama knows that you can be taken very seriously as a woman professional without donning pantyhose. (Read her confession on *The View* before a nationwide television audience.) And about those signals you are sending . . . the signal may be that you are "hot" from the high temperatures, but make sure that the signal is not that you are "hot" sexually. It might be fun, but it is highly inappropriate and you will regret it.

However, when the mercury climbs, it is a tad more complicated than that because the weather outside may be 20 degrees hotter than the inside office temperature. Layer, layer, layer is the key. The jacket or little cardigan can be ditched in the miserable subway and on the walk over sizzling concrete to the office, but it will come in handy for the supercharged AC that most law firms demand—even though cost-cutting should be on their minds these days.

And finally, what about exposed arms? Although there seems to be some debate on this, I think that sleeveless can be very professional. Again, check out the sleeveless shifts that the First Lady favors. And, if you had her arms, why not! However, at least one law firm banned sleeveless attire last summer when in the presence of clients, so beware of the dinosaurs that still roam the earth.

So, no pantyhose required, sleeveless can be professional, layer, layer, layer and apply a generous dosage of common sense. That's what should be in your summer survival kit.

From www.bestfriendsatthebar.com

So, always remember that you need to dress professionally and act professionally. No exposed cleavage and thighs at the office, and please do not turn up in what could pass for lingerie. In addition, you should not indulge in "girl talk" at length in the sacred corridors of the law firm any more than your male colleagues should Monday morning quarterback the Big Game until mid-day on Tuesday. You have work to do, and you do not want to be perceived as someone who does not take the requirements of the job seriously. I also would not recommend that you sit around your office reading *InStyle* or surfing your favorite fashion web sites any more than I would recommend that the men do the same with their manly magazines and ESPN channels of choice—for the very same reasons.

You also need to use your femininity appropriately. It is understandable that women lawyers today do not want to be tied to stereotypes that correlate their successes with their dominant personas as "women in men's suits." Women recognize that they are different and bring different skills and attributes to the table than their male counterparts, and women have an opportunity today to expand the model, find their own brands and make it work for them and for their organizations. Although there is an accepted wider range of behavior models for women attorneys today than in the past, as pointed out by panelists at the National Association of Women Lawyers (NAWL) Conference in New York City in July of 2011, pushing the limits can present a whole new set of problems.

The NAWL panelists emphasized the need for women to develop their individual identities without overplaying their feminine and sexual attributes, to pick their moments of gender challenge carefully, and to be authentic. Women are typically nurturing, and that can work to their advantages in certain situations of high anxiety and extreme discord, but those attributes must be used positively and effectively without compromising professionalism. In the same way, women lawyers have opportunities to find where they connect best and to create synergies in their practices more than ever before, but they must learn to use these new opportunities judiciously and without a negative display of femininity.

42

In some respects, it is a double-edged sword. Your feminine characteristics can be extremely effective in enhancing your practice opportunities, but, if used in the wrong way, they can become weapons that have the potential to be used against you.

Here is a recent blog entry from my web site that makes the point.

July 27, 2011

Hot Temps and Hot Topics for Young Women Lawyers

Last week was hot on the East Coast for a number of reasons. Yes, the mercury was off the charts, but things also were "hot" at the National Association of Women Lawyers (NAWL) conference at the Waldorf Astoria Hotel in NYC. There were hot topics from some leading authorities on issues affecting women in the law. You can imagine my excitement to discover that all of the topics discussed are included in my book, *Best Friends at the Bar: What Women Need to Know about a Career in the Law*, and are expanded on in my new book, which will be released in 2012.

However, my books have twists that go beyond just reframing the issues. I actually propose some solutions! Novel, indeed! Stay tuned for more on the second book. It addresses the New Woman Lawyer— Gen Y. They are not their mothers' lawyers! Not by a long shot, and we should be happy about that. What is that definition of insanity: Doing the same thing over and over and expecting a different result? We need a different approach *and* a different result.

The conference focused on implicit bias and had some interesting perspective from Jerry Kang, Professor of Law and Asian American Studies, UCLA Law. I was particularly interested in his comments, and those of fellow panelists, about the implicit bias that some senior women lawyers have against some younger women lawyers. This can be based on appearance, dress, demeanor or just because the young women have a different approach to practicing law and living their lives at the same time. These biases exist even when the young woman lawyer is doing an excellent job and meeting all of the deadlines. This is not exactly Women Helping Women, a theme I stress in both my book and the new manuscript. I really hope that one day soon we will become enlightened and able to stop talking about this over and over.

Too often the senior women lawyers show bias toward their young, dynamic women colleagues with attitudes that are shocking. The senior women seem to be saying, "We worked for you to have these opportunities, but we *do not want you to take advantage of it.*" One of the panelists pointed out the irony that the Baby Boomer women lawyers have raised their daughters to be powerful and independent women, and many of their daughters now are lawyers. However, no matter how much those senior women support their own daughters, they cannot tolerate other similar young women in the workplace. It reminds me of what I tell young women about having children. Yes, you may not think that you like little kids—in fact they may annoy the heck out of you—but that does not mean that you should not have some of your own. It is ALL different when they're yours. You cannot get enough of them!

You will be happy to know that I spoke up for you. I suggested to the group that young women lawyers are deaf to our haughty conversations about how it was "in the day" and are offended by the wagging of fingers while hearing that we can tell them "a thing or two." Yes, we have a lot to share that will help you, but we need to find voices that will appeal to you and that you will listen to. Those voices cannot be judgmental. Those voices cannot be condescending, and those voices cannot be preachy. Those voices must be authentic. Those voices must be sincerely caring, and those voices must be helpful. You young women know the difference, and you have a right to more.

Young women lawyers today are expanding the model and redefining who they are. They are NOT willing to hinge their success on being "men in skirts". Rather, they believe that there is a wider range of behavior attributes that can be defined as professional. They are young women modeling success while pushing the limits to fit their own generation and lifestyle. However, they too often are met with resistance from the very women who should be cheering them on.

You know that I am your biggest cheerleader, as long as you use your femininity appropriately, always act professionally, and be the best lawyers you can be. I think that there are actually many more senior women lawyers just like me. They just need to take the time to think it through!

Keeping all of that in mind, remember who you are and protect that identity. If you are one of those young women who thinks it is wonderful being a girl, go for it! Do it discretely and wisely and let it bring greater happiness to all parts of your life, including your professional life.

So, whether you are a Girly Girl Lawyer or an athlete lawyer or a history buff lawyer, ask yourself, "What makes me happy?" "What feeds the 'essence' of me and what will keep me getting out of bed every day and going to a very challenging and demanding law practice?" Once you have the answers, you will know what to protect.

As you might have suspected all along, I am a bit of a Girly Girl Lawyer myself—albeit of the older variety! It is who I am, and I have no intention of changing it. Do not even think of getting between me and my new issue of *Architectural Digest* or *Veranda*. And, I will fight you for first dibs on *Vogue* magazine. I believe that an afternoon of shopping in Georgetown can cure most ills, and I love to watch the Academy Awards just to see the fabulous gowns. I could not wait to see the royal wedding and what Kate Middleton would wear—even if I had to get up at 5 AM!

This does not make me any less of a lawyer. I was a pioneer as a woman lawyer in construction litigation, and I know more about tunnel boring machines and cofferdams than most of my male colleagues. I refused to embrace the oxford cloth shirts, little bow ties and pinstripe suits that were popular for women lawyers when I started practice, and I wore silk blouses and pearls to the job sites. I am published on issues of constitutional law, and I have stared down more than one opposing counsel in depositions (including the one who asked me to define "sexual intercourse" during a deposition in one of the first toxic shock syndrome cases taken to trial in this country). I have threatened to lie down in front of a bulldozer to save my client's building from destruction, and I know how to handle people who are unfair to me in the workplace. Being feminine did not interfere with my career because I did not let it. I was good at what I did, and I maintained my professionalism.

As a result, I have absolutely no problem with Girly Girl Lawyers—in fact, I wish there had been more of them around "in the day." They work hard and play hard, and they understand the value of laughter. They know what makes them happy, and they run with it. I want to be sure that they stick around to enrich the next generation of lawyers and spread their happiness and *joie de vivre* around to some of the less joyful types. It can have great value in taking the edge off a very stuffy profession. I count them among my best friends—along with many other women who are not girlish types at all. I am proud to have a variety of friends, and I appreciate them all equally.

So, in the process of being true to yourself, remember the example of the Girly Girl Lawyers. Also remember the biker, the mountain climber, the kayaker, the bird watcher and the musician or whichever description fits you best. Let the delight of being your own person buoy you up so that some of that joy can spill over to your professional life. Then you will be in a position to keep your life in balance—the *new* balance—to get the most out of your law career. It is all about authenticity. You will know who you are and who you want to be. So, be it!

Accomplishing the *new* balance also is a lot about confidence. Being confident about who and what you are is critical in our profession. The legal business is full of both sharks and bottom feeders, and you want to be up near the surface swimming in the clear water without exhibiting negative shark-like behavior. It is a confidence game, and you need to garner your strength from a variety of sources. Trying to be someone you are not only robs you of precious time and ultimate happiness. Be content with who you are and what makes you happy, try to fashion your life with those things in mind, and you will be ready to take on the challenges of your profession.

As you continue to be who and what you are, stop making excuses and explaining yourself. If you want to go out for a manicure in the middle of the workday afternoon, do it. If the kayak sale at the REI store starts at 10 AM, and you want to be first in line, do it. If you want to take in the cooking show at the Convention Center for an hour in the afternoon, do it. No one needs to know where you are going and where you have been. No one asks the guys where they are going—and we probably do not really want to know!—and the men typically do not volunteer the information. A simple, "I will be gone for the next hour" will do nicely.

It is *your* professional time to manage, and you are perfectly capable of managing it. If getting your nails done will make you feel more confident as you sit around the settlement table the next day, do it. You can make a great settlement presentation or you can make a killer settlement presentation because you feel good about your appearance. It is your choice and no one else's.

AND, don't forget that another way to put the annoying "lightweight" feminine perception to rest is to beat the pants off the male opposition. That will gain you positive attention and should quickly change the subject to something more appropriate. And, it will feel so good!

To read more on the importance of being who and what you are, I recommend the following. I hope that you will have the time to explore some of these authors as the need arises.

Craddock, Maggie. *The Authentic Career: Following the Path of Self Discovery to Professional Fulfillment.* **New World Library, 2004.**

Craddock believes that identifying authentic career goals and strategies requires a careful examination of one's inner life. She outlines a therapeutic process that carefully separates what the reader wants and needs from the often-frustrating demands of family and work.

Giardina, Ric. *Your Authentic Self: Be Yourself at Work.* **Beyond Words Publication, 2002.**

Giardina explains that by honoring our authentic self at work, we open the doors to hidden gifts, including creativity, intuition, and innovation. The end result is greater clarity of insight and better on-the-job performance, expanding our opportunities for advancement even as we enjoy more fulfilling work relationships.

Robbins, Mike. *Be Yourself, Everyone Else Is Already Taken: Transform Your Life with the Power of Authenticity.* **Jossey-Bass, 2009.**

Robbins, a highly visible motivational speaker/coach/author/guru, delivers a primer on authenticity: what it means, what it can do, and how to achieve it. With questions, exercises, action points and sound practices, Robbins provides a map to transforming fear, gaining self-knowledge and celebrating your authentic self.

Valentis, Mary, and John Valentis. *Brave New You: 12 Dynamic Strategies for Saying What You Want & Being Who You Are.* **New Harbinger Publications, 2001.**

While young girls generally have high levels of self-confidence, many adult women downplay their own desires in deference to others. This book inspires women (particularly in the workplace) to blend the curious, risk-taking, independent spirit of youth with the self-possessed maturity of adulthood. Each chapter presents a specific issue and guides the reader in making changes and gauging progress.

You *Really* Need to Put Yourself First—At Least Part of the Time

Notice the tag line here—"At Least Part of the Time." Putting yourself first is a matter of knowing when to do it and when you need it most. If you put yourself first all of the time, you probably will eliminate sharing your life with others and most chances of being happy in any part of your life. Although it is not all about you, it needs to be about you part of the time when you really need it.

Putting yourself first is not easy for most women, and it is especially difficult for women who have responsibilities as weighty as practicing law. However, the experts who study stress will tell you that you work most effectively if you have daily exercise and eat and sleep well, and you should always keep that in mind. Your physical health depends on it, and you are not going to be much of a lawyer or a caretaker if you are the one lying in the bed after collapsing from a stress-related illness. You cannot succeed at your profession or help others if you are broken, so you need to keep yourself in good shape, both physically and mentally.

To put yourself first, you must get over the idea that there is some shame in choosing yourself. There is not. You deserve to be first some times, and you need to get to the point where you feel comfortable with that concept. We are a long way evolved from the taboo against voting for yourself for class president or crossing guard captain when it is clear that you are the best choice. Let's leave those notions where they belong, somewhere in grade school.

This does not mean, however, that you should ignore the needs of others. You need to become proficient at assessing the nature of your needs *vis-a-vis* those of others, and you will discover that it is not unusual that the needs of others are exaggerated. If that is the case, then your needs may be paramount. Learn to tell the difference, and it will take you a long way toward finding your emotional and physical comfort zone. It is only then that you will be happiest, do your best work and have the greatest opportunity for success.

At all cost, avoid the resentment that comes with having fallen into the trap of being all things to all people. Resentment creates a lot of negative energy, and that is not the kind of energy you need to meet the demands of your personal and professional lives. If you are feeling deprived of your personal time, take that time back and revel in it. The people around you would rather have you happy than resentful, and you don't need to take a poll to find out the truth in that.

When you give time to yourself, give it freely. Enjoy those experiences and create good memories and feelings about your life. It may just be a walk in the park or an outing at your favorite shops. It may be a night at a concert or an afternoon at the movies. It may be a trip to the spa or a weekend at the beach relaxing with friends. You will get the most out of those experiences if you start with the premise that you deserve it and you concentrate on the experience and not on what is on your desk at the office. You will come back from the experience refreshed and ready to go at the job.

The same is true when you give time to others. Do not keep checking your Blackberry or iPhone when you are supposed to be enjoying an afternoon with your friends or family. Just as you want to feel that your personal time is valuable, your family and friends want to feel that you value time that you spend with them. It is fundamental, really, but we very often forget the interconnection.

It is surprisingly easy to fall into the habit of giving everything you have to your work. After all, you are surrounded by people who would have you believe that your role as a lawyer should totally define who and what you are. These are the case managers and supervising attorneys who want 100% of you and who know that, if you are eaten up by the system in the first five years, there are plenty of others behind you. However, once you are around them long enough, you very often will have a window into their personal lives and know that you want something different.

There also are the clients who want what they want when they want it and who do not have any interest in your happiness or the balance in your life. This does not make them bad people, it just makes them what *they* are—clients who have big problems, demanding jobs and lots of responsibility at their ends. If you allow your life to be taken over by people with agendas different than your own, you will get further and further removed from what makes you happy. If you want a different and more healthy and balanced approach, you will have to fight for it.

How do you do that? You do it by realizing what it is you need and making sure you get it *when the time is right*. That is a very important concept. You know that you will have to work hard as a lawyer—there is just no getting around that. It is why you are paid the big bucks. If you are not prepared to work hard, you should not have gone to law school. I think we covered that in Book One. However, working hard and working smart are two different things. Working smart includes maximizing your efforts when you have to and taking time off to feed your personal side when the schedule is less hectic. It is all about energy depletion, burnout and pacing yourself. You will have to take good care of yourself to survive in this profession and gain the payoff of having a satisfying and successful career.

Take that vacation that you have been putting off because there is always a new matter on your desk. The new matter will be there when you get back.

Take time out for the opening day at the ballpark if you are a baseball fan. Have a beer and relax. You have been waiting for opening day throughout the dismal winter.

And the sample sale you have been waiting for? Go to it! It will not only make you feel good but it will probably make you work harder at the office to put away a nest egg for future bargains.

For those of you with families, make sure that you take time out for family events and occasions and that you prioritize them. Your first grader will only star in that first grade winter holiday program one time. Be there.

If these attempts at carving out some personal time from your professional life do not meet with the approval of your employer and become an impediment to making partner in a law firm, for example, maybe that is exactly what you needed to know. As we explored in Book One, there are many more definitions to being a success as a lawyer than just being a law firm partner. You may find that you are in the wrong place for you, and you will have to consider your options and the alternatives. We will look at those alternatives and the issue of making transitions in the second half of this book.

Putting yourself first is not a bad thing as long as it is balanced against the other responsibilities in your lives. Make sure that you give it a try, and do not succumb to the feelings of guilt and insecurity that will be gnawing at your heels. After all, this is a critical component of the *new* balance that ultimately will help you in achieving satisfaction in both your personal and profession lives.

Of course, there will always be exceptions. My litigator husband and I have both canceled our share of family vacations for professional reasons because it was absolutely unavoidable. Sometimes work at the office must come first, and you have to learn to accept that. Having a supportive mate or spouse or family helps immeasurably in those circumstances. But, remember that the exceptions should not become the rule. You must learn to distinguish between a real crisis and a manufactured crisis, which is usually the product of insecurity. Do not make your time at the office your security blanket because that would be false security. You are more likely to gain security from having a healthy approach to work and producing the best work possible.

Happiness is not the only reason to take time out for yourself. The other reason is your health. Failing to take time out for yourself very often results in stress, and excess stress is very bad for you. We need to talk about stress for a moment to make sure that you know what to avoid.

Women lawyers often are "high achievers," particularly as that phrase is used by psychologists. According to Dr. Harriet Braiker in "The Type E Woman: How to Overcome the Stress of Being Everything to Everybody (Lincoln, NE:iUniverse, Inc. 2006) and as quoted in a recent *Ms. JD Blog* ("High Achieving Women Need More Than a Bubble Bath," December 19, 2011), the phrase refers to characteristic ways of thinking about achievement, rather than how high on the career ladder a woman may be. High-achievement traits that Dr. Braiker identifies are: a drive to excel and seek new challenges; competitive and serious nature; perseverance; high level of responsiveness; recognition of performance; and passion for work. She also identifies assumptions that are possessed by high-achieving women. Those assumptions are particularly interesting. They include the following:

- I have to be perfect and do things perfectly;
- I should be able to manage it all and accomplish it without feeling stressed or tired;
- I have to prove myself to everyone;
- I can't relax until I finish my task;
- I should be able to accomplish more in a day;

- I can handle it all on my own; and
- I have to be a people pleaser.

Does this sound familiar? Did I just describe you? If so, you really need to listen up because, according to Dr. Braiker, these are flawed assumptions that drive a lot of stress-producing behavior in high-achieving women who overextend their time and resources, fail to delegate, are not assertive in saying "no," don't ask for help, and evaluate themselves harshly and often. According to *Ms. JD*, high-achieving women lawyers are particularly susceptible to this type of stress because they work in environments that provide the women with very little control over their schedules, the cases and projects that they work on and the outcomes. In addition, the law firms are slow to adopt the flexible schedules that these women need and alternatives to the billable hour for measuring competency and determining upward mobility. The end result it that the very traits that are attractive to law firms in hiring high-achieving women lawyers are the very traits that the law firms are failing to address, and the high-achieving women become discouraged and take their talents elsewhere.

It sounds like classic mismanagement, but we know that it is a little more complicated than that. However, firms would be well-advised to take a close look at what the high-achieving women need to be satisfied with their work-life "balance." Dr. Marcia Reynolds identifies those factors as:

- Frequent new challenges to stretch their talents and to grow;
- Flexible schedules;
- The opportunity to collaborate and work with other high-achievers;
- Recognition from the firm; and
- Freedom to be themselves.

(Dr. Marcia Reynolds, "Wander Woman: How High-Achieving Women Find Contentment and Direction," San Francisco, CA: Berrett-Koehler Publishers, Inc. 2010)

Having said this and identified the kind of stress and expectations that we need to eliminate, we also need to remember that some degree of stress can actually be good for you. Stress can keep you focused and make you very productive. I know lawyers who are classic procrastinators and who thrive on the effects of the last minute adrenaline rush. They are also very good lawyers. However, more often than not, stress can be very bad for you and make you unable to focus, to make a decision or to produce your best product.

Medical doctors Stephanie McClellan and Beth Hamilton are experts on stress, and they have written a very important book on the subject and the negative effects on high-achieving women. In their book, *So Stressed: The Ultimate Stress-Relief Plan for Women* (Free Press, 2009), they address the consequences of long-term stress for women. Here are some of their findings.

Women are more likely than men to report stress and report a wider range of stress inducers, including time constraints, the expectations of others, marital relationships, children, and family health. Women are almost three times more likely than men to develop the following autoimmune diseases as a result of stress: Type 1 diabetes, multiple sclerosis, lupus, rheumatoid arthritis, thyroid disorders, and inflammatory bowel disease.

In addition, McClellan and Hamilton report that stress-induced heart disease is the number-one cause of death in women, in spite of the fact that less than 15% of women consider heart disease a health threat, and stroke kills more women than men (women represent 61% of stroke victims). They also report that stressful events, including loss of a loved one, are linked to an increase of breast cancer in women within two years after the event, and they identify the manifestations of stress that specifically impact women to include the following:

- A general calm that turns into a highly agitated state when stress hits;
- A feeling that you are living in a bubble and watching life pass you by;

- A constant state of overdrive; and
- The ability to respond positively to stress for as long as you have to—which is then followed by a crash.

The conclusion is that chronic stress can make you really sick, but the book also includes ways to prevent stress and make yourself feel better, look better, slow the aging process and lower the risk for disease. Some of these are:

- Think like an athlete and pace yourself;
- Rejuvenate and renew your energy often—as often as every two hours when you are at work. This can include taking a break away from your desk or just stretching at your desk. You also need to rejuvenate in a larger way outside of work, and that involves physical exercise and taking time to enjoy things you really like to do with some degree of regularity; and
- Pare down the number of choices that you have so that your decisions will be simpler and not lead to stress. In other words, do not allow yourself to indulge in the "scorched earth" policy every time you pick a restaurant or a swimming suit. Do a fair sampling, and make a decision. Get on with it or it can become a lengthy, frustrating and very stressful situation.

In addition to controlling your stress, watching your weight so that it does not cause health issues and eating right are very important. You all know about the health benefits of the various food groups and all that good stuff, but eating right at the office can become a challenge. Avoid skipping lunch because you are too busy. Avoid working through the dinner hour only to leave the office late and going home to "drink your dinner" and go to bed without eating. Eating and drinking wine and alcohol too late at night is also another bad habit and has the additional side effect of interfering with sleep—and we know how important sleep is to job performance and reducing stress.

It appears that these issues are not restricted to the American lifestyle and our issues with stress. According to Kaizen Lifestyle Management— Coaching for Continuous Improvement, which is based in Toronto, it also is a problem for Canadians. In a recent on-line article entitled "Women Lawyers Need Healthy Boundaries for Work-Life Balance," Kaizen outlined the competing roles of women lawyers to juggle as: Lawyer; mother; spouse; daughter; housekeeper; colleague; associate; and friend.

The article also cited the Ontario Lawyers Assistance Program statistics that "lawyers have higher rates of divorce, illness and suicide than other professionals; are twice as likely to succumb to alcohol abuse; are three times more likely to suffer depression and other forms of mental ill health." In response to these statistics, Kaizen offered seven strategies to improve work life balance. They can be summarized as:

- Learn to manage stress and feelings of panic;
- Set healthy boundaries with your clients, associates, family and self;
- Build healthy lifestyle practices;
- Practice self-care—quiet the mind and calm the emotions through mindfulness, meditation, and reflective practice;
- Network regularly with colleagues employed in a wide variety of legal capacities to share insights and explore career opportunities;
- Cultivate a social circle outside of your legal network to dream up new ideas and take risks; and
- Partner with a life coach and transform stress and let go of feelings of guilt and remorse; define sustainable success, set goals and priorities, and improve life satisfaction.

Putting yourself first can also mean getting advice on financial management so that you do not live beyond your means and fail to plan for your future. My experience tells me that lawyers are not great planners when it comes to their own finances. Whether it results from lack of interest or lack of time can be debated, but the importance of the issue is fairly undebatable. Put that on your list as well.

This is really serious stuff, and I hope you will take it seriously. Do not make the mistake of thinking that you are too young to have to worry about this. Not so.

Habits start early, and you want to choose good habits and routines and continue them throughout your career. It is much harder to start them after the crisis has hit.

So, put yourself first in every way that will make you better and more effective in your personal and professional lives and that will keep you healthy. You cannot be good for others unless you are good for yourself. It is all about the *new* balance.

A recent edition of *Slaw*, Canada's online legal magazine, included a list of New Year's resolutions to choose from to improve your well-being. Fortunately, a bubble bath was not suggested, but there were some thought-provoking suggestions. My personal favorites for all women lawyers can be summarized as:

- If you never get time with your husband or partner, hire a sitter for a regular date night or for three hours on the weekend so that you can have the time you need for your relationship;
- Book a weekly massage or yoga class or hire a coach at the gym or club of your choice; and
- For women with children, do something to help yourself unwind and create separation between you and the office before you arrive home and meet the kids. Studies show that kids' first choice isn't more time with parents. Their first choice is less grumpy, stressed out parents for whatever time they get.

(*Slaw*, October 6, 2011)
It sounds like they have things right in Canada!

Putting yourself first is not a new concept. Here are some additional resources for you:

Benson, Herbert, and Eileen M. Stuart. *The Wellness Book: The Comprehensive Guide to Maintaining Health and Treating Stress-Related Illness*. Simon & Schuster, 1993.

In 24 chapters, the reader is introduced to the essentials of healthy lifestyle, including the relaxation response, nutrition, exercise, and stress management. The workbook format includes short patient histories, space for write-in exercises and personal data, charts, and diagrams.

Bowden, Johnny, Ph.D. C.N.S. *The Most Effective Ways on Earth to Boost Your Energy: The Surprising, Unbiased Truth about Using Nutrition, Exercise, Supplements, Stress Relief, and Personal Empowerment to Stay Energized All Day*. Fair Winds, 2011.

Nationally known health expert Johnny Bowden presents small changes anyone can implement up front for big energy—such as what to eat for all-day endurance, when to time a workout for the biggest brain boost, or how working with (or against) natural light cycles can make your sleep restorative. Energy starts with attitude—readers learn how to "think" like a high-energy person and use breathing techniques, meditation, and exercise to bust stress, beat fatigue, and boost stamina.

Hall, Dawn. *7 Simple Steps to a Healthier You: A Busy Woman's Guide to Living Well*. Harvest House, 2006.

The author provides firsthand advice for handling weight issues, hectic schedules, unhealthy behaviors, and the hurdle of excuses as she shares why healthy living starts with choosing the best food and exercise plan for you. The book includes meal plans and recipes to be successful.

Kelly Newsome, Director/Instructor, Higher Ground Yoga, www.highergroundyoga.com

Kelly Newsome is an attorney turned yoga instructor and counselor serving the Washington, DC metropolitan area. Her company motto is "Helping Busy Women Breathe Easier." She can be reached at Kelly@highergroundyoga.com.

Jampolis, Melina B. *The No-TimeTo-Lose Diet: the Busy Person's Guide to Permanent Weight Loss.* **Nashville: Nelson, 2007.**

Busy people see to everything and everyone—except themselves. The author's approach to weight loss embraces the hectic lifestyle and provides realistic strategies for staying on target, including helpful dining options for eating out, healthy, flavorful, and FAST menu ideas for eating in, and timesaving strategies to maximize results.

Kornblatt, Sondra. *A Better Brain at Any Age: The Holistic Way to Improve Your Memory, Reduce Stress, and Sharpen Your Wits.* **Conari, 2008.**

Kornblatt, along with the experts she interviews, helps readers put their heads on straight through healthy activities for the body (exercise, healthy food consumption, and relaxation) and through specific activities to boost brain power like movement, eye rolls, supplements, and making environmental changes.

Rath, Tom, and James K. Harter. *Wellbeing: The Five Essential Elements.* **Gallup, 2010.**

This book will provide you with a holistic view of what contributes to your wellbeing over a lifetime. Written in a conversational style by #1 New York Times bestselling author Tom Rath and bestselling author Jim Harter, Ph.D., it contains novel ideas for boosting your wellbeing in each of five areas: career wellbeing, social wellbeing, financial wellbeing, physical wellbeing, and community wellbeing.

You *Really* Need to Gain Perspective

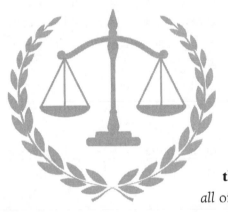

To illustrate this point, I must harken back to a very important theme of Book One: You cannot have *all* of it *all* of the time. To grasp the total meaning of that theme, you must have a firm foothold in reality. As stated in Book One, you can have some of it all of the time, all of it some of the time, but it is the rare woman lawyer who can have all of it all of the time. In other words, you cannot be the best lawyer all of the time, the best mother or caretaker all of the time, the best hostess all of the time, the best room mother all of the time . . . and the list goes on.

Here I suggest that you check out a new book, *Good Enough Is the New Perfect—Finding Happiness and Success in Modern Motherhood* by Becky Beaupre Gillespie and Hollee Schwartz Temple (Harlequin, 2011). Although it is not specific to women lawyers, the book is a primer for women looking for professional fulfillment and personal happiness. It is an extension of the authors' blog, TheNewPerfect.com, and their columns on related topics for the ABA Journal, and it is worthy of your consideration.

Rather than striving for perfection, what you are likely to find is that you have to strike a balance that works for you. In my conversations with women about this issue, I have come to realize that balance in its pure sense—whether it is the old model or the new model—may be an unattainable goal. Many women will say that there is no real balance and that you will have to be satisfied with things being out of balance some of the time with the understanding that it will even out in the end. In other words, one week may be heavily weighted toward the work side, but another week may be heavily weighted toward the personal side. According to this theory, rarely will you find a period of time that is in true balance.

That seems to square with reality, and I accept the nuance. I think it is what you will find to be true. It is important that you anticipate this situation and that you do not expect too much of yourself during any one period of time and assign success or failure on that basis. It is a long career that you hope to have. There will be times when you are completely satisfied with what you give to one component of your life, and there will be times when you will be sorely disappointed with another result. But, give yourself time to figure it all out and do not become easily discouraged.

Take time to get some perspective. Talk to women professionals around you and take advantage of their experiences. Book One offered you advice from many experienced women lawyers who had faced your same dilemmas, and there are many other such women surrounding you in your workplaces and in your professional organizations. These women are typically not only willing to talk to you but they *enjoy* talking about their experiences. Even though their work-life model may not be the exact balance that you are seeking, their experiences will be valuable.

Another wonderful way to get perspective is to take a vacation— something we talked about in the previous chapter. Taking vacation is not only critical to your personal time but it also helps to gain perspective. Most of you know that. However, as you progress in your practice, you will start to think that you are indispensable to the client and to the outcome of matters you are handling. That is rarely true because your firms and practices have hired other talented lawyers, and the world will not come to an end if you take a few days off. Besides, today's technology can keep you in touch as much or as little as you like when you are physically away from the office.

There is nothing like standing on the top of a mountain or walking on the beach contemplating the great beyond to give you perspective. Make sure that you do it often enough to make a difference in your life and the lives of those who depend on you to have the perspective you need. In addition to helping you to understand what matters, this kind of perspective will help you to identify what you really want and need. And, that is what this book is all about.

Other cultures know the value of extended vacations—something more than just a few days—but it can be a hard sell in the American workplace. As a result, you will have to be wise about how you approach it. However, you will be the keeper of your sacred billable hours—along with someone in the management dungeon who also has committed your personal statistics to memory!—and you will know when you are in "good shape" to take the vacation that you were promised. When that time comes, take it. Next year you may be in trial for six months without the possibility of an odd day off, much less an entire week or two. There is definitely a "make hay while the sun shines" component to our profession.

When you are contemplating a vacation, you would be well-advised to discuss it early with your case managers. You need to make them aware of your plans and to work with them to create as little disruption to client services as possible. This is completely doable and very important to your future relationships with your colleagues.

Gaining this healthy perspective needs to include pacing yourself. If you are fortunate enough to find the *new* balance, you will have a long career ahead of you. If you do not pay attention to the needs of your body and your mind, you will burn out early and never reach the time when you have practiced long enough to reap the real benefits of your own feeling of expertise and the other rewards of being a competent lawyer. There are plenty of stories about professional burnout in lawyers, and I know you have heard some of them. You do not want to become one of those statistics. Pacing yourself is very important to avoiding this result, and you need to pay attention to it. Ask any long distance runner, and the benefits of pacing yourself will become very clear to you, or watch the racehorse at the back of the pack overtake other horses in the last lap. It is all about timing and saving your strength for both the long run and the sprint.

Another important part to gaining this perspective is letting yourself enjoy and appreciate the practice of law. The law can be as interesting and exciting as you let it be. However, you will not understand this by reading the popular legal blogs that have gained their popularity as "gripe" sites. Although it is entertaining to read some of these complaints, it can lead to a very jaded attitude about the law. In my experience, this is unnecessary and not accurate. I know many lawyers who are very happy and content in their work, but they also understand that it is called *work*—and not *play*—for a reason. It takes a lot of effort and dedication, but it also includes a great deal of satisfaction and reward. To have the greatest chance for a similar result, avoid the temptation to connect to legal gripe sites to calculate how happy you are.

To enjoy and appreciate the law, you will have to challenge yourself. It is no surprise that people who do the same types of things all the time become bored. Branch out and experience some new things in the law. Volunteer for a case that you know will be a challenge but has the potential for very valuable learning. Take a risk and experience the ecstasy of having succeeded against the odds.

I recall one particular case that I had as a young attorney that illustrates this point. The case involved the appointment of a conservator for an elderly person who would not voluntarily commit herself for the medical treatment she needed. I had brought the case to the firm, and I had a lot at stake in making a success of it. However, it represented a risk because it was not in my area of expertise. As I prepared for the hearing to appoint the conservator, I could not have known how unprepared I would be. After the judge convened the hearing and asked me to 'call my first witness,' the gravity of my lack of preparation became clear to me. I thought that it was a non-evidentiary hearing! Although I was very prepared with my oral argument and case citations, I was not prepared to put on evidence, much less call my client as a witness! So, I asked to approach the bench and requested a five-minute recess to explain the situation to my client and make her feel comfortable about testifying. The judge obliged, and the rest of the afternoon went very well.

I can still remember vividly my feeling of accomplishment as I left the courthouse knowing that I had stretched myself, overcome the odds, and surprised myself with my competence. That feeling made me understand that risk, change, and accepting new challenges would be important to maintaining a high level of interest throughout my career.

Gaining the perspective that you need to keep your professional and personal lives in balance will be uniquely personal to you. We all are different and have different needs. However, it is undeniable that you need to continue to pursue that healthy perspective throughout your practice years. It will be a very good investment in your future. It is a long career.

Here are a few resources on gaining perspective that I think will be helpful to you.

Elwork, Amiram. *Stress Management for Lawyers: How to Increase Personal & Professional Satisfaction in the Law.* **Vorkell Group, 2007.**

When you practice law, stress comes with the territory. Such stressors as time pressures, work overload, conflict, and difficult people can rob you of a satisfying career and personal life. It doesn't have to be that way, however. You can take effective action and this book, written specifically for lawyers, shows you how.

Levit, Nancy, and Douglas O. Linder. *The Happy Lawyer: Making a Good Life in the Law.* **Oxford UP, 2010.**

The Happy Lawyer examines the causes of dissatisfaction among lawyers, and then charts possible paths to happier and more fulfilling careers in

65

law. Eschewing a one-size-fits-all approach, it shows how maximizing our chances for achieving happiness depends on understanding our own personality types, values, strengths, and interests.

Melcher, Michael F. *The Creative Lawyer: A Practical Guide to Authentic Professional Satisfaction.* **American Bar Association, 2007.**

Written in a fun and inspirational way, this book will help lawyers find a way to happiness in their careers and personal lives. Starting with self-examination, readers will be able to analyze their personal values and then create their own personal fulfillment plan.

Molloy, Andrea. *Stop Living Your Job, Start Living Your Life: 85 Simple Strategies to Achieve Work/life Balance.* **Ulysses, 2005.**

Packed with interactive tools, this book empowers readers to control their responsibilities instead of having their responsibilities control them. It offers realistic and practical solutions to everything from decluttering space, managing finances, staying committed, and pursuing dreams.

Schreiter, Larry. *The Happy Lawyer: How to Gain More Satisfaction, Suffer Less Stress, and Enjoy Higher Earnings in Your Law Practice.* **Shiloh Publications, 1999.**

The author presents simple principles to enable lawyers to increase happiness, such as how to choose the right clients, whose work will bring satisfaction and fulfill professional goals, and how to develop a niche to distinguish oneself from the mass of generic legal service providers.

6

You *Really* Need Time—And All the Help You Can Get!

What a segue! You not only need time to reflect and to get much-needed perspective, but you simply need time. Time to do all the things in your life that seem to be on collision course. Remember that song phrase from the Jim Croce classic, "If I could save time in a bottle . . ."? If that were possible, we all would be drinking from that bottled elixir. It seems that time is the commodity that we just never have enough of.

How do you get more *time*? Actually, you don't. Time is finite. But, what you do get is help that frees up more of the time that you do have. You have to pay for help, but, as a lawyer, you are a pretty highly paid professional, and you can afford it within reason. In doing this, try to discount all of the finger wagging by people who do not understand your life. Your mother, your aunt, your grandmother, your father—they all came up in a different era. Sure, getting a washing and folding service for your clothes may be an enigma to them, but it may be a lifesaver for you.

Take a look at all the things you have to do in your life. Now, apply a few management concepts and figure out ways to reduce the personal hands-on in your life and increase the help from others. I understand that you have to live within a budget, but think how much happier and content you will be if you are not always running behind the clock and showing up late for everything, hassled and worn. It is all a function of time, and time is always running out.

In addition to needing help to create the illusion of extra time, you also need help just to keep sane. Let's look at the kinds of help that you can get from those at home and at work that really can make a difference for you. Help from people who understand and respect your life is invaluable to protecting your personal time.

Here are some examples of the kinds of help that you may need in your personal life to provide you with extra personal time and make your professional life go smoother. Help like maids and house cleaners, nanny services, laundry service—even the pick up and delivery type—errand runner, service "sitter" (remember that sofa that had to be delivered on a day that you were in court?), hired car, etc. How much help you need depends upon you and your personal roles as professional and home-maker. When you do need help, there are resources out there for you to access:

Find reputable sitters and nannies online (including petsitters!) by searching for caregivers in your area at sites like:

www.care.com
www.sittercity.com

Make doctor, dentist, or spa appointments using services like:

www.lifebooker.com
www.zocdoc.com

Find an errand runner or service sitter at websites like:

> **www.bestfrienderrand.com**
> **www.myerrandservice.com/directory.htm (a national directory)**

Order your groceries online from places like:

> **www.peapod.com**
> **www.schnucks.com**
> **www.albertsons.com**
> **www.ethnicgrocer.com (ethnic foods)**
> **www.diamondorganics.com (organic foods)**

Sign up for a weekly menu sent by email and a grocery list, categorized by aisle, sent to your inbox from a menu planning service like:

> **www.savingdinner.com**
> **www.dinewithoutwhine.com**

Get meals delivered to your home from:

> **www.familychef.com**
> **www.artiko.com**

Get stamps delivered to your mailbox from the United States Postal Service's Postal Store, at:

> **www.usps.com**

Find repairmen, contractors, and maids on directories such as:

> **www.angieslist.com**
> **www.servicemagic.com**

The demands on your time are not always obvious, and there are so many of them.

Time and happiness are related. Although women, like people in general, are responsible for their own happiness, women typically also have the lioness' share of the responsibility for a healthy relationship with their spouse or significant others. As a result, it will often be up to you to take care of your romantic/love relationship as well as taking care of yourself. This all takes *time*.

Most men do not focus on the health of a relationship—in fact, most of them shy away from the word "relationship" altogether!

That reminds me of a story—in fact, I am willing to bet that it reminds most women of a story!

I was amused years ago when my daughter told me about her experience interning during college for a consulting group that coached companies on making sales presentations. Most of the client companies were being coached on making presentations to government panels, and those panels consisted mostly of men. As a result, the clients were counseled to avoid using words like "relationship" and "commitment" because many men have an aversion to those words. The clients were told that it could mean the difference between a successful presentation and a not-so-successful one. True story. I was amazed at the time, but I can certainly see the wisdom of that advice.

In fact, it is women who keep most relationships going. It typically is the women who work hard to stay connected to their friends and family, who set up social events, and who understand the value of friendships in keeping them grounded. This all takes *time*, but it is critically important to most women and their relationships. In order to have the time necessary to feed this need, you will have to have help in other parts of your life from sources like those cited above.

Just as you need help to free up time and keep you balanced in your personal life, you also need help in your professional life to create the time that you need to keep all of the balls in the air.

Good staff support at the office is critical to saving you time. First, make sure that you choose good support—to the degree that you have a say in the matter. Do not "settle" or continue to overlook incompetence

70

just because you do not want to make waves or have the tough conversations. It will catch up with you in the end. Good help at the office can make or break your career.

The way you treat your staff is also critically important to getting the help you need. If you create a team and treat your support staff as important members of the team, it will pay huge dividends to you. You must respect them to get them to respect you. If you do it right, your team members will be fiercely loyal to you, and they will make your life so much easier. Leadership should not be taken for granted, and you must work to be a good and benevolent leader. Remember that it is the tyrants who get the blade in the back by "trusted" colleagues. Et tu, Brute!

The obvious things that your staff can do for you are get your work out *on time*, get the memos to the partner *on time*, get the pleadings filed at the courthouse *on time*, get your correspondence to your client *on time* and the many other things that your secretary and paralegal do to make sure that your law practice is getting executed in the best possible way. It is the staff that often makes you look the best, and you cannot forget that. I cannot emphasize enough the value of making your staff feel appreciated and proud of the work that they do. If you feel that your staff members do not deserve that kind of treatment and praise, you probably need new staff.

I never forget, however, that there is another philosophy. I recall years ago a partner in one of my firms who had the best secretary I ever had encountered. This secretary had a college degree from a major university in the day when that was not the norm. She was exceptionally professional, she was a great grammarian, and she was very pleasant, gracious, and gregarious and always made a good impression on clients. In other words, she was a real keeper. I would have given up part of my salary for her! But, her boss's approach was to make her cry! He said things to her with the intention of making her insecure about her job, and he rarely praised her because he said that he never wanted her to feel like he could not do without her. Sounds like spousal abuse! Well, you guessed it. She finally had enough of him and left for a better place. What a waste! There is something fundamentally true about getting better results with honey.

71

There also are some not-so-obvious ways that your staff can make your life easier and provide you the extra *time* you need. Let's take lunch for instance. You may very likely find yourself falling into the pattern of skipping lunch. That is not a good idea because you are probably also a person who skips breakfast. Our bodies need fuel to run on, and we start to wane in the afternoon without fuel. So, lunch of some kind or another is a good idea, but what if you have back-to-back conference calls and no time to get out to grab a bite to eat?

If you have fostered a good relationship with your staff, you will be comfortable asking them for help. If you have not, you may be out of luck. In most cases, if you treat your staff as important and valuable people in your life, the occasional request to pick up a sandwich for you will not be received as an offense. In fact, if you offer to get a sandwich for them once in a while, it can hardly be taken that way. Many of the problems between attorneys and staff are the result of how staff is perceived and treated and not the specifics of what is required of staff. Everyone wants to be appreciated and treated well, and your staff is no exception. It will work to your benefit to treat them well—and you might just get lunch out of it!

Working overtime is another issue. Some times you just cannot get the job done during regular working hours, and you must call on staff to put in extra time. You need to remember that you are a salaried employee, and that you are expected to get the job done no matter what the time demands are. This is not true of your staff. Your staff works by the hour and is expected to work a certain number of hours a week. Anything more is up to them. They are within their rights to turn down overtime work, and there is usually some kind of a word processing pool for you to turn to in those circumstances.

However, if you are like most attorneys I know, you want *your* staff to be working on *your* cases. You may or may not even know the person in the word processing pool—in fact, that person may be in a location half a world away. To get the best result, you want to have a good relationship with your staff so that they feel like part of the team. As part of the team, they are much more likely to agree to stay after regular hours and come in on weekends to make sure that the job is done right. This will reap great benefits for you in terms of *time*, and it will only cost you a little kindness and generosity. You are a woman with womanly ways. Don't scrimp on the charm when it comes to the people who work for you.

That charm will also go a long way with people you have to rely on outside your workplace. For instance, the people in the clerk of court's office can make or break you as a lawyer. Be nice to them, and they will go out of their way for you and save you time. Treat them like hired help, and they are likely to be fast on the trigger with the date stamp. This makes me remember a lovely woman in Charleston, South Carolina.

I had a case in Federal Court in Charleston years ago. This is the heart of the South, and it was not real comfortable territory for a young woman lawyer from the North in the early 1980's. As a result, it was one of the most challenging experiences of my career. My job was to prepare an appellate brief, and I spent a lot of time at the courthouse looking through the record from the trial court for material to support our appellate efforts. The supervising lawyer on the case was accustomed to showing up in his Washington DC-style three-piece suit to impress someone—himself, perhaps—and he was perceived as an irritant by both the judge and courthouse staff. This was getting us nowhere. The judge's annoyance was palpable, and he did not hesitate to make it clear that Mr. Three-Piece-Suit was not welcome in his courtroom. Since I was the newcomer to the case and needed background and documents, this put me in an untenable situation and often brought the judge's wrath down on me.

So, I tried a different approach. I knew that I was not going to win over the ladies in the clerk's office or the judge's chambers with a demonstration of my intellect and ability—especially as a young woman lawyer. The time and the place just wasn't right for that. However, I was not above flashing a big smile and discussing the lovely courthouse gardens and the charm of Charleston. As I suspected, it went a long way toward making them feel comfortable with me and gaining me the access to files that I needed in a timely manner. In the law, time is money and this new approach was a blessing for me and for my client.

In addition to help from your staff and outside folks, you also will need help from your colleagues to provide the *time* that you need so desperately. As noted earlier, most lawyers will be willing to counsel you and help you and share their own experiences as examples. This can save you hours and hours of time in reinventing the wheel. These colleagues will be much more willing to help you if they see that you are trying very hard to do your job and to learn what it takes to be a good lawyer. Slackers rarely get the positive attention that they want. So, make the best impression that you can with your supervising attorneys as early as possible. Once you create value, people will want to help you even more. You also will find out that they are much more likely to forgive mistakes if they know that you are sincere and trying your best.

Face time also is a very important kind of time in a law firm. You need to have face-to-face interaction with your supervising attorneys and management. Come out of your office and actually talk to people who can be very important to your future and to your promotion in the firm or other legal setting. Talk to them about what they are working on and how their matters are progressing. Keep the dialogue going so that when you have something serious to discuss about your own career, the lines of communication will be open.

When you ask for help from your professional colleagues, be prepared for responses you may not want to hear. Be prepared to hear that your approach is wrong, and accept it and learn from it. This will not be easy in our current political and social environment. We live in a "my way or the highway" society, and, as pointed out by newspaper columnists David Brooks and Peggy Noonan (who represent different political perspectives) on a recent airing of *Meet the Press*, our society no longer pays a lot of attention to wrongdoing, and collectively we lack humility.

This kind of discomfort with criticism seems to be very prevalent in our new generation of college students, and, presumably, in the continuing education of those students. We hear stories about students demanding that college professors change their grades and being unwilling to look at their own responsibility for results. Consequences do not seem to be in vogue any more.

Unwillingness to take responsibility for your decisions and actions will not serve you well in the law profession. The law is all about assignment of responsibility for wrongdoing. You will have to be a part of that process and learn to accept positive criticism and learn from it to adjust your behavior and your approach. Hopefully, your superiors will understand the power of helpful criticism and positive reinforcement, and you will benefit from their assistance and understand that it ultimately will save you *time* and keep you from repeating the same mistake.

Finding a good mentor can also save you *time*. You know from Book One that I put a lot of emphasis on mentoring. I believe that mentoring is the responsibility of senior lawyers, and I think that is especially important for young women struggling with the challenges of a male-dominated profession. It is important that these young women have both male and female mentors to help them through some of these challenges and short-cut some of the *time* that would be necessary to learn it all on their own.

However, I do not always see the kind of mentoring that I would like to see, and this can be disappointing. I do not see practitioners seizing the teaching moments that they should in order to bring the younger generations along. I am sure that this has to do with the billable hour requirements and the stressful nature of the profession, but it is regrettable. Conversely, I am always impressed when I see lawyers taking the time to teach and mentor, and I admire them for understanding the importance of it.

I am particularly disappointed when I do not see women come forward to help other women, and I regret to report that I see it a lot. I see old jealousies and resentment get in the way, and there is no place for that in our profession. If women are going to stay in the profession and reach the highest levels, experienced women will have to reach out to their female colleagues to offer assistance and mentoring. This will take work because too many women in our profession are still playing the competition and envy game. They are still undermining each other over petty grievances and jealousies, and we still have senior women in the practice who would rather compete with young women lawyers than mentor them.

This is wrong. Cat fighting may sell reality TV like the Housewives of Wherever, but it has no place in our profession. Until we wipe out this negative behavior, we will not have done our jobs well enough. At the risk of repeating myself, I will quote again—as I did in Book One—former Secretary of State Madeleine Albright when she said, "There is a place reserved in Hell for women who do not help other women." I hope the day will come when I do not have to keep saying this.

Another positive resource for help to save you *time* around your office is the group of fellow associates and junior lawyers. They are experiencing some of the same things that you are, and some of them have "been there, done that" before. They very often can steer you in a direction you have not thought about or share an experience they had with the same "difficult personality" that is currently the bane of your existence.

The key to whether your fellow associates will be a source of help to you will depend on your relationship with them and how you treat them. Unfortunately, the aura of competition among associates is cemented from Day One of the summer associate experience. Try to get beyond this and realize that you are all trying to survive. Be your best person, and do not let the competition eliminate this source of help that can be very valuable to conserving your time. Also, do not let it prevent you from giving the help that someone else needs. What goes around comes around!

For other help that you need in your professional life that will save you *time*, get down to basics. Some things that come to mind are: On-site child-care for emergency situations, at least; law firm and company cafeterias to make eating on a regular schedule easier; office locations in buildings with amenities like dry cleaners, convenience stores and, yes, even nail salons! How about that car service to drive you home in the wee hours of the night after you have completed the project, met the deadline, are exhausted and need to get home safely and in *time* for at least a few hours of sleep before returning to the office for an early meeting? The list goes on according to what you need in your life to meet the challenges to your *time*.

The bottom line is that we save *time* by getting the help we need. In addition to all of the help available in your workplace from colleagues and staff, you also will need help from the managers in whatever legal setting you choose. You will have to go to your managers about a variety of matters over the life of a career. It may be about salary, hours, flexible time, problems with supervisors, problems with staff or other issues that will surface over time. To get the most out of these "discussions," you should think about developing a rapport with these people before you have problems. You should also consider taking the high road and being reasonable and pleasant. You do not have to be disagreeable to have a disagreement. Tone down the rhetoric and give people a chance to help you. Make allies of the people you need for support, and resist picketing management. It rarely ends up well.

Some of the things that are most important for a positive workplace for women lawyers may become topics of conversations between you and management. This is no place to scrimp on *time*. Give some thought to them in advance, take the time necessary to articulate them effectively, and promote them whenever you can.

Here is my web site blog entry that addresses this and related topics.

Mar 28, 2011

What Women Should Look for in a Law Firm

For you third-year law students, soon your biggest challenge will be finding a job after graduation. That seems daunting, I know, especially in these economic times, but your hard work will pay off and soon you will be looking critically at firms and other employers and evaluating them for your future needs.

When you are considering that job offer—and you will be—here are some suggestions about what should be important to women lawyers in the workplace. The information is directed to the law firm employer, but it could just as well be a judicial clerkship or another practice type.

Every time I share this information with the students I speak to at law schools, they urge me to put it on my web site so that they will be able to access it easily when they need it. So, here it is.

Things to Look For in a Law Firm

- Pay attention to the dynamics of the firm.
- Who controls the conversations and are women included?
- Is there a respectful environment for women?
- Are women represented at the management level?
- Is there a Women's Initiative and does the firm take it seriously?
- Are both men and women mentoring women?
- Are women represented at all levels of the firm and not just on "mommy track"? Are they getting quality work?
- Do the women of the firm support each other?
- Do the lawyers at the firm appear to be happy and enjoying their practices?
- Check out the different work models of the firm and the potential for flexible schedules and reasonable billable hour requirements. You may need arrangements like that in the future.
- Ask yourself whether you got constructive criticism and feedback during and at the end of your experience.

Enhance Your Law Firm Experience

For others of you, you are either already employed or you are about to join a firm as a summer associate. Here are some useful pointers to get the most out of your employment experience.

- Meet and dialogue with as many partners as possible—they will determine your future at the firm.
- Get out of your office or cubicle! You must make your presence known. Sitting at your desk with earphones on will not help you when your name comes up at the partnership table.
- Find both a mentor and a sponsor. A mentor will teach you the ropes, and you need both male and female mentors. A sponsor will go to bat for you for promotions. Both mentors and sponsors are critical to your professional future.
- Talk to attorneys about what they do in their various areas of practice. Ask yourself how you would fit into that practice.
- Go to EVERY social event! Even if you have to go back to the office afterward to finish your work—that is what the other lawyers do.
- Volunteer for committees and become involved in the organization of the firm.
- Embrace constructive criticism and accept it as a learning experience. This is especially difficult for some women when the critic is a man. Get over it.
- AND, if you are an associate attorney, learn how to network and get involved in every networking opportunity you can. Do not automatically choose billable hours over networking. Networking is the foundation for generating clients, and developing clients is what upward mobility is all about.

Good luck in putting these tips to work for you!

From www.bestfriendsatthebar.com

Some of these need a little more definition:

- Access to quality work—even for alternative work schedule lawyers. You do not want to be "mommy tracked" with less interesting and important work just because you are on a flexible schedule.

- A respectful environment that does not marginalize women. Women should not be willing to put up with sexist attitudes and behavior for the sake of advancement and to keep from rocking the boat. It ultimately is bad for them and for the women to follow.

- Constructive criticism and feedback. This is very important, and you must remember that to get constructive feedback you must be willing to take constructive criticism. I sometimes think that this is harder for women than for men, especially when the critic is a man, and we must get beyond our own gender issues.

- A Women's Initiative or program.

- Women *and* men mentoring women. This is very important. Most lawyers would agree that typically male and female lawyers have different work styles. Of course, there are many exceptions. It is important that young women lawyers experience good role modeling from female mentors but it also is important that those same young women learn from male mentors whose style may be different but instructive and equally as valuable.

- Flexible schedules including reasonable billable hour requirements. This is not just a female issue, and it should not be treated as one. The need for flexible schedules is not gender specific, but it is more likely that women will need alternative work schedules in connection with childcare and family responsibilities at some points in their careers. It is very important that the billable hour requirements for these alternative work schedules are reasonable and that those expectations can be met. If not, you are setting yourself up for failure. Do not reach too high with the expectation of cutting back. It usually sends wrong signals and results in dissatisfaction. Face the issue straight on with management, be reasonable and keep your promises to the best of your abilities.

- Exercise and childcare facilities. A healthy body is a healthy mind, and childcare facilities, especially for unanticipated office hours, is a must to help you stay on course in your career.

- Generous maternity/adoption leave. Most of you are probably familiar with the federal laws on these issues, and there is an expanded discussion of the Family and Medical Leave Act (FMLA) in Book One. Many firms go beyond that minimum requirement, and you should encourage your firm to do the same. A happy employee is one who is confident that he or she has covered the needs of family and is not distracted by family issues and guilt on the job. Generosity in addressing these issues works to the benefit of the employer and the employee.
- Openness on the part of management and responsible partners to discussions and to creating solutions that are good for women and good for the organization.

This is just the shortlist for a positive workplace for women lawyers, and I am sure that you will add others of your own along the way. I hope that you will take *time* for these discussions and will have success in reaching mutually satisfactory results from your pursuits.

One of these items, flexible schedules, deserves particular attention. Getting the *time* you need to reach the balance that is right for you may require that you practice part-time or have an alternative work schedule for at least a few years during your career. That is understandable, but you need to be skeptical about some information that is currently in the mainstream that can give you false hope and unrealistic expectations about these types of flexible practices. Your antennae should go up when you read assertions that flex-time and part-time practice are going to become the *rule* rather than the exception in this "reordering" of law firms. It just isn't the case, and I do not want you to be led down that primrose path.

Although it is widely recognized that alternative work schedules are very important as interim solutions to serious work-life issues, a theme that I explored in Book One and one that I very much support, the thought that law firms will soon become full of lawyers working alternative and flexible schedules belies an understanding of what law firms do. Large law firms represent clients with big problems and fast-paced criminal matters, civil litigation and transactional needs. Those clients very often need 24-7 dedication to their matters, and a preponderance of alternative work schedules typically is not compatible with those requirements. It is the clients who need full-time attention, and it is the clients who pay regularly and in full to keep the law firm afloat. Law firms need a high percentage of those types of clients to make business run smoothly and meet overhead and salary demands, and, as a result, law firms must cater to the needs of their clients. Anything less is unrealistic.

A radical shift to a part-time workforce of women attorneys also would not accomplish women's goals in reaching the top of the profession where they can influence policy and management decisions to improve the working conditions for all women in our profession. We need to have a critical mass of women reach those corner offices, and a preponderance of women lawyers working part time will not get them there.

A 2006 report by Wellesley Centers for Women study, titled "Advancing Women to the Boardroom," and reported by *Newsweek* magazine in the August 30, 2010 issue, underscores the importance of the presence of women in decision-making settings. That report identifies *three* to be the magic number for women in the boardroom to create a critical mass where women are no longer seen as outsiders and are able to influence content and practice.

Based on information like this study and the opinions of the many law firm practitioners who I have consulted, I see neither the possibility nor the wisdom of any cosmic shift to a part-time legal workforce. Rather, my prediction is that the hard charging 24-7 alpha lawyer will continue to be the rule and not the exception and that, as long as the policies of law firms are driven by demanding bottom lines, the transition in favor of alternative work models is not a likely scenario.

So, it is important that you do not fall victim to empty promises and that you stay focused on good choices, good plans, and a new work-life balance that will support a happy life—not a radically changed professional model to meet your needs. That would be betting on a dark horse and wasting a lot of valuable planning time.

For more on this theme, sit back and enjoy two of my web site blog entries on this and related issues. Make a new friend of Sheryl Sandberg and be inspired by her prophetic words about advancing women in business.

May 24, 2011

Young Women Lawyers—Do Not Leave Before You Leave

I hope that you all are familiar with Sheryl Sandberg, former VP of Google and the current COO of Facebook. She also is the mother of two preschoolers, and she has identified an interesting concept that I include in my speeches to young women lawyers. Although Ms. Sandberg is not a lawyer, the concepts that she discusses with young women in business are equally as pertinent to all young women in the law, especially those who are involved in the work-life struggle.

Her concept of "Leaving Before You Leave" is discussed in this video, http://thecareerist.typepad.com/thecareerist/2011/01/facebook-coo.html, where Ms. Sandberg speaks to a group of women about advancing in business. It is one of the most valuable resources that I can recommend to you. Check it out!

As you will see and hear from the video, Ms. Sandberg is very concerned about the future of young women in business. She sees fewer women than she would like on the path to the corner office, and she provides good, sound advice to increase those numbers. In that respect, she and I are very much on the same page in encouraging all of you to have a plan that works for you and keeps you in the game, in one way or another. That will result in more women in positions of power and decision making on policy issues that are so important to the future of women in business and law. That result depends on YOU YOUNG WOMEN AS THE KEY TO SOLVING THE PROBLEM. You can control the outcome and do not have to leave decisions about your professional futures to others with separate agendas. Women have the ability, through careful planning and good personal and professional choices, to have satisfying and successful careers. Here is my personal take on the subject of "Leaving Before You Leave" as it relates to all of you.

To avoid leaving before you leave, think about how your future is likely to unfold earlier than you might have expected to do—before the pressure is on. Discuss it with your spouse or significant other, have a plan in mind, become comfortable with that plan and then get it over with, put it on the back burner and continue to throw yourself into your practice until the things you anticipate are on the horizon.

At that point—when you actually are faced with putting a plan into action and after all of your hard work in the first years of your practice—hopefully you will be indispensable in your job and you will have the bargaining power that you will need to work out a solution with your firm or other employer that is satisfactory to you and to them.

The key is for you to accept the responsibility early so that you are not like a deer in headlights at year five of your career and make a hasty and unnecessary departure from practice. It is a process, and it ideally starts long before your first billable hour, particularly for women who desire to have children, women who are devoted to family and home, and women who have responsibilities for aging, ill or disabled family members.

It will take time and attention, but you really have no choice unless you are willing to play Russian Roulette with your career. All of this is discussed at length in my book, *Best Friends at the Bar: What Women Need to Know about a Career in the Law*. Check it out, too!

Here's the bottom line:

At all costs, be the best lawyer that you can be and do not leave before you leave!

May 26, 2011

Women in Business—and Law Is a Business–Must Learn to Lean In

I promised you more on Sheryl Sandberg, and here it is. I might have mentioned that I admire this woman a lot, and here is more to make you understand why.

Recently, Ms. Sandberg, former VP of Google and current COO of Facebook, delivered the commencement address at Barnard College, the esteemed women's college at Columbia University. Her theme was that today's young women need to close the ambition gap before they can close the achievement gap. She contends that her generation (and mine, for that matter) has blown it.

She reminded the graduates that they are all privileged on a day when they graduate from college—privileged because the future is full of boundless opportunities. She asked the graduates to contemplate what in the world needs changing and how they were going to change it. She also reminded them how lucky they are to be equals with men under the law and then added the sobering fact that the promise of equality is not equality. The truth is that men still run the world, and she quoted these facts to support her assertion: Of 190 heads of state, nine are women; Of all the parliaments around the world, 13% of the seats in parliament are held by women; Of corporate America's top jobs, 15% are held by women; And of full professors around the United States, only 24% are women. Even more sobering, these numbers have not changed in nine years.

Sandberg is saddened by the lost opportunities for her generation of women, many who were raised by women who told them they could be anything they wanted to be. However, thirty years later, women do not have an equal voice about the decisions that affect all of their lives. So, the only thing that she can do is place her hope in the next generation of women—YOUR generation—to do better—to change the dynamic, to reshape the conversation and to make sure that women's voices are "heard and heeded, not overlooked and ignored." To do this, Sandberg says that you will have to "lean way into your careers." Find something that you love doing and do it "with gusto." If all young women start to "lean in," we can close the ambition gap here and now, according to Sandberg.

Sandberg emphasizes the importance of believing in yourself. She cites studies which show that, when compared to men, women underestimate their performance. Here it is worth quoting directly.

"If you ask men and women questions about completely objective criteria such as GPA's or sales goals, men get it wrong slightly high; women get it wrong slightly low. More importantly, if you ask men why they succeeded, men attribute that success to themselves; and women, they attribute it to other facts like working harder, help from others. Ask a woman why she did well on something, and she'll say, 'I got lucky. All of these great people helped me. I worked really hard.' Ask a man and he'll say or think, 'What a dumb question. I'm awesome.' So women need to take a page from men and own their success.'

Sandberg acknowledges her own failures on these issues along the way. We all have them. The important thing is that we recognize this and do something about it so that we are not held back by our own bad habits. According to Sandberg, you must believe in yourself and start acting like you, too, are awesome. Raise your hand when you have an opinion. Your opinion is just as important as the guy sitting next to you in your class in law school or at the meeting at the law firm.

Sandberg also acknowledges the external forces that work against women, things like a positive correlation between power and success and likeability for men as compared to a negative correlation for women. You all know that old saw. However, Sandberg says the way through that is to put your head down and just keep on working.

She wants you to think big and to own your successes. She understands the work-life struggle and the compromises that you will have to make. She gets very practical in suggesting, as I do in my book, that who you choose as your life partner makes a real difference. If you choose the person who supports your career and the burdens and successes of your personal life, you will have a greater opportunity to go further and change the world into what we need it to be. She also recognizes that jumping into the work force and rising to the top is not the only way to make a difference. However, she also believes that, if you pick the right job—a job that is compelling— you are going to be far less inclined to walk away from it. Something that stirs your passion may be worth the rat race. She states, "If you want to make a difference, you better think big and dream big, right from day one."

This is all great food for thought, and I discuss these same concepts, as they specifically relate to women lawyers, in *Best Friends at the Bar: What Women Need to Know about a Career in the Law*.

Sandberg closes by encouraging the new Barnard graduates to "aim high"—something that you know I want for all of you. She reminds them that the world needs them in positions of leadership— women throughout the world need them in positions of leadership. She asks them to ask themselves the question, "What would I do if I weren't afraid?"

The answer is in each and every one of you.

For the full text of Sheryl Sandberg's speech, see www.business insider.com/facebook-coo-sandberg.

From www.bestfriendsatthebar.com

To advance in business and leadership, women will have to get help in all aspects of their lives to provide more precious personal *time* for themselves. Personal time is critical to your happiness and to the *new* balance, and I hope that you will fight very hard for it. You will be doing yourself a huge favor, and you ultimately will be doing your family and loved ones a huge favor, as well.

You may want to check out some of the following resources to help you get this right.

Cottrell, David, and Mark Layton. *175 Ways to Get More Done in Less Time!* **CornerStone Leadership Institute, 2000.**

A handy and quick read, this book is loaded with ideas about how you can better utilize your day to accomplish all of your long-term goals. It includes 175 suggestions to help you get things done faster and more effectively.

Louden, Jennifer. *The Woman's Comfort Book: A Self-Nurturing Guide for Restoring Balance in Your Life.* **HarperOne, 2005.**

Louden encourages you to assemble and draw on personal rituals, journals and sanctuaries that can add comfort and breathing space to your life. Her point is to pick and choose what works best for you, but do take some actions to make your life happier.

Righton, Caroline. *The Life Audit: A Step-by-Step Guide to Taking Stock, Gaining Control, and Creating the Life You Want.* **Broadway, 2006.**

In this brisk, sensible book, British broadcast journalist Righton lays out a plan she calls the Life Audit. "The Life Audit is all about assessing your life and then analyzing everything so you can become an informed player in your own existence," explains Righton. Part of the task is figuring out how to streamline time spent on must-do's and whittle down unnecessary or draining activities and relationships.

Wieder, Marcia. *Doing Less and Having More: Five Easy Steps for Discovering What You Really Want, and Getting It.* Quill, 1999.

Essential to Wieder's program is learning how to access "ease": "using a small amount of energy to get what you want effortlessly." First, look at where you waste energy and when you feel uneasy. Wieder presents many techniques you can use to shift energy, focus, recognize your style of coping with stress, and look at ways you may be making life more difficult.

7

You *Really* Need Your Friends

We all know that friends make a huge difference in our lives, and I touched on this earlier. However, I cannot emphasize this enough, and the subject deserves a more expansive discussion.

I know personally how important female friends are to my happiness and well-being, and I was reminded of it as I watched the events following the tragic assassination attempt on Arizona Congressman Gabrielle Giffords unfold in January 2011. At a time when the Congresswoman remained in a coma and was surrounded in her hospital room by her close women friends from Congress, including Senator Kirsten Gillibrand of New York and Congresswoman Debbie Wasserman Schultz of Florida, Gabrielle Giffords opened her eyes for the first time. It was reported that her friends were describing their recent pizza outing and future plans to get their families together during the summer months when Congresswoman Giffords regained consciousness. Afterwards, Congresswoman Wasserman Schultz stated that she considered that minor miracle to be the result of the "power of girlfriends."

Here is my take on the importance of friendship from my web site blog entry.

May 17, 2011

Young Women Lawyers Need to Remember the Importance of Friendships

It is time for me to come clean with you. I was just *slightly* less than honest with you last week when I told you that I was MIA for a week because I was doing community projects. That *was* the truth but not the whole truth. I also was out playing with my girlfriends at the Picasso exhibit at the Virginia Museum of Fine Arts in Richmond, and the significance of this will become more clear in a moment.

The exhibit, by the way, is excellent and is on loan from the Musee National Picasso in Paris where I first saw it years ago. It is on tour while the Paris museum is being renovated, and Richmond is the only east coast venue on a seven-city world-wide tour. Richmond is the closest venue for my friends and me, so off we went for two days of art, shopping, eating really good food, and acting like Thelma and Louise times two and without the harsh overtones. Just the fun.

The significance of this is the value of friendship and how important it is to protect your friendships no matter how busy you become in your professional lives. Friends are what ground you. They are the ones you can laugh with and cry with and the ones who give you great advice because they have known you "in thick and in thin" and they understand what makes you happy. They are the ones you will call on in your future when you need a babysitter at the last minute to make that critical meeting with clients, when your mother becomes ill, when you lose a family member and when you are on the edge from the weight of all your responsibilities. And they will call on you, and you will do the same for them.

Holding fast to who and what you are is very important in this demanding, project-oriented and time-consuming profession you have chosen. It is very easy to stray from the things that make you happy, and friends help you from straying. They help to keep you on a straight course, they nurture you, they rejoice at your successes, and they help you through your losses. Without them you simply can cease to be who you really are and who you were meant to be.

I hold fast to my friends. They are my college friends, my law school friends, my professional friends, my book club friends, my dinner club friends, my community friends and, now, my Picasso Troupe friends. They also are the friends who have dropped into my life unexpectedly over the years and renewed my faith in new beginnings and endless possibilities. Those are the ones I call my "bosom buddies"—who can forget Anne of Green Gables! I will do just about anything for my friends, and I think they feel the same way about me, and that is both fortunate and comforting.

You must make time for your friends if you expect your friendships to last. That does not mean that you always should choose your personal life over your professional life because that would be bad career advice. And sometimes keeping that lunch appointment or movie date with a good girlfriend may not be possible because the senior partner or the agency head is breathing down your neck for yet another revision. However, it is important that you throw your friendships a life line often enough to make your friends know how important they are to you. Your friends know what you are going through—especially in the first years of practice when you are on a steep learning curve and everything seems to be about work—and it will not take much to let them know that you are still there for them. And, it is not all about them. It is about you. Friendship is a two way street—you give and you get. That is the beauty of it.

This is why I tell you that making friends is more important than making money. That is why I tell you to keep in mind who and what you are and what you need to be happy as you develop your career plans.

Of course, friends are not the only people who keep you happy. Family is also very important, and I do not want you to think that I am somehow denying the value of your love relationships in all of this. The relationships with your spouse, your mate, or your significant other are very important, and that is not lost on me. I have been married for over 40 years—to the same man! (Do not hold the applause!) My relationships with my children and my extended family also are precious to me, and I fully understand the value of these relationships to my happiness and to my successes. But, those relationships are different than the relationships that I have with my girlfriends. No one talks 'girlfriend' but a girlfriend. No one understands the healing powers of chocolate, a good cry, a shopping spree, or a pedicure like a girlfriend. It is not better, it is just different, and most of us need all of these relationships to get us through the challenging life we have chosen.

I hope that you will nurture your friendships and find time to sustain them. As with most things in the lives of young women attorneys, it will not be easy. But it will be worth it.

So, if this sounds a little soppy to you, so be it. That is my story and I am sticking to it. For me, there is no question that giving time to my friendships is critical to keeping the *me* in *me*. It is critical to reminding me who I am and what makes me happy. It is critical to striking an acceptable balance between my professional life and my personal life, and it is critical to me being willing to work countless hours at my job in anticipation of time out with friends.

So that should set the record straight. I know you understand. Who can resist a road trip with the girls!

From www.bestfriendsatthebar.com

As illustrated by this blog entry, friends are very important to my happiness, and I work hard at keeping them in my life. I stay in touch with my friends from college, from law school, from law practice and from all of the community activities that are an important part of my life. It was not always easy to do that because my generation did not have the benefit of cell phones (where the numbers do not have to change no matter how many times you move), *Facebook* and other social media (where it is almost impossible to hide) and the other computer magic that you have available now to assure continuity with friends.

However, even without the benefits of modern technology, many of us who prioritized it, made it happen. Recently, a female friend who was in my first year law class and who I did not see again for almost 20 years, introduced me at a law school speaking event. She told the audience that I am the only person she knows who will keep up with someone after only knowing them for a year! I plead guilty, and I am glad that is the case. Clearly, that person had a very positive impression on me, and I did not want to lose her in my life. In fact, she is a Contributor to Book One.

I do not keep up with friends to create an impression. I do it because it is such a great benefit to my life. There is truth to the old adage: "New friends are silver and old friends are gold. Hokey, maybe, but it is true.

You will also learn that the law is a jealous mistress, and the demands of law practice can make it difficult to find *time* to spend with your family and friends. As a result, unless you are careful, you can find yourself drifting away from your friends at a time when you may need them the most.

Your first years in law practice will be demanding and difficult, and those are the times when you may need your friends the most. It is the time when your confidence is likely to be challenged. Think back to the time that you started law school, and magnify it many times over. Everything is new, a lot of what you are doing is confusing, you are not used to putting in the long hours that are demanded of you, and you are being asked to put your reputation on the line by actually making recommendations for *real* clients. This all can be quite overwhelming for law firm associates and for those who choose to practice in other demanding legal settings. Your confidence may begin to erode, and you may start thinking that you have chosen the wrong profession. It can be a slippery slope, and you do not want to begin the slide.

What you need most at times like this is a whole lot of faith in yourself and people around you who will remind you who you are and what you have accomplished in the past. Those people are likely to be family and friends, but it is often the friends who will buoy you up the most. You can tell them almost anything without worrying about putting too much stress on them. Your friends are the ones who have been there for you during both the highs and the lows, and they also recognize your melodrama. They can talk you back from the edge just like you have done for them in the past. You do not have to be embarrassed about what you tell them because real friends have no memory that will hurt you. They just know how to be there when you need them.

So, make sure that you take good care of your friendships. If you never can find *time* for coffee or *time* for a drink or dinner with your friends, you just might find that they will find other friends. If all that you can talk about during dinner is your work, your friends may look for people who are more interested in them and who want to laugh, have fun, and play a little.

Although it is important to have both male and female friends, your girlfriends—yes, believe it or not, it is now OK to call them your "girl-friends" even in the U.S. Congress!—can be invaluable to your happiness, your well-being and the *new* balance you are looking for in your life.

Nobody "gets it" like another woman. Nobody else understands that a shopping spree with girlfriends can go further than antibiotics in curing your ills. In fact, tracking down the perfect pair of shoes with a girlfriend or an evening of chick flicks with your female friends may be some of our most powerful weapons in raising spirits and spurring us on to greater accomplishments. Witness all of the new "girl talk" shows on television—all spawns of Oprah and most of them very successful. The energy from supportive friends is without equal, and we all need to foster such wonderful resources.

We all need to know that others appreciate the difficulties we face, and your girlfriends will be there like the Welcome Wagon. They know that, as a young woman lawyer, you have a lot on your plate and that you very often have to be all things to all people, which is very difficult. They will know how to give you the support you need when you need it.

I know that you have a lot of balls to juggle, and I hope that you will always remember the power of friendships. In addition, I hope that you will look to your professional colleagues, who have the potential to become trusted new friends and give you great support.

For example, women's initiatives at your law firm can be a source of important information and solidarity, and Women's Bar Associations and women's committees of your local bar associations can provide the same kind of support. Most of the challenges and problems that you will face have been experienced by others, and they should be willing to help you. Most states and major cities have Women's Bar Associations or comparable groups. The national Women's Bar Associations and groups are the following:

Association of Black Women Lawyers

Legal Momentum: Advancing Women's Rights

Lex Mundi, Women in the Law

National Asian Pacific Women's Forum

National Association of Minority and Women Owned Law Firms

National Association of Women Judges

National Association of Women Lawyers

National Bar Association Women's Division

National Conference of Women's Bar Associations

National Women's Law Center

There also are similar groups at the state level throughout the country. For a comprehensive list of all US-based WBAs, see http://www.american

bar.org/groups/women/resources/directory_of_associations_of_women_ lawyers/state_local_associations.html# and the American Bar Association Commission on Women in the Profession, Directory of Associations for Women Lawyers, on the ABA web site at www.americanbar.org..

In addition to needing help from your friends, you will also need help from your best friend. This most often is your spouse or your significant other. The help that you need from a mate cannot be underestimated in our quest for the *new* balance, and it takes the form of physical help, psychological help and emotional help. It is not only important throughout your life, but it also is essential.

There is one time when the support from your spouse becomes especially important, and that is when you expand your family. It is when you have a child and experience the responsibilities of childcare that are completely overwhelming in addition to all of your other personal and professional responsibilities. That is when you need to learn to accept the help of a friend—your best friend—in a way that you never have before. And that is exactly what I mean. You must learn to *accept* the help.

This sounds easy, because you are exhausted and you really need it. Right? Not so fast. Too many women, particularly first-time mothers, think that they are the only ones who can care for a newborn properly. They set childcare standards so high that no one else feels comfortable performing the tasks. Perhaps it is because these mothers think that their babies are so fragile. However, I think it is more than that. I think that it is the perfectionists in so many of us—especially the Type A lawyer moms—and we do not want to entrust the job to anyone who will not do it *exactly* the way we would.

That attitude is on a collision course with getting the help you need. After a few episodes of chastisement for holding the bottle at the wrong angle or applying too much baby lotion, the helper is chilled. Gone is the helper and the help.

So, if you want help from your mate with childcare—or the housework for that matter—be receptive to the help. Do not be too picky about your standards, and do not forget to compliment the helper on the quality of the help. Make a big deal over how well the mate can rock the baby to sleep for instance, and maybe the mate will be volunteering to do it for the 3 AM feeding. Compliment the mate for the great job cleaning the kitchen, and it may get cleaned for you more often. Resist the temptation to point out the grease on the range! If you do it right, it could become the gift that keeps on giving.

Here is my web site blog entry on the changing roles for women lawyers and the men in their lives that may shed some additional light on this subject.

May 19, 2011

Changing Roles for Women Lawyers—and the Men in Their Lives

The roles of women and men in our society and in our profession are changing, and we need to embrace the opportunities presented by those changes. As women lawyers and law students, you have chosen a profession that will result in success and power, and this has the potential to interfere with the relationships that you have with men—many of whom may be threatened by these new roles for you. It is important to think about these changes and to anticipate the future dynamics to give yourself the best chance at a positive outcome. Here is some food for thought. There is no real news in the fact that the roles of women have changed. It has been going on for decades, and much has been written on the new roles for women as professionals, executives, entrepreneurs, managers, and power brokers. Women entered the workforce in record numbers during this time, and there was bound to be plenty of change for them.

We also know that the roles of men have changed and that many of those changes are related to the changing roles of women. Many men are more involved in caring for their children, in the details of home life and in supporting the work their spouses do outside the home. Some men have enthusiastically embraced these new responsibilities and involvements and some have done it more reluctantly because it needed to be done. It has not been easy for the men any more than it has been easy for the women, but very often financial and economic concerns have driven the result. We now have many more stay-at-home fathers than ever before, and it is not unusual for a law firm to provide paternity leave as well as maternity leave.

This is common knowledge, but I recently read a new take on this familiar story that I think will interest you.

First the backstory. You may have seen the April 26, 2011 front cover of *Newsweek* magazine and the accompanying inside story titled 'The Beached White Male.' The gist of the article is that unemployment during the current recession has many men feeling defeated, shamed and powerless as the roles of breadwinner have shifted and the male confidences are eroded. It is a despairing article and paints a very dismal picture of the future for men in America. The author predicted that we will not be getting back to the 'way things were for men' any time soon.

The new take that interests me is provided by a response to that article written by Dan Mulhern, husband of former governor of Michigan Jennifer Granholm. The response appears in the May 9, 2011 issue of *Newsweek*, and is captioned 'How to Be a Real Man.' It is written as a letter to Mulhern and Granholm's 13-year-old son and is summarized as follows: "The old rules don't work—as I've learned being married to a powerful woman. Here's what I am telling our son about modern manhood."

Mulhern goes on to describe the role reversal for him when his wife became governor—instead of him, as he had expected—and his insecurities about his strength and manly contributions to the family. He describes extreme doubt followed by a realization of the great opportunities in becoming comfortable with himself as a caregiver, lead parent, and supporter. He found a new and deeper meaning to treating his wife as an equal and in learning new skills for communicating, negotiating, showing emotion . . . and even sacrificing. In summary, he found that it is "a great time to be a man."

Think about this and then file it away for another time when you may want to share it with someone who is feeling uncomfortable in his new role. It is positive and hopeful and inspiring, and it may just go a long way toward making the transitions to these new roles and perspectives less painful.

So, the message is to cherish your friendships, always remember to be a good friend, and let the love and support of your friends positively affect the balance in your life and your ultimate happiness. This one should be easy!

On the subject of the effect of positive relationships in your life, you may want to check out the following:

Dobransky, Paul, and L. A. Stamford. *The Power of Female Friendship: How Your Circle of Friends Shapes Your Life.* **Plume, 2008.**

A recent study has shown that women have fewer friends than they used to. In the years after college and before children (and even after that), many women find that they have fewer friends, and new ones are harder to make. Dr. Dobransky breaks down the primal codes of friendship that many women aren't even aware of and gives scientifically grounded advice for understanding how to be a better friend and how to cultivate new friendships.

Ferrazzi, Keith. *Who's Got Your Back: The Breakthrough Program to Build Deep, Trusting Relationships That Create Success—and* **Won't** *Let You Fail.* **Crown Business, 2009.**

Ferrazzi offers a strategy to execute on your most ambitious plans without costing your happiness, well-being, or sanity—in fact his program promises to enhance them by building deeper, more supportive relationships.

He offers a nine-step approach to building what he calls "lifeline relationships," an inner circle of deep, trusting peer support partners who serve as advisors, cheerleaders, and accountability watchdogs.

Paul, Marla. *The Friendship Crisis: Finding, Making, and Keeping Friends When You're Not a Kid Anymore.* **Rodale, 2005.**

Embraced by some of the most popular women's magazines, this book has struck a chord with women everywhere who know that finding close friends as an adult isn't easy. Marla Paul brings together the moving personal experiences of many different women with the keen insights of psychologists and other relationship experts.

Rath, Tom. *Vital Friends: The People You Can't Afford to Live Without.* **Gallup, 2006.**

Rath explores the inherent value of friendships and says that the need for friends goes beyond commonality or companionship; in particular, he devotes a section to friendship at work, which, unlike many companies and managers, Rath sees as a positive force. Rath's research shows that employees who have a best friend in the office are more productive, more likely to engage positively with customers, share new ideas and stay longer in a job.

Slotkin, Jacquelyn Hersh, and Samantha Slotkin. Goodman. *Sharing the Pants: Essays on Work-Life Balance by Men Married to Lawyers.* **Vandeplas, 2009.**

This book of essays focuses on work-life balance from the male perspective. Subjects include prioritizing time as a spouse and parent, acceptable working arrangements, and being an effective team. The book explores the pressures faced by men and their spouses; describes work-life balance issues and the satisfactions and difficulties of a dual career marriage; gives advice on how to do it; and explains the frustrations, disappointments, demands, and compromises—from the husband's perspective.

Yager, Jan. *Friendshifts: The Power of Friendship and How It Shapes Our Lives.* **Hannacroix Creek, 1999.**

"Friendshifts" is the word that sociologist Yager invented to explain how friendships change throughout life. Drawing on her own research, Yager discusses how friendships develop and how changes such as relocation, marriage, or a new job often provoke changes in relationships. Yager sees making friends as a skill that can be learned, but she cautions that each friendship is unique, with its own rules and privileges. Yager ably demonstrates how friends can improve the quality of our lives, enhance our self-esteem, provide encouragement, and compensate for family defects.

8

You *Really* Need to Live Within Your Means to Keep Your Options Open

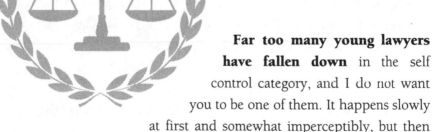

Far too many young lawyers have fallen down in the self control category, and I do not want you to be one of them. It happens slowly at first and somewhat imperceptibly, but then one day, WHAMO, you are faced with the consequences of no self control. The biggest consequence of a lack of self control can be the loss of professional options, and that can be very bad.

Here's how it works. Many young lawyers, men and women alike, start their law practices at big firms for big salaries. These young lawyers work hard over time and advance in the firm, and they convince themselves that they are entitled to some really expensive lifestyle trappings for their pain and suffering—the fancy car, the big house, the designer clothes, the vacation home, exotic trips—and soon they feel like they cannot live without these things. They look around the law firm and see senior members of the firm with extravagant lifestyles, and they want the same thing. They consider it a statement of importance and having "arrived," and soon these choices become automatic.

As you know, choices like this come with big price tags, and the biggest price tag typically turns out to be the house mortgage. While it is true that the big salary can support the big house mortgage, that scenario only works until the job that supports the big salary is no longer desirable or available. There comes a time for many of these big earners when they either are burned out or they experience a change of heart about what they want to do professionally. There also comes a time for some, especially during an economic downturn, when the job is no longer there. Very often the choice or the solution is to go to a job that pays less.

Sometimes that can be good—less stress and more job satisfaction. Who needs that big salary anyway? That's the rub. Make sure you don't!

It is fundamental that you need a certain amount of income to support the overhead of your lifestyle. When you scale back the income, you also have to scale back the lifestyle. Even if you are OK with that and it is possible, there are other things to consider. Maybe *you* can live without the big house and the country club membership, but what about your mate? Has your acquired lifestyle become so much a part of what you are as a couple or a family that you cannot give it up? Are the Golden Handcuffs locked so tight that you must forgo the options and the happiness that you might otherwise have had?

And, what about the fact that it can be a little out of your control to scale back? Consider the fact that houses—especially expensive houses—do not sell in a down economy and that there most certainly are going to be similar challenging economic times again in the future. Recession is like the boomerang. It always comes back if you wait long enough.

It is never too early to start thinking about these things. How about the decisions that relate to your family and raising the children you may have one day? Will your mate work or not? What if he or she needs to be home with the children, can you afford to do without that second income? Or have you lived such a lavish lifestyle to make that option impossible?

Remember that you cannot predict the future. Who knew that the economic collapse of 2008 would catch so many people without adequate nest eggs to stem the tide? Who knew that the credit crisis would ruin so many dreams and that the stock market losses would change so many visions of retirement?

You do not want this to happen to you. You want to live within your means and save enough to provide the security you need against an uncertain future.

So, here's my advice. Exercise self control. Do not overextend yourself. Concentrate on what you need and not what you want—at least most of the time. Emphasize simple pleasures.

To do this, you will need to learn to say "no" to yourself and to others. You will need to use credit sparingly and within reason. You will need to resist the temptation to keep up with the next door neighbors—or the partner in the firm.

It sounds harsh, I know, but preserving your options and being the mistress of your own destiny will pay off in spades. Deny the Golden Handcuffs! You will be doing yourself a huge favor.

Another issue that relates to your future financial security has to do with your debt from student loans, which many of you will have by the end of law school. You have to plan for the repayment of these student loans, and the future of those loans and the repayment provisions are not totally settled. The truth is that student loans are far from a free ride, and they may not even be a good deal—especially for the U.S. Government, which makes all of the loans these days. As pointed out in a recent article in the *ABA Journal*, entitled "The Paradigm Shift: The Law School Bubble," written in part by Professor William Henderson, Director of the Center on the Global Legal Profession and Professor of Law at Indiana University's

Mauer School of Law, repayment of some student loans for law school will represent 15% of a lawyer's income over more than half of his or her career span. That is a severe burden, especially if the sought-after gains in earning power fail to materialize. (*ABA Journal*, January 2012, pp. 30-35.) The article cited figures from *U.S. News & World Report* indicating that in 2010, 85% of law graduates from ABA-accredited schools had an average debt load of $98,500, and this is something that definitely affects the future of most law students. What used to be viewed as "easy credit" may not be that any more, and you need to be an informed consumer when it comes to your borrowing and your ability to repay debt. Professor Henderson's article will do just that for you, and I recommend that you take a look at it. Although there may not be any options in terms of financing a legal education for many of you, that does not mean that you should not prepare yourself for what lies ahead.

In addition to concerns about controlling debt, to really keep your options open, you need to become savvy about matters of budgeting, taxes, inheritance planning, retirement plans, and investments, to name just a few. Here are a few resources that may help you gain and retain the financial self-control to protect your future:

Bach, David. *Smart Women Finish Rich: 9 Steps to Achieving Financial Security and Funding Your Dreams*. Crown Business, 2002.

Bach's approach to money management is rooted in years of investment seminars for women and his work as senior vice president of investments at Morgan Stanley Dean Witter. He addresses tax strategies, wills, insurance, retirement plans, and investments in a highly accessible manner.

Haunty, Thomas A., and Todd D. Bramson. *Real Life Financial Planning for Young Lawyers: A Young Lawyer's Guide to Building the Financial House of Their Dreams*. Aspatore, 2006.

Practicing law today brings many challenges that prevent lawyers from adequately addressing their own finances. This book will give you a blueprint to help you get your financial house in order. Practical steps are presented on how to build a solid long-term financial plan that addresses every level of your finances from budgeting and insuring to investing and taxes.

Orman, Suze. *The Money Class: Learn to Create Your New American Dream.* **Spiegel & Grau, 2011.**

Suze Orman, the woman millions of Americans have turned to for financial advice, says it's time for a serious reconsideration of the American Dream—what promise it still holds, what aspects are in need of revision, and how it must be refashioned to fit our lives so that we can once again have faith that our hard work will pay off and that a secure and hopeful future is within our reach.

Orman, Suze. *Women & Money: Owning the Power to Control Your Destiny.* **Spiegel & Grau, 2010.**

In this book, Suze Orman addresses the complicated (and often dysfunctional) relationship women have with personal finance. Orman's direct, non-condescending style is perfect for this subject matter. She begins with the premise that "Women can invest, save, and handle debt as well and skillfully as any man" and then tackles the important question—"So why don't they?"

Ramsey, Dave. *The Total Money Makeover: A Proven Plan for Financial Fitness.* **Nelson, 2009.**

"Winning at money is 80 percent behavior and 20 percent head knowledge." So states Ramsey, author and radio show host, offering a comprehensive plan to get out of debt and achieve financial fitness. His seven-step plan includes paying off all debts except the home mortgage at an accelerated speed, creating a financial safety net that covers three to six months' expenses, investing 15 percent of income in a retirement fund, and saving for children's college expenses.

Thakor, Manisha, and Sharon Kedar. *On My Own Two Feet:*
A Modern Girl's Guide to Personal Finance. **Adams Business, 2007.**

By offering women the key 20 percent of financial advice (minus the complex mumbo jumbo) that drives 80 percent of a person's financial wealth, the authors will show women that the sooner they learn to apply basic financial strategies, the more likely they are to achieve the typical lifetime financial objective of owning a home. Along with other financial objectives, it provides for oneself and/or a family, being able to take fun vacations (and yes, wear designer labels), and retiring in comfort.

9

You *Really* Need to Take Credit for What You Do

Women typically do not take credit for their successes, and this can be a big problem in business. That does not mean that you should be running around the office bragging about your accomplishments, but it also does not mean that you should hide your light under a bushel. You need to make people aware of the good things that you do because it is quite likely that no one else will.

Here is an example. I have a lawyer friend on the West Coast who has several young associates working for her in her litigation practice. On motions days, she typically sends these young associates, both male and female, to court to argue motions in her cases. After court, they return to the office and report the results to her. The difference in their manner of reporting the results is very instructive.

My friend describes the female associate who comes into her office and starts reporting all of the things that she could have done better in court that morning. The female associate says that she could have argued the equities stronger or she could have put more emphasis on the XYZ case or that she forgot to mention an important legal precedent in her oral argument and more. It is not until my friend interrupts to get to the bottom of things that the young woman attorney discloses that she *won* the motion.

Now, fast forward to the young male associate making his report. My friend says that the young man usually does not even really enter her office. Instead he leans in through the doorway and says something simple like "I won." Not even, "We won." That's all, and he is off to lunch!

These are very different approaches. Neither one of them is perfect or ideal, but they demonstrate completely different styles. It is hard to be certain of the cause, but I think it has a lot to do with confidence. You have to have confidence in yourself to feel comfortable taking credit for things. While it is true that a lot of confidence in the law profession comes off as false *bravado*, that should not keep you from adopting a very acceptable and non-offensive way of taking credit for your accomplishments. Sometimes you just have to toot your own horn if people are going to notice you and realize what good work you do.

We all have heard the stories about the woman lawyer's comments during a meeting that are totally ignored only to be followed by a male lawyer saying the exact same thing and being treated like some kind of a genius for his incredible wisdom and insight. Not only is it wrong for that to happen, but it is also wrong for the woman to sit there and *let it happen* without calling attention to it. Eleanor Roosevelt is often quoted as saying, "No one can humiliate you without your consent."

We must get to the point where we call out people on this bad behavior and let them know that we are keeping score. Our efforts cannot be allowed to receive less recognition than the efforts of the men we work with.

I am not trying to suggest that this is easy, and I made some real mistakes at this along the way. Having my accomplishments ignored while the accomplishments of others—usually male colleagues—were played up made me very angry and even resentful at times. But the thing that should have made me madder was my reluctance to set the record straight even though it would have been uncomfortable.

So, learn from my mistakes. When you score a win, let it be known in good taste. When you publish that article, get that new case, speak at the bar event, or appear on a panel, do not hesitate to make sure that you get recognition in the law firm newsletter. You have to make your accomplishments known so that you have all of the material you need to compete for promotions and the most desirable cases and matters. There is nothing wrong with taking credit where credit is due, and your future may depend on it.

Taking credit is very closely associated with asking for opportunities. You have to be able to say that you are the best person for the job in order to get the job. You have to be able to confidently promote yourself, not only within your firm but to potential clients.

Promoting work is particularly critical to your success in practice. In today's law firm and the law firm of the future, your survival will depend on your ability to promote work and generate new clients for the firm. Gone are the days when senior lawyers "fed" work to junior lawyers because there was so much of it to go around. The law has become a very competitive business, and everyone in it is expected to be competitive as well.

However, that does not mean that you have to promote work in the traditional ways, which can include typical male choices like a round of golf or a game of squash at the athletic club. There are many other more women-friendly ways to promote work, and you must always be on the lookout for them. It can be as simple as talking to your fellow parents at the daycare center or the preschool about what you do and how well you do it. Some of them are likely to be CEOs of companies or represent businesses that could use your services.

Lauren Stiller Rikleen, of the Rickleen Institute for Strategic Leadership, had some interesting tips on business development in her article "Millenials: Tips for Building a Foundation for Success," which first appeared in the *ABA Practice Management Magazine*, January/February 2009. According to Ms. Rickleen, "It is critical that young lawyers understand early in their careers the relationship between their future success in the profession and their ability to attract and retain clients. . . . Effective business development is really all about relationships. Classmates from law school go on to become clients and sources of referral business. The same is true of your colleagues at work and other friends in the legal profession. Maintain these relationships throughout your career."

Some women practitioners think that development is harder for women than for men. They say that women were raised to be more "mannerly" as a rule, and men were raised to push each other around on the field, outbrag each other and go to war. As a result, many women do not feel as comfortable with calling attention to themselves in the business setting as men.

I am not sure that I totally buy into that because I see women as great communicators, and development is just another manner of communication. However, I do understand that much of client development is still done in typical male settings, and that presents a separate challenge.

However, you need to get over such reluctant behaviors. It is the 21st century. You need to become assertive and confident in the way that you deal with people who could become clients or who could recommend clients. You need to find those settings that are comfortable for you and talk about business instead of the weather. Have your business cards "at the ready" and offer them without being asked. Everyone understands the game and the need to generate and promote clients—including the potential clients. They may not say "yes" the first time, but keep on trying. AND, do not take "no" personally. The men mastered this the moment they were born!

You *can* do this, and you need to practice at every opportunity. To do it well, you may have to stop looking at yourself as women lawyers and start looking at yourself as lawyers who happen to be women. THINK ABOUT IT!

Here are a couple of blog entries from my website to get you started.

May 13, 2011

Women Lawyers Need to Learn to Generate Work in Their Communities

I know. You have not heard from me this week. Hope you missed me! I tried to work in a "Thought For the Day", but even that was hard. You see, I was working on two projects for my community, and it took up most of my time.

But I was thinking of all of you. Volunteering on behalf of your community is a really good thing for young women lawyers to do, and you need to start thinking about it. First, it is a great way for you to give back to your community. We all live very hectic lives these days, but the volunteer work in our communities still has to be done—even more so in a "down" economy like this one. Government services have been curtailed in some areas, and there is just more work that needs to be done by volunteers.

Second, and maybe the more important reason for my purposes here, is the great networking opportunities for all of you through community work. You know my mantra about generating work—that it is your path to freedom and options in your practice. The way to get the attention of the partners and management in your practice is to bring in work. Do that, and you will find that you have a great deal more control of your practice, options in your practice and respect from your colleagues. That all converts to upward mobility and job security. One way to generate work, which is very often overlooked, is through involvement in your community. This is particularly important for women lawyers, who often are the ones volunteering in the schools, the churches, and the community organizations—including the sports leagues. (Those are not just for Dad any more, thank goodness!) These community groups are full of CEOs of companies, people with legal entanglements and people who just plain know other people with legal problems. Unfortunately, too often, women lawyers do not take advantage of these opportunities.

The key is to let people know what you do. Let people know about your practice and your specialties. Stop thinking of it as unsavory self-promotion and start thinking about it as selling a great product—YOU. There is nothing wrong with talking business, and women need to get used to it. Men do it all the time on the field, in the athletic club, on the golf course, at the ball park, while cruising the Bay—you name it. It is the way business is run, and, as I tell you repeatedly, law is a business.

So, sell your product. Strike up a conversation with your fellow volunteer while you are licking envelopes or raking leaves, and give them something professional to remember about you. Do it enough times, and you will begin to realize the benefits. One major client can change your practice and your life. Make a new friend and fellow volunteer in your community, who trusts you as a neighbor and as a professional, and see where it leads you.

I hope you will remember this and put it into action next week. It is never too soon to start.

As for me, I must go now. The proposed two-lane bridge in my bucolic neighborhood needs to be defeated, and the landscape beautification projects need to be installed while weather permits. Letters need to be written, agreements need to be drafted and meetings need to be attended. Yes, it is work, but there are so many rewards—both personal and professional.

Happy generating!

From www.bestfriendsatthebar.com

Jun 17, 2011

Learn to Play Golf FORE Business and Pleasure

I am a golfer, and I like to play golf. It is an enjoyable, but sometimes frustrating, sport, and it is nice to play with friends. However, the benefits of golf go far beyond recreation and have long fingers into business development.

The benefits of golf in business were illustrated at some length in the *Washington Post* today in an article titled, "Leader of the Tee World." This was not about some guy who owns a T-shirt shop. It was, however, about some guy—specifically a young lawyer/lobbyist in DC named Tony Russo—who has perfected his golf game to the point where presidents and vice presidents—of the United States, that is—like to shoot a round with him.

The recent buzz about Tony Russo is because the US Open Golf Tournament is being played at Congressional Country Club in Bethesda, Maryland this week. That is right in my backyard, so I take particular notice. Well, it is not exactly "right in my backyard" technically because I live on the Virginia side of the Potomac River, but it is close enough. "Right in my backyard—or front yard, as it is" would more accurately refer to the residents of homes surrounding the golf course who are renting out parking spaces in their front yards for early-bird tourney watchers. But, not all for profit, you understand. In fact, one groundskeeper told the press that his boss, the doctor/homeowner, was only charging money for parking on his lawn so that he could donate the money to charity. Sure! And we wonder what is wrong with health care in this country. But . . . I digress . . .

Back to Tony and his perfect backswing that makes heads of state want to golf with him. Tony not only has a perfect backswing, but it seems that he has a perfect lobbying practice as the head lobbyist for

117

T-Mobile. Tony apparently has found a comfortable way to gain access to people with power and to make them seek out his companionship and expertise—both on the golf course and in the board room. A rather fine recipe for success in business, if you ask me.

So, when you read in my book that golf can open up some doors for women in the law—just as it has opened up doors for men—listen up and remember Tony. Or for a female to show you the way, check out Hilary Fordwich, who I discuss in Chapter 4 of my book. She is the CEO of business consulting firm Strelmark, LLC in Washington, DC, and, as an excellent golfer and contributing editor on ABC affiliate News Channel 8's *Capital Golf Week* and the *Washington Post's Metro Talk,* she has helped build her business around golf expertise.

But I understand that golf is not for everyone, and I have received some push back from female colleagues who do not think that women should have to pursue traditionally male methods of business promotion. I respect that view, but I do not see how embracing golf can hurt, especially when combined with the other kinds of business promotion that may be more comfortable for women. I say use what you can. There is no reason to have to choose. Just get out there and promote work and network with people at every opportunity. We all know what gets the attention in law firms—clients and a book of business. If you have that, you have real independence. It is hard to put too high a value on that.

Oops, gotta go. I need to get up early in the morning to snag one of those charity parking spaces on the doc's lawn. Can't get up too early for a fantasy like that!

From www.bestfriendsatthebar.com

Here are a few other resources that may be helpful to you in learning to take credit for your accomplishments and develop work:

Harrington, Mona. *Women Lawyers: Rewriting the Rules.* **A.A. Knopf, 1994.**

Drawing on interviews with more than 100 female lawyers, most of them graduates of Harvard Law School, attorney Harrington presents an absorbing mosaic of the issues impeding advancement of her subjects. She describes the professional, legal and social strictures that hamper women at corporate law firms.

Holtz, Sara. *Bringin' in the Rain: A Woman Lawyer's Guide to Business Development.* **ClientFocus, 2008.**

In *Bringin' in the Rain*, Holtz taps into her experience as a business development coach to lawyers to offer practical advice on the most effective and efficient ways to generate business. You'll learn how to focus your marketing efforts, engage in high-payoff activities, employ effective follow-up, build strong revenue-generating relationships, and more.

Rikleen, Lauren S. *Ending the Gauntlet: Removing Barriers to Women's Success in the Law.* **Thomson/Legalworks, 2006.**

Rickleen focuses on the institutional impediments to women's success in the practice of law—the challenges and roadblocks women face as they struggle to succeed in law firms. The book sets forth recommendations for change, describing concrete actions which law firms can implement in order to enable women to take their rightful place as equals in the legal profession.

Slotkin, Jacquelyn H., and Samantha S. Goodman. *It's Harder in Heels: Essays by Women Lawyers Achieving Work-Life Balance.* **Vandeplas, 2007.**

This book contains essays by and about women lawyers: stories about women practicing (or choosing not to practice) law, about hitting the glass ceiling, about amazing lawyer-mentors, about professional achievements, about personal and professional hardships, about the stress of juggling multiple roles, about meeting the demands of work and family, about being Superwoman, and about hitting the maternal wall.

Thalacker, Karen. *The New Lawyer's Handbook: 101 Things They Don't Teach You in Law School.* **Source, 2009.**

This book touches on a little of everything that a new lawyer needs to know as she enters a firm: from how to handle your clients and how to work with people in your office, to why it pays to learn to play golf.

10

You *Really* Need True Grit

No, this chapter is not about movies and popcorn! It is about the difficulties of the practice of law, especially for a woman. It is true that the business of law is hard work, but you are up to the task. You got through law school, and many of you found jobs in a difficult economy. You are not shrinking violets. But, you are going to have to realize what you are up against and learn to protect yourself and your future. Success in your professional life is integral to the *new* balance, just as success in your personal life is, and you need to know how to safeguard both.

You must have True Grit to safeguard your professional life and survive. That means getting tough when you have to and having courage. It does not mean playing dirty or turning up the *machismo*, but you have to learn to access your thick skin and to "push back" when you are sure of your position and are challenged.

Fortunately, the Gen Y women have learned to push back better than prior generations. But, if you do not fit that description, you may have to ratchet it up a bit. Always remember that you can disagree without being disagreeable, a theme that runs throughout my books.

True Grit also means protecting your turf. Always protect your work product, and if someone is trying to pass it off as his or her own, confront them about it. If that person is superior to you, it will be difficult, but you have to do it. You cannot let people take advantage of you in your personal life or in your professional life.

You also cannot let others take work away from you. If you believe that you are in line for work that has gone to someone else, get to the bottom of it. I once was overlooked for work that I knew should have been mine, and I made a fuss about it. Turns out that the partner on the case did not want to travel with me because I could not go to the gym and shoot hoops with him on the road. True story. I made a fuss and got the work. Fortunately, there are laws against that kind of discrimination now, but it still happens in much more subtle ways today, and you have to be on the lookout for it.

True Grit also means protecting your future in the firm. I have heard it said that the four most important words for any lawyer are *Portable Book of Work.* You must always be striving to get clients who will be loyal to you and will follow you if you decide to relocate. You cannot do that if you do not become skilled at promoting yourself and giving those clients a reason to have faith in you and be loyal to you. Sometimes this means moving out of your comfort zone and being a little more assertive than you would like. That is understandable, but you have to do it. It is a tough world out there, and the competition for work is fierce. But, you have everything you need to be successful. Just give yourself a little push.

My own personal twist on the four most important words is *Personal Book of Work.* The distinction is that you need to control work to have a secure future *in your firm* as well as to take that work somewhere else. The more work you control, the more flexibility and latitude the firm will allow you. As long as you have clients and work and are bringing money into the firm, folks tend to leave you alone to allow you to become even more successful. They do not ask as many questions, and they do not scrutinize your behavior as much. This can really help with that *new* balance you are looking for. You want to go to the Nordstrom shoe sale in the middle of the work day, no questions asked!

However, both versions of the four most important words may be too simplistic. A trusted colleague reminds me that in Big Law, especially, it is very often unrealistic to have your own book of work. Too often the work is controlled by senior attorneys, who will have to retire or die for you to ever "control" it.

That does not mean that you cannot prove yourself indispensable in a subordinate role. Proving yourself indispensable often means having the True Grit to take on the challenge of becoming an expert in some area of the law that is highly regarded by senior lawyers and clients. It can be hard work, but it also can be an insurance policy of sorts against the uncertainty of your future.

Sometimes having True Grit means setting boundaries. These kinds of issues are examined in the new book *Nice Girls Just Don't Get It: 99 Ways to Win the Respect You Deserve, the Success You've Earned, and the Life You Want* by Dr. Lois Frankel and Carol Frohlinger (Crown Archetype, 2011). In that book, the authors explore themes like overextending yourself by taking on all the unpleasant tasks no one else wants to do—just because you want to be liked by others—and they describe how to politely decline when a friend asks you to do an unreasonable favor without feeling the need to apologize or explain yourself. They also encourage women to set boundaries for pushy, meddlesome friends and relatives and to confront colleagues who are shirking responsibility. This is all good advice, and I know that you will benefit from reading more about it.

I remember well when I discovered this particular meaning of True Grit. I was a second year associate and the first and only woman litigator in my practice. I was scheduled to travel with a male partner on a case, and this started a "buzz" in the firm about men and women colleagues traveling together. (Are you detecting a theme here?) It became very uncomfortable for me, and I knew that I had to put a stop to it. The way that I did it took all of the True Grit that I could muster at the time.

I walked into the office of a partner who was the source of the gossip and confronted him. I told him that I knew what he was saying, that I thought it was highly inappropriate and that I wanted it to stop. I told him that it was not only an insult to me and to the partner that I would be traveling with, but that it also was an insult to my husband. Remember now, he was a senior partner, and I was a second year associate!

His response was to tell me that he was sorry that I did not have a sense of humor, to which I replied that I was sorry that he did not have a sense of propriety. End of discussion.

His little game stopped, and I never had to put up with that from him again. Fortunately, I did not have to depend on him for work. If that had been the case, it would have been a whole lot more complicated.

True Grit also can mean exercising restraint. Talking to your colleagues, your superiors, your clients and your adversaries is not the same as talking to your friends. You will have to assess your audience and temper your tone and approach accordingly. You do not talk to clients the same way that you talk to your girlfriends—even when the client is yelling at you or making false accusations. It will get you into a heap of trouble because clients support the business. They pay the bills, and associate lawyers are expendable, as compared to clients.

This is particularly true when it comes to representing corporate clients where the case is being managed by in-house counsel. Those in-house lawyers direct the caseload for their companies, and they parcel out the work to outside counsel. You need to treat them with kid gloves. If you are experiencing difficulties with those counsel, button your lip, smile and report it to your supervising attorney. He or she gets paid the really big bucks to deal—or NOT deal—with these situations.

This does not mean that you should allow yourself to be abused by clients or anyone else. But, let's face it, women, like men, often can be strident in their approaches. Unfortunately, sometimes, even an unintended strident approach by a woman can be interpreted as "bitchy" by male colleagues and clients. Recognize this, and watch out for it in the way that you relate to colleagues, clients and, of course, the court. Judges have little patience with lawyers on high horses.

Restraint is particularly important for women because men still rule the profession. The vast majority of you will have to find a way to stay in the profession and get to management levels to change that result. You certainly do not want to short-circuit those efforts by indulging in imprudent behavior. As good as getting on your high horse may feel at the time, there can be a big price to pay for that fleeting pleasure.

Having True Grit also means coming to terms with decisions that you make in your life. Some of the decisions that you will have to make in terms of choosing between your personal and professional lives will be very painful and will take real courage. Trust me, I know. I remember getting so discouraged by the relatively little time that I had to spend with my children in their early years. It seems like just yesterday when I spent the afternoon of my daughter's fifth birthday in the office preparing for trial. Sometimes there is not much of an institutional heart in law practice, and you have to be tough to live with that reality. Often you have no choice, and beating yourself up about it does not help. Have the strength of your own convictions and move on knowing that there are many other opportunities to do the right thing up the road. The key is making sure that you take those future opportunities. As discussed earlier, balance does not mean the *same* balance all of the time. It is more of an *average* concept.

Having True Grit also means not complaining openly—even when you are right. Complaining openly and presenting a negative *persona* is not a good strategy for the office or most places, for that matter. Even if you have every good reason to complain, people do not want to hear it. They have their own problems, and your complaining brings them down. They do not want to become associated with your problems because they often fear reprisal if they appear to be in agreement with someone who is balking establishment and management. As a result, you may find them avoiding you. If this sounds a little too much like a Big Brother scenario out of George Orwell's *1984*, understand that it is. Corporate mentalities and corporate politics can be very unforgiving, and you do not want to put your friends and colleagues at the office in a position where they have to choose. Too often, the choice will be to your detriment.

Deal with your problems with trusted family, friends, and colleagues only. Do it behind closed doors, not in the hallways and open to the public. Keep a stiff upper lip, and do not show your weak side. Walk tall and draw from the strength of knowing that you are capable of handling things without making a victim of yourself. The victim mentality is never a good approach, and it certainly does not work in business because so much of the workforce is already insecure. Your insecurity makes them feel vulnerable, and no one wants to feel vulnerable.

Ironically, having True Grit also can mean allowing yourself a good cry now and then. It can clear your head, and it can be cathartic! It takes a certain toughness to know when you need it.

If someone told you along the way that only sissies and weak people cry, that is unfortunate. We have seen plenty of famous people in the public arena cry over the recent years, including then Senator Hillary Rodham Clinton during the 2008 presidential primary season, and House Speaker John Boehner after his ascendance to that position, and few assorted burly professional athletes when they did not make it to the Final Four or the playoffs. A few tears now and then do not make you a lesser human being, and it does not make you unprofessional.

However, crying openly at the office about your problems is never a good idea. As pointed out in Book One, most men do not feel comfortable with tears, and you will rarely accomplish your objective. You will start reminding them of their mothers and their wives, and that is not a comparison that will work to your advantage in the professional setting. Sometimes a public tear or two cannot be avoided, but it usually is not advisable. Try to keep that in mind. Office doors are made for opening *and* closing.

To help develop the True Grit and thick skin that can be a real benefit to you, I suggest that you take a look at the following resources:

Evans, Gail. *Play Like a Man, Win Like a Woman: What Men Know About Success That Women Need to Learn*. Broadway, 2000.

Evans argues that women enter the business game disadvantaged, having been taught to be cooperative rather than competitive, to enjoy the process rather than simply the result, and to seek approval rather than assume success. She provides instructions on how men play and teaches women to play smarter and win on their own terms. She supports her observations with both personal and professional anecdotes and covers the gamut of women's experiences on the corporate path.

Frankel, Lois P. *Nice Girls Don't Get the Corner Office: 101 Unconscious Mistakes Women Make That Sabotage Their Careers.* **Warner Business, 2004.**

Dr. Lois Frankel reveals why some women roar ahead in their careers while others stagnate. She discusses a unique set of behaviors—101 in all—that women learn in girlhood that sabotage them as adults. She helps you eliminate these unconscious mistakes that could be holding you back—and offers invaluable coaching tips you can easily incorporate into your social and business skills.

Kolb, Deborah M., Judith Williams, and Carol Frohlinger. *Her Place at the Table: A Woman's Guide to Negotiating Five Key Challenges to Leadership Success.* **Jossey-Bass, 2010.**

This book is a practical guide for any woman dealing with a demanding professional role. Drawing on extensive interviews with women leaders, the authors isolate five key challenges: Intelligence; Backing; Resources; Buy-In; and Making a Difference. The three expert authors reveal what women have to teach us about the challenges and opportunities of leadership.

Mindell, Phyllis. *How to Say It for Women: Communicating with Confidence and Power Using the Language of Success.* **Pearson Professional Education, 2001.**

Phyllis Mindell, an expert on professional communications, teaches women how to transform themselves by shedding weak phrases, gestures and words, in order to command respect, motivate, establish authority, and make a difference.

11

You *Really* Need to Be the Best Lawyer You Can Be

I cannot emphasize this enough. It is a part of every speech that I give and everything I write. I addressed this in Book One, and I repeat some of it here. It is the keystone for everything else in your career.

Being the best lawyer that you can be is fundamental. It should be your goal every day of your practice, and following that objective will make everything else easier. Knowing that you are doing a really good job and making a valuable contribution to your profession will give you the confidence to continue to be who you are and to take the time you need for yourself to achieve the *new* balance that is critical to your success as a person and as a lawyer.

Being the best lawyer you can be will open doors. You will gain a reputation for trustworthiness and a good work ethic, and you will find

129

yourself being sought out for interesting work by those who need to trust you. Fast forward that reputation a few years into your practice, and you will have put yourself in a position to negotiate from a position of strength when you need to ask for special practice accommodations to get you through some of the challenging years of your personal life. You will have proven a value to the firm that the leadership will not want to lose.

Being the best lawyer you can be does not start and stop with being a good researcher, being a good analyst and being a good writer. Yes, memoranda and briefs and settlement proposals are very important, but they are only a few aspects of what a good lawyer does.

A good lawyer looks out for her client and her firm by always conforming to the rules of the court and being prepared for every meeting, motion, settlement conference or other opportunity to represent the client. A good lawyer looks out for her staff because they are the ones who make her look good by taking care of all the *minutia*. A good lawyer understands the political issues at the law firm and learns to maneuver among them to get the best opportunities for her practice. A good lawyer understands the structure of the law firm and how to successfully work within that structure or how to go about changing it effectively.

A good lawyer serves on committees and initiatives to improve the law firm and keep it economically healthy. A good lawyer finds time to mentor less experienced lawyers and becomes a sponsor to those she wants to see advance in the firm. A good lawyer takes networking and promotion seriously, understands that it is critical to the future of the firm, and commits to making significant efforts to get new clients and new work. A good lawyer takes care of her health and fitness and understands that she has a responsibility to herself and her clients to do that. A good lawyer takes time out for herself to create the balance between her professional and personal lives to keep her happy. A good lawyer always is learning.

A good lawyer can also be defined by what a sponsor looks for in a young lawyer that he or she chooses to support and nurture. Some of those attributes were pointed out by panelists at the July 2011 National Association of Women Lawyers conference and included innovation, drive, interest in the subject matter, and sincere concern for the client and the firm. According to the panelists, those are the qualities that set certain young lawyers apart and make them particularly attractive to firms and to mentors and sponsors.

A good lawyer is enthusiastic about the profession. Enthusiasm is infectious, as pointed out by Laura Stiller Rikleen in her article on tips for Millennials in the ABA *Law Practice Management Magazine*, January/February 2009. People enjoy being around those who love what they do. Enjoy your work and share that enthusiasm in a way that lets others know that you are the perfect person to handle their future matters."

There is a lot to being a good lawyer, and you should strive to be a good lawyer in each of those categories. You then will be the best lawyer that you can be. It is all that you can ask of yourself and all that others can ask of you. It does not mean that you have to be the next Edward Bennett Williams or David Boise. It just means that you need to be the best that YOU can be.

I was lucky to have a great role model in my father. He was the best lawyer I could imagine for all of the reasons mentioned here and more. Some of you may have a similar role model in your life, and I hope you do. Where you do or not, you can access great role models through reading biographies of great lawyers and modeling the behavior. Examples are biographies of Melvin Belli, Thurgood Marshall, Sandra Day O'Connor, Ruth Bader Ginsburg, and the new biography of Clara Folt by Barbara Babcock, to name just a few.

Make it your goal to be the best lawyer you can be and watch the doors open for you!

Here are a few good resources for helping you be the best lawyer you can be:

Anders, Kelly Lynn. *The Organized Lawyer*. Carolina Academic, 2008.

The Organized Lawyer is designed to address the needs of all types of lawyers—corporate, nonprofit, government, private, academic, and solo practitioners. Whether you're in a cubicle, corner office, or working out of your home, this book will help you develop and maintain a more organized space.

Hermann, Richard L. *The Lawyer's Guide to Finding Success in Any Job Market.* **Kaplan Pub., 2009.**

With 25 years in legal career counseling, Hermann helps attorneys deal with downsizing in a precarious economy. The book provides a savvy outlook on the current job scene, with specific topics that include: opportunities impervious to economic flux; beating "recession depression"; using a law degree outside the "mainstream"; combining career opportunities; maximizing contacts; nailing an interview; and relocation considerations.

Herrmann, Mark. *The Curmudgeon's Guide to Practicing Law.* **American Bar Association, 2006.**

This collection of essays written by The Curmudgeon, offers practical, honest and "you need to know this" advice for surviving and thriving in a law firm. The book covers the basics of law practice and law firm etiquette, from doing effective research and writing to dressing for success, dealing with staff and clients and building a law practice. Concise, humorous and full of valuable (albeit curmudgeonly) insight, this is a must-read for every newly minted law school graduate or new lawyer.

Levit, Nancy, and Douglas O. Linder. *The Happy Lawyer: Making a Good Life in the Law.* **Oxford UP, 2010.**

The Happy Lawyer examines the causes of dissatisfaction among lawyers, and then charts possible paths to happier and more fulfilling careers in law. Eschewing a one-size-fits-all approach, it shows how maximizing our chances for achieving happiness depends on understanding our own personality types, values, strengths, and interests.

Lund, Morten. *Jagged Rocks of Wisdom: Professional Advice for the New Attorney.* **Fine Print, 2007.**

A new job is scary for anyone. A new job as an attorney is scary times two: the challenges are both substantive (as in actually knowing the law), as well as procedural (as in knowing how to act like an attorney). In this professional transition, many new attorneys fall by the wayside. This book is a guide to keep the new attorney on track. It includes advice for the new law firm associate, written by a Yale Law School graduate who made partner in a national law firm. Written in a first- and second-person tense and filled with no-nonsense guidance from someone actually in the mentorship role in a real-world law firm.

Messinger, Thane J. *The Young Lawyer's Jungle Book: A Survival Guide.* **Fine Print, 1999.**

The Young Lawyer's Jungle Book is a survival guide for the new attorney, with in-depth advice on law office life, including working with senior attorneys, legal research, memos, drafting, mistakes, grammar, email, workload, time-sheets, reviews, teamwork, deportment, attitude, perspective, working with clients (and dissatisfied clients), working with office staff, using office tools, and, well, not just surviving but thriving in a new career.

You *Really* Need to Think About Career Transitions

Sometimes, no matter how hard you try, you just cannot find that right balance. It may be because of work-life issues or it may be because the subject matter of your practice does not interest you and will never make you happy in your professional life. Stuff happens, and you have to be resilient. As a result, from time to time in your career, you will need options and strong practice models for transition. No matter how well you follow the advice in books like this, sometimes it just does not work out where you are and you need to be prepared for that.

Let's face it, knowing who you are and finding time to protect that identity and creating happiness in your life while billing 2200 hours a year at a law firm may not work out for you—or it may, depending on the circumstances. If you are one of the women who finds the perfect mate and the perfect nanny, you may be able to soar in private practice, and you will not be in the market for options. Or, you may be a woman who finds the perfect law firm and very acceptable flexible work arrangements. For others of you, options will become very important as your career advances and your personal circumstances change in ways that make the work-life struggle increasingly difficult. That is when you need to revisit the personal definition of success that was addressed in Book One and become comfortable with what defines success for you at specific times in your career.

You cannot get that kind of information too early. There are so many unanticipated circumstances in the course of a career, and you always want to be ready to meet the challenges that arise and map out a new route. That flexibility is critical to survival in a profession as dynamic as the law has become, and getting this kind of information early will put you in a preferred position when the time comes.

Always remember that it is a long career if you let it be. You will have to make some adjustments to your personal definition of success as you are presented with different circumstances. Often those changed circumstances involve children. It will help you to remember that staying in your profession in one way or another will protect you from the feelings of abandonment that you are likely to experience when the kids get wings and take flight—and it happens much sooner than you would expect. Kids grow up, and you will want to have something meaningful and satisfying in your life to fall back on when that happens—something more productive than crying your eyes out and looking behind every nook and cranny for that woman lawyer you used to be. It is better to keep a hand in your career so that, when that day comes, you can jump back in with renewed energy and enthusiasm. Who knows what you can accomplish then? If you need a change, it is important that you rely on yourself as the change agent and do not let others define who you are.

So, we have come nearly full circle and are back to the topic we explored in Chapter 3. Always remember who and what you are and BE that person. If one practice setting is not working for you, pursue another.

Successful transitions take research and reflection. There are many definitions of success, and certain definitions will fit better at different times in your career. The definition of success needs to work for you and not just for firm managers with agendas separate from your own.

Here is a blog entry from my website to further explain this personal definition of success.

May 5, 2011

The Male Definitions of Success in the Law May Not Work for Women Lawyers

News flash: The male definitions of success in the law many not work for women lawyers. I always include this message in my speeches at law schools and law firms, and I want to share it with you here.

This statement, of course, is a reference to the work-life struggles that are so difficult for women lawyers who have responsibilities for home, family, and aging and disabled family members. I emphasize that young women lawyers are all different and that you must make choices that will work for you. I also emphasize that for those choices to be good, they must be made by you and for you and be tailored to your personal circumstances. I always include a Power Point slide that presents the various practice options, from full time to part time and including both public and private sector settings. I do not make any value judgments about individual choices and career plans, and I emphasize that the only bad choice is no choice and the only bad plan is no plan.

The male definitions for success in the law are a big part of this dilemma for women, and young women lawyers must stop buying into these male stereotypes for success. You must remember that, for the most part, those men have wives, and you do not. The male definitions of success only work if you have no greater responsibilities in your personal life than the men you work for and the men you compete against. For the rest of you, it will be an uneven playing field, and you will have to throw off the time-honored stereotypes and chart your own course to success.

Does that mean that I want all women to work part-time or flex hours? No! Of course not! What it means is that I would rather have you work those alternative schedules than give up being a lawyer entirely. In fact, I tell my audiences that I hope that enough of them find the perfect nanny or a mate or family member who is willing and able to assume a large share of the childcare responsibilities to allow the young women lawyers to continue in full time practice to help accelerate women to the top of our profession.

So, in reporting about my speech at Marquette University Law School recently for the *Ms. JD* blog, Marquette Law Professor Lisa Mazzie included the above remarks. Her blog was great, and I hope you caught my post about it earlier on this blog. What interested me also was a comment to Professor Mazzie's post where the writer pushed back by saying that we should not be making new definitions of success for women and that women should be competing on the same terms as men because they could—or something to that effect. I think that comment begs the point, and here is why. Sure, it would be great if all women stayed in the profession full time and competed with the men for those positions in management and control at the top of firms. But, we know that, because of the work-life struggle alone, that is an unrealistic expectation. The truth is that, if we do not give women lawyers other alternatives, many of them will drop out.

Keeping women in the profession is necessary to support, elevate and promote other women. It is as simple as that. Aim for it and do not be steered off course by those who want to be short sighted or are unwilling to take a practical approach to a complicated issue for the sake of posturing. It gets us nowhere.

From www.bestfriendsatthebar.com

Although Book One was all about career planning and choices, it made no pretense to guarantee that your personal choices would be either the right choices or would last throughout your career. The discussion in Book One was designed to prepare you to make the right choice, but the right choice at the moment does not always work out in the long run. There always are unexpected circumstances, contingencies and opportunities that result in changes that alter careers. Nothing is carved in stone, and many of you will arrive at a time when your chosen career path either no longer works for you or a better opportunity presents itself. This chapter addresses those times and those changes—changes from one form of practice to another—changes that hold promise for risk-taking attorneys and changes that not only are good and advisable but also lead to great success and professional satisfaction.

"Careers in Transition" is a fascinating subject to me, and I hope it will be for you. Transition is often associated with flexibility, and flexibility in the legal profession is often associated with women lawyers. "Flexible Time" is the popular jargon, but that is only the beginning. While it is true that many of the career decisions for women lawyers are rooted in the need for flexible time to respond to the needs of their personal lives (childcare, responsibilities of home, etc.), a study by Columbia Business School and the University of Amsterdam indicated that women tend to embrace flexibility and take risks associated with career change more often than men in their professions. (http://thegrindstone.com/strategy/what-is-a-social-risk-and-are-you-taking-one/)

The reasons for this are not clear, but it is indeed fortunate that women possess the kind of risk taking that often is necessary to salvage their careers. Some commenters contend that this risk taking is the result of women having the "luxury" to take these alternative routes because their husbands or mates will continue to toil away as the primary breadwinners. They also point out that, in many cases, the couple is heavily in debt from the "Golden Handcuffs" of large incomes and acquired life styles and that the men are limited in their options.

Whatever the reasons—and I will leave that for another discussion— women lawyers are spending a lot of time in transition because of the work-life struggles and the challenges of a male-dominated profession with rules based on male stereotypes. These transitions are often difficult and can result in not only career-altering experiences but also life-altering experiences.

However, that does not mean that transitions are bad. Transitions can be excellent adventures—even the ones that do not turn out as well as the others. You can learn valuable things from each of these transition experiences, and, hopefully, with the right research, you will find a place that works better for you in achieving the necessary balance in your life.

There is a whole lot more movement in the law profession than ever before (lawyers changing law firms readily and often). Some of that movement is the result of the down economy and law firm cutbacks, but a lot of it is just representative of the global economy, the faster pace and the greater fluidity of the world today. The old attitudes of loyalty and devotion to the "law firm family" are often just that—old attitudes. The law profession has become much more competitive, and the players also are much more competitive and self-interested than ever before. The law has become a very "dynamic profession," in the purest sense of the word, and the movement applies to all lawyers, women and men alike. To get a feel for the magnitude of the movement activity, google "lawyers on the move" and be prepared to see a lot of lawyers changing jobs in all major employment areas.

Transitions, if they are to be successful, must include good choices and good planning, and for that you need good information. To help you with those personal decisions, let's look at some typical transitions through profiles of remarkable women lawyers, including what these women have to say about where they came from, where they went, the need for the transition and the challenges of change.

As with most things, first we have to look at the facts. Statistics from the National Association for Law Placement (NALP) show that approximately half of young women law school graduates will start out in the private sector as associates in law firms. (http://www.nalp.org/classof2010_

salpressrel). Law firm practice is a big draw for graduating law students because of the high salaries and perks and the prestige of private practice. Fortunately, this career path works out for some women. Although statistics show that 76% of women law graduates who take jobs in Big Law leave the firm by their fifth year of practice (*Working Mother* online, "Focus on Best Law Firms—Part-Time Practice," November 16, 2008), that means that 1 out of 4 of them sticks with the law firm model at least for some time beyond those first five years. Those young women who stay in law firm practice either achieve and remain on partnership track or they find ways to combine the needs of their professional lives and their personal lives in one or another of the alternative practices that have become popular—alternatives like flexible time, part-time practice, job sharing and other blended models.

Most often, these alternative practices require that the attorneys transition to non-partnership tracks. Although non-partnership tracks work for some women lawyers, other women feel like they are relegated to less important practices and treated like second-class lawyers under those circumstances. As a result, many women, who are engaged in the work-life struggle or who are not enchanted by law firm practice, look to alternatives outside of the law firm setting.

As young women law students and young women lawyers, I know that you have questions like:

What are those alternatives to private practice?

Do those alternatives provide more flexibility than law firm practice?

Do those alternatives satisfy the needs for quality work and reasonable opportunities for promotion?

How difficult is the transition?

Are you locked in once you make the change or could you go back to private practice at some point?

And myriad other questions that will become important during the decision-making process.

I cannot answer all of those questions for you, even though I have done my fair share of transitioning and reinventing myself during my career. As you may know from my first book, my own legal/legislative career of more than 25 years includes private practice with three law firms and years in the public sector in a legislative setting. I have been a law firm associate, a part-time law firm practitioner, a law firm of counsel, a law firm partner and an Administrative Aide in government. Although I gained a lot of experience from these transitions from private practice to government and back again, I do not pretend to know all of the answers about transitions to corporate practice, to academia, to public interest, to the judiciary and other models that will be examined here.

But, I *do* know the women who can give you clear pictures of what those transitions are all about. Those women, my new contributors, are a remarkable group, and it is my pleasure to bring their stories to you.

In addressing transitions, you need to understand that transitions can be scary. Facing your fears is generally the best antidote to fear itself, and the testimonials and experiences of these women will help you to do just that. Failing to make a decision because you are afraid is like making a bad decision, and my Contributors and I will give you the information that you need to avoid that result. My goal is to take the scary out of the process of decision making so that you have full range to take advantage of opportunities that may enhance your experiences, achieve the balance that you are looking for, and lead to even more satisfying and successful careers.

The information will be presented to you as profiles of women who have gone before you to address those issues and contemplate those transitions. You will "meet" and get to know women attorneys who successfully made those transitions. You will find out what precipitated those changes and what important considerations went into the decision to make the career change. You will learn the importance of "creating value" to give you the flexibility that you need to address change. You also will discover the differences between the various practice settings and what may make one setting preferable to another. You will acquire role models and practice models that will become permanent fixtures in your lives, and you will become familiar with women attorneys who will give you the true scoop and will not sugar coat for the sake of making themselves look good— women attorneys who know the meaning of effective mentoring and are willing to take the time to mentor you.

What a find! I have interviewed all of these women specifically for this book. They were all given questions in advance to contemplate in an attempt to provide the best information to you. They were generous with their time, and they gave me the flexibility that I needed to tell their stories in my own way. I am grateful to each of them, and I am excited about introducing them to you.

So, let's explore those Careers in Transition. Meet my new *Best Friends at the Bar* and let them share their experiences and wisdom with you. For those of you contemplating a change, you will get a bird's eye view of what to expect. You can be the judge of whether a particular career move meets your expectations or fits your life plan.

And for those of you who are trying to choose an initial career path, this information will help you to make those first choices with confidence and positive expectations. What an opportunity for you as well.

For a general discussion of career change and empowerment of women in the workforce, I recommend Caroline Dowd-Higgins' book, *This Is Not the Career I Ordered: Empowering Strategies from Women Who Recharged, Reignited, and Reinvented Their Careers* (Reinvention Press, 2010) and her career transition blog by the same name, which feature women who are thriving after career transitions. Ms. Dowd-Higgins is also the Director of Career and Professional Development at the Indiana University Maurer School of Law, and, as you would expect, her comments often are tailored to the legal profession.

So, let's have some fun. Roll out the possibilities. Explore Careers in Transition!

Where We Are and How We Got Here

Past as prologue—you already know how much I value history as a teacher. As we discussed earlier, the statistics are discouraging for women in the law today. We have a dropout rate (women leaving the profession mid-career) of over 40%—and a very high percentage of women attorneys leave Big Law—76% within the first five years of their practices.

How did we get to this point of serious dilemma or near crisis? To answer that question, we must look back at the messages that have been sent to women over the last 50 years. It is often hard to know where you are going if you do not know where you have been. So, we need to go back to the 1960's, a time before many of you were born.

In the 1960's and 1970's young women were told by leaders of the women's movement like Gloria Steinem and Betty Friedan, among others, that they could have it all—family, home, profession and anything else that they desired—because men could have it and, therefore, women were entitled to it also. This was the first wave of feminism, and I certainly respect all that these women did to raise awareness of issues affecting women and holding them back from their true potential. Unfortunately, in that dialogue, someone forgot to point out that women will always bear the children and that the likelihood that the greatest degree of responsibility for childcare would fall to anyone but women was unrealistic. However, any attempts to send that message had been drowned out by the outcries from euphoric and liberated young women who were busy burning their bras and celebrating their new-found freedom. By the late 1970's and early 1980's, women were enrolled in law schools in record numbers as a result of these new attitudes and also as a result of the court decisions that assured them greater access to the bastions of legal education.

These heady times were followed by the 80's and 90's when these same young women became practicing lawyers and clung to the belief that they could have it all. Soon, however, many of these young women lawyers began to have children and came to grips with the differences between themselves and their male colleagues.

As we marched through the 80's and 90's, it became a more and more desperate situation. Young women lawyers found that they could not achieve their professional and personal goals simultaneously, and they began to feel inadequate—inadequate as lawyers and inadequate as caretakers of their children and families.

Women's initiatives sprung up at law firms throughout the country in response to this frustration. Although these groups had little power and little influence, they did provide forums for discussion and solidarity and, on occasion, led to new more flexible work models. However, some women did not feel content with these new alternative work schedules, which usually included non-partnership tracks, and they became discouraged. Many of these young women dropped out and never returned to the profession. As a result, the attrition rates for women in the legal profession have been on the rise for the last decade.

Looking back, we realize that the Women's Liberation Movement of the 1960's ostensibly freed women from the expectations of others and gave them choices about their futures. It opened up many new opportunities for them in their personal and work lives. However, in their enthusiasm for this new power of choice, fueled by the Movement's leadership, these young women believed that they could "have it all." In doing so, they traded one set of stereotypes for another and adopted the male stereotypes for success in their work lives. Women in the law profession were no exception, and the myth of having it all juxtaposed to the realities of the work-life struggle have had women professionals, especially, reeling ever since.

Flash forward to today. We now have the opportunity for another kind of liberation. That liberation is to free ourselves from the male stereotypes of success and to chart our own courses and decide what truly makes us happy. We now must ask the important question, "Is it what I want or is it what I think people expect of me?" We must develop our own personal definitions of success and throw off the constraints and expectations of others, which have not worked so well for many women, to truly be successful in a way that will make us happy.

We have proven through the yeoman's efforts of the Women's Liberation Movement that women *can* achieve like men. But, the real questions become, "Do we want to achieve like men? Does success mean the same thing to women that it means to men? And, DOES IT HAVE TO?"

Women today are at the threshold of great expectations, both *for* themselves and crafted *by* themselves. Many women do not want to be partners in law firms. However, that does not mean that they do not want to be lawyers. There are plenty of other paths to follow in our profession that will bring great satisfaction, and we need to start viewing those alternative paths as something besides fallback positions. The only real question for each of us is not, "Are those alternatives worthy pursuits?" but, rather, "Will those alternatives bring me the satisfaction and happiness that I am seeking?"

It is true that we are now in control and that we hear the message, but often we are not believing the words. However, we can change that.

So, with this as the background, I hope that you recognize the need for a serious discussion about transitions. If law firm practice is not meeting your needs, what are your options? There must be alternatives to declaring defeat, throwing up your hands and abandoning the profession that you studied hard for and invested in heavily. The ability to transition from a law firm to another practice setting—or to transition from another practice setting to a law firm—is becoming more and more important as time marches forward, and particularly in these dire economic times.

Today, women need to have jobs more than at most times in history. According to the United States Census, the divorce rate for the past decade has remained around 50% (46% for 2012, Divorce Fact Sheet 2012, http://www.separation.ca/pdfs/divorcefacts.pdf). Women cannot count indefinitely on a spouse's income any more. The cost of housing is high, and it typically takes two substantial incomes for a young couple to purchase a starter house to allow them to get into the equity market. Parents are living longer, their retirement accounts have shrunk, and they often need

146

financial help from their children to get them through retirement and elder care. Gone are the days when most women had the latitude to choose to stay home with the children without serious repercussions to their lifestyles and life choices.

This all sounds pretty grim. However, the good news is that at least one major obstacle has been removed and that men are no longer keeping women out of the profession of law. We have come a long way from the turn of the last century when women were not allowed in law schools and law practices. Young women lawyers today have the opportunity to have satisfying careers in the law and to make substantial salaries, which will allow them to contribute significantly to assuring the lifestyles that they desire for themselves and their families.

But, there also is bad news. The bad news is that today women are keeping themselves out of the legal profession because of their failures to anticipate the future needs in their personal lives and to have realistic expectations about their careers, failure to craft personal definitions of success, and failure to make good choices and good career plans. That result is bad for the individual attorneys, and it is bad for the profession. Women attorneys have unique talents and skills that are very valuable to the profession, and losing women at the current rate of over 40% is like robbing the profession of important natural resources.

However, women can control the outcome and do not have to leave the decisions about their professional futures to the whims of others with separate agendas. Women have the ability to craft satisfying and successful legal careers, and the key to reaching that goal is to accept responsibility early so that they are not overcome by unanticipated circumstances and do not make hasty departures from practice. A large part of that strategy has to do with making successful transitions if and when the need arises.

What follows is the most valuable information on transitions that I can provide to you. Its high value derives from the fact that it comes straight from those who have accomplished transitions successfully. You will hear from women of stature in the profession who are willing to share their stories with you to help you to make good decisions in your professional life.

Women helping women is the theme of this book, just as it was an important theme of Book One. Here are the mentors you need. Pay close attention to their stories and use their wisdom and insight to the best advantage in your career to help you make good choices about transitioning your practice. Then, assume your own responsibility as a mentor and Pay It Forward. Mentor another young woman lawyer in your future. It is critical to the survival of women in our profession, and it is the right thing to do.

The Starting Point

The U.S. Bureau of Labor Statistics Occupational Outlooks Handbook, 2010-11 Edition, gives us a starting point in defining "lawyers" and what they do as follows:

"Lawyers may specialize in a number of areas, such as bankruptcy, probate, international, elder, or environmental law. Those specializing in, for example, environmental law may represent interest groups, waste disposal companies, or construction firms in their dealings with the U.S. Environmental Protection Agency and other Federal and State agencies. These lawyers help clients prepare and file for licenses and applications for approval before certain activities are permitted to occur. Some lawyers specialize in the growing field of intellectual property, helping to protect clients' claims to copyrights, artwork under contract, product designs, and computer programs. Other lawyers advise insurance companies about the legality of insurance transactions, guiding the company in writing insurance policies to conform to the law and to protect the companies from unwarranted claims. When claims are filed against insurance companies, these attorneys review the claims and represent the companies in court.

Most lawyers are in private practice, concentrating on criminal or civil law. In criminal law, lawyers represent individuals who have been charged with crimes and argue their cases in courts of law. Attorneys dealing with civil law assist clients with litigation, wills, trusts, contracts, mortgages, titles, and leases. Other lawyers handle only public-interest cases—civil or criminal—concentrating on particular causes and choosing cases that might have an impact on the way law is applied. Lawyers sometimes are employed full time by a single client. If the client is a corporation, the lawyer is known as "house counsel" and usually advises the company concerning legal issues related to its business activities. These issues might involve patents, government regulations, contracts with other companies, property interests, or collective-bargaining agreements with unions.

A significant number of attorneys are employed at the various levels of government. Some work for State attorneys general, prosecutors, and public defenders in criminal courts. At the Federal level, attorneys investigate cases for the U.S. Department of Justice and other agencies. Government lawyers also help develop programs, draft and interpret laws and legislation, establish enforcement procedures, and argue civil and criminal cases on behalf of the government.

Other lawyers work for legal aid societies—private, nonprofit organizations established to serve disadvantaged people. These lawyers generally handle civil, rather than criminal, cases."

With this as a starting point, we now can examine transitions from one practice setting to another.

Typical Transitions

The Law Firm Practice Model

Law firm practice will be our base for this discussion, so let's start by defining it. Most of you are familiar with lawyers who practice as a group and under one firm name, like ABC Law. All of the lawyers at ABC Law work on the business of the firm, and all of the profits from the business are used to pay wages and expenses first and then are distributed to partners or shareholders as salaries after that.

Within the law firm, there are likely to be various practice groups (litigation, corporate, commercial transactions, estates and trusts, real estate and land use, etc.), and there is usually a head of each practice group. There are committees in the firm to address issues like recruitment, collections, business development, etc., and generally there is one all-important management committee that is responsible for things like partnership recommendations, partnership decisions, and compensation. The members of the firm typically fall into categories like associates, of counsel, partners, contract lawyers and a few blends that have popped up as a result of the recent economic downturn and the challenges to law firm budgets. At the helm of all of this there is usually a managing partner, who steers the firm and tries to keep an eye on both the day-to-day matters of the firm and long-range strategy.

That pretty well describes mid- to large-sized law firms. In addition, there are small law firms, and those are much less complicated. Just scale down the numbers and the committee structure above, and you have some idea of what a small law firm is and how it operates.

Opportunities for part-time practice and flexible practice are available in law firms, but they are not as common as in some of the alternative practice settings. There are many reasons and justifications for that, but suffice to say that making a profit in a service industry lies at the heart of most of those reasons and justifications. However, part-time work and flexible schedules are becoming more commonplace at law firms, and here is some general information that will help you in determining whether law firm practice will meet your needs.

Part-time or flexible hours are different models for addressing the needs of employees who, for personal reasons, do not desire to work full time. Part-time practice generally involves fewer hours of work per week, whereas flexible time generally involves reduced hours and/or is a rearrangement of the daily schedule of hours spent in the office. These alternative work models may be attractive for women lawyers because they can provide more time for home and family, and, according to statistics, 73% of attorneys who work part-time are women (2009 Study by the NALP. http://www.nalp.org/parttimesched2009).

Although law firms have not embraced the part-time and flexible schedule models to the degree that many commenters think advisable, firm managers are beginning to recognize that making accommodations in terms of alternative work schedules makes very good business sense. For starters, the merger and acquisition activity of the new millennium has produced larger firms that have an increased ability to be more flexible in terms of work models and continue to meet financial obligations. In addition, an increasing number of firms understand the advantage of having a growing number of talented women lawyers to meet the increasing diversity requirements of clients. It has become typical for corporate clients, where diversity is much greater than in law firms, to require firms to respond to Requests for Proposals (RFPs) as part of the process for competition for legal services, and most RFPs require detailed information on firm diversity and diversity within the particular legal teams that will work on client matters.

The issue of law firm succession also presents another motivation for law firms to pay closer attention to retention issues. As mentioned earlier, succession plans are a big topic of discussion at law firms across the country these days. Law firm managers are concerned about who will take the law firms into the future after the Baby Boomers have retired. The answer of course is Generation X and Generation Y, and the retention of talent, including female talent, will play heavily into those succession plans. Firms that approach this subject in a prudent manner will recognize that providing flexibility for the years when women struggle with work-life issues the most will help to assure that those women will remain with the firm and lend significantly to the talent retention that will play heavily into successful succession plans.

Although flexibility seems to be more attainable these days, you cannot take it for granted. It is always important to ask for flexibility in the right manner, as I pointed out at some length in Chapter 3 of Book One. Approaching it as an entitlement is not the right approach. The better approach is to go to management with a detailed plan that includes what you need, how long you will need it, how it will benefit both you AND the firm, and what your plan will be for returning to work full-time, including details of timing and transition. Try to craft a plan that will be realistic and also will give you the kind of salary satisfaction that will not lead to resentment, and make sure that the work that you are assigned as a part-time lawyer will be of the quality and interest to keep you happy during this difficult transition. It must be a win-win for you and for the firm to be successful.

If the request for alternative work arrangements is made correctly and earnestly—and with an intention to make it work for both you and the firm—management's response should be either "yes" or "goodbye." If the female attorney is worth keeping, the answer should be "yes" because a negative response eventually will drive the attorney out of the firm. If, on the other hand, the attorney is not highly valued, the answer should be to say goodbye and let her leave for a place where she can be more successful. As a business decision, the firm should calculate the costs of attrition in this analysis and try to avoid these costs wherever possible if the attorney is highly valued. If it is handled correctly, the job satisfaction among part-time attorneys can be high, and the talent is retained.

Because there are pitfalls to part-time practice (less prestigious work, longer hours than anticipated or promised, departure from partnership track, in most cases), women need to be prepared to demonstrate their commitment to the profession while working part-time. It will help those women to remember that they are not part-time lawyers. They are lawyers who happen to work part time. They need to make it clear that they are committed to their clients 100%; they just happen to have fewer clients for the time being.

Here are some resources to consult on part-time and flexible-time practices:

Solving the Part-Time Puzzle: The Law Firm's Guide to Balanced Hour Programs (Project for Attorney Retention, 2004);

Balanced Hours: Effective Part-Time Programs for Washington Law Firms (Project for Attorney Retention, 2001); and

Balancing Work and Personal Life—Developing Flexible Work Options for Lawyers (www.wisbarlorg/.AM/Template).

To fully understand the law firm model and how issues like flexible work schedules and alternative work arrangements are viewed, you must understand "overhead." Overhead will play into any salary and work arrangement negotiation that you have, whether it is for full-time or part-time work. Here is a mini-tutorial on overhead that your law firm likely will never give you and that will put you light years ahead of the pack when you need to know it.

As a rule of thumb, firms use a 1/3, 1/3, 1/3 formula in determining salary. One third of the total potential revenue earned through your work as a lawyer goes to you as salary, one third goes to the law firm to pay for expenses that can be broken down as direct and indirect expenses, and the last third goes to the firm as profit to be distributed to the partners. Although the percentages may vary sightly from firm to firm, it is a good general rule of thumb to know in developing strategy.

Here is an example. Mary is hired by ABC Firm and is paid a salary of $100,000. She shares a secretary with two other lawyers and has full health care, 401(k), and vacation benefits. It is projected that she will bill 1750 hours a year, working full time. Using the formula above, in order to collect $300,000, which is three times her salary, Mary will have to bill at a rate of at least $172 per hour for 1750 hours a year and collect $300,000 ($172 per hour × 1750 hours) to "break even" financially. If the market will not support a billing rate of $172 or more for an associate of Mary's experience, either the minimum billable hour requirement would have to increase or the salary would have to decrease for the formula to work. It is all about simple arithmetic, and the law firm managers are experts at this formula. In addition, all of Mary's billables would have to be collected in the first year of Mary's employment to make the formula work. This usually does not happen because there is at least a two month to three month delay between the time that bills are sent out and the time when the money is collected, and, therefore, the formula simply does not work for first-year associates. However, law firms typically do not want to increase billable rates or decrease salaries in ways that would affect the firm's competitiveness in the recruitment and hiring market, and, for that reason, law firms know that they most likely will be losing money on first-year associates. They understand that the formula is valid and works for the more experienced lawyers in the firm, and the law firms are willing to write off the losses for first-year associates as investments in the future of the firm.

So that is generally the way the formula works. However, once you advance in seniority in the firm to the point where you are able to carry the burden of your salary and the direct and indirect expenses through your billings, the billings/salary model will break down again when you introduce the concept of part-time work. Quite simply, when you reduce your hours and therefore the revenue from hours billed, you reduce your ability to carry your share of the overhead, both direct and indirect, and the burden to cover those expenses is then shifted to other lawyers in the firm.

When you are negotiating for part-time work, the issue of overhead becomes especially important. As a part-time lawyer, the revenue from your time spent billing clients for work will be reduced. You may not think that is a significant problem if you can demonstrate that the revenue from your work is enough to cover your own salary and direct expenses like the wages paid to your secretary and the other expenses that you consider directly connected to your practice. However, that most likely will not account for the indirect overhead like lease costs for your office space, accounting costs, IT costs, salaries of management staff, utility costs, equipment rental costs, country club memberships, key man insurance policies, and many other hidden costs that keep the law firm operating every day.

So, does that mean that part-time work and other alternative work models cannot work? No, it does not. What it means is that you have to understand the impact of what you are asking for and prepare to advocate for your worth to the firm in spite of it. If you take the approach that, even as a part-time lawyer, you are still a productive lawyer, that may not be persuasive. You most likely cannot make that argument work because of the hidden costs of indirect overhead that you are responsible for. So, you will need another approach.

An alternative approach is to recognize the burden that management has in making the numbers work and emphasize the value that you bring to the firm. Value such as client relationships, unique practice skills that are important to the firm and represent an investment, and trustworthiness and reliability that work to the advantage of the firm. This is what I referred to earlier as "creating value" in your early years of practice to give you leverage in negotiating work arrangements to meet your needs in the future.

So, remember the important concept of overhead in any discussions with management. Most young associates do not understand it, and you will have an advantage if you do. Overhead, direct and indirect, represents a huge number in any business, and it has to be covered one way or another.

Now that we have a general definition of a law firm practice and have developed a baseline, let's look at the alternatives. Let's see what these other job descriptions entail and if any of them might appeal to you and better fit your circumstances.

The alternatives to law firm practice are replete, but we will look at the most popular and most widely utilized alternatives first. Those practice alternatives are:

- In-house lawyer at a corporation or other business;
- Government Lawyer;
- Public Interest/Non-Profit Lawyer;
- Solo Practitioner;
- Academic;
- Judge;
- Alternative Dispute Resolution (ADR) Practitioner; and
- Law Firm Consultant.

Other interesting alternatives, which are becoming popular today, are non-traditional practices like women-owned law firms and virtual law firms. Those practices often are the results of special interests and the need for flexibility that other more traditional practices cannot provide.

Examining these practice types and having the information that you will need about alternatives to law firm practice at your fingertips is important to your future. Become familiar with the information early so that you have the confidence of knowing that there *are* alternatives and which ones might fit you best.

Although the model set out here is the progression from law firm practice to alternative practices, it also is possible to move from the alternative practices to a law firm, but it is a less likely scenario. It also is possible to move among the alternatives, for example, from the government to the judiciary, from the judiciary to private practice and other similar progressions.

The transition from government lawyer to private practice in a law firm is not uncommon. This is a transition that law firms can both embrace and view skeptically, depending upon the circumstances. The experience gained by a government lawyer, particularly those in general counsel's offices, in the offices of elected officials, and in prosecutorial positions, can be very valuable to law firms. Those lawyers come with significant practice skills, first-line trial experience, and contacts that often cannot be duplicated in private practice without many more years of experience. They also come with in-depth knowledge of government tactics and strategy that can be invaluable to law firms, which are adverse to the government in their practices.

However, those lawyers also come without clients, and law firms are businesses with bottom lines that depend on new business generation—as I hope you learned from Book One. So, it is often a mixed bag, and knowing how particular law firm managers think about this kind of transition and how difficult the transition can be are critically important to your decision to pursue this kind of transition.

It also is possible to move from being a government lawyer to being a judge. By midcareer, many government lawyers have amassed the kind of prosecutorial and litigation experience that makes them very attractive as jurists. You may have watched television coverage of past Senate confirmation hearings for federal court and United States Supreme Court nominees, and you understand the depth of questioning. The process is different for elected judges, but there are very similar issues to the transition itself.

And then there is the very interesting transition from the judiciary to private practice in a law firm. This transition can result from an unsuccessful election run for those judges who are subject to voter approval, but it can also be a voluntary move, as demonstrated by the profile of Marianne Short below. Her story, although unusual, is inspiring.

The careers in transition and the profiles of women practitioners are included below. In asking the women who are profiled about their experiences at these alternative practices, I specifically requested that the contributors respond to questions similar to those addressed at the beginning of this chapter and that they contrast their various practice experiences.

They came through with flying colors, and I want to take this opportunity to thank these women from the bottom of my heart. Reading their responses and personal statements made me understand how much thought and care they had put into those materials to give you as much good information and guidance as possible. I also thank them for telling me their very personal stories. I was moved by much of what they shared, and I consider it a real privilege to have the opportunity to take their materials and craft them into the narratives I present here. In doing that, I hope that I have captured their passions, their hopes, their dreams and their disappointments accurately. They are outstanding mentors, and their stories are remarkable. I hope you enjoy these profiles as much as I enjoyed writing them for you.

From Law Firm to In-House Corporate Practice

The American Bar Association Lawyer Demographics reports that the number of licensed lawyers in the United States in 2010 was 1,225, 452. (ABA Market Research Department, 2011) The ABA and the ABA Foundation statistics do not distinguish between 'practicing' and 'non-practicing' lawyers, and, unfortunately, another source has indicated that there is no accurate way to assess this information. (World Direct Law, http://www.worldlawdirect.com/forum/attorneys-legal-ethics/26278-how-many-lawyers-licensed-practice-law-united-states.html)

The ABA document lists the percentage of licensed lawyers practicing in "Private Industry" in the United States as 8% in 2000, and the *Princeton Review* reported that more than 10% of lawyers in America in 2006 were "corporate" lawyers. (Bernstein, Alan, "Corporate Lawyer: Guide to Your Career," *Princeton Review*, 2006) As a result, we can assume that there were somewhere between 98,000 and 122,000 lawyers in private industry/corporate practices in the U.S. in 2006. (More recent figures breaking down the areas of practice are not available. The ABA reports these figures only periodically and reported its last figures in 2004 for the year 2000.)

These corporate lawyers are employed as in-house counsel by public utilities, banks, insurance companies, real estate agencies, manufacturing firms and other businesses (U.S. Department of Labor Bureau of Labor Statistics Occupational Outlook Handbook 2010-2011 Edition, www.bls.gov/ocol/ocos053.htm#emply). A recent survey by the Association of Corporate Counsel (ACC) shows that 39% of these corporate lawyers are women. (http://www.acc.com/vl/public/Surveys/loader.cfm?csModule=security/getfile&pageid=16297 page 76)

Although some of these lawyers joined in-house corporate practices directly upon graduating from law school, the more typical scenario is for lawyers to join corporations from other practice settings. Often those lawyers were members of law firm teams that represented the corporations, and it was advantageous for the corporations to have them "in house" for a variety of reasons.

Going "in house" traditionally has been a very popular alternative to law firm practice. The culture of a corporation or another similar business entity is different from the culture of a law firm, and that is attractive to some lawyers. Corporations tend to be much less traditional and formal than law firms, and there is less emphasis on competition and more emphasis on teamwork in the corporate setting. Often, there are also increased opportunities for flexible work schedules that attract many women to these positions. Although the competition may be reduced in corporate settings, there are other "political" considerations within the corporate culture that may be more challenging.

Lawyers in a corporation have to function as more than just lawyers who understand the law and can apply the facts. In-house corporate lawyers must understand the company's business, including the underlying product or delivery of services, and they must become business partners with management to help advance the company in the marketplace.

At the same time, the business side of companies can see in-house counsel as an impediment to what the business side wants to do, and the necessity for "going to legal" (meaning taking the issue to counsel's office for a legal review of business decisions), can be seen as a negative. Although corporate management understands that the lawyers provide a support service, the leadership also wants to feel that the company's goals are also the lawyer's goals. As a result, the in-house lawyers do not want to find themselves in the position of saying "no" to management all of the time. Instead, the lawyers want to be perceived as helping management achieve their business objectives, and any contrary ideas from the lawyers must be expressed respectfully and cautiously.

These concepts were discussed and debated at a District of Columbia Women's Bar Association Initiative on Advancement and Retention of Women event at Hogan Lovells on January 19, 2011 in a program entitled "Navigating the Corporate Matrix—Advancing Women in Corporate Law Departments." It was a very candid discussion, which included the following panel members: Claudette Christian, Co-Chair, Hogan Lovells US LLP; Maureen Del Duca, Deputy General Counsel-Litigation, AOL LLC; Robin Sangston, General Counsel, Cox Communications; and Laura Thomas, Chief Financial Officer, XO Communications.

The panel featured discussions of the relationship between in-house counsel and their in-house clients, and between in-house counsel and outside counsel. Specifically, the panel focused on issues impacting the advancement of women, especially how women outside counsel can help advance women in-house counsel and vice versa.

Here is some excellent advice from these seasoned in-house lawyers for those of you considering a transition to in-house.

Get in there and roll up your sleeves and learn the business metrics for your company. Management must see that you are trying to learn the business side. It is as if you have two jobs—one legal and one business. Attorneys are lifelong learners, and you must demonstrate your curiosity and desire to conquer new territories. In this process, you will need to transition from being a lawyer to being a leader.

Continue to "connect back" with others in your business, including others with your same job in other companies. It is a good reality check and familiarizes you with the benchmarks that are important to your success. Have lunch with these people and be helpful to them in ways that are meaningful and establish the relationship of trust that you need to learn and progress in your business. Attend conferences—especially those away from home where there are no work-life issues to distract you. Women, especially, need this kind of networking time. That's where the people that you need to meet with will be, and you need to be there, too. However, there are budget constraints for those kinds of events, so you will have to choose wisely among the opportunities and make a good case for why your attendance will benefit your company. To do that, you will have to carefully research the conference and the attendees.

Networking is key to your success in most businesses, and there are many different kinds of networking opportunities for in-house counsel. Charitable events can provide good networking opportunities to promote your company, and other networking opportunities can be as casual as weekend time in the office. This kind of good casual interaction can build an *esprit de corps* with fellow workers, break down barriers and lead to work opportunities. Social networking, like *Facebook* and *LinkedIn,* also can be effective, but the conference participants cautioned that *Facebook* should only be used for personal networking and that *LinkedIn* is the appropriate choice for professional networking.

It will not surprise you to hear that there are some additional challenges for female in-house counsel. Many women report little contact with male business leaders, both inside and outside the company, and this is perceived as a real problem. The recommendation of the panel was to actively seek out male mentors to try to bridge this gap. Men with children—especially daughters—can be very helpful as mentors because they seem to "get" some of the gender issues more than others.

Sometimes it is necessary to network to find mentors that are not readily available. You may have to cross functional lines within a corporation and volunteer for special projects to have contact with a desirable mentor. Often there are many opportunities outside your area of expertise, and you should pursue them. You also should look for mentoring outside your organization. According to the panelists, sometimes everyone on the inside has "drunk the Kool-Aid," and you may need an outside perspective.

To be effective, networking should be strategic. You should not forget to network among your peers because they are likely to be in the business longer than your bosses. Remember that even those below you in the corporate hierarchy may be very talented and could end up being your bosses in the future. Knowing that there may come a day when your boss is younger than you are should be incentive for you to be pleasant and supportive in your interactions with these colleagues. Also remember that there are four generations in the workplace now. They communicate differently and have different priorities, and you must be sensitive to that. Show your value and learn to communicate at all levels without wasting the time of the business leaders—they will recognize that value and start reaching out to you and provide the mentoring that you need.

These are some of the things that you will have to remember to be a successful in-house counsel. Making the additional move from pure legal counsel to a supervisory role on the management side can be difficult, and it helps to avoid legalease that non-lawyers find annoying. Having confidence and demonstrating business savvy is important, and you need to remember that you are not expected to know all of the answers, but you do need to know how to find the answers.

Most of these skills are universal. The skills that you develop at one business can be valuable in another business. You do not have to come to a company knowing everything that is unique to that business and its operations, but having the universal skill set will put you on the road to success.

Getting the "top legal job" in a corporation creates even more challenges. If you have your eye on becoming General Counsel, your opinion must be valued at a lot of different levels. You need to be cross cultural to gain the confidence of both the legal and the business types throughout the company. You must engage, manage and stay cool in a crisis, and you need to be able to absorb, deal with and promote the corporate culture.

Understanding the corporate culture is key to the way business gets done. As an in-house attorney, you need to be true to yourself and have a high degree of ethics. As a result, you will not always have good news for management, but understanding the corporate culture will make it easier to deliver the message and have it taken seriously. Having an ally in outside counsel can be a great assistance in this.

As in-house counsel, knowing what you want from outside counsel is very critical. Some in-house counsel want outside lawyers to help assess risk and reorganize the business model, if necessary, in a way that reduces risk and makes good business sense. This can be an interesting process for both sides: The in-house counsel get the benefit of the opinions of outside counsel, and outside counsel can become involved on both the legal side and the business side of these issues.

To conduct this kind of risk assessment, outside counsel must be familiar with the risk tolerance of the client company. Outside counsel must understand, that there may be other things on the horizon for the client that make it wise to take a pass at risk for the moment and look forward to the next opportunity when circumstances are different. In-house counsel needs to share these perspectives with outside counsel to increase effective legal representation.

To be effective at this, both in-house and outside counsel must read the trade press religiously to know what competitors are doing and what is going on in the industry as a whole. This will give outside counsel the opportunity to be proactive and to educate clients and in-house counsel about business models gone wrong. Being familiar with the formal complaints that have been filed by government agencies against companies and the resulting enforcement actions will give both in-house lawyers and outside counsel opportunities to get the attention of management on issues related to these actions. The message is "We are not making this up. It is for real."

In-house counsel also should call on outside counsel to help educate junior in-house lawyers and make up for skill deficits. For instance, in-house lawyers may be strong on the law but weak on communication. Outside counsel should see this as an opportunity and should offer assistance. This will make the junior lawyers look good to the General Counsel and to management. Praise for these junior lawyers is very important, and taking an interest in these junior members of counsel staff will benefit all parties. Building a loyal staff of junior lawyers at the client is a good investment in your future as outside counsel. Those junior lawyers will be senior lawyers before you know it. Caring for the client is an investment in the future.

Of course, it should go without saying that in-house lawyers expect outside counsel to have the expertise that is needed to address the legal issues, but they also expect you to know the judge, know the court rules and know the "lay of the land" for the type of dispute the company is facing. They expect you to appear self-confident and to ask the right questions.

As strange as it may sound, in-house lawyers also expect outside counsel to ask for business. This was emphasized at the Women Legal-Ark 2011 Conference in New York City. The speakers and panelists were very insistent that women are more reluctant to ask for work than men, and they encouraged the attendees to get over that reluctance and to treat any rejection as a pure business decision and not as a personal rebuff. They also discussed the ways that lawyers can continue to correspond with potential clients, like offering CLE programs at the corporate offices, sharing critical new legal development information about the client industry, among others.

In-house counsel appreciates these efforts and understands the desire to get their work. They know that these efforts are still part of the "pitch" for their work, and they are accustomed to sales personalities because they are surrounded by a lot of them on the management side. As a result, they understand "the sell" and associate it with the kind of assertive and competent counsel they would want to retain when the time and circumstances are right.

It is all about relationships, relationships, relationships and building those relationships.

For those lawyers already retained by corporations, in-house lawyers expect outside counsel to stay present and provide valuable information even when it has not been requested. In-house counsel welcome these casual visits from outside counsel as long as the time is not billed. And, the participants in both the conferences emphasized that in situations when you are "on the clock," you must make that clear and not indulge in small talk and later charge the client for that time.

163

For more information on women general counsel, I recommend a new book, *Courageous Counsel: Conversations with Women General Counsel in the Fortune 500*, by Michele Coleman Mayes and Kara Sophia Baysinger. This book celebrates the achievements of successful women GCs and also serves as a mentoring tool for lawyers in law firms seeking to understand the challenges experienced by in-house counsel clients, for mid-career lawyers mapping paths to GC's offices and for young lawyers looking at career options.

For more on women corporate lawyers, both in-house and in law firms, see the ABA online article "Panel of Wisdom: Women Corporate Lawyers Share Strategy and Insight for Success," February 14, 2012, http://www.abanow.org/2012/02/panel-of-wisdomwomen-corpo.

As you can see, there are many interesting aspects of practicing in-house. Let's hear from a woman who has transitioned from private practice to in-house and done it very successfully.

Sally Blackmun, until recently, Senior Associate General Counsel at Darden Restaurants, Inc. (the largest casual dining restaurant owner and operator in the country) is one of those in-house lawyers. As the daughter of Supreme Court Justice Harry Blackmun, Sally Blackmun comes to the law very honestly. However, she plotted her own course. Here is her story.

Profile of Sally Blackmun

When Sally Blackmun was growing up and coming of age, she heard a lot about the law and learned a lot about being a lawyer. That was to be expected as the daughter of a lawyer, Federal Court of Appeals judge and, later, Supreme Court Justice. Sally had a unique opportunity to view the law from a perspective that most young people do not have. She spent considerable time at the Supreme Court over the years and heard many oral arguments and decisions announced. She also had the unique experience of meeting and interacting with other Justices and Court staff.

Sally attended Skidmore College and graduated Phi Beta Kappa from Wilson College and from Emory Law School where she was a member of the Emory Law Review. Her first job out of law school was a clerkship on the Georgia Supreme Court, followed by a career as a commercial litigator with a construction law firm in Atlanta. She was very successful as a trial lawyer, and her litigation career was highlighted by a $1.2 million jury verdict in the U.S. District Court in Portland, Oregon. Although she found private practice both interesting and challenging, she also found the stress of putting in the required time and hours at the firm and spending many days each year on the road, while trying to raise two daughters and maintain a healthy marriage, to be very demanding. She contemplated a career change as she rose through the ranks to partner, and then circumstances intervened which gave her an opportunity to reassess her career and decide the next best steps for her and for her family.

When Sally's husband had an opportunity for a new job, which would require relocation of the family, Sally resigned her partnership after ten years with her law firm and took some time to re-examine the direction of her legal career and the tradeoffs that would be necessary in raising her daughters, then 3 and 5 years old. She concluded that she needed a better work-life balance, and she knew that meant a different type of practice. However, she also knew that she wanted a meaningful and rewarding legal career.

Sally was thoughtful about her future and took her time in choosing her next career move. She took a year off to get settled in a new city, spend quality time with her children and study for and take the Florida Bar. When she was ready to re-enter practice, Sally was protective of her family situation and she did not jump back into a full-time schedule. Although she interviewed with several law firms, her objective was to try something different.

The opportunity with General Mills Restaurants, Inc., a wholly-owned subsidiary of General Mills, Inc., a Fortune 500 company based in

Minneapolis, came along at exactly the right time. Sally returned to work as a part-time in-house lawyer for General Mills, and, after a year, she joined the company as a full-time attorney in 1989. Six years later, Darden Restaurants was spun off as an independent Fortune 500 company in 1995, and Sally became a part of the new company as counsel to Darden. Sally's husband was supportive of her career decisions, which was very important to her, and her new practice was a better fit with her responsibilities on the home front.

Sally ended her career as Senior Associate General Counsel at Darden. She retired from Darden in June 2011, after nearly 24 years. During most of her career with Darden, she oversaw and managed commercial disputes and litigation for Darden's restaurant support center and its more than 1850 company-owned and operated restaurants, including Red Lobster, Olive Garden, Bahama Breeze, Seasons 52, LongHorn Steakhouse and Capital Grille. As the largest casual dining restaurant company in the country, Darden was an exciting place to be, and Sally thrived.

The things that appealed most to Sally about an in-house counsel position were being a part of a well-respected corporation, excellent corporate benefits, use of her litigation background and expertise without personally handling the litigation, more regular hours, and control of her travel schedule. There were, however, challenges to this new practice.

Learning the corporate culture was one of the greatest challenges. The inter-workings of a huge public company can be daunting, and Sally spent a great deal of time learning and understanding the corporate structure and key players in the business. Developing an open line of communication with the General Counsel was also critical, and it took time and finesse. Sally needed to have this open line in order to alert the General Counsel about potential newsworthy events related to litigation matters she was managing, and she worked hard to develop a direct and continuous dialogue with her superiors.

She found a great teacher and mentor in the first General Counsel she served. With the help of her mentor, she developed the skills that made her successful as an in-house attorney: Excellent communication, organization, legal expertise, and carefully developed working relationships with internal business clients, insurance adjusters, and outside attorneys handling the company's litigation matters. She must have been a good student because she went on to serve three other General Counsels in the 24 years that she worked for the corporation.

Sally Blackmun's best advice to young women lawyers who are interested in in-house positions is to start at a law firm or public sector position and develop an expertise that is valuable in the corporate setting. She points out that many corporations do not typically hire inexperienced attorneys, and she recommends at least five years of practice experience in another legal setting before attempting the transition to in-house. She believes that the most valuable practice experiences as preparation for in-house counsel positions are in employment, litigation, corporate/SEC, benefits, contracts, real estate, and international trade and related matters.

As you might imagine, Sally Blackmun has no career regrets. She says that she had "a good ride." There were challenges and bumps along the way, but she stuck to her dream of having an interesting and challenging career. Her career decisions worked *for her*. She listened to her heart and also to her young children. In her own words:

"I found it very difficult to balance a national litigation practice out of Atlanta and raise children at the same time. I knew that I had to make a change after spending most of six months away from my 3- and 5-year-old daughters while I was preparing for and trying a case in Federal Court in Portland, Oregon. When I returned from that trial, I asked my younger daughter if she remembered who her Mommy was. She pointed to her Daddy (he loved it, and I cringed). The second zinger came when my husband left for his new job in Florida, and, on the first night he was gone, my older daughter asked me whether I knew how to babysit!"

From the mouths of babes . . . sometimes we need to listen to more than just our hearts.

Sally Blackmun is a frequent speaker regarding her father Justice Harry Blackmun's legacy to women through his Roe v. Wade decision. For more information on Ms. Blackmun, see her introduction to *The War on Choice: The Right-Wing Attack on Women's Rights and How to Fight Back* by Gloria Feldt (Bantam 2004).

For another view of the transition from private practice to in-house counsel at a much earlier point in a law career and in a much smaller corporate setting, meet Amy Yeung, Assistant General Counsel of ZeniMax Media Inc. Amy spent two years in private practice at one of the largest law firms in the country before transitioning to a small corporate legal environment in a cutting edge industry, and her experience is very different from Sally Blackmun's. Amy brings the perspective of a young woman lawyer on the rise. Like her company, she is assertive and innovative. Let's hear her story.

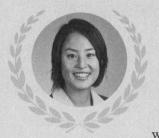

Profile of Amy Yeung

Amy Yeung is a high achiever. She graduated from the University of Chicago with honors and from Duke University School of Law, where she was Managing Editor of the *Journal of Comparative and International Law* and Student Body President of the Duke Bar Association. She also served as the Editor of the *Harvard Journal of Law and Policy* while at Duke Law, was the Chair of the Duke Law Young Alumni Association, and became a moot court quarterfinalist in the Dean's Cup competition. And, she had summer associate clerkships with two prestigious law firms. I think that you are beginning to get the picture. Excellence is something that Amy Yeung expects of herself and of others.

After law school graduation, Amy got a highly-coveted clerkship with the Delaware Court of Chancery, and, after that, she took a job in Big Law with WilmerHale for "the experience," although she acknowledges that she "was never really sure what that meant." She heard it from mentors and senior attorneys, who emphasized "proper credentialing," which involved joining the best law firm possible, learning to multitask successfully, demonstrating the commitment and dedication that defines a successful career, and becoming comfortable working under extreme pressure.

It sounded good to Amy at the time, and Amy understood that bypassing the Big Law experience might lead to the incorrect conclusion by prospective employers that she either was not qualified for that practice setting or that she had some sort of "fit issue" that precluded her from obtaining a Big Law offer. Amy is very analytical, so she was looking at it from all angles. She also was told that large law firms have sophisticated practices that center on the cutting edge of law and business, and she was intrigued with being in an environment where she could contribute to "pushing the boundaries of law and policy." She also liked the idea that a large law firm would provide exposure to a broader framework of skills, teamwork and analysis that would be consistent with her future career goals. She wanted to learn how to interact with lawyers at different levels of practice, what to expect from other lawyers, how to appropriately respond in different meeting settings, and how to "be both proactive and reactive at the right times."

Most of all, Amy wanted to be an attorney with close ties to business—being part of the overall business strategy of a client or entity—and she knew that could be from the law side or from the business side. She knew that she wanted to participate in initiating, driving and pushing forward on business decisions and negotiating and developing long-term strategies and that she might be able to achieve those goals better from within a company than as outside counsel. But, she was not sure where those goals would lead her, and she forged ahead at the law firm, learning as much as possible and preparing herself for whatever the future held.

That is when fate intervened for Amy Yeung. We know that our past experiences help shape our futures, and that was more than true for Amy. All of her life she enjoyed a passionate interest in video games. She and her siblings spent hours as children playing video games, and she understood the great market potential for the product. So, after two years with

WilmerHale, when Amy learned of a job opening as in-house counsel for a company on the cutting edge of that industry, she knew that it was time to activate her long-range career plan. She worked hard to research and compete for that position, and, as anyone who knows her would have predicted, she was successful.

Amy is grateful for the help that she received from law firm colleagues in making the transition to in-house. They recognized her unique professional needs, and they served as excellent sounding boards. She emphasizes the importance of maintaining positive professional relationships with colleagues and co-workers from various career settings, and she works hard at it. Her involvement in young lawyers associations and other professional groups, like her experiences as the Immediate Past Chair of the Bar Association of the District of Columbia Young Lawyers Division and her active memberships and leadership in the ABA and the Asian Pacific American Bar Association of DC, enhance her mentoring opportunities. Amy appreciates the help that came her way, and she knows the meaning of "pay it forward" and practices it regularly.

At Zenimax Media Inc., Amy serves as entertainment law counsel and handles a variety of intellectual property, regulatory and corporate projects. As one of only four in-house attorneys at her company, she has the opportunity to work on a wide variety of legal and business issues. Amy was willing to take considerable risk in leaving Big Law, and it has paid off for her. She found a very collaborative environment and one where she gets to wear many different hats in a day's time. Her experience is different from the traditional in-house position, where there are hundreds of attorneys and many individuals working on the same general business operations. Because of the smaller setting, Amy also has an opportunity to use her proactive problem-solving skills earlier in her career than she would have been able to in a law firm. In a small in-house counsel setting, even junior attorneys have significant contact with management and other corporate players and need to hone strong communication skills with a variety of professionals to develop comfortable dialogue and build long-term rapport.

Amy is very realistic about the challenges of her new setting. The legal resources are sometimes limited, and there is little opportunity for the training that exists in larger corporate settings and in law firms. Although her company definitely recognizes the value of the legal group, she understands that there is continuing competition for dollars between the legal services group and the dollars spent on business development group. In approaching this new setting, Amy has had to become comfortable with addressing issues that are not always familiar to her or at her level of expertise. When an issue is not important enough to warrant the cost of bringing in outside counsel, the pressure to come up with the right solution on short notice can be especially challenging. That is when Amy has to remember that it is rare to have a perfect answer or a perfect response in her new setting. She readily acknowledges that becoming comfortable with incomplete facts or a lack of time to fully research the issues will always be a challenge for her.

One of the skills that Amy identifies as most valuable to achieving success as an in-house lawyer is being able to identify what you don't know about the business and where to go to get the answers. Understanding business risks also is a big part of the job, and Amy knows that you cannot assess risks unless you thoroughly understand the facts. Other valuable skills include being able to work with a variety of personalities, being a team player, and always being professional. Amy also emphasizes the value of having a positive attitude, recognizing how much others have 'on their plates,' and being a part of the solution and not a part of the problem.

Amy now views law firms from the outside and as service providers. From that vantage point, she encourages law firms to recognize the value that women bring to positive client contact and good, efficient management. She regrets that women lawyers often are undervalued by law firms, in terms of opportunities and promotion, and she sees that as negative personal service that can adversely impact law firms in the marketplace.

Amy's best advice to young women lawyers is not to approach the in-house option as a 'knee jerk' reaction to dissatisfaction with the large law firm setting. The preferred lifestyle often associated with in-house—fewer hours, better hours, no billable hour requirement, the ability to raise children more comfortably, and a greater likelihood of job stability—are not specific to the corporate setting, and young lawyers should not overlook the opportunities that may exist in government service or in a smaller law firm or a smaller geographic setting to achieve the same goals.

For those genuinely interested in transitioning from private practice to an in-house position, Amy recommends thorough background research on the industry to determine whether "the fit is right." She also encourages women attorneys to aspire to jobs that they think they *can* do rather than always for the jobs they know they are qualified for. To do that, she points out that women must learn to think more like men and have confidence in their abilities.

Amy also has strong opinions about the job search involved in transitioning from one practice setting to another. She used the services of a headhunter, and she has valuable insight into that relationship. She says that working with a headhunter is delicate and that you should choose someone who understands your background and your desires and who also understands the business of the companies you are interested in. The greatest benefit from a headhunter is as an advocate for you, not as an aggregator of job opportunities (you can do that for yourself). Being really familiar with your skill set allows the headhunter to advocate for you in the most effective way possible. However, engaging a headhunter does not mean that your work is over—far from it. To be successful in your job search, you need to be introspective and identify what you really want and need in a new legal setting and research and evaluate the types of companies that that you think would meet your identified needs, both personal and corporate. This work will be very helpful to your headhunter and may help justify the significant cost of the services associated with your placement. As Amy puts it,

> "If you are reading this book, you probably are trying to be proactive in managing your career (hooray for that!). Challenge yourself to be an introspective and critical thinker *about you*."

So, that pretty much sums it up. Amy Yeung has used her skills as an introspective and critical thinker to find a professional setting that fits her like a glove. She loves her new practice, and recently she was named the Outstanding Young Lawyer of the Year by the Bar Association of the District of Columbia. Her star is definitely rising, and there is much more to hear from Amy Yeung.

Stay tuned.

For more information on Amy Yeung, please consult www.linkedin.com/profile/AmyYeung.

From Law Firm to Public Interest/Non-Profit Lawyer

This is another career path that has become particularly popular for women lawyers. There are so many societal issues that are being addressed through the non-profit and public interest practices, and those issues very often involve families and children and education and preservation of natural resources on global scales and are logical extensions of the passions of many women. However, there are multiple trade-offs in this decision, and you need to be aware of them all.

These public interest and not-for-profit practices can be very professionally rewarding and address issues in our society that present compelling needs for underrepresented constituencies. As more thoroughly discussed in Chapter 4 of Book One, public interest law addresses gaining justice for disadvantaged and underserved individuals or communities; promoting the interests of the public through the protections of the agencies of government; protecting and preserving the world's health and resources for the public good; and preserving, protecting, and defending human rights, civil rights and civil liberties.

Public interest law can be practiced in government agencies or in public interest organizations, which are typically not-for-profit entities, and in public interest law firms. Those firms are generally smaller in

173

scale and focus on individual plaintiffs or class actions and policy that impacts litigation.

Not-for-profit organizations include nongovernmental organizations (NGOs) and charities. The roles of lawyers in these settings include reviewing the laws of the jurisdiction where the organizations and charities solicit contributions and assuring compliance with laws and regulations throughout the organization. This practice also has a high concentration of regulatory oversight and constant monitoring of the rules and regulations and laws affecting the organization.

An excellent summary of public interest law is provided in Book One, and I repeat it here for your convenience.

> People commit to public interest work for many different reasons: it is part of their core identity, it gives greater meaning and significance to their lives in a way that capitalizes on their professional skills, they want to make a real difference in someone's life by reducing human suffering, righting a wrong, stopping an unfair practice, or ensuring that justice is not just for some but for all. In addition to any of these motivations, public interest law demands a higher level of creativity, hard work and devotion than any other professional undertaking, and can provide the greatest professional and personal satisfaction and rewards you will ever know. Add to this the privilege of working with social justice-motivated colleagues with whom you will share a treasured bond, and you have a winning combination of factors leading to a lifelong commitment to public interest law no matter where your legal career may take you. There is always a contribution you can make, a role you can play in the furtherance of justice.
>
> From the Seattle University School of Law website.

It has to be obvious from that description why lawyers, who are jaded from representing big corporations and being on the side of the wealthy and influential, often choose to transition to this practice. For more on practitioners who have found great success and satisfaction in this practice, see Section 1: Protecting Civil Liberties, Civil Rights, and the Environment in *Beyond the Big Firm—Profiles of Lawyers Who Want Something More* by Alan B. Morrison and Diane T. Chin (Wolters Kluwer Law & Business/Aspen Publishers, 2007) and *Lawyering from the Heart* by Deborah Kenn (Wolters Kluwer/Aspen Publishers, 2009), where the author/law professor presents interviews with twenty-two talented law school graduates who stayed true to their dreams of practicing law for the benefit of society and embarked on careers as public interest lawyers. These interviews include candid discussions of what can be a downside of making much less money than in private practice, and that discussion underscores the need to budget and exercise restraint, as discussed earlier.

Bonnie Brier, formerly of the Ballard Spahr law firm and currently Senior Vice President, General Counsel and Secretary of New York University, is an excellent example of a not-for-profit lawyer. Here is her story.

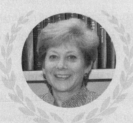

Profile of Bonnie Brier

Bonnie Brier considers herself to be extraordinarily lucky, both professionally and personally. She describes her life as "more wonderful than anything I could have imagined." She appreciates the role that women lawyers before her played in forging a path that made her career possible, and she recognizes with incredible gratitude that she "stands on their shoulders."

Ms. Brier had experiences growing up that marked her future and her legal ambitions. She grew up in Florida in absolute segregation— bathrooms and water fountains were marked "colored" and "white," people of color were not allowed in public accommodations, and there was pervasive discrimination for jobs and opportunities. In grades 7 through 9, every public school day began with a Christian prayer and the singing of *Dixie*. There were no people of color in the schools she attended until she was a senior in high school. That year two busloads of black students arrived at her public school of 3,700 students. She remembers thinking that the black students must have been "so scared."

Women who Bonnie Brier knew growing up also faced discrimination, and that had more of a direct effect on Bonnie. She came from a poor, single parent family, and she needed to work. Every day after high school and all day on Saturday and into her college years, she worked for minimum wage (or less, as her work as a children's counselor at a motel was exempt from the minimum wage laws). Minimum wage in those days was $1.25 an hour and increased to $1.60 an hour when Bonnie was in college. Although the best summer job for college students was as a substitute "mailman" for mail carriers taking vacation at that time of year, Bonnie could not get that job because the U.S. Post Office did not hire women.

Bonnie did well in school and went to college at Cornell on a near full scholarship. It was a whole new experience for her, and she remembers both the challenges and overcoming them. While she was at Cornell, she experienced some of the most "heady times" in the history of college education in this country. Male students were burning draft cards, and female students were protesting for women's liberation. All she knew about the law in those days came from television shows like *Perry Mason*, and she was interested. She had never known a lawyer, much less a woman lawyer, but she did not let that stand in her way. Bonnie knew that the world was changing for women, and she wanted to be a part of it.

She graduated from Cornell, *magna cum laude*, received a half scholarship and loans from Stanford Law, and off she went to California. At Stanford, Bonnie was a member of Order of the Coif and an editor of the *Law Review*. Stanford's only woman full-time faculty member at that time was Barbara Babcock, the former head of the Public Defender's Office in Washington, D.C., and the future Assistant Attorney General for the Civil Division in the U.S. Department of Justice. Barbara Babcock soon became a strong role model for Bonnie, and Bonnie set her sights on becoming a public defender.

Bonnie got excellent and diverse legal experience working during her law school years, including at California Rural Legal Assistance, the Miami Public Defender's Office one summer, an internship at the Center for Law and Social Policy in Washington, D.C. one semester, and a summer split between law firms in Miami and New York City. She recalls interviewing for a job with a Miami law firm and being told that the firm was very "anxious to hire a woman attorney" but that she should understand that she could not wear pants to work. The male senior partner explained that, although she might look "cute" in pants, that wardrobe choice "was not suited to all women" (all delivered in a deep Southern drawl, she recalls). Those were the times.

Bonnie met her husband in law school, and they both ended up with judicial clerkships in Philadelphia. Later, Bonnie switched sides and became a criminal prosecutor as an Assistant U.S. Attorney in the Eastern District of Pennsylvania. In the first 18 months, she handled six felony trials and began to wonder what she thought she liked about litigation. In a period of turmoil in the office due to a change in leadership, she left the U.S. Attorney's office and joined a Philadelphia law firm, where she specialized in tax matters. She wanted to be in an environment of excellence, and she wanted to be trained by outstanding lawyers.

She was not disappointed in her choice of law firms. She found lawyers at Ballard Spahr, who had been classically educated at the best boarding schools and universities and who were "elegant writers and thinkers." They would debate esoteric grammar rules and considered Strunk & White's *The Elements of Style* to be pleasure reading! She learned to be a good writer and a clear thinker in ways that the economies of practice in Big Law do not allow today.

That is when serendipity took over. At the law firm, Bonnie volunteered to work for a *pro bono* client, a sort of United Way for women's groups in the Philadelphia region. She learned the laws related to charities and became the firm expert in that area of law. She also developed a specific expertise in non-profit work related to hospitals and universities, and she honed her skills for eleven years at the firm, half as an associate and half as a partner (having two children as an associate and a third as a young partner along the way).

The non-profit practice was not much of a revenue-producing practice in the 1960's and 1970's, but it soon took off as hospitals restructured and entered into joint venture agreements for delivery of medical services, universities became involved in complex transactions, and charitable giving developed sophisticated nuances. Bonnie's expertise positioned her to become the first general counsel at Children's Hospital of Philadelphia and, after almost 20 years of practice, to become General Counsel at NYU.

At Children's Hospital of Philadelphia, Bonnie found herself a part of something especially meaningful. She valued knowing her hospital client from every perspective and turning that familiarity into better lawyering on behalf of the institution. She was devoted to the hospital that she served and respected the wonderful caregivers. The institution grew by four or five times while she was there, which kept her intellectually stimulated. She learned to love children born with deformities and disabilities and admired the incredible courage and fortitude they and their parents displayed in meeting those challenges. Her experiences made her appreciate each day in a profound way and to view the glass as half full. She describes this as "the substantial measure of peace" that is not characteristic of most legal practice.

But, there also were challenges for Bonnie in the new non-profit setting. An academic medical center presents myriad legal issues in which she had no prior experience. Learning the players and the politics of a non-profit organization is always challenging, but learning it within the context of life and death situations or where physicians are being scrutinized by malpractice lawyers or government regulators can be stressful. Bonnie found that doctors don't like the law or lawyers very much, although it is easier when you are "their lawyer." Although billable hours was not a concern, finding time to get all the work done was another significant challenge.

In meeting those challenges, Bonnie learned that one of the most significant differences between being an in-house lawyer and being an outside lawyer is that you can take legal/business risks as in-house counsel. She explains that an outside lawyer is under more pressure to protect the firm from being sued and often must opt for the conservative view, and an in-house lawyer needs to be ethical and legally compliant but can take more business risks. Here is a case in point in Bonnie Brier's own words.

"One poignant moment involved a dying child. The child's parents were not married but they had lived together until a year prior to escalation of the child's illness. The father had psychiatric problems and was dependent on medication. When he did not take his medication, he could become violent. The mother had obtained a restraining order against him, and ultimately the father was institutionalized. In spite of the restraining order, the hospital managed to allow the father one supervised visit to say good-bye to his son the day before the little boy died."

Moments like that are rare in private practice, and Bonnie clearly appreciates the difference. She identifies the skills most valuable in non-profit work as good judgment, practical problem solving, working collaboratively with diverse groups of people, seeking out common ground, a willingness to make tough decisions, learning from your mistakes and taking responsibility for them, learning from the mistakes of others, knowing how to apologize, and leading by examples of hard work, ethical practice and excellent lawyering.

Her best advice to young women lawyers is to enjoy your work and your colleagues, appreciate what you accomplish, see the humor in life, and get as much varied practice experience as possible.

In reflecting on her law firm days, Bonnie Brier commends her employer for being "committed to having women lawyers find success in the firm," but she recognizes the "historic baggage" that could interfere. In Bonnie's experience, that historic baggage manifested itself in many ways. Women were not mentored in the same way men were. She saw this as an almost innocent "birds of a feather flock together" result and understood that male partners saw themselves in the young male associates more readily than in the female counterparts. Women also carried most of the responsibilities for family and childcare, and that had the potential of becoming a huge impediment to success at the law firm. Once when she was admonished during her associate review for not dressing more professionally, she responded that she had been up early in the morning with her baby and she felt it was quite an accomplishment just to be fully clothed!

There were no part-time policies for women in her law firm when she started working there and, later when they were implemented, some male lawyers complained about the lack of commitment by the women who worked part-time and the economic unfairness of those arrangements to the firm. The firm leadership in her time also could be insensitive to the vestiges of discrimination. It was not uncommon in those days to hold firm meetings at private clubs that required women to enter through the back stairway and eat in the ladies' dining room—or at clubs that discriminated against blacks and Jews—and to address all letters as "Dear Sir" or "Gentlemen."

Even though Bonnie Brier recognizes that women have made great strides in the law since her law firm experiences, she believes that firms often do not offer the collaborative and team-oriented environments that women prefer and thrive in. She notes that firms today are more likely to provide role models and mentors for women, but thinks that many firms could do a better job in mentoring women more effectively (including teaching them to generate work) and in providing a broader array of alternative work arrangements that are economically satisfactory for both the lawyer and the firm. She sees the continued disproportionate responsibility that women bear for childcare and household duties as impediments to finding success in a law firm.

However, Bonnie Brier is not looking back with any regret. Quite the contrary. Her experiences were overwhelmingly positive, and she feels fortunate to have had the opportunities. Those experiences and opportunities also increased her awareness of what she wanted to do in law practice and led her to the non-profit world that she loves. According to Bonnie, "It doesn't get any better than what I have had."

For more information on Bonnie Brier, please consult her bio on the New York University web site at www.nyu.edu.

I close this discussion of non-profit practice with the words of Professor Philip Schrag upon his installment in 2009 as the first Delaney Family Professor of Public Interest Law at Georgetown University Law Center:

Public interest lawyers make huge differences in the lives of many people, whether through keeping them housed, limiting the amount of time they spend in jail or improving the conditions of their confinement, helping them to become employed or re-employed, enabling them to go to school, preventing them from being cheated, enabling them to enjoy physical security or an unpolluted environment, and in so many other ways. Public interest lawyers also help clients to understand how to exercise power, to advocate effectively for themselves even when the lawyers are no longer representing them.

So I say to my students who are here today: whether you do public service as a part time pro bono activity or as a life's mission, I hope that many of you will experience the incredible satisfaction of providing service to people who need it and cannot pay for it.

Philip Schrag, Professor and Director for Applied Legal Studies, Georgetown University Law Center, www.law.georgetown.edu/news/documents/ Delaney professorship speech.pdf.

From Law Firm to Government Lawyer

The transition from being a law firm practitioner to a government lawyer is a road less traveled, but it has been a successful model for many women attorneys. According to the NALP, approximately 7 percent of the women who leave private firms go to government jobs. (Judith S. Kaye and Anne C. Reddy, *The Progress of Women Lawyers at Big Firms: Steadied or Simply Studied?*, 76 Fordham L. Rev. 1941 (2008), http://ir.lawnet.fordham.edu/flr/vol76/iss4/1)

Just getting away from billable hour requirements can make this transition look very attractive to women with significant home and family responsibilities. However, the need for flexibility is only part of the story. Being a government lawyer has its own cache, and it can be a very exciting and satisfying practice. Even though government attorneys function much the same way as lawyers in private practice—just from the other side—there is no requirement that government lawyers have a "portfolio of work" to sustain them and to impress their employers, and this can be a very important difference. The client is the United States Government, and there is always plenty of work. This transition often comes with a much lower salary, but it can be worth it for those who do not want the responsibilities of developing work and clients and just want to concentrate on interpreting and enforcing the law.

It is hard to describe what government lawyers do because the experiences are so broad. There are so many agencies of government and so many other legal positions within government that pinning down a general description is almost impossible. But, here is some information to get you started.

One typical career path in the federal government is counsel's office at departments of government like the Office of Transportation, the Office of Homeland Security, and the Securities and Exchange Commission, to name just a few. The function of these agencies is enforcement, and the lawyers there have the role of enforcing the rules and regulations of those divisions of government. The regulations are codified in the U.S. Code, and those regulations govern how business is done and how the rights and privileges of U.S. citizens are enforced. The lawyers at the various agencies investigate alleged wrongdoing and noncompliance complaints, respond to interrogatories and handle all other administrative issues associated with the complaints.

They work with attorneys from the Justice Department when the cases go to trial and assist at trial as well.

Here is a list of some of the top departments and agencies of the federal government that have counsel staffs.

Social Security Administration

Department of Treasury

Department of Veterans Affairs

Department of Justice

Department of Defense

Department of Homeland Security

Department of Labor

Department of State

Securities and Exchange Commission

Department of Commerce

Department of Health and Human Services

Department of the Interior

For a complete list, see: http://www.makingthedifference.org/federalcareers/law.shtml (via Fedscope).

The government also offers many opportunities for part-time practice. For example, the Securities and Exchange Commission provides flexible work schedule options and also offers backup childcare to employees with children if the regular childcare options fall through (http://www.sec.gov/jobs/jobs_worklife.shtml). At the Department of Justice, two part-time employees may opt to "job share" and voluntarily share the duties and responsibilities of a full-time position. This job share concept is discussed more thoroughly below.

Another benefit of government practice that cannot be ignored is the excellent retirement and benefit packages. Although private law firms also can provide excellent benefit packages, private practice attorneys generally pay for their own coverage plans. A counterbalance to those expenses, of course, is the higher pay in private practice, which can make affording those plans easier.

However, the government may have defined benefit plans, sometimes known as pensions, which are funded by the government, and there is nothing in private practice to compare with those benefit plans. Although there are opportunities for 401Ks and matching funds, and partnership accounts and other similar mechanisms in private practice, most of those funds are made up of earnings put aside by the practitioners.

As a result, some of the government retirement programs are envied by private practitioners. Many of us know high-level government lawyers who retired with pensions that came close to the levels of their salaries when they were still working. That alone would be worth considering! You should keep in mind, however, that the nature of these defined benefits plans at the government are changing, and those benefits may be a thing of the past by the time that you are interested in government practice.

In addition to the career opportunities at the government agency and department level, the Department of Justice is another option. Justice Department lawyers are the trial lawyers for the various departments of government. For instance, if a matter that is being investigated by the Federal Aviation Administration ends up going to trial, it is the lawyers at the Justice Department in the Aviation and Admiralty Section of the Torts Branch of the Civil Division who will be the lead attorneys on the case. Similarly, if a matter that is being investigated by the Department of Labor goes to trial, it is the labor law practitioners at the Justice Department who will be the lead trial counsel. The Solicitor General, who represents the United States of America in cases before the United States Supreme Court, and the Attorney General, who is the federal government's top lawyer, are both a part of the Department of Justice. Working for the Department of Justice has a lot of prestige, and Justice Department attorneys invariably describe the pride in standing up in court and saying, "I represent the United States of America."

The Justice Department is made up of the departments and divisions in the chart on the next page. Each of the divisions functions somewhat independently, and they all report to the Attorney General. (http://www.rff.com/justice_orgchart.htm)

Lateral hires at the Justice Department are not unusual. Lawyers in private practice, who have gained excellent trial experience, can be very attractive to the DOJ. However, the Justice Department is an elite department of government, and the chances of landing a lateral position there may be fewer than transitioning from law firm practice to another department of government. This does not mean that you should not "go for it," but it means that you have to be realistic about the possibilities. Knowing exactly what kind of experience the Department of Justice is looking for in any one practice section and getting as much of that experience as possible prior to your attempt to relocate is very important, and you cannot start too early with that kind of planning.

In addition to all of these opportunities for lawyers at the federal government level, there also are similar opportunities within each state and local government around the country. Working for state and local governments can be very exciting because you can see the results of your work "in your own backyard." On the state level, the breadth of issues is almost as broad as at the federal level, and the benefit of the local level is that the issues and interest areas are not as compartmentalized on the smaller scale, and a lawyer may have opportunities to gain experience in a greater variety of areas.

And there is more. Quite apart from the typical government lawyers described above, there are lawyers who are involved in the more political functions of government. They are the lawyers who serve on the staffs of elected officials. They are the "Hill" practitioners—as in "Capitol Hill"—, and there are similar practitioners at the state and local levels. There also are White House Counsel and staff lawyers who advise the President of the United States, and governors and local supervisory boards and committees

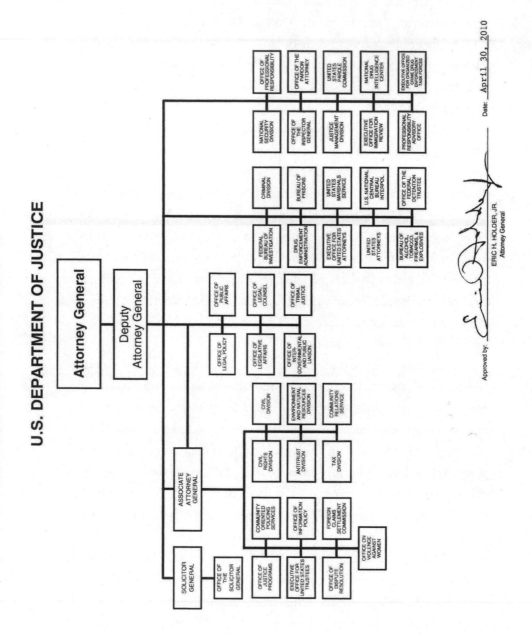

have similar legal staff at the state and local levels. There also are lobbyists, many of whom are lawyers in private practice, whose job it is to educate and influence lawmakers on behalf of their clients. Most of these lobbying practices are located at the seats of government around the country, and many of them are concentrated in Washington, D.C. Sometimes referred to as "K Street" practices because the lobbyist law firms traditionally have been located along K Street in D.C., it can be a very fast-moving and demanding practice, especially when Congress is in session. Although these lobbyists are in private practice, they are so closely associated with legislation that I include them here.

I have some experience that might be helpful here. I served as the Chief of Staff for an elected official for eight years during the time that I needed greater flexibility in my career to accommodate my responsibilities for children and family. My boss was one of only ten members of a county Board of Supervisors, and the county had over 1 million people—one of the most populated counties in the United States. As a result, our office represented over 100,000 constituents, and we dealt with a panoply of issues. My job description was "legislative and administrative aide," and I had a close working relationship with the county attorneys and senior county administrators. It was one of the most interesting jobs I ever had. It was part policy, a lot of legislation and a front-row seat on the day-to-day workings of a very sophisticated local government.

As stated earlier, a major downside of government practice can be compensation. Instead of starting out in practice at six figures, as in some private law firms today, government lawyers start out for much less money and they do not have the same potential for increased earnings as those in the private sector. However, if you paid attention to my earlier admonishments on avoiding the "Golden Handcuffs" of excessive lifestyle that often accompanies private practice, you will be able to make those adjustments. It is all about keeping your options open.

Here is a woman who can tell you all about transitioning from private practice to government practice. Kathleen Tighe is the Inspector General of the U.S. Department of Education, and she loves her job and is happy that she made the transition. Just recently, following the President's State of the Union address in January 2012, the White House announced that President Obama has appointed Kathy Tighe to chair the Recovery Accountability and Transparency Board (RATB), which was established after the economic downturn beginning in 2008 and became a model for government oversight. As you will see from her profile below, Kathy was an excellent choice for the job.

Kathy Tighe participated in this interview in her personal capacity, and the views expressed do not necessarily represent the view of the Department of Education or the United States of America.

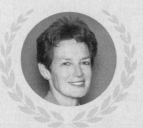

Profile of Kathleen Tighe

Kathy Tighe views government from a very high perch. As Inspector General of the U.S. Department of Education, she provides leadership for a 300-person office and has a staff of auditors, criminal investigators, and lawyers that report to her. Her government career included other significant stops along the way, and she faced work-life issues that, fortunately, most of us will never have to face. Hers is a true success story, and, as her friend and former colleague, I am happy to share it with you.

Kathy's plans after graduating from law school *always* involved work in a law firm. She had attended law school in the night program at George Washington University Law School, where she graduated with honors. She also had a Masters Degree in International Relations and was *Phi Beta Kappa* at her undergraduate *alma mater*, Purdue University. She clerked for a large Washington, D.C. law firm as a law student, and she decided that a medium-sized firm was probably the best fit for her and would provide more responsibility and valuable experience for junior associates. She found exactly what she was looking for, and her experience at a mid-sized Virginia firm in the D.C. metropolitan area was just what she expected. She experienced good mentoring by partners and acquired a strong background in government contract litigation and related matters.

Everything seemed to be going well until the surprising dissolution of her law firm in the 1980's, leaving 50-some lawyers without jobs. By that time she had married another associate at the firm and was pregnant with their first child. The dissolution of her law firm had been hard on all of the attorneys involved, and Kathy was no exception. She decided that she was ready for something different.

Five months after the birth of her baby, Kathy took a job as an attorney at the Department of Justice Civil Frauds section. She was lucky to have worked on a fraud matter while in private practice, and, based on that experience, she received a strong recommendation for the position at DOJ. With the exception of the expected "pay cut," Kathy made a smooth transition, and she does not recall any particular difficulties that she had in moving from law firm practice to public service. She had spent five years in private practice before making the career move, and she thinks that made a big difference in her successful transition.

Kathy enjoyed the heightened level of responsibility she experienced in government practice, especially being in charge of her own cases. She worked hard to turn this experience into an expertise in False Claims Act cases, and she particularly enjoyed working for the taxpayers and trying to make government more efficient and effective. Kathy explains it like this: "Seeing justice done in civil fraud prosecutions brings money back to the U.S. Treasury. I like that result, and it is very rewarding."

Kathy took that experience and built on it in the Federal Government. It is a testament to her competence that her career was meteoric, and you may need a flow chart to keep her career steps straight. However, it is fairly representative of government careers that end up as successful as Kathy Tighe's, so hang in there!

As a trial attorney in the Civil Frauds section, Kathy was responsible for the litigation of multimillion dollar civil fraud cases, and, after three years and the birth of her second child, she left DOJ and joined Counsel's staff at the General Services Administration (GSA) Office of Inspector General. While at GSA, Kathy worked part-time for five years to accommodate her family responsibilities, particularly the special needs of her second child, who had been born with a physical disability. She eventually was able to return to full-time work, but, prior to that time and while she still was working part-time, she was promoted to Counsel to the Inspector General in the Office of Inspector General for GSA. In that position, she supervised an office of eight employees and handled a range of legal matters that included overseeing procurement fraud cases referred to DOJ by her office, and subpoena issuance and enforcement of ethics and personnel advice. After 14 years in that job, Kathy left GSA to become the Deputy Inspector General of the Department of Agriculture. In that position, she was effectively the chief operating officer of a 600-person office, supervising the audit, criminal investigative and management functions.

Then, in 2009 Kathy Tighe was nominated by President Barack Obama, and later confirmed by the U.S. Senate, as the Inspector General of the Department of Education. She assumed the responsibilities of her new position early in 2010, and in that role, she works to make the Education Department's programs and operations more efficient and effective and to combat fraud, waste, and abuse.

Most recently, on December 23, 2011, Kathy was appointed by President Obama to be the Chair of the Recovery, Transparency and Accountability Board. Today, she continues to do her job as the Education Department Inspector General in addition to this new position.

At various points in her government career, Kathy faced significant challenges. She had to learn to navigate huge government organizations, learn to be a good manager, learn the programs and operations of new agencies so that she could speak authoritatively about them (including while testifying before Congress), and learn how to keep tabs on and oversee the day-to-day operations of hundreds of employees. In meeting these challenges, Kathy learned to study hard, rely on her good instincts, compromise when advisable, see the "big picture," and remember the power of laughter. For those of us who have experienced Kathy's infectious laugh and wonderful sense of humor, it is not at all surprising how valuable that has been to her success.

Kathy's best advice to young women lawyers is to work hard, seek advice when you have questions, be flexible, and find good mentors. She would like to see law firms look to the Federal Government as a role model for recruiting, generating positive morale, providing flexible work schedules and teleworking, and allowing limited leave for family care purposes. Kathy particularly benefitted from the latter, and the government would have lost out on her talents without it. As a response to Kathy's superior work ethic and skills, Kathy's superiors happily recommended her for advancement at every turn and even sought out positions for her, which would allow her to meet the needs of her personal/family life circumstances.

Kathy considers herself lucky in her career, but she also knows that she made much of her own luck. "People can help you along the way, but it is up to you to live up to their expectations." Of course Kathy Tighe did all of that, and it is why she is protecting our tax dollars from her high perch at the Department of Education Office of Inspector General and as Chair of the Recovery Accountability and Transparency Board, where she functions as the Recovery Act's "top watchdog" according to Vice President Biden when he announced her appointment.

Kathy may consider herself lucky, but I think we are the lucky ones!

For more information on Kathy Tighe, please consult her bio on the U. S. Department of Education web site at www2.ed.gov/news/staff/bios/tighe.html.

From Law Firm to Solo Practice

Solo practice presents another option. There are 271,000 solo practitioners in the United States (Bureau of Labor Statistics http://www.law.harvard.edu/programs/plp/pages/statistics.php#wlw), and it is the ultimate in independence for a practicing lawyer—independence in terms of what clients you chose to represent and what hours you work—but it is still a demanding practice. A case that looks like it will not be much work can grow into an octopus of a case, and there is only one of you to do all the work.

There are several solo practitioners in my family, and they have what I call the "real lawyer" practices. They live in small towns and represent clients in diverse legal matters. They draft wills for their clients, represent them in bankruptcy court, help them with refinancing their homes, and make sure that they have good representation when a family member has an accident or gets into trouble with the law. They get to know their clients well, and they experience great reward in helping the people of their communities get through difficult times.

However, this route can seem a little scary for those of us who are used to caucusing with colleagues over issues on a case. In law firm practice, there usually are at least a few fellow attorneys who have "been there, done that" when it comes to most legal matters. "Going solo" does not have those same benefits, and it is usually a good idea to get some firm experience before hanging out your solo shingle. However, in the current depressed economy, getting law firm experience first may not be possible, so solo practice right out of law school may be for you. Keep up your contacts with your law school and bar association friends if you choose that route. Often they can be counted on for the caucusing you need, and they also may become sources of work, especially in conflict of interest situations.

Law firm administration, even for a solo practice, can seem daunting if you do not have any background in it. I recommend you take a crash course on that subject if you are considering the solo practice option. Most law schools do not teach it, and, unless you have experience on the management committee of a larger firm, you probably do not know much about it. However, that can be an easy fix. There also is a lot of information about solo practice and tutorials available on the Internet today, and there is more being written about it in the bar association journals.

Blogs about going solo include:

www.myshingle.com
www.soloinminneapolis.com
www.startingasolopractice.com

Articles and books about solo practice:

"The Real Reason Women Are More Likely to Fly Solo When It Comes to Work," Huffington Post on-line, May 7, 2012, http:www.huffingtonpost.com/Shannon-kelley/women.

Elefant, Carolyn. *Solo by Choice: How to Be the Lawyer You Always Wanted to Be* **(LawyerAvenue, 2008).**

Solo by Choice contains 300 pages packed with down-to-earth, well-organized advice on everything from making the decision to set up your own law practice, to deciding if and when to expand your solo practice. It includes appendices on everything from writing a business plan to creating a forms library. "Solo's" author tackles everything from alternative billing methods to finding good suppliers, all with common sense and good humor.

Foonberg, Jay G. *How to Start and Build a Law Practice* **(ABA, 2004).**

A classic ABA bestseller, you'll find over 100 chapters packed with techniques for getting started.

Huss, William W. *Start Your Own Law Practice: A Guide to All the Things They Don't Teach in Law School about Starting Your Own Firm* **(Sphinx, 2005).**

After years of school and maybe even after some years of practice, you are ready to be the boss. You want to hang out your shingle and open an office of your own. But running a profitable business takes more than just being a great attorney. *Start Your Own Law Practice* provides you with the knowledge to be both a great lawyer and a successful business owner.

Lockwood, Karen, editor, *The Road to Independence: 101 Women's Journeys to Starting Their Own Law Firms* **(ABA, 2011).**

The Road to Independence is a collection of 101 letters from women who have taken the courageous and difficult step of creating a law firm of their own, either as a solo or with others. Focusing on the experiences, challenges, and opportunities of women-owned law firms, these women, in their personal voices, reiterate key themes: of becoming businesswomen; of choosing a practice area true to their passion and the high character they bring to the bar; and of controlling not only their days but their destinies.

Pfeifer, William L. *How to Start a Successful Law Practice: The New Lawyer's Guide to Opening an Office as a Solo or Small Firm Attorney* (Pipers Willow, 2006).

From an attorney who started his own practice, this book explores several key components to a successful solo practice, such as how to develop your personal identity as an attorney, what to consider in choosing a legal specialty, and even what office equipment and supplies you need to get started.

Here is a blog entry from my website about going solo.

June 30, 2011

Good Advice for Women Lawyers Going Solo

Going solo is an interesting concept and one that is gaining more popularity during these tough economic times when law firm hires are down. A new book has just been published by the American Bar Association addressing the issue after a three-year study by the ABA Commission on Women. The book is based on letters written by women lawyers addressing their experiences in launching their own firms. According to a recent description on the ABA web site, the reasons for women going solo have nothing to do with work-life and family pressure. That seems to make sense because a solo practice can't be any less demanding than a firm practice—at least not in the formative years. Rather, the reasons most often cited are control, ambition, success and challenge.

The book, *The Road to Independence: 101 Women's Journeys to Starting Their Own Law Firms*, seems to me to be a bit like *Best Friends at the Bar*. It gathers the advice and wisdom of established practitioners and puts it at your fingertips. Although I have not read the

ABA book yet and I never practiced solo, I can identify a little with the issues from my own experience starting a small business. The *Best Friends at the Bar* project, including the book, speaking engagements and consulting services, is part of my company LegalPerspectives, Inc. Sounds easy, right—researching, writing, speaking and consulting? Piece of cake if you know what you are writing and talking about. And that would be correct—that *is* the easy part. The not-so-obvious parts that are really challenging are the PR, the marketing, the technical issues that will either make you or break you, and the cash outlay for all of the incidental expenses of setting up a small business—web site designers, lawyers to handle the IP issues, techies to make sure that the equipment does not break down and, if it does, that it is fixed before the next deadline, and PR folks to make you look good and get your name out, to name just a few. And, believe me, I have come to appreciate the old days when I had "people" who were at my beck and call in a law firm at a moment's notice. Not having people will define the importance of having people in a nanosecond.

That must be what it is like to go solo in law practice. It must be pretty scary at first, but it also must be really satisfying to be your own boss, set your own goals and objectives, make the rules and practice law the way you want to—instead of the way the Management Committee tells you to. So, hats off to all of you who decide to make the leap, for whatever reasons. But, first, before you leap, it seems like a good idea to check out some of the excellent web sites on going solo and/or reading the new ABA book on the subject. Trust me, you can never be too prepared for what lies ahead.

There are two solo practitioners in my family, and one was my Dad. He practiced solo for 50 years. That is a really long time, and I can honestly say that he loved what he did. He was a fiercely independent type, and it served him very well. He also was the most ethical lawyer I ever knew, and he was able to steer clear of anything that had the "appearance" he did not like. I know that meant a lot to him, and it was one of the things I admired most about him. He was a great sounding board for me, my brother and my husband when we were starting in practice, and I miss his wisdom.

However, I do not think I could have done what he did. I am too social an animal, and I think that I would miss the human interaction that a firm or company environment provides. But, to each his own, and it sure worked out for my Dad.

As for me, I could not be happier in what I do today. This is the most gratifying work I have ever done in my life, and I thoroughly enjoy meeting all of you along the road as I travel the country giving speeches and helping young women lawyers and law students. There is no manual for what I do, and that is part of the appeal. I make it up as I go, and it is never dull or boring. I could not ask for more, and I do not take your support and interest for granted. Never will.

From www.bestfriendsatthebar.com

There certainly are benefits to solo practice, and Laura Oberbroeckling knows them all. A Harvard-educated attorney who left Big Law to operate a solo practice out of her home, Laura knows the ins and outs and shared her story with me recently for an article about Book One that was published in the February 25, 2010 edition of the *LA Daily Journal*. Here is Laura's story as it appeared in that article.

Profile of Laura Oberbroeckling

I went to law school because I had strong interest in public policy and wanted an intellectually challenging, financially-secure career. Growing up in Dubuque, Iowa, during the farm crisis in the 1980s, I saw what dire economic conditions could do to individuals. A legal career fit my interests and needs. My substantial educational debt made a career outside of a private law firm impractical, so after graduating from Harvard Law School, I started my career in a general litigation practice in a Washington, D.C., law firm. I was fortunate to work with many good people, including mentors who delegated substantial responsibility to junior associates, such as me. I gradually shifted my practice from general litigation to health care litigation, and moved firms to make this shift, eventually focusing on health care law more generally. Although my shift from a more litigation-based practice to a more general health care practice fit with my early career goals, the shift really happened because I needed to move away from a practice with unpredictable hours and frequent travel, to one that allowed me to spend more time with my growing family.

After making partner at a national firm and having my first child around the same time, I realized that I could not have it all. I could not have an active litigation practice and grow my client base and be active in firm administration without sacrificing a significant amount of time with my family. I chose to have children (they didn't choose me) and I wanted to be a significant part of their lives; I did not plan to outsource the tasks associated with raising my family to "good help" as more senior attorneys had advised years before I had children. It became quite clear to me that "having it all" was a fiction—for men and women.

As I was due to have my third child, and dealing with chronic health issues with my other two children, I decided to leave the large firm setting and focus on my family. I already had tried working reduced hours and gave up most of my non-billable commitments. I worked every day, but shorter days and with limited travel, but I still felt that I was not dedicating enough time to either family or career; there was only so much of me to go around. I remembered an attorney telling me a story of his daughter's school essay—she wrote that she wanted to be a client when she grew up. She knew that as a client, she would get her father's attention. I did not want my kids to wish that they were my clients. When I explained my decision to leave the practice to clients, some asked if they could continue to work with me. At the same time, one of my colleagues, with whom I had worked at three firms, was leaving the large firm practice to establish his own small firm and asked if I could support his practice. At my clients' suggestion, and with the option of continuing to work with my long-term mentor, I decided to establish my own practice and work from home, allowing me to be the primary caretaker for my children and attend to their health. As a result, I continue to have a satisfying career and fulfilling personal life. Instead of feeling like I was giving neither my career nor my family the proper amount of attention, I struck a balance that allows me to continue to have the intellectual challenge of a legal career and provide quality legal services to my clients, and to be the kind of parent that I want to be for my children. My choices are not ones that everyone would or could make, and I have had to sacrifice many things along the way, including my role as a partner in a major firm, the bulk of my litigation practice, the satisfaction of collaborating with other attorneys on large matters, and, of course, the financial rewards of working at a large firm. But I have not had to sacrifice my happiness, nor have my children had to sacrifice theirs.

I have been able to have a satisfying career and personal life in large part because of the amazing people in my life. My husband, also a lawyer, has always been supportive. My mentors (interestingly, mostly male attorneys) have taught me much about not only the practice of law, but also the need to retain your self-identity and values. My clients have been tremendously understanding about the odd hours I keep and the fact that they may hear the sounds of a preschooler vying for my attention at the other end of a conference call or that they may need to call back after I have made sure that my kids are home and have had their after-school snack. I have learned along the way that it is important to reevaluate career goals, and not to be afraid to make career path changes as career choices may (and probably should) change as your life changes. Undoubtedly my career path will lead me to bends around which I cannot yet see, but as long as I stay true to my self and my values, and continue to search for intellectually challenging work with people that I enjoy and admire, I will be proud to be a lawyer. And, perhaps most importantly to me, my children are happy and proud that I am a lawyer. My daughter has told me that she wants to be a lawyer just like me when she grows up; she did not say that she wants to be a client. I must be doing something right.

More on Laura and Her Transition

After this article was published, I had greater opportunity to talk with Laura, and I found that she had interesting views, not only on the work-life struggles, addressed in the article but also on the changing nature of law firms and what law firms should be doing to retain talent. In fact, Laura identifies the changes in law firms in the early to mid 1990's as one of the reasons that she left law firm practice. She talked about the effect of law firms growing exponentially as the result of the dot.com bubble and the advent of new technology practices. She witnessed the results of this growth, which included expansion of office locations, additional lease obligations and raising associate salaries to outbid other firms for talent. These new realities, in turn, led to changes to increase revenues to meet the new expense obligations, changes like raising hourly rates and increasing the number of required billable hours.

As a conscientious and responsible lawyer, Laura had trouble implementing those changes at her level. It was difficult for her to justify charging clients high hourly rates for associates, who still needed her supervision, and she found herself either doing the work herself or not billing some of her time to reduce the size of the bill. However, this was not a very good strategy because it was not an efficient use of her time, and her firm did not approve of cutting the client's bills this way.

Eventually, these changes, together with all the responsibilities for administrative non-billable work and marketing and new client development, created the kind of economic and work-life pressure that caused her to leave private practice—but not until she had experienced four different law firms!

Laura's reluctance to leave large firm practice might have been related to her recognition of the excellent training and good mentoring she received at law firms, including Piper & Marbury (predecessor to DLA Piper), Proskauer Rose, Mintz Levin and Reed Smith. She always wanted to be an exceptional lawyer, and the close association with mentors and the availability of diverse opinions from colleagues and benefits from their experiences were attractive to her. Even with the success that she has experienced, Laura wonders whether she gave up on firm practice too soon. She recommends exhausting the possibilities that might be worked out with the firm to accommodate needs as preferable to leaving prematurely. She experienced the disappointment of leaving one firm for another, including sacrificing status and relationships, and she knows that transition decisions must be thought out very carefully.

Not surprisingly, Laura identifies the inability to consult colleagues about legal judgments as the most challenging thing about her move from law firm practice to solo practice. Although she has been supported in her moves by former colleagues and understands the importance of that support to her success, she also knows that she cannot take undue advantage of those colleagues for consultation. She only calls on her network of colleagues on rare occasions out of respect for their time constraints and because of concerns for client confidentiality.

Laura attributes her success in solo practice to her 15 years of law firm practice before making the move. She cautions young lawyers to make sure that they have adequate training and preparation to be able to make the change successfully. In Laura's words,

"A solo practice really only makes sense for seasoned or experienced professionals. You must be financially able to make the transition from receiving a regular paycheck to investing in a solo business and waiting for revenues to exceed expenses and result in profits, which can be converted to income."

The skills and circumstances that Laura thinks are most valuable to achieving success as a solo practitioner are the ability to work independently, the availability of a defined workspace that allows you to work without distraction, and an existing client base. She also recognizes that the Internet is invaluable to a solo practitioner for research and background information and says that she could not have been as successful as she has been without the existence of this technology.

So, you can see that Laura Oberbroeckling sees both sides of the coin. She values the large firm experience but understands that it does not fit all lifestyles. In fact, she would like to see law firms pay much greater attention to the workplace environment as it affects both women and men. She does not think that there is anything particularly unique about the law firm setting that drives young women away except for the "crushing hours and the effect that it has on personal and family lives." According to Laura,

> "It has the same effect on men. . . . The issues are not women's issues, and law firms should recognize everyone's life outside the office and the value of that life to make real progress retaining talent—both male and female talent."

Hear, hear.

For more information on Laura Oberbroeckling, please consult www.linkedin.com/pub/laura-oberbroeckling/23/5b1/84.

From Traditional Law Firm to Non-Traditional Law Firm

Women-Owned Law Firm

Hats off to the women who have forged ahead with this model. It is really the flip side of, "If you can't beat them, join them" and instead it is something like, "If you can't beat them, band together and beat them better!" As actress Drew Barrymore said in an interview with *InStyle* magazine when addressing the subject of women helping women, "One person is a force. A tribe is unstoppable." (October 2009, *InStyle* magazine)

Women banding together to form their own law firms is an example of that tribe mentality. It does not have to be exclusive, however, and I always caution young women not to repeat the sins of the past. Just because men historically have excluded women in our profession, it is no time for women to become exclusive toward men. Fortunately, that is not the motivation behind this model of practice, which is typically attractive because it gives women some of the flexibility they need for home and family and provides back-up and assistance from colleagues who understand the work-life struggle.

Here is a young woman who sought out a woman-owned practice to help deal with the work-life issues that she had encountered. She loved her women-owned practice experience, and she will tell you why. Meet Kathryn Smith Spencer, formerly of the women-owned law firm Patrick Law Group LLC in Atlanta and currently Corporate Counsel for AGL Resources Inc. in Atlanta.

Profile of Kathryn Smith Spencer

Kathryn Smith Spencer is an excellent example of a young woman lawyer in transition. Kathryn began her legal career in a large private law firm and later transitioned to a small woman-owned boutique firm where she could practice in the convenience of her own home. Private law practice initially appealed to Kathryn because she believed that it would provide her with an opportunity to learn the practice of law from talented, respected and well-trained lawyers with diverse legal backgrounds. In addition, Kathryn knew that practicing in a large law firm would open doors for her in the future if she "paid her dues" and cultivated contacts in the legal field that she could carry with her to the next phases of her career.

Growing up with a father who practiced law in private firms, Kathryn had been familiar with the ins and outs of private practice, and her expectations were soon met. After graduating from the University of Virginia and Wake Forest Law, Kathryn started her legal career in litigation. However, Kathryn quickly realized that litigation was not the best fit for her personality and that she needed to make a change. It was at this time that Kathryn considered moving into the transactional field where her efforts could assist on the front end of deals and actually "help business get done." Kathryn and her husband also wanted to start a family, and she knew that a transactional practice would allow for some additional flexibility and less travel time.

Although Kathryn knew that she needed to make a change, it was very important that she make the *right change* at the *right time*. As luck would have it, a woman partner at the firm, who Kathryn liked and admired, offered Kathryn an opportunity she couldn't refuse. After the woman partner left the firm to start a women-owned boutique practice, she asked Kathryn to join her in this new venture. Kathryn knew that a position with the Patrick Law Group was the opportunity she had been waiting for. Kathryn accepted the offer and, although it was "scary" to give up the comfort and benefits of a large firm, she was excited to start something new and work for someone with tremendous passion for her work and clients. Kathryn also hoped that a women-owned firm would provide an environment that was particularly supportive of women. And, she could work at home, which appealed to her as she contemplated adding to her family.

Although Kathryn was confident about her decision to transition into a smaller law practice, her decision had its challenges. Initially, it was difficult for Kathryn to adapt to having fewer resources and a limited staff with no paralegals or full-time administrative assistants. Working from home also had its complications. Kathryn no longer had a large group of attorneys inside her office to consult with or an extensive law library at her fingertips.

However, she quickly adjusted to her new position and became self-reliant and resourceful. By taking the time out to seek alternative research methods, Kathryn learned that there are significant and inexpensive resources through the professional bar and other organizations that are available to practitioners in small practices. In addition, Kathryn leveraged available technology and reached out to the firm's founder, who continues to be a valuable resource and teacher.

Kathryn came to love her new practice, and she found that there were fewer distractions working from home than there were working in an office environment. Gone were the mandatory group meetings and recruiting lunches, and colleagues did not drop in on a whim just to chat. As a result, Kathryn was able to get her work done more quickly and efficiently and had more time to attend to the other aspects of her life that were important, like family, friends, and church. Maintaining and fulfilling life outside of work led to a more balanced lifestyle, and Kathryn is extremely grateful for those opportunities and experiences.

Katherine has since had another "offer that she could not refuse." She has traded the women-owned law practice for an in-house counsel position for some of the same reasons that you read about earlier in the profiles of Sally Blackmun and Amy Yeung. Katherine's career is still a work in progress, and she is enjoying each and every experience.

Now a mentor herself, Kathryn advises young women lawyers interested in transitioning from private practice. She tells them not to be afraid to take a chance on something new. Kathryn advocates that young women lawyers must "make and maintain contacts with former classmates and colleagues [and] strive not to burn bridges." Further, she cautions young women who are unhappy in their practices not to "make a change just for the sake of change" but, rather, to get to the source of the unhappiness first and use that information to make the right change. She also encourages law firms to get serious about accommodating those young women in the profession who want to transition into part-time or flextime positions.

In all of this, Kathryn is "paying it forward" and emulating the mentor that she so admired and who changed her life.

For more information on Kathryn Spencer, please consult her bio at kspencer@aglresources.com.

Virtual Law Firm

Technology is freeing lawyers as well as business types. Virtual law practice (meaning online law practice) has liberated many women from the constraints of traditional law practice and allowed them to work when and where it fits their lifestyles. In that respect, virtual law firms may be the way of the future.

According to an *ABA Journal* article virtual law firms typically hire seasoned lawyers and allow them to work at home, and they allow partners to keep somewhere in the range of 80-85% of their billings. The lawyers who work for these virtual law firms can earn more money than in traditional practice, even while working less and billing at lower rates ("Another Virtual Law Firm Allows Lawyers to Work Less, Earn More," in the *ABA Journal,* "Law News Now," October 7, 2010). One lawyer interviewed for the article started his career at Big Law and moved to increasingly smaller firms but never found the "right fit." Eventually, he found his way to a virtual law firm in Atlanta. He describes spending part time working at home and part time working in other settings, and he considers it a good mix. He also reports that he has more time to spend with clients now because he has to bill fewer hours. "I had to bill 160 hours per month in a law firm, and now 80 hours per month is great, and that's generally what I'm doing," he said.

However, some virtual law firm practitioners point out shortcomings of this practice. One commenter on the *ABA Journal* article observed that the virtual practice only works if the firm has a small book of business. He noted that, in matters that require additional manpower, the virtual model is not workable because the 15% (the portion of the billables retained by the firm) does not cover the costs of distributing work to others. He additionally noted that other essential costs like marketing and retirement also make the 85/15 split unworkable. His conclusion was that the virtual model is a good working platform for semi-retirement or solo practitioners who want to create the appearance of being part of a bigger firm.

Stephanie Kimbro is someone who knows all about virtual law practice and is very successful as the founder of Kimbro Legal Services, LLC. Stephanie was described recently in *Forbes* online as a "young lawyer, mother and budding technology maven [who] embraced the concept of a virtual (online) law practice long before it became part of the practice mainstream." In fact, the *Forbes* article described her as *the reason* that the practice is in the mainstream at all and heralded her efforts helping her husband develop one of the virtual law practice platforms used by many virtual practitioners today. I am fortunate to have her as a contributor, and here is her very *au courant* story.

Profile of Stephanie Kimbro

You may recognize Stephanie Kimbro's name. She is very active on legal Internet sites, and she has published extensively on the subject of virtual law practice and the delivery of "unbundled legal services" (also known as "limited scope representation"), which is generally confined to consultation, document preparation, and limited representation in court.

Stephanie graduated from Miami University in Ohio and from the University of Dayton School of Law. In 2006, she founded Kimbro Legal Services, LLC, and she continues that practice today while also working with Total Attorneys in Chicago. In her virtual law practice, Stephanie works from a home office and does not meet with clients in person. She delivers legal services to her clients through a secure online client portal.

Stephanie, however, did not go straight to this innovative practice directly out of law school. She followed the more conventional path and worked at two law firms before leaving the traditional law firm setting to work for a virtual law firm in Wilmington, NC.

Ms. Kimbro puts a high value on the mentoring she received at the traditional law firms where she worked. She was mentored by partners and even by paralegals and legal assistants in her office. However, after five years of law firm experience, Stephanie decided that she needed a legal setting where she would experience more challenge and responsibility, and she wanted flexibility in her hours and no responsibility for the "face time" that is associated with upward mobility in law firms. The desire for flexibility became even more important when her baby was born.

The new virtual law practice seemed to fit the bill for Stephanie. She would be able to plan her work around the baby's schedule—working in the mornings and at night when the baby slept and spending time with the baby during the day.

Stephanie also saw a market for legal services to be delivered to individuals of low to moderate means in this new form of practice. These clients also needed flexibility, and most of them could not take time off of work during the day or pay for childcare to physically visit a law office. The virtual practice gave Stephanie and her clients the chance to work together outside normal business hours.

Stephanie believed in this new practice, for herself and for her clients, but she also knew that she would be taking a large financial risk to make it happen. However, she always had been an independent worker, and she was motivated to prove the value of virtual law practice.

The founding of Kimbro Legal Services, LLC, enabled Stephanie to reach her goals. Most of Stephanie's colleagues from the local legal community were skeptical, and they did not offer much support. However, Stephanie found wonderful mentors online from both the small business and entrepreneur worlds and from solo practitioners on the ABA's SoloSez listserv.

It was an exciting venture, but there were challenges that Stephanie needed to overcome. She had to educate members of the legal profession and prospective clients about virtual law practice as a *bona fide* alternative form of legal service delivery. However, she soon learned to give an "elevator pitch" about the benefits of virtual practice and to tailor her website to explain the process in greater detail. She also found the isolation difficult and sometimes yearned for colleagues to talk with about cases and matters. Overcoming that took a lot of self-confidence, but, after a few years, Stephanie "stopped cringing every time she pushed the button to send something out to the client."

Stephanie considers being technologically savvy and being conversant with the rules of professional conduct to be the two most valuable skills for her practice. She keeps current on security issues for both her hardware and cloud-based applications, and she employs best practices for the use of technology to ensure that she is compliant with ethics rules requiring her to protect the confidentiality of her clients' information.

Stephanie's best advice to young women lawyers, who are interested in virtual law practice, is to be highly self-motivated to build a brand around themselves and their services and to use social media and other forms of online networking on a daily basis.

"You need to be comfortable communicating online or in person through web conferencing tools, and you have to be compliant with your state bar's ethics rules. You need to be confident that your clients are purposefully coming to you for something different than the traditional law practice.

It is best to develop an expertise at a law firm before establishing a virtual practice of your own. If all of your legal background is general, you will need to do a lot of self-learning to be successful. The types of matters that my clients come to me with are quite specialized. It is not cost-effective in this practice to spend days researching a matter. Get the expertise first."

Stephanie also warns young women about listening to the naysayers. She thinks this is particularly hard for women because women are raised to trust, to seek out approval, and to please. She emphasizes the importance of good research, but she also values intuition.

"It's a hurdle to get over that initial jump, but once you realize your ideas are worthwhile, the hurdles are not so difficult. Take that first jump or you'll just end up running on the sidelines your whole career."

That is excellent advice, and you can feel the power of Stephanie's convictions. She has found her niche. She firmly believes that she is filling a need, and it is working for her and for her family and for her clients. She says that unbundling legal services works very well with the alternative billing models that are being considered today, even by large law firms. According to Stephanie, fixed fee and value billing provide a great way to serve an untapped market for legal services.

Stephanie Kimbro took a big chance and lives the rewards. She is a true entrepreneur.

For more information on Stephanie Kimbro and her legal services and publications, please consult her web site at www.virtuallawpractice.org.

For more on Virtual Law Practice, see Forbes *She Negotiates* on-line, "Women Lawyers Without Borders Rock Legal Practice," January 9, 2012, http://www.forbes.com/sites/shenegotiates/2012/01/09/women.

From Law Firm to Law Firm Consultant

There is a recent trend toward law firm consulting by lawyers who have "been there and done that." These consultants are assisting law firms on issues of productivity, hiring, management and many related issues, including diversity.

Karen Kaplowitz, of the legal consulting entity The New Ellis Group and the founding member of the first women-owned law firm in Los Angeles in the 1990's, is a woman lawyer who has been at the forefront of issues affecting women in the law for decades. She is recognized in legal circles as "The Goddess of Networking," and she writes and speaks frequently on leveraging professional and business networks and building clientele. Here is her story.

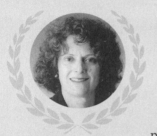

Profile of Karen Kaplowitz

Karen Kaplowitz is a woman with a vision and a re-vision. Her education at Barnard College and the University of Chicago Law School prepared her well for the challenges of the law profession and taught her to seize opportunities. Although she began her career in a law firm as a litigator, her career has undergone three major transitions that have led to her current position as President of The New Ellis Group. As a consultant, Karen shares her experience and expertise as a rainmaker with law firms and other professional organizations, and she is a woman with a lot to teach you.

Karen began her career in the Los Angeles office of O'Melveny & Myers. Although she attended law school with the expectation of becoming a public interest lawyer, she knew from experiences working as a summer law clerk that she needed training in private law practice to become a first-rate lawyer. Karen was fortunate to have several mentors at the firm to learn from and who encouraged her to pursue *pro bono* work, and, as a first year associate, Karen had the opportunity to organize a large group of ACLU lawyers to investigate and sue the Los Angeles Women's County Jail. This may have been the beginning of her dedication to women's rights that she has continued throughout her career.

At O'Melveny, Karen also represented small business clients. These same clients followed Karen when she left O'Melveny to form Bardeen Bersch & Kaplowitz, one of the first women-owned law firms in the country. At the new firm, Karen was responsible for generating work and was fortunate to tap into a strong market for women lawyers in Los Angeles. When the Bardeen firm dissolved, Karen joined the small boutique law firm of Alschuler Grossman & Pines and, based upon her experience running her own law firm, she became Alschuler's partner in charge of marketing. In that role, she provided support to lawyers who were interested in rainmaking, and that experience led her away from practice and into the world of consulting.

After a combination of practicing law and providing marketing leadership for over 27 years, Karen decided that she wanted to focus on the business side of the law, and she founded The New Ellis Group, a consulting firm that advises law firms and other professional organizations on issues related to marketing and developing new clients. Alschuler supported Karen's decision and even asked her to remain in the firm with the ultimate hope that her interest in consulting would be short-lived and that she would return to the practice. Karen, however, embraced her new consulting role and soon was off and running on a new phase of her career.

The transition from lawyer to business development strategist was challenging for Karen. Although she had a reputation for strong networking and rainmaking skills, she now had to establish herself in a new area of competency. She worked hard at building a reputation as a business strategist, trainer and coach, and the rest is history. As always, Karen was very successful in this new venture.

Despite the obvious differences between law practice and consulting, Karen sees overlap. In both settings, she has been responsible for problem solving and organizing teams of people to tackle large projects. Karen's core competencies of "building networks and helping others to do the same" and her ability to "connect the dots, understand how things relate to each other, and how to create pathways to business opportunities" have been invaluable components of her success. The opportunity to help others build significant client and referral networks has been rewarding for Karen, and she is very satisfied with her latest career transition because she now can do what she truly loves—"to help lawyers and other professionals find their core strengths, develop business plans and execute those plans with success."

Karen spends a lot of time inside law firms in her new role as consultant, and the low retention rates for young women lawyers in many of those firms concern her. To improve these retention rates and conditions for women at law firms, Karen recommends that law firms give young women lawyers challenging assignments to provide them with the best opportunities to grow and be successful. Karen also suggests that law firms encourage young women to build client relationships to help the firm generate work. Lastly, Karen urges firms to create family-friendly environments for both men and women so that they can devote time to their careers and their families without stigma. With two adult children of her own, Karen has learned a thing or two about these issues along the way.

Karen's best advice to young women lawyers interested in transitioning from private practice to a new practice setting is to begin building a network of contacts from day one of practice. Karen encourages young women to engage with fellow professionals both inside and outside the law firm and to build relationships that are based on mutuality. To do so, young women lawyers must show interest in the firm's business dealings and offer to help more senior lawyers initiate and maintain client relationships. Young women lawyers also should strive to seek out mentors to help sustain their careers. Karen has found mentors in law partners, in clients, in friends, and in family members whose encouragement and wisdom have led Karen to overcome obstacles and manage her career transitions.

Karen also urges young women to search within themselves to discover hidden passions. A continuous thread in Karen's life has been her passion for attacking inequality for women and, although the nature of her work has changed over time, she has channeled this passion in different ways and in different settings. As proprietor of The New Ellis Group, Karen continues that passion. She has worked with Legal Momentum, the Women's Legal Defense and Education Fund, to create the Aiming High awards to honor leading women in the business community, and she also has worked with Vision 2020 to create a network of national groups representing over 25 million women and girls who support that project.

Young women and young women lawyers owe a big "thank you" to Karen Kaplowitz, a woman with a vision and a re-vision and a woman who takes women's causes and women's rights seriously. Her biweekly newsletter "*Monday Monday*" is a very valuable resource for young women lawyers on networking and developing clients. You can access her newsletter at www.newellis.com.

For more information on Karen Kaplowitz and her services and publications, please consult her web site at www.newellis.com.

From Law Firm to Academia

There are myriad examples for this model, and many of the transitioning attorneys make a change to academia at the middle or end of the private practice years. It is far less typical for a law firm attorney to transition to academia during the early practice years, but it is certainly done and done successfully.

An article on Vault's Law Blog, entitled "The Other Side of the Socratic: Tips for Pursuing a Career in Legal Academia," May 25, 2011, described the hurdles of attaining a job in legal academia because of the competition and the paucity of information in the mainstream about pursuing this career route. The article quotes the Columbia Law School's Careers in Law Teaching Program website to explain the difficulties.

Traditionally, getting excellent grades at a distinguished law school, being a law review member or (preferably) officer, and having a prestigious clerkship after graduation have been the most important factors [for a career in academia], especially at the top schools. In recent years, however, scholarly achievement—not just potential—is increasingly required. By the time you are applying for tenure-track teaching jobs, you should have at least one polished piece of work ready to be submitted to prospective employers and use as a "job talk." A paper already in the publication pipeline can serve these purposes well. Better yet is to have something published already, and a second project suitable for presentation to schools. **Most law faculties still value candidates who have practiced law, so a few years of experience (particularly if you have been able to write as well) can be useful** (emphasis added).

So, you can see that there is a lot of preparation necessary if you are interested in transitioning from law firm practice to academia. That preparation will have to begin while you are practicing, and "publish or perish" still seems to be the law of the land in academia. Publishing law review articles or legal treatises when you are also practicing law is challenging, but it is not impossible. I have experience with this, and I lived to tell the story!

In a recent entry on the Marquette University Law School Faculty Blog on September 14, 2011, Lisa Mazzie, a professor at the law school, expressed some interesting views about how the current trend toward a greater emphasis on practical skills in law schools may benefit women. (http://law.marquette.edu/facultyblog/2011/09/14/the-making-of-a-law-professor/) She pointed out that the number of women on law faculties has improved in recent years but that it still does not reach half, particularly at the associate professor and full professor level. She cites statistics from the Association of American Law Schools showing that two-thirds of lecturers and instructors, which are non-tenure track positions, are women. According to Professor Mazzie, "a large number of women are found on the often lower-paying, lower prestige clinical and legal writing faculty, many of whom are not eligible for tenure." However, as the practical skills of legal writing and clinical practice experience are increasingly emphasized in law schools, it stands to reason that the tenure opportunities for women may increase as well.

Professor Mazzie also is concerned that, as the number of women in law school decreases, the number of women with the credentials for law teaching also will decrease. She considers that particularly problematic because it is important to her that women maintain a presence in the legal academy. Often those professors are the first women lawyers that women law students ever meet, and they become strong role models for what it is to be a woman lawyer.

Deborah Burand, a clinical professor at the University of Michigan Law School and former Vice President of Legal Affairs and General Counsel of the Overseas Private Investment Corporation (OPIC), is one of those academics who presents a particularly strong role model for young women lawyers. From law firm to non-profit sector to government to academia to government and back to academia again, her story underscores her commitment to following her dreams.

Be prepared to take a journey. Deborah Burand's story will give you valuable insight into not only academia but law firm practice and the world of non-profits. She has done it all and learned a lot. Consider yourself extremely lucky to have Deborah share her story with you.

Profile of Deborah Burand

Deborah Burand has done so many things in the private and public sectors that it is hard to keep all of them straight. She is a recognized expert on microfinance and most recently headed up the legal department of OPIC, the U.S. Government's development finance institution. However, most of all, she wants to be known as a professor of law. She has accomplished much in other arenas, but teaching is her calling and where she feels she makes the most impact. Those who have served her and those whom she has served may disagree, but, when you talk to Deborah Burand, she makes it clear where her priorities lie.

She has come a long way from a small town in the Midwest. After graduating *cum laude* from DePauw University, Deborah attended and graduated from Georgetown University with a joint degree combining a JD with a masters degree from the School of Foreign Service. She knew that she wanted to practice with a global law firm, and that is what she did. She wanted that experience because it could open up so many doors in other practice areas, and she met senior lawyers at Shearman & Sterling, who had enjoyed extraordinary careers that she could model. She accepted them as great mentors and learned all that she could from them.

New York City was a very different place than small town middle America, especially in the mid 1980's, and Deborah had to adapt to her new surroundings. Even the taxi cabs were a challenge until she learned that she needed to sit in the back seat, and revolving doors were a little intimidating, too. But, Deborah figured it all out in record time and developed as a young lawyer at that same pace. In her words, "I was growing at time-warp speed, such that the lawyer I was on a Friday was more skilled than the lawyer I had been on the prior Monday."

It was not long after joining Shearman & Sterling that Deborah began to reinvent herself, and, to date, she has reinvented herself multiple times. All of the shuffling started when she was a third-year associate and her client, a non-profit, wooed her to the client organization to help save diverse ecosystems. Deborah was so intrigued that she took a non-legal position to be a part of the cause. In that job, she helped conduct the first debt-for-nature swap in the world, and she went on to structure other similar transactions using Wall Street-like deal structures to support conservation finance needs.

Her job was fascinating for other reasons as well, and she hiked through rain forests and spent time with some of the world's most knowledgeable and inspirational conservationists. She held spider monkeys in her hands—and she was paid for all of these incredible experiences. However, the bubble burst when she saw her learning curve start to flatten out. In the end, she calculated that both she and the organization would benefit by her departure. Coincidentally, at the very same time, several of her mentors at Shearman & Sterling were in the process of recommending her for a job with the Federal Reserve Board. She took the job, and she was forever grateful that she had left her law firm on good terms and was in a position to get the recommendation.

Deborah spent five years at the Federal Reserve Board and later returned to Shearman & Sterling for three years before leaving to work for the Department of Treasury and, later, for two non-profit organizations focused on microfinance. Her experience can be categorized as private law practice, government, and non-profit, all in nearly equal measure in terms of time, and she is a wealth of information about all three. When asked what appealed to her about each professional setting and what were the greatest challenges of each, she responds

"Law firm: I really enjoyed the people I met at the law firm. I am a better lawyer because of their mentoring. The challenge for me was the crush of the long hours. One day, my secretary asked me why I had quit laughing at work, and I said that I was too tired to laugh any more. That response got my attention, and I did not last long at the firm after that.

Government: I have worked as a civil servant and, more recently, as a political appointee in the federal government. My most brilliant 'clients' were the people I worked for in government. Not only were some of them extraordinarily smart, but I often admired their value systems as much as their intelligence. For me the most challenging thing about government service was that I always wanted to be at the table when policy was being developed; however, the lawyers are not always invited to those discussions. I was disappointed when I was not invited, but I was euphoric when I was. Making good public policy can be extraordinarily rewarding.

Nonprofit: Although I have worked at three non-profit organizations, none of those positions has been as a lawyer. However, that is one of the things I enjoyed most about that work. I was able to stretch and develop skills that were far outside my legal talents, background and expertise. I had opportunities to manage and lead people that I would not have gotten in private practice, and I was able to travel far and wide and develop a global network that has benefitted me in so many other aspects of my personal and professional life.

The downside to nonprofit work is the emotional toll it can take on you because you expect so much from your job. You accept that you are not being paid well, so you put so much more stock in what you are accomplishing (what I call the "psychic income") to balance it off. Often in the non-profit sector, however, there is a shortage of not only financial capital but human capital. Matching grand visions to limited resources can be frustrating and emotionally draining. Downsizing dreams to what is achievable is hard—especially when the dream has the potential to change millions of lives for the better."

Change and more change. You see the pattern. Deborah says that change became a coping mechanism for her. She changed jobs frequently, but, in retrospect, she knows that shifting from job to job is not a very good way to advance professional growth. She says that, at some point, vertical growth is sacrificed for lateral growth. Deborah's salvation was that, although she had many jobs, she often followed colleagues from organization to organization. In the end, she is very satisfied with the skill-building, loyalty-driven trajectory that has characterized her career.

Deborah is particularly influenced by Malcolm Gladwell's book, the *Outliers*. Reading it made her realize that the keys to achieving extraordinary success are: 1) to be smart enough (not necessarily brilliant); and 2) to get others (bosses, peers, subordinates, other stakeholders) to invest in your success and growth. For her, that has meant providing as much support as she can to others. Deborah believes that investing in others has a boomerang effect and that, eventually, the fruits of that investment come back to you.

Deborah's best advice to young women lawyers is to "start where you are." A small step on behalf of something that interests you can set you on a course widely divergent from your peers. The step she took as a third-year associate at Shearman & Sterling taught her that legal skills, which are developed to serve corporate clients, can be put to use and become just as valuable in the service of a much wider range of organizations and missions.

With all the twists and turns in her career, would Deborah Burand do anything different? Her answer is "no." She might tweak some things, but she is very satisfied with the result. She wishes that she had learned earlier that "who" you work for is the most important career decision you can make. "What" you do is next in the order of importance, and "where" you do that work is a distant last. Deborah says that she would concentrate more on the "who" the next time around.

Most importantly, Deborah saved the best for last. Four years ago she joined the faculty of the University of Michigan Law School, and she believes it is the best job she has ever had. She is still passionate about changing the world, and now she is doing it from a different platform. She enjoys sharing her experiences and helping to nurture the abilities and interests of her students "as they too touch the world." She teaches in a clinical setting (an international transactions clinic—the first of its kind in the world) and feels that she is growing right along with her students. Her experience in microfinance and nonprofits is a perfect fit for the position. Initially, she had to be cajoled to consider academia, but she never looks back. Returning to the Midwest after 25 years and to a more traditional legal setting was not on her dance card, but fate intervened.

> "While I was debating the pros and cons of the faculty position, I decided to go to church to quiet myself. Sitting behind me in a pew was a woman who I recognized but could not place. I turned my head to get a closer look and, yes, I knew it—she was my contracts professor during my first year in law school. She was my only female law professor that year and the first female lawyer I had ever met at the time. She showed me that a girl from small-town Indiana could achieve her dreams. I scribbled a message on the offertory envelope and handed it to her—only to find that she remembered me after so many years, including my full name!
>
> When I finally had an opportunity to talk to her after church, I told her how lucky I was to meet her again while I was in the throes of this big decision. Her response was, 'This is not luck, Deborah. This is divine. It was meant to be.'"

Divine, indeed. Deborah Burand took that job, and she considers herself blessed. She has come full circle.

For more information on Deborah Burand and her publications, please consult her faculty bio on the University of Michigan Law School web site at www.law.umich.edu.

Law school administration and student services is another popular landing spot for lawyers transitioning from private practice. For some insight into that world and those experiences, meet Markeisha Miner, Assistant Dean of Outreach and Career Services, University of Detroit Mercy School of Law.

Profile of Markeisha Miner

Markeisha Miner can easily light up a room with her warm smile and effervescence. That has served her well in her role as the Assistant Dean of Career Services and Outreach at the University of Detroit Mercy School of Law, an administrative position she assumed in 2008. Detroit has been a challenging venue since the economic collapse of that same year, but Markeisha loves her city and remains positive and supportive, and that attitude carries over to her students, colleagues, alumni, and prospective employers. She is a woman who knows how to make a difference, one small step at a time.

Markeisha broke some molds growing up in Detroit. She is "a first"— the first person in her immediate family to graduate from college and the first to attend professional school. She graduated *magna cum laude* and Phi Beta Kappa from Mount Holyoke College and then from the University of Michigan Law School, where she was an editor of the *Journal of Race and the Law*. She also had an externship at the Commission on Gender Equality in Durban, South Africa during law school, and she worked with Michigan's Legal Assistance for Urban Communities Clinic on community development projects in Detroit. She continued on this road of excellence and earned a clerkship with a Federal Judge in Michigan, and she landed summer associate positions with two prestigious law firms. She received associate attorney offers from both and chose the Dickinson Wright firm based in Detroit. For Markeisha, home was very important, and Detroit was home.

She enjoyed experiences that she never dreamed she would have, and she did not take anything for granted. As an associate at a top law firm, Markeisha worked hard. She appreciated the depth and breadth of practice areas, the sophisticated legal issues, the diversity of the client base, and the capable and seasoned lawyers who were her colleagues and who served as excellent resources. She invested an incredible amount of time in not only her practice but in the activities that contributed to "the life of the firm." She understood that those non-billable activities are important to the business side of firms, but she also came to realize that those activities can consume young associates, especially attorneys of color and women, and that the rewards are not measured in the same way as billable hours.

After four years in private practice, Markeisha began to contemplate something different. She knew that it was time to do something for herself and for others in the tradition of her family. Taking the first step, however, was not easy because her accomplishments got in the way. The law firm leadership had assured her that she soon would be nominated for partnership at the firm, where very few minority women had risen to that level, particularly those who came from the ranks of summer associates. She was being given greater responsibility for cases, her client contacts were increasing, and the litigation opportunities were coming her way. She was in such a desirable position that her confidants thought she was "crazy" for even thinking of leaving the firm.

Her decision became easier when an opportunity in law school administration came along. It was "a natural fit" for her. She had spent many years in volunteer activities involving students, from being the youth director of her church to serving as her college's alumnae recruitment representative for the Detroit area. Working in law school administration was an extension of some of those experiences, and Markeisha knew she would love it. She would be in a position to help students articulate and achieve their career goals, and Markeisha knew that you could not put a price on those kinds of experiences. The University of Detroit Mercy Law School had announced bold, innovative initiatives that were receiving national attention, and Markeisha wanted to be a part of that wave.

Markeisha's family also played an important role in her decision. Although she was single with no dependents when she began the transition from law firm to academia, Markeisha wanted to spend more time with her father than her life in private practice had allowed. Her father passed away less than a year after she assumed her new position at the law school, and she always will be grateful for the increased time that she was able to spend with him during that year. At about that same time, Markeisha's family life also changed in another very positive and wonderful way when she married a widower with two children. She had the time she needed to devote to her new family, and she was certain that she had made the right choice for all of the right reasons.

Markeisha's time at the University of Detroit Mercy Law School has been every bit as exciting and rewarding as she knew it would be. She left her law firm with the blessing of her colleagues, although they had tried hard to convince her to stay. She has not burned the bridges to law firms that she knows are so important to the work that she does at the law school, and she can use her experience as a litigator to help her students choose the right course for them. She knows that she is in a position to make a difference for students and for the legal community, and that is what Markeisha Miner is all about.

Markeisha finds the energy, enthusiasm and optimism of the students and the entrepreneurial faculty and administration at the law school to be invigorating. She loves the opportunity to be in a scholarly environment, and she has an outlet for her love of writing. Continuing her relationships with former colleagues in private practice is good for business, and she enjoys the work that she does with local and national bar associations that are part of her work on behalf of the law school. She now has more time to build relationships with students, attorneys, and administrators—both on the employer side and on the academic side—without the demand of billable hours.

However, there have been challenges to the new position. Markeisha has found that the resources in academia are not as extensive as those in private practice, and she has had to gain new skills in the areas of marketing, gathering and reporting statistics, and event planning. She has learned to maximize the resources available to her, and she has become skilled at partnering with bar associations and other departments at the law school and at the university to deliver key programs to law students. She also has learned to utilize the information published by industry-specific organizations to enhance legal recruitment opportunities.

Among the skills that Markeisha considers most important to success in career services are developing and maintaining relationships with students, with employers, with faculty, with alumni, with other administrators, and with other career services professionals. Quality client service, efficient time management, attention to detail, and enthusiastic advocacy for students and for her department are also skills she values. Being attentive to the cost of services and being able to justify expenditures are also critical to success.

Markeisha Miner's best advice to young women lawyers is to 'find your voice' by listening to your 'inner self' and to follow your dreams. For those who are interested in transitioning from private practice to law school administration, Markeisha advises them to talk to others who have made the transition. She describes career services professionals as congenial, welcoming, helpful and willing to share experiences and ideas. She also suggests researching information about the current state of the law profession and employment markets that are published by the American Bar Association and the National Association for Legal Career Professionals (NALP). She cautions that compensation and bonuses for law school administrators are not as flexible as in private practice and that it is important to negotiate the best salary and benefits package at the beginning without much expectation for future adjustments.

Markeisha has learned a lot from her experiences. She has learned that a law degree leads to a vast array of opportunities and that law firm practice is only one of them. She also has learned that law firms need to protect the talent that they have and let the young attorneys know that they are

223

appreciated. She would like to see institutionalized objective means of tracking the types of work that attorneys are assigned so that there is some control on the quality of work given and completed to assure equal opportunity for upward mobility. She believes that the practice of assigning work based on the assigning attorney's "comfort level with individual attorneys" should be eliminated.

She also thinks that it is imperative for law firms to make greater efforts to recognize the value of women lawyers. Markeisha knows that the best-qualified female lawyers, especially women of color, are in high demand and that, if those women do not receive fulfilling, stimulating work at one firm, they will leave to go to another. Firms will lose out on their talent investment unless they are willing to open a dialogue with the women about what the women want and how the firm can work with them in achieving their goals. Markeisha also reflects on her own experience in practice and knows that diversity must be a "top-down mandate" implemented and demonstrated by the firm's leadership. If diversity is valued, then activities promoting diversity should be shepherded by attorneys from all backgrounds, both women and men.

It is apparent that Markeisha Miner is a tireless advocate of her city, her profession, her law school and her students. She accepts the challenge at all levels and faces each day with enthusiasm and a winning smile. She is doing what she loves, and she is very good at it. She knew enough to grab the brass ring, and she works hard to pass that same attitude and confidence on to others. Without question, she has found her calling.

For more information on Markeisha Miner, please consult her bio on the University of Detroit Mercy School of Law website at www.law.udmercy.edu.

From Law Firm to the Judiciary

Fortunately, this transition is not so uncommon for women any more. We now have many more women lawyers on the bench, including on the highest court of the land where one-third of the United States Supreme

Court Justices are women. A recent study by the University of Albany shows that women in 2011 held 23% of all federal judgeships and 27% of all state-level positions in the judiciary. This number is growing: the 2010 levels were 22% and 26% respectively. (http://www.albany.edu/womeningov/judgeship _report_partII.pdf). Although membership in the judiciary at all levels is highly regarded, you will find that there are many important considerations to this particular transition. We, as women in the profession, are grateful for the women lawyers who make these critical transitions to bring the female perspective to the rule of law.

The Honorable Marianne Short, Managing Partner of Dorsey & Whitney since 2007 and a former judge and prosecutor, is a recognized mentor and role model for young women lawyers. Ms. Short left private practice for the bench and then returned to private practice after a star-studded career as a judge in state court.

When I heard Marianne Short deliver the keynote address at a Women's Legal Conference in New York City in the Spring of 2011, I felt like there was an echo in the room. Everything she said made perfect sense to me, and it was like she was reading my mind on the subjects of women in the law, how we are going to advance them, and the talent drain that law firms are experiencing. It is one thing to know the right things to say; it is quite another to have lived them all. It was clear that Marianne Short not only "talked the talk," but also "walked the walk."

As the Managing Partner of Dorsey & Whitney and a former Minnesota state appellate judge, Marianne Short has experienced the law from a variety of perspectives. She is a no-nonsense woman with a great sense of humor and a winning smile, and she excels as a storyteller. She hails from a big Irish family, and I think storytelling comes naturally for her. I also think that her nurturing and caring ways have their beginnings as a part of that family and later in her experiences raising her own two children while practicing law. When she looks back on her career, Marianne says that one thing she might do differently is to have more children, and it is clear that she really enjoys the ones she has. Her bio says that she is an avid distance runner and Alpine skier "to keep up with her boys."

Distance running and skiing also may give her the energy to achieve at such a high level in the law. She has been recognized as one of "America's Leading Business Lawyers" by *Chambers USA*, as the "Top 10 in Minnesota (2010) Super Lawyers," and the "Best Lawyers 2010 Minneapolis Bet-the-Company Litigator of the Year," to name just a few accolades.

Not surprisingly, Marianne Short's personal philosophy is "Reach for the stars and if you end up on the moon, you will be happy." It is exactly what you would expect from someone with the kind of positive attitude that she exudes. She describes herself as someone who "thinks big and believes in miracles. I encourage everyone to be bold." Here is her remarkable story.

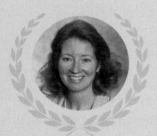

Profile of Honorable Marianne Short

Although she is a Minnesota native, Marianne's march to the top of her profession all started in and around Boston. That is where she spent her college years (Newton College of the Sacred Heart—before it merged with Boston College) and that is where she attended and graduated from Boston College Law School.

After graduating from law school, Marianne went to work for the Minnesota Attorney General. She was given hands-on courtroom experience and worked with bright, young colleagues and for a "dedicated and decent AG." She left public service several years later because she "wanted to learn how to try cases from more experienced litigators and to benefit from in-house experts in numerous areas of the law." For her, Dorsey & Whitney, with its home office in Minneapolis, fit the bill.

Her expectations for private practice were met immediately. She joined a seasoned, specialized and robust trial department and, during her associate years, she was able to observe, model and adapt her work habits, courtroom styles and client relationship skills from all of the partners in the firm. Marianne thrived in this fast-paced litigation environment, but her personal circumstances initiated a detour in her career—if you can call a Gubernatorial judicial appointment a detour at all!

As it happened, closing the window on the career of one pioneer woman jurist opened the door for another. With the death of Judge Suzanne Sedgwick, the Governor of Minnesota chose Marianne to replace Judge Sedgwick on the Minnesota Court of Appeals. Marianne was more than happy to agree to this appointment because she had a new baby, another child entering kindergarten, and her husband traveled a lot in his work. The work-life challenges were likely to be fewer with this judicial appointment, and off Marianne went to the bench where she stayed for more than a decade.

Although the work-life challenges proved to be more manageable, the transition to the bench was very difficult. Marianne had become accustomed to a much quicker work pace in private practice, and the slower pace at the court did not suit her as well. She experienced feelings of isolation in chambers and missed the "give and take" among professional colleagues. She also felt "smothered" by being in the public eye—or the "public fishbowl" as she refers to it. On the other side of the scale, Marianne liked serving the public and had great respect for her fellow public servants.

At the end of nearly twelve years as a Minnesota Court of Appeals judge, Marianne was ready to return to a more fast-paced legal position. Her older son was leaving for college, and her younger son was entering junior high school. She was delighted to be enthusiastically welcomed back to practice at Dorsey & Whitney, which, by that time, had become a national law firm. However, Marianne soon discovered that the practice had changed dramatically while she was away. The advent of computers alone was "scary," not to mention e-mail correspondence, and there were new management systems and processes to master, and a whole new set of faces. Marianne spent many days and nights wondering what she had been thinking! During some of those moments of doubt, she found herself missing the civilized life of an appellate judge.

However, as time went on, Marianne readjusted to big firm litigation, and she particularly enjoyed working with clients again on challenging legal matters and setting strategy for the firm. She learned how to balance the various requirements of the job, including mentoring, business development, and keeping current on expertise and management responsibilities.

Seven years after Marianne returned to Dorsey & Whitney, she was elected Managing Partner and became the first woman to serve in that leadership position in the firm's history. As Managing Partner, she manages the operations of the law firm's 650 attorneys and 19 offices in the United States, Canada, Asia, Australia and England. She chairs the Management Committee and serves on the Policy Committee. Prior to being elected to Managing Partner and now in that position, Marianne takes her managment responsibilities at her law firm very seriously, particularly on matters including compensation, professional reviews, and recruiting. She has since become a popular speaker on these and other subjects at legal conferences throughout the country.

When Marianne Short speaks, people listen. She is succinct and gets to the point. She understands the value of time, and she makes sure that everyone in the audience walks out with valuable "take aways." In many of her speeches, she advises women lawyers on leadership and divides her advice into three stages (early, middle and senior practice years).

In the early practice years, which she describes as "Positioning for the Spotlight," Marianne recommends the following. Know yourself and identify your strengths and weaknesses. Do this annually and figure out what "makes you tick" and gives you energy. Identify opportunities for improvement and act on them. Set your personal vision and goals and make sure that they are authentic. She also advises you to work hard and absorb (observe what works for others and mimic it) and seize opportunities and take risks. Aspire to and campaign for positions of leadership. Take it easy, and don't burn out. She also emphasizes building relationships and developing a leadership style, and she points out the need for good judgment and compassion to achieve these goals. Her best recommendations for developing a good leadership style are to collaborate, empower others through delegation and trust, avoid micromanaging, be liberal with thanks and praise, and make work as much fun as possible.

In the middle years, "Earning the Spotlight," Marianne suggests increased focus and adjusting personal vision and goals. Make your mark through leadership during these years, thrive on challenges and stretch to meet them. Don't be afraid of change, and avoid comfortable and stagnant positions. Renew relationships, seek advice from trusted colleagues and mentors, and give advice to reach your potential. Look forward and take advantage of other work opportunities if your expectations are not met. And, finally, network, network, network.

In the senior years, the theme is "Sharing the Spotlight." Marianne recommends that you stay relevant by inspiring others to continue your vision and goals, remain humble and acknowledge your own past mistakes in counseling others. Never rest and always make room for growth. Listen, encourage and assist others. Do not play favorites, nurture leadership in colleagues, and give back.

Marianne ends most of her speeches by reminding her audience that, "Life is a motion picture, not a still frame. Be bold. Reach for the stars." She wants all young attorneys to know that the profession is worth the tremendous efforts required. She says she wishes that she had relaxed more along the way, but, then, I wonder about that . . . I really can't see her happy in a hammock. She is a bundle of energy, and you can't help feeling energized when you are around her.

So, there you have it. A roadmap to success! Marianne hopes that at the end of her career someone will think that she "succeeded in making a difference."

I don't think there is a problem with that!

For more information on Ms. Short and her publications, please consult her partner bio on the Dorsey & Whitney web page at www.dorsey.com.

From Law Firm to Alternative Dispute Resolution

Hopefully you all know how helpful alternative dispute resolution (ADR) can be to resolving controversies and reducing docket overcrowding in courts throughout this country. The Alternative Dispute Resolution Act of 1998, 28 U.S.C. §651 et seq. describes alternative dispute resolution as "any process or procedure, other than an adjudication by a presiding judge, in which a neutral third party participates to assist in the resolution of issues in controversy, through processes such as early neutral evaluation, mediation, minitrial, and arbitration. . . ." Almost every jurisdiction has adopted such a practice to help speed along dispute resolution and unclog court calendars.

The alternative dispute resolution practice in this country has grown exponentially within the last ten years, not only because of the burden on court calendars and the desire to achieve more speedy resolution of disputes but also because some parties view the alternative processes as more cost effective than resolving issues in a court of law.

Today, it is estimated that there are as many as 6,920 legal practitioners who are involved in mediation and arbitration practices. (http://www.bls.gov/oes/current/oes231022.htm#(1)). Although many of those practitioners transition to the ADR practice after retiring from law firms and other legal practice settings, it is becoming more and more popular for practitioners in the middle years of practice to choose this alternative.

One person who knows all about this process and can tell you how her work as an Alternative Dispute Resolution expert evolved from her years in litigation is Victoria Pynchon, principal at *She Negotiates* and contributor to *Forbes Woman* on line. She also is a weekly host on New Day Talk Radio's "Negotiating Women" show, and she has been featured on National Public Radio's "All Things Considered." She excelled as a litigator and loved the thrill of it. Why did she leave the world of Big Law after all that success? Read on for the answers and to get to know Victoria Pynchon.

Profile of Victoria Pynchon

Victoria Pynchon was a model student. She even was valedictorian of her Junior High School class, something that may be unique to California. She graduated from the University of California San Diego and received her law degree from University of California Davis School of Law, where she was Order of the Coif. She went on to receive a Master of Laws degree from the Strauss Institute of Dispute Resolution at Pepperdine University School of Law.

After law school, Victoria followed her dream to be a trial lawyer. Her father was a lawyer, and trial work had always interested her. She did not go to Big Law at first, but, instead, she took a job with a two-man law firm because she wanted to learn how to try a case to a jury. The firm promised her that experience and made good on the promise, and after two years Victoria felt that she could represent "anyone, anytime, anywhere in response to any type of injustice." However, hard times hit the law firm, and Victoria lost her position in the cutbacks. But, she bounced back and landed a job with a prestigious commercial litigation firm that was more in line with her law school ambitions. Her practice areas included antitrust, securities fraud, intellectual property disputes, environmental insurance coverage law, and general commercial litigation in the finance, professional practice, manufacturing, health care, consumer product, and technology industries.

Over the next 25 years, Victoria practiced with three more law firms and took two years away from practice to explore teaching business law to undergraduates at the California State University at Northridge. She found that teaching lacked some of the intellectual challenge and stimulation that she needed and concluded that she actually liked the stress of practice. Her journey gave her a clear view of the upsides and downsides of law practice, and here is the way she sees that tradeoff.

On the benefits side of law firm practice, Victoria identifies: Stimulating intellectual work; collaborating with bright, ambitious, hard-working, creative and boisterous people; representing bright, hard-working, interesting, creative, ambitious, and entrepreneurial, managerial, and executive clients; constant challenge and expectation for improvement; financial security; prestige; autonomy; and the thrill of the chase. Detriments include: All consuming professional life leaving little time for personal life; unbounded adversarialism that sometimes interferes with relationships with colleagues; pressure to develop work; boring tasks like discovery and document review; unprepared judges; and clients with unrealistic expectations.

Victoria also recognizes the shortcomings of law firms in terms of eliminating gender bias. She looks forward to the day when law firm managers develop programs that are reflective of the consciousness of bias and the desire to eliminate it in the workplace—programs that respect the difficult choices that women professionals have to make and accommodate motherhood without judgments about dedication, reliability and priorities. Although these bias issues do not seem to have been limitations for Victoria Pynchon, she hopes for better days for all women in the profession.

Eventually, Victoria applied her introspection and analysis to a decision that shaped her future. She traded in the adversarialism that had become a burden to her in private practice for the cooperation inherent in an ADR practice. After three years as lead counsel on a huge antitrust litigation matter, which settled before trial, Victoria was exhausted from the adversarial process. She decided to take a course on "Mediating the Litigated Case," and she had an epiphany. As she describes, "It was as if the heavens were torn open and the angels descended." It felt right to her from the beginning, and she threw herself into it.

However, there still is room for improvement in the dispute resolution system, and Victoria Pynchon knows it. She looks forward to the day when the adversarial system is modified to accommodate the speed of commerce and include adjudicative and dispute resolution procedures that are sufficiently efficient and effective for the needs of 21st century business enterprises.

Transitions can be hard, and Victoria encountered challenges in the new practice. A solo ADR practice of the kind that Victoria fashioned was not likely to generate profit for a while. Fortunately, Victoria had resources to get her through the initial stages of the practice, and that put her in a "blessed position." Learning to market her services, to manage cash flow, and to develop and stick to a business plan were additional challenges and involved new skills that she had to acquire. The change from self-described "adversarial zealot and Queen of the Jungle" to neutral, impartial mediator was particularly difficult. "These are very disparate situations—one focusing on protecting rights and seeking remedies on behalf of a client and the other focusing on understanding the various parties' desires, needs, fears, preferences, priorities and constraints and reaching a solution that is more mutually beneficial. The total transition took six years." Victoria was fortunate to have the support and help of ADR practitioners, who generously shared their wisdom, knowledge, insight and skills with her.

She was drawn to Alternative Dispute Resolution because of "the efficient, effective, collaborative resolution of disputes in which the parties' resources go directly to solving the problem not into the *process* of solving it—or failing to solve it." Victoria's new practice setting is similar to a solo practitioner, even though she sits on an ADR panel (ADR Services, Inc.) and mediates for the American Arbitration Association in Los Angeles. She finds it a much lonelier practice than being in a law firm, and she misses having colleagues and working in teams. However, she loves the autonomy and the entrepreneurial opportunities her new practice allows for her professionally. She has developed a training and consulting business (*She Negotiates*), she is the author of two books, and she also writes for *ForbesWoman* online with her "She Negotiates" column.

Victoria Pynchon is very busy, but she loves what she does. She was more than happy to trade the rush of litigation for the interesting future prospects she found with her new choice of practice. Although it appears that she has been very successful, Victoria has this to say about success.

> "You're never successful. The day I'm successful is the day I drop in my tracks. I continue to address the challenges of running my own business, generating clients, improving my skills and being the calm center of any dispute people have asked me to help them resolve."

Among the skills that Victoria considers most valuable to an ADR practice are empathy, creativity, persistence, listening more than talking, and searching for answers more than giving answers. She also values a fairly deep understanding of business and business people, which helps her build trust with clients, humility in the face of conflict, and belief that any problem is solvable.

Her best advice to young women lawyers who are interested in ADR is to follow your heart, be the best in your field, pay close attention to the adequacy of your financial resources, build a network of people who support you in your goals, join professional organizations and work hard. She also emphasizes the value of being generous of spirit and learning to accept advice you do not want to hear. "Be authentic, be passionate about what you do and communicate that passion to the people you meet. Most importantly, have fun with whatever you choose."

Twenty-five years is a long time to practice law, and you do not have to wait that long to make a transition if you need one. However, we all should be grateful that Victoria Pynchon took her time. During her long law practice career, she forged paths for all women attorneys. Her legacy is two-fold: As a litigator and as an ADR specialist. We owe her a debt of gratitude for introducing new pathways for women attorneys.

For more information on Ms. Pynchon, her services and her publications, please consult her web site at www.victoriapynchon.com.

So, that's a wrap for Careers in Transition—at least for this book. In addition to these models, there are many other opportunities for lawyers outside the practice of law. You may be aware of some of these opportunities, but they are worth mentioning here.

By now you know that my goal is to keep you *in* law practice where I think you bring the greatest benefit to the profession and take the greatest advantage of your background and education. However, the main goal is to see you happy, and some of the opportunities outside of law practice may suit you best. The bottom line is that a law degree is a terrible thing to waste. Use it inside the practice or outside the practice. Just USE IT!

The opportunities for lawyers in business and entrepreneurship are replete, and it is not at all uncommon to encounter business moguls who also are lawyers. To get your research started, below is a list of some common areas of opportunity for lawyers outside law practice.

Government administration and politics

Lobbying

Human resources

Education and academic administration

Financial planning and advising

Journalism

Banking and finance

Agency representation for artists, writers, performers and athletes

Legal writing, editing, and publishing

Legal headhunter

Foreign service officer; and

Special agent (FBI, CIA, DEA or DOJ)

For more information about opportunities for lawyers outside of law practice, consult the following online sources:

Options for Unhappy Lawyers

www.martynemko.com/articles/options-for-unhappy-lawyers_ id1270;

From Lawyer to Law-Related Position

http://www.infirmation.com/articles/one-article.tcl?article_id=922;

Career Alternatives for Lawyers

http://www.cba.org/cba/practicelink/careerbuilders_advancement/ alternatives.aspx; and

Create a New Career Outside the Law

http://www.thecompletelawyer.com/create-a-new-career-outside- the-law.html.

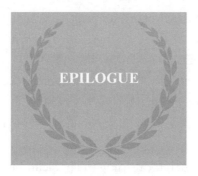

From a Queen of Reinvention

This concludes what I think you REALLY need to know about the *new balance* of work/self/home and family and how to be happy and have satisfying careers in the law, which may include successful transitions. There is much more to be explored, and I hope this will be only the beginning of the journey for you.

In reading and digesting this material, please remember that Rome was not built in a day, and a satisfying and successful career and personal life do not develop overnight. You will have ups and downs, and it is important that you keep your eyes on the end game. Sometimes the best and most effective lessons are the products of mistakes. Mistakes are not inherently bad. They only are bad when you refuse to acknowledge them and learn from them.

Take the time—there is that word again—TIME!—to examine your personal and professional lives and to explore the possibilities for making changes that will benefit you on both sides of the ledger. It will make you a happier person and a more satisfied lawyer if you achieve the *new balance* that is premised on modern young women lawyers.

Some of my friends and colleagues have called me the Queen of Reinvention. It is a title that I am proud of, and I have had a very interesting career as the result of all the twists and turns and interesting transitions. I have practiced law with three law firms, headed up a legislative office in public service, and raised record amounts of money for charities in my off-ramp years. Some of these changes in direction were more difficult than others, but they all were worthwhile and achieved my goal at the time.

Most recently, of course, I left law practice to concentrate on writing and speaking and consulting to help young women lawyers like you. It has been the highlight of my career. I love meeting all of you as I travel around the country, and I learn so much from you.

Thank you very much for reading the book and lending support to the *Best Friends at the Bar* project in so many ways. You are doing a great service to your profession by spreading the word that women can be in control of their own destinies, and you are following the model of the book. You are Paying It Forward, one woman lawyer at a time. Truly, I could not have asked for more.

I hope that you will keep in touch. Let me know if I can help you, and follow me on my web site at www.bestfriendsatthebar.com. Blog with me—I would love to hear from you. Put my information on your Facebook, your LinkedIn, and Twitter about it. Stay in touch with your women colleagues and offer them assistance. Become someone else's Best Friend at the Bar!

In addition to speaking at law schools, law firms and law organizations, I also provide individual counseling and group services, and I consult to law firms and law organizations about issues of balance, retention and advancement.

God's speed. I look forward to seeing you along the road. You will recognize me because I will be the one cheering you on.

TRANSFORMING

Violence

TRANSFORMING
Violence

Linking Local and
Global Peacemaking

Edited by Judy Zimmerman Herr
and Robert Herr

Foreword by Konrad Raiser

A Pandora Press U.S. Book

Herald
Press

Scottdale, Pennsylvania
Waterloo, Ontario

Library of Congress Cataloging-in-Publication Data
Transforming Violence : Linking Local and Global Peacemaking / edited by
Robert Herr and Judy Zimmerman Herr ; foreword by Konrad Raiser.
    p. cm.
    "A Pandora Press U.S. book"
    Includes bibliographical references and index.
    ISBN 0-8361-9098-X (alk. paper)
    1. Peace. 2. Peace—Religious aspects—Christianity. 3. Peace move-
ments. 4. Political violence—Prevention. I. Herr, Judy Zimmerman, 1952-.
II. Herr, Robert, 1948-.
JZ5582.094 1998
261.8′73—'dc21   98-27615
                                                   CIP

The paper used in this publication is recycled and meets the minimum
requirements of American National Standard for Information Sciences—
Permanence of Paper for Printed Library Materials, ANSI Z39.48-1984.

TRANSFORMING VIOLENCE
Copyright © 1998 by Herald Press, Scottdale, Pa. 15683
        Published simultaneously in Canada by Herald Press,
        Waterloo, Ont. N2L 6H7. All rights reserved
Library of Congress Catalog Number: 98-27615
International Standard Book Number: 0-8361-9098-X
Printed in the United States of America
Book design by Michael A. King, Pandora Press U.S., in consultation with
Jim Butti, Herald Press
Cover design by Gwen M. Stamm, Herald Press

07 06 05 04 03 02 01 00 99 98 10 9 8 7 6 5 4 3 2 1

*To Reverend Michael Robert Zigler,
A Church of the Brethren delegate to the 1948 Amsterdam
inaugural meeting of the World Council of Churches.
An early member of the WCC Central Committee, Zigler
frequently asked, "When will Christians stop killing each
other?" At one meeting he formally moved that
"We eliminate war among us as Christians."
His motion failed for lack of a second . . . but his witness
continues to call all of us to a life of peacemaking.[1]*

ACKNOWLEDGMENTS

Chapter 2, "Jesus' Third Way," originally appeared in Walter Wink, *Violence and Nonviolence in South Africa: Jesus' Third Way* (Philadelphia, Pa. and Santa Cruz, Calif.: New Society Publishers, 1987). Used by permission of the author.

Chapter 3, "Mysticism and Resistance," was translated from the German by Mark Janzen.

Chapter 5, "The Politics of Forgiveness," is based on the Gandhi Memorial Lecture, organized by the Gandhi Smriti and Darshan Samiti on August 21, 1993, in New Delhi, India. The lecture was subsequently published under the title, "The Politics of Forgiveness: Islamic Teachings and Gandhi's Thoughts," in *Gandhi and Global Nonviolent Transformation*, edited by Dr. N. Radhakrishnan (New Delhi: Gandhi Smriti and Darshan Samiti, 1994), and in a revised form in *The Nonviolent Crescent: Two Essays on Islam and Nonviolence*, No. 3 in the Patterns in Reconciliation Occasional Paper Series (Alkmar: International Fellowship of Reconciliation, 1996). Used here by permission of IFOR, the Gandhi Smriti and Darshan Samiti, and the author.

Chapter 7, "Cultures of Peace and Communities of Faith," was first given as a talk at the UNESCO Conference on "The Contribution by Religions to the Culture of Peace," Barcelona, Spain, December 1994.

Chapter 11, "Churches in a Planet-Sized Peacemaking System," is based on a presentation, "The View from UN Plaza," presented to the Quaker Peace Round Table, Pendle Hill, Pennsylvania, 1996.

Chapter 15, "Providing Space for Change in Mozambique": the author would like to express his thanks to Emily Marino, a writer of many qualities, for her invaluable help with this article.

Contents

Foreword by Konrad Raiser • 9
Preface • 11
*Introduction: Crisis and Opportunity, by Robert Herr and Judy
        Zimmerman Herr* • 13

FOUNDATIONS FOR A JUST PEACE • 21

Chapter 1 Soldiers of Christ • 23
            Jim Forest

Chapter 2 Jesus' Third Way • 34
            Walter Wink

Chapter 3 Mysticism and Resistance • 48
            Dorothee Soelle

Chapter 4 Just Peacemaking • 53
            Duane K. Friesen & Glen H. Stassen

Chapter 5 The Politics of Forgiveness • 68
            Chaiwat Satha-Anand

Chapter 6 Reconstruction: Healing a Nation's Soul • 79
            Gerald J. Pillay

A LOCAL CULTURE OF PEACE • 91

Introduction by Judy Zimmerman Herr • 93

Chapter 7 Cultures of Peace and Communities of Faith • 95
            Elise Boulding

Chapter 8 Neighbors in the Bosnian Tragedy • 105
            Doug Hostetter

Chapter 9 Building Community Peace in South Africa • 119
Andries Odendaal & Chris Spies

Chapter 10 Breaking the Cycle of Violence in Wajir • 133
Dekha Ibrahim & Janice Jenner

A GLOBAL CULTURE OF PEACE • 149
Introduction by Robert Herr • 151

Chapter 11 Churches in a Planet-Sized Peacemaking System • 153
David Jackman

Chapter 12 Exploring Civilian Peace Teams • 161
Lisa Schirch

Chapter 13 Applying Civilian Peace Teams • 168
Kathleen Kern

Chapter 14 Remember and Change • 177
John Paul Lederach

Chapter 15 Providing Space for Change in Mozambique • 190
Andrea Bartoli

Chapter 16 Human Rights: Dignity, Community, Freedom • 203
Martin Shupack & Rachel Brett

PEACEMAKING IN ECUMENICAL PERSPECTIVE • 217
Chapter 17 Theology for a Just Peace • 219
Lauree Hersch Meyer

Notes • *231*
Bibliography • *243*
Index • *245*
The Contributors • *251*
About Herald Press, Pandora Press, and Pandora Press U.S. • *256*

Foreword

A book on local and global strategies for Christian peacemaking comes at the right moment. With the end of the Cold War and the first steps towards effective disarmament, the issue of peace seems largely to have disappeared from the public agenda. At the same time, after removal of the restraints imposed by the balance of power and mutual destruction, there seems to be an explosion of violent conflicts and of brutal fighting, especially within national boundaries. The development of effective strategies for peacemaking is therefore more urgent than ever.

The World Council of Churches has a particular reason to welcome this book. Three years ago, at a meeting of its Central Committee in Johannesburg, the WCC launched a "Programme to Overcome Violence." Lest this formulation seem too presumptuous—as if the churches or the WCC knew how to overcome violence and could teach everybody else—the objective of the program was stated positively, as contributing to the building of a "culture of peace." The present publication operates in this same dialectic: overcoming violence and Christian peacemaking.

The historic peace churches and the Fellowship of Reconciliation have been committed to peacemaking long before this was affirmed as an ecumenical imperative. When the mainline churches were still concerned with asking the question whether and under what circumstances war could be considered an "act of justice," the historic peace churches had long since begun to work on the basic elements of the theory and practice of a "just peace."

With the apparent convergence of agendas, a new phase in the relationship and cooperation between the WCC and the peace churches has begun. This book builds on the long experience with local and global strategies for peacemaking and can therefore serve as an important re-source for all who want to help build a culture of peace. It also evaluates critically the political, theological, and spiritual lessons learned by those who have been engaged in the task of peacemaking already for decades. It is my hope, therefore, that this valuable publication will find a wide and attentive audience.

—Konrad Raiser,
General Secretary,
World Council of Churches

Preface

We live facing a new millennium, in an age of new hopes but also great fears. The last ten years have seen changes in political configurations, economic structures, and information flows. In such times, an important discipline is to focus on the lives of real people and their work. Stories like these can anchor us in the life of the church as it is experienced, through times of hope and optimism as well as a through fears and crises.

The practical peacemaking work of Christians has expanded considerably in recent years. A decade ago the focus of a book such as this would almost certainly have been on the constant threat of nuclear war. Today the emphasis is on the need to build a just peace in more direct and tangible ways. The large issues and threats are still with us, but our response is led by the stories of communities mobilizing to resolve problems through immediate and direct participation.

The Historic Peace Church and Fellowship of Reconciliation Consultative Committee has often, since its beginnings thirty years ago, produced books and study documents to further understanding of and commitment to peacemaking. Its primary mandate has been to place this discussion on the agenda of the ecumenical movement. This book is another contribution to this process, looking toward the December 1998 World Council of Churches Assembly in Harare, Zimbabwe. These accounts, contributed to the larger effort of the Programme to Overcome Violence, present a picture of people effectively and successfully responding to the call to build communities of peace.

The book grew out of a meeting called by the Historic Peace Churches/Fellowship of Reconciliation Committee in December 1993.

One year after the international military peacekeeping intervention in Somalia, the meeting struggled to understand the changes taking place with the end of the Cold War and the role of peace churches and fellowships in the new world we were facing. In a world entering a new millennium and grappling with new configurations of power, what could we share that would contribute to peace? As we reflected on such questions, the idea was born to pull together readings to form a book that would include spiritual and biblical bases and practical stories of peacebuilding.

We are especially pleased with the generous response from the numerous authors that contributed to this work. When the Committee initially envisioned putting together such a book, we listed possible writers from within our own confessional circles. However, as we talked further, we realized that work for peace is happening across the divides of denominations and faiths. It then became our goal to include as writers persons from a variety of traditions, all of whom share with us a commitment to peacemaking that grows out of faith. In this way, the book itself can be a sign that peace requires the involvement of all.

The authors whose works are included here graciously worked with us through various stages of editing, deadlines, and requests. We thank them all for their contributions to the collection and trust that in our editing we enabled their voices to come through. Our thanks also to others who helped with the process, including Roger Epp and Ernie Regehr, and to the members of the committee: Lamar Gibble, Duane Friesen, Doug Hostetter, Lauree Hersch Meyer, Helen Wiegel, Tom Paxson, and Gene Hillard. Their contributions are evident in these pages; where there are gaps or errors, the responsibility should be assigned to us.

The world is replete with examples of people of faith who are working at various levels for peace. One book cannot hope to do more than point to a few examples. But such illustrations are important. They can expand our awareness of possible responses to the dilemmas we face and push our imaginations in new directions. The Programme to Overcome Violence of the World Council of Churches is one channel for sharing of such examples and possibilities. We hope this book contributes to ongoing ecumenical discussion as Christians from many contexts and traditions find ways to be peacemakers.

—*Judy Zimmerman Herr*
and Robert Herr, Directors
Mennonite Central Committee
Peace Office

Introduction:
Crisis and Opportunity

Robert Herr and Judy Zimmerman Herr

During the late 1980s, a young Mennonite church worker from the United States, Mark Jantzen, was living and studying in East Berlin. He was a Christian ambassador from the West to the "enemy" in the East. His assignment was to support East German churches and participate as a student in the life of the university, especially in discussions and dialogue between Christians and Marxists.

On the evening of November 9, 1989, Mark was with the crowds of East Berliners who first crossed over the broken-down Berlin Wall to visit and socialize with people in West Berlin. That event sent shock waves around the world and marked the end of an era. Mark reflected that the fall of the Wall took away people's certainties about how things worked. Suddenly everything looked new.

We live in an age preoccupied with endings and beginnings. We often attach the prefix "post" to the words we use, including "postmodernism," "post-Cold War," and increasingly, "post-twentieth century." The end of a millennium features centrally in our discussions, sometimes giving us a feeling of being in crisis. But we also live in a time of great hope and expectation. The Chinese symbol for *crisis* is made up of the symbols for danger and opportunity. A time of change and crisis carries dangers but also opportunities for new thinking and possibilities.

The fall of the Berlin Wall marks a time of world change, change which has included both dangers and opportunities. The breakup of the

Soviet Union paved the way for reduced fears of nuclear war between the great powers, but nuclear weapons still pollute the world. The year in which South Africans of all races voted together for the first time was also the year in which massive killing and displacement erupted in Rwanda. Nations have made progress in developing systems of international negotiation, but conflicts within nations have increased. Even though a decade has passed since the world first celebrated the end of one era and the beginning of another, both the powerful and those without power still struggle to know how to respond to the end of a bipolar world power structure.

We refer to these bipolar years as the Cold War—"cold" in that a major clash, such as World War I or World War II, never erupted between the alliances of the West and the East. The years since the end of this Cold War have been uncertain ones, as the world struggles to develop new relational systems and organizations. To be sure, there is cause for optimism, as proxy wars in Angola, Mozambique, El Salvador, Nicaragua, and Guatemala stumble to an end.

But there is also ground for pessimism. Conflicts of local origin have split nations in Somalia, ex-Yugoslavia, Rwanda, and Congo. Both for those who control military power and look to it to bring order or control, and for those who seek to be peacemakers in new ways, the world continues to be confusing. Even the term "Cold War," which carried so much meaning only a few years ago, now seems parochial. At a conference in 1994, a participant from Colombia posed the question: "Why do you call this war cold? For us in poor countries, who bore the brunt of East and West proxy struggles, this war felt very hot!"

This volume is the result of conversation in the Historic Peace Church/Fellowship of Reconciliation Consultative Committee based in the United States. Christian peace theology and peacemaking have been the heart of this group's existence since its formation over thirty years ago. But commitment to peace cannot remain a static idea. The end of the Cold War era requires that as people of faith we once again look at our situation and think together about responding to the new world we see around us.

The need for peacemakers seems obvious. The easing of nuclear tensions between Moscow and Washington has given way to growing fears that nuclear, chemical, and biological weapons of mass destruction may spread to additional countries. The gap between the world's rich and poor is growing. Environmental problems spurred by overconsumption, resource shortages, pollution, and burgeoning populations threaten unprecedented violence to God's creation. They stimulate selfish, warring rivalries among those created in God's image. Ethnic, national, and religious prejudices, inflamed by political leaders who incite citizens to hate and fear, spark violent conflicts, and fragment societies.

In this context the Christian church, and all people of religious faith, face difficult questions. Is peace possible in our world? What today is the role of national governments and of international institutions? How can we as people of faith respond to large-scale systems of globalization and economic forces which seem so powerful? And, how can we build communities of peace with our neighbors?

Historic peace churches and the Fellowship of Reconciliation have a long history of thinking about and working for peace. Throughout the Cold War era, these groups and other churches continued ecumenical conversations on peace. On one level, such work is theological--understanding the nature of God's will for peace and God's calling of people to peace. But such work has also always found practical expression in the lives of individual people as they work at making peace in their community and in their world.

This book surveys some current thinking and presents examples of activities on these three levels. The fact that its contributors include writers from a variety of traditions reflects the ecumenical nature of the peacemaking task.

The first section, "Foundation for a Just Peace," includes writing from various traditions and locations. Even in a new context, we can find a basis for our peacemaking in past experiences and examples. In this light, Jim Forest points to the earliest history of the church and the teachings of Jesus. Walter Wink finds in Jesus' command to turn the other cheek some practical advice for people in situations of oppression. Dorothee Soelle examines the life of eighteenth-century Quaker leader John Woolman, whom she sees as providing an example of the necessary connection between spirituality and working for justice.

Changed contexts also call for new ways of thinking, however. Glen Stassen and Duane Friesen suggest a new paradigm for peace conversations that moves beyond the just war and pacifist debates to ask what is being done to make peace. Their "just peacemaking theory" proposes normative activities that can guide actions of churches as well as governments and international bodies. Chaiwat Satha-Anand, a Muslim peace scholar from Thailand, reflects on the usefulness for politics of the concept of forgiveness which he finds in Christian, Muslim, and Gandhian teachings. Finally Gerald Pillay, writing from a context of rebuilding after a long struggle against apartheid, explores the notion of a theology focused on the need to reconstruct the basis of society.

Building a culture of peace begins locally but also includes awareness of work at a global level. These two levels exist in a dynamic interaction, so separating them may seem artificial. Yet while skills at one level may transfer to the other, there will also be differences. The remainder of this volume focuses on direct accounts of such work, locally and globally, with stories from a variety of persons and places.

The practical stories recounted here grow from a commitment to peace as the heart of the Christian message. In the final chapter, Lauree Hersch Meyer, of the Historic Peace Churches/Fellowship of Reconciliation Committee, reflects on these examples and activities in the light of a peace church theology.

Being a peacemaker today takes place in a world that is changing rapidly. Before we turn to specific examples, it is important to reflect on the forces that shape the world in which we live and to ask what these may mean for the task of making peace.

One obvious change in the past ten years is the breaking up of global military balance-of-power blocs. The old bipolar world, with two superpowers vying for influence and smaller nations positioning themselves as clients, is gone. Wars still erupt—sometimes it seems with increasing frequency—but they are smaller. Nations break up. Boundaries take on new meaning and are sometimes redrawn. Some analysts fear we are returning to a more feudal, city-state polity. At the same time, new global networks are developing which function outside of the control of established government structures and international associations.

As national and ideologically based relationships give way, the world is characterized by "globalization." Economic power replaces military power as central. Economic self-interest carries more sway with governments than do the former political relationships and alliances. Free trade is the prevailing value, in contrast to the previous era with its walls of tariff control and currency restriction. Questions of fairness and justice abound in this new climate, but countries continue to jump onto the bandwagon of the free movement of capital, information, and, increasingly, even people.

Philosophically, we are described as living in the postmodern era. This is a time characterized by many choices and options as well as individualized, decentralized authority. Throughout the world, peoples' organizations and nongovernmental organizations (NGOs) now do things that once were the sole responsibility of governments. States and international bodies such as the UN struggle to maintain program continuity and stability with this new and assertive NGO phenomenon.

We are witnessing a revolution in systems of communication which is changing the world. Instantaneous and inexpensive communication networks open the world to new discussions. Technology such as cellular satellite phones and computer e-mail linkups reach corners of the globe bypassed by earlier technological developments. We may regret the standardization that comes with worldwide television networks channeling the same sanitized news and advertisements into every country, but this communications revolution also gives to those previously isolated a world platform from which to share ideas and solicit support.

These trends—open trade, free movement of capital, increasing mobility of people, importance of nongovernmental organizations, growth of communications technology—all change the management and organizing systems available to nations. Governments no longer have the ability they had even recently to set terms and define boundaries of international relationships. International agencies also struggle to define their roles in this new world. Although these trends hold promise, there is a great deal of uncertainty about what they will deliver.

Relationships among nations have traditionally relied strongly on the principle of national sovereignty. This established and often wise pattern provided a measure of international legal protection for smaller countries. Outside interference in the internal affairs of countries needed to contend with especially high legal hurdles. But here too there has been great change, beginning with the development in the past fifty years of international Human Rights Law, which has enlarged the moral and legal ground for international intervention. New legal understandings are developing, based on Human Rights Law, that question sovereignty by calling states to abide by international standards in their treatment of people.

These developments can place strains on older foundations for national identity. As identities change, others form or resurface, often in the guise of older categories—ethnic group, religious affiliation, or clan/family structures. And from this comes the new cliché that wars are now fought *in*—rather than *between*—nation-states.

What do these trends mean for peacemakers in this new world of the twenty-first century? Although many of the developments summarized here are threatening, they also present opportunities. This "opening up" creates new possibilities for citizen networks. International bodies such as the UN, regional bodies such as the OAS (Organization of American States), OAU (Organization of African Unity) and EU (European Union), and some nations as well, recognize that peoples' organizations and NGOs play a vital role.

On February 12, 1997, three international NGOs (Medicins Sans Frontiers, CARE and Oxfam), all sponsoring humanitarian relief work in Eastern Congo, were invited to address the UN Security Council. This was the first time NGOs were invited to participate at this level. The willingness of governmental and international structures to engage these unofficial networks in dialogue varies, but they are listened to in ways that did not happen a decade ago. Boundaries between "public" and "private" are less precise than before.

One example of the growing recognition given to unofficial actors is in programs for peacemaking. "Track-one diplomacy" is traditional international diplomacy, carried out by country ambassadors and international state negotiators. "Track-two diplomacy" is a new term which describes peace negotiation that takes place away from the official negotiation tables. International agencies and diplomats now speak of the need to use multiple tracks to broker international relationships.

Religion, culture, and local identity are increasingly recognized as important components of a peace process. Peoples' organizations and nongovernmental groups participate in the mediation of conflicts in or among nations. An alternative track-two approach can fill a void in the connection to resolving conflict at community or grassroots levels.

Changes in communications technology and the growth of peoples' groups and NGOs make it possible to hear from people in less advantaged situations. This can offer a new voice to the Christian church outside its traditional centers. The strength of the church in the world's poorer areas gives a new urgency, and often a new definition, to peacemaking, mission, and service. Christian theology is called to respond in new ways to communities facing distress.

In light of these challenges, Christians are looking again and with new eyes at the calling to be peacemakers. This task, which requires a strong spiritual base and attention both to the local and the global, is marked by experimentation.

Peace requires more than achieving a cease-fire or a political settlement. To enable people to truly live at peace with one another, valuing one another and seeking the welfare of all, is a monumental task, especially where war or oppression have been the norm. Such peace will not be built quickly and cannot only be based on changing structures. It also requires changing people. To be genuine, peace must reach into people's basic identity structure; it must include spiritual change.

In the latter part of the 1980s, peoples' movements brought rapid changes to government and national structures in Eastern Europe and the former Soviet Union. At the same time, movements for democracy culminated in multiparty elections and new systems for governance in many countries in Africa and Latin America. Euphoria was widespread. This was the dawn of a new era of democracy and freedom! Now, at the end of the century, it is clear that change in society does not happen quickly or easily. Many of the countries which saw this rapid change are struggling to hold their societies together. Building peace is long, slow work.

So building peace indeed requires spiritual resources for sustenance. But this is the essence of the Christian faith! Jew and Greek will no longer see each other as foreign. Slave and master will be reconciled. Male and female will work as equals. Above all, loving enemies will become the hallmark of the new humanity. This vision that has sustained Christians through the ages is particularly relevant for the world we live in today.

This book grows from Christian traditions which throughout their history have been committed to peace as God's will for Christians and for the world. These traditions have understood the practical implications of working for peace in different ways at various times in their history. But their commitment to a faith which sees peace as a central aim undergirds their practical efforts.

In a world characterized by both globalization and a resurgence of local identity, peacemaking will be both local and global. Tools for working at peace will begin in homes and communities, in schools and neighborhoods. At the same time, peacemaking will form networks reaching around the world. Thus the stories in this book include accounts of both local and international peacemaking.

Finally peacemaking is marked by experimentation. There is no one right way to go about creating peaceful communities and a peaceful world. Working for peace will differ according to the context. In some cases, it will include nonviolent interventions. In others, it will include building new structures to ensure peace. A culture of peace will be marked by variety and diversity. Thus what we have to share are examples, not formulas. This book is one attempt to share both theological resources to undergird and examples to inspire and encourage.

Foundations for a Just Peace

1

Soldiers of Christ

Jim Forest

Jesus Christ was not simply a great rabbi whose splendid teaching and exemplary but ultimately tragic life inspired the creation of a new religion. We who are Christians know him as the incarnation of the second person of the Holy Trinity, the Son of God, who gave his life for us and was raised from the dead. Everything about the incarnation is significant to us. It was no accident Jesus was born of a certain Jewish mother in a certain Galilean village at a certain time two thousand years ago. He entered history purposefully, at an exact and chosen moment, as the Son of Mary.

What sort of place and moment? Not the starlit dream world of the modern Christmas card, but a humiliated, overtaxed land kept in the Roman Empire by brutal, bitterly resented occupation troops. Jesus Christ, Son of God, Savior, was born, lived, was crucified, and was raised from the dead in a land of extreme enmity—a country resembling much of Europe during German occupation in the Second World War.

Think of what we might call the primary characteristics of Christ's life in the years recorded by the Gospel authors. On the one hand, there are the many healing miracles. On the other hand, we hear Jesus condemning those who pile burdens on others they would never carry themselves. He wasn't simply doing good deeds while keeping silent about a corrupt and violent social order. It was not for his healing miracles that the religious and political authorities decreed his execution.

Despite his opposition to the rulers, however, Jesus never became part of the Zealot movement of violent opposition to the Roman presence. Neither did he bless anyone joining the nationalist groups which were using violent methods to seek recovery of national independence. Jesus did not help the Romans—nor threaten their lives. We see in him a third way, a way neither violent nor passive but centering on conversion.

Consider Jesus' encounter with the Roman centurion who came seeking his help (Matt. 8:5-13). Jesus not only responded positively to the centurion's appeal for help but also openly admired the centurion's faith, describing it as being greater than those of his own people. Some who heard Jesus express respect for an enemy's faith no doubt spat on the ground and muttered to themselves, "Traitor! These Romans are all filth!" But we can also wonder whether, given his encounter with Jesus, the centurion's life afterward may not have taken a turn. Might he have been among the first Romans to place himself under the rule of Christ rather than Caesar?

Not once in the Gospels do we find a deadly weapon in Christ's hand. His most violent action involved using a whip of cords to chase money changers out of the temple because their activities were profaning a place of worship. The action was fierce but endangered no one's life except his own. It was after this event that those religious leaders who profited from trade inside the temple decided this troublemaker from Galilee, the alleged Messiah, must die.

Again and again we see Christ healing people. Think about the last miracle before his crucifixion. It is the most surprising healing miracle in the Gospels. He mended the wound of one of the men who came to arrest him in the garden of Gethsemane, an injury caused by the apostle Peter, who was only trying to defend his Lord. Consider what Jesus said to Peter at that frightful moment: "Put away your sword, for whoever lives by the sword will perish by the sword (Matt. 26:52)."

"Put away your sword." These words of Jesus were taken to heart in the early church. From the time of the apostles until the beginning of the third century, we find no sign of Christian participation in military service but rather many accounts of Christians refusing to serve in the army.

In a criticism of Christians written in A.D. 173 by the pagan scholar Celsus, Christians were sharply condemned for their refusal to serve in the army. "If all men were to do as you [Christians] do," wrote Celsus, "there would be nothing to prevent the Emperor from being left in utter solitude, and with the desertion of his forces, the Empire would fall into the hands of the most lawless barbarians."[1]

In the same century, St. Justin the Hieromartyr explained the Christian attitude: "We who were filled with war and mutual slaughter and every wickedness have each of us in all the world changed our weapons of war . . . swords into plows and spears into pruning hooks." Elsewhere he writes, "We who formerly murdered one another now not only do not make war on our enemies but, that we may not lie or deceive our judges, we gladly die confessing Christ."[2]

At the heart of these and similar writings from the early church is the conviction that we are, through baptism, people under the rule of God, obeying the rulers of this world only insofar as their regulations are not in conflict with God's law. As St. Euphemia, a martyr of the early fourth century, declared, "The Emperor's commands and [those of anyone in authority] must be obeyed if they are not contrary to the God of heaven. If they are, they must not only not be obeyed; they must be resisted."[3]

In the Church in Asia Minor in the early fourth century, it was declared,

> Let a catechumen . . . if he desire to be a soldier, either cease from his intention, or if not, let him be rejected. For he has despised God by his thought and, leaving the things of the Spirit, he has perfected himself in the flesh, and has treated the faith with contempt."

One finds similar declarations in other parts of the Church throughout the Empire in the pre-Constantinian era.[4]

Beginning in the late second century, there are indications of soldiers who had been baptized. The oldest known Christian grave marking indicating the deceased had been in the army dates from 197. What about those who came to Christian faith while in the army? They were told they must never take anyone's life. "Anyone who has received the power to kill . . . in no case let them kill, even if they have received the order to kill," stated the Canons of Hippolytus of the Church in Egypt in the mid-fourth century.[5] This is similar to St. John the Baptist's instructions to soldiers: "Do violence to no one, accuse no one falsely, and be content with your pay (Luke 3:14)."

One must keep in mind that in the Roman Empire soldiering was not a period lasting only a few years but was normally a lifetime career with no right of resignation. One either was born into the military profession because one's father was a soldier or entered the army as a young volunteer or conscript.

Anyone guilty of actually killing another person was subject to grave penances and prolonged exclusion from the Eucharist. The Canons of Hippolytus state that "If anyone has shed blood, let him not take part in the [Eucharistic] mysteries, unless he has been purified by a punishment, by tears and groans."[6] We notice that even today canons sur-

vive from the Ecumenical Councils which require that priests and iconographers be persons who have never shed human blood.

Records survive of Christians martyred for their refusal to accept
military service in a period when other Christians were willing to accept
conscription. For example, in 295 a young Christian, St. Maximilian, was
brought before Roman Proconsul Dion in North Africa. His testimony is
recorded in the ancient Acts of the Saints. "I will not be a soldier of this
world," Maximilian said, "for I am a soldier of Christ."

"But there are Christians serving in the army," Proconsul Dion replied.

"That is their business," said Maximilian. "I too am a Christian,
and cannot serve." Condemned to death, he proclaimed, "God lives!"[7]

A generation later, in 336, we find St. Martin of Tours, an army officer who later became a missionary bishop, applying for discharge. "I
am a soldier of Christ," he declared. "It is not lawful for me to fight." As
his request was made on the eve of a battle, Martin was accused of cowardice. He responded by volunteering to face the enemy and advance
unarmed against their ranks. Caesar instead ordered Martin imprisoned, but soon after this he was permitted to resign from the army.[8]

Late in the fourth century, St. John Chrysostom compared the violent to wolves:

> It is certainly a finer and more wonderful thing to change the mind of
> enemies and bring them to another way of thinking than to kill them, es-
> pecially when we recall that [the disciples] were only twelve and the
> whole world was full of wolves. . . . We ought then to be ashamed of
> ourselves, we who act so very differently and rush like wolves on our foes.
> So long as we are sheep we have the victory; but if we are like wolves we
> are beaten, for then the help of the shepherd is withdrawn from us, for he
> feeds sheep not wolves. . . . This mystery [of the Eucharist] requires that
> we should be innocent not only of violence but of all enmity, however
> slight, for it is the mystery of peace.[9]

How strange all these texts seem to Christians in our age—even those
of us in the Orthodox Church, known for our preservation of the ancient liturgy and for maintaining many other traditions of the early
Church. We are scandalized and saddened when we notice new distor-
tions of the faith. Yet there is much from the Church's first centuries
that we have completely forgotten.

When did the change begin? Perhaps the crucial year was 313,
when Emperor Constantine ended the persecution against the Church
by issuing the Edict of Milan. No longer the object of suppressive actions
by the state, Christianity soon became the most favored religion of the
empire—and in time the only legal religion. Those who wanted to ad-

vance in the world first had to accept the Emperor's religion. They quickly lined up for baptism, though it is instructive to notice that Constantine delayed his own baptism until he lay on his deathbed.

The relationship between church and state was drastically changed. Before Constantine, Christians had, in effect, either been barred from the army or permitted to serve in areas where their work was what is today done by police and firemen. Within a century of Constantine's death, all non-Christians were excluded from the army. As St. Jerome wrote from his cave in Bethlehem late in the fourth century, "When the Church came to the princes of the world, she grew in power and wealth but diminished in virtue."

In the Orthodox Church, for the past fifteen centuries only monks, priests, and iconographers are seen as having a vocation which, by its nature, bars them from bloodshed. They are required to live by a standard once normal for all followers of Christ.

Late in the fourth century the foundations of the "just war theory," as it has come to be called in the Western church, were laid by St. Ambrose of Milan and St. Augustine of Hippo. While both maintained the traditional view that the individual Christian was barred from deadly violence in self-defense, they proposed that armed defense of one's community was a different matter. Yet they maintained that Christ's command to love one's enemies remained in full force even for the soldier. I doubt any historian would argue that the just war doctrine has had much influence on war in actual practice. We may wonder if any wars ever satisfied all the conditions, but modern war especially discards many of the limitations, most strikingly in using weapons and methods which cause many noncombatant deaths.

Development of the just war doctrine occurred entirely in the West; gradually it became well-established. Some Orthodox bishops have supported war, but in the Eastern church just war theory never acquired doctrinal status. In researching patristic sources, Byzantine military manuals, and Orthodox declarations about war, the respected Orthodox theologian Father Stanley Harakas was startled to discover

> an amazing consistency in the almost totally negative moral assessment of war, coupled with an admission that war may be necessary under certain circumstances to protect the innocent and to limit even greater evils. In this framework, war may be an unavoidable alternative, but it nevertheless remains an evil. Virtually absent in the [Orthodox] tradition is any mention of a "just" war, much less a "good" war. The tradition also precludes the possibility of a crusade. For the Eastern Orthodox tradition . . . war can be seen only as a "necessary evil," with all the difficulty and imprecision such a designation carries."

Nonetheless, he continues, "the pacifist emphasis is retained in liturgy and in clerical standards."[10]

We find what Father Harakas describes as a gradual "stratification of pacifism" in the church. "Clergy were to function as pacifists, uninvolved in any military activity, even prohibited from entering military camps."

Despite the gradual acceptance of military service that followed Constantine's act of peace with the church, Christianity and war have never been happily joined. The great majority of Christians came to regard war as the lesser of two evils and military service as an honorable calling. Nonetheless, there has never been a period in Christian history without its nonviolent teachers and witnesses, nor a time without those who taught Christianity as a way of love rather than coercion.

Reflecting on the word and example of Christ, we can identify seven aspects of spiritual life that are essential aspects of Christian peacemaking: love of enemies, prayer for enemies, doing good to enemies, turning the other cheek, offering forgiveness, breaking down walls of division, and resisting evil in ways which may lead one's enemies toward conversion.

Love of enemies. As used in the Bible, love has first to do with action and responsibility; the stress is not on how one feels at the time. To love is to do what you can to provide for the spiritual and physical well-being of another, whether you like that person or not. What Christ does is love. In explaining his Father's love, he talks about what God gives to all.

An act of love may be animated by a sense of delight in someone else or, more significantly, it may be done despite anger, exhaustion, depression or fear, done simply as a response to God, our common Creator, "who makes the sun rise on the evil and on the good, and sends rain on the just and the unjust" (Matt. 5:45).

Paul taught that the greatest gifts of God are faith, hope, and love, and, of these, the greatest is love. Genuine love, he wrote, is patient and kind, without jealousy or boasting, without arrogance or rudeness; it doesn't demand its own way, does not rejoice at wrong but rather in the right, and endures everything (1 Cor. 13).

Prayer for enemies. Inseparable from the love of others is prayer for them. "But I say to you, love your enemies and pray for those who persecute you" (Matt. 5:44). Without prayer for enemies, how can we love them? In fact the only love we can offer anyone, friend or enemy, is God's own love. Prayer can help us gain access to God's love for those we would otherwise regard with disinterest, irritation, fear, or active hostility.

We are given a witness to the power of prayer in the life of Saint Silouan of the Holy Mountain. He was a Russian peasant, born in 1866, who fell asleep in the Lord on Mount Athos in 1938. He devoted the whole of his adult life to prayer. Earlier he had had an intimate experience of his own violence, nearly killing a neighbor in his village. In his many years of spiritual combat as a monk, Saint Silouan learned that the love of enemies is not simply an aspect of Christian life but

> the central criterion of true faith and of real communion with God, the lover of souls, the lover of humankind. . . . Through Christ's love, everyone is made an inseparable part of our own, eternal existence . . . for the Son of man has taken in himself all mankind.[11]

Doing good to enemies. Jesus calls us not only to prayer but to action: "Do good to those who hate you, bless those who curse you" (Luke 6:27, 28). Prayer is not an alternative to action; in fact, prayer may empower us to take personal responsibility for what we wish others would do. In his Letter to the Romans, Paul says,

> Bless those who persecute you; bless and do not curse them. . . . Repay no one evil for evil, but take thought for what is noble in the sight of all. If possible, so far as it depends on you, live peaceably with all. Beloved, never avenge yourselves, but leave it to the wrath of God; for it is written, "Vengeance is mine, I will repay, says the Lord." No, if your enemy is hungry, feed him; if he is thirsty, give him drink; for by doing so you will heap burning coals on his head. Do not be overcome by evil, but overcome evil with good. (Rom. 12:14-21)

Overcoming evil with good was what the Samaritan did when he found the enemy dying on the side of the road in Jesus' parable (Luke 10). In offering help to an enemy in his distress, the Samaritan transformed the wounded Jew's idea of Samaritans. That Jew could never again think of Samaritans simply as enemies. If we were to tell the story in modern terms, it could be a Turk helping an injured Greek, a Christian helping a Muslim, a Jew helping an Arab, an Iraqi reaching out to a U.S. soldier.

Turning the other cheek. Jesus says to his followers, "If someone strikes you on the cheek, offer him the other also" (Matt. 5:39). How different this is from the advice provided in the average Hollywood film or politician's speech! There the constant message is, "If you are hit, hit back. Let your blow be harder than the one you received. In fact, you needn't be hit at all to strike others." Provocation, irritation, or the expectation of attack is warrant enough.

Turning the other cheek is often seen as a suspect doctrine, even dismissed as masochism. We see it as Jesus at his most unrealistic. "Human beings, but especially my enemies, just aren't made that way." For a great many people the problem can be put even more simply: "Turning the other cheek is for wimps!"

The conversion of the ancient world had much to do with Christians turning the other cheek in many acts of courageous witness that should not be forgotten. In our own century such witness was offered again by countless believers persecuted in the Soviet Union, where literally millions of Christians were shot, tortured to death, or left to die of hunger and cold in the Gulag Archipelago.

Forgiveness. Every time we say the Lord's Prayer, we ask God to forgive us only insofar as we ourselves have extended forgiveness to others: "And forgive us our debts, as we also have forgiven our debtors" (Matt. 7:9-13). Christ also says

> "Judge not, that you be not judged. For with the judgment you pronounce you will be judged, and the measure you give will be the measure you get. Why do you see the speck that is in your brother's eye, but do not notice the log that is in your own? (Matt. 7:1-3)

On another occasion, Peter asks Jesus how often he must extend forgiveness: "As many as seven times?" Jesus responds, "I do not say to you seven times, but seventy times seven" (Matt. 18:21, 22). It is such teaching that inspires the verses we sing every Easter: "Let us call brothers even those who hate us, and forgive all by the Resurrection."

The Desert Father Abbot Moses was once asked to take part in a meeting in which the community was planning to condemn a certain negligent brother. Abbot Moses arrived at the meeting carrying a basket from which sand was pouring out through many openings. "Why are you doing that?" he was asked. "You ask me to judge a brother while my own sins spill out behind me like the sand from this basket," he replied. The embarrassed community was moved to forgive their lax brother.[12]

Nothing is more fundamental to Jesus' teaching than his call to forgiveness. He invites us to give up debts, let go of grievances, pardon those who have harmed us. We need to seek forgiveness, offer forgiveness, and accept forgiveness. We are followers of Jesus who taught us forgiveness even when his hands were nailed to the wood of the cross: "Father, forgive them. They know not what they do" (Luke 23:34).

Breaking down walls. In Christ enmity is destroyed, Paul wrote to the church in Ephesus.

> For he is our peace, who has made us both one, and has broken down the dividing wall of enmity . . . that he might create in himself one new person in place of two, so making peace, and might reconcile us both to God in one body through the cross, and thereby bring enmity to an end. (Eph. 2:14-16)

Jesus often exemplifies such reconciliation himself, as in his encounters with the Roman Centurion and the Samaritan woman at the well.

We live in a world of many walls of separation: racism, nationalism, all sorts of tribalism. Nothing is more ordinary than enmity. Far from living in communion with others, we tend to flee from it. Metropolitan John of Pergamon comments,

> Communion with the other is not spontaneous; it is built on fences which protect us from the dangers implicit in the other's presence. We accept the other only insofar as he does not threaten our privacy or insofar as he is useful to our individual happiness. . . . The essence of sin is the fear of the Other, which is part of the rejection of God.[13]

Resisting evil in ways which may help convert enemies. We are obliged to oppose evil. As we are both flesh and spirit, we must use both flesh and spirit in our acts of resistance. But how ought we resist? Certain kinds of resistance are clearly rejected in the gospel: "You have heard that it was said, 'An eye for an eye and a tooth for a tooth.' But I say to you, do not resist the one who is evil" (Matt. 5: 38, 39).

Responding to evil with its own weapons, though it can seem the best option, results in a life centered on evil. Often people who fear violence become violent themselves. They take up the same weapons and even adopt characteristics and hated practices of the adversary. When the Nazi forces bombed cities in World War II, there was immense revulsion in Britain and the United States. In the end, however, the greatest destruction of cities was perpetrated by Britain and the United States.

Then what are we to do? Are Christians supposed to do nothing more than pray in the face of injustice and oppression? Are there not warriors as well as pacifists among the saints?

We see in the example of many saints that our choice is not limited to passivity on the one hand and bloodshed on the other. There is the alternative of unarmed resistance. This is a form of combat which begins with the refusal to collaborate with injustice. Then it actively helps the victims of oppression, protests evil, and finally prays and works for the conversion of adversaries.

Among the saints of this century is Mother Maria Skobtsova, an Orthodox nun who came to France as a refugee. Her house of hospitality became a place of refuge for Jews and others in Nazi-occupied Paris. She finally perished in a gas chamber at Ravensbrück. In her we see that nonviolent, spiritually rooted struggle is not without risk and great suffering.[14] It can easily cost us our lives, just as happens in armed struggle. But we prefer courageously to put our own rather than others' lives at risk.

This approach to conflict begins with a conscious aspiration to find solutions rooted in respect for life, including the lives of our enemies, and our hope that they too may be saved. We cannot be sure we will always discover a nonviolent solution, but what we fail to seek we certainly will fail to find. As expressed in the membership statement of the Orthodox Peace Fellowship,

> While no one can be certain that he or she will always find a nonviolent response to every crisis that may arise, we pray that God will show us, in each situation, ways of resistance to evil that will not require killing opponents.

This is a way of life that many men and women witnessed in the great Russian saint, Seraphim of Sarov, who lived in peace with everyone around him and who sometimes fed a wild bear from his own hands. "We cannot be too gentle, too kind," he said.

> Shun even to appear harsh in your treatment of each other. But remember, no work of kindness or charity can bring down to earth the holy breath, unless it be done in the name of Christ. When it is, joy, radiant joy, streams from the face of him who gives and kindles joy in the heart of him who receives. All condemnation is from the devil. Never condemn each other, not even those whom you catch committing an evil deed. We condemn others only because we shun knowing ourselves. When we gaze at our own failings, we see such a morass of filth that nothing in another can equal it. That is why we turn away, and make much of the faults of others. Keep away from the spilling of speech. Instead of condemning others, strive to reach inner peace. Keep silent, refrain from judgment. This will raise you above the deadly arrows of slander, insult and outrage and will shield your glowing hearts against the evil that creeps around.[15]

Let us return to the Beatitudes. There are only eight of them. We dare neglect none. One is the Beatitude of peacemaking. In the early centuries of the church's life, the whole world was astonished at how Christians witnessed to the peace of Christ, not only refusing to shed the blood of their enemies but trying in every possible way to save their enemies. The Beatitude of peacemaking invites us to do all in our power to renew such faithful witness in our time.

How desperately we need peacemakers! We need them not only in places where wars are being fought or might be fought but in each household, each church, each parish. Even the best and most vital parishes often suffer from deep divisions. And who is the needed peacemaker? Each of us. Often it is harder to forgive and understand someone in our own parish or community than an abstract enemy we see mainly in propaganda images on television. We can see in the church that we don't simply disagree with each other on many topics, but that often we despise those who hold an opposing view. In the name of Christ, who commanded us to love one another, we engage in a war of words in which, far from loving opponents, we don't even respect them. But without mercy and forgiveness, without love, I am no longer in communion either with my neighbor or with Christ.

At the deepest level, peacemakers are used by God to help heal our own relationship with God. We get no closer to God than we get to our enemy—that is, to any person regarded as "different" and "a threat."

The challenge comes in these words of Mother Maria Skobtsova of Paris:

> The bodies of fellow human beings must be treated with greater care than our own. Christian love teaches us to give our brethren not only spiritual gifts, but material gifts as well. Even our last shirt, our last piece of bread must be given to them. Personal almsgiving and the most wide-ranging social work are equally justifiable and necessary. The way to God lies through love of other people and there is no other way. At the Last Judgment I shall not be asked if I was successful in my ascetic exercises or how many prostrations I made in the course of my prayers. I shall be asked, did I feed the hungry, clothe the naked, visit the sick and the prisoners: that is all I shall be asked.[16]

Jesus' Third Way

Walter Wink

Many who have committed their lives to working for change and justice in the world simply dismiss Jesus' teachings about nonviolence as impractical idealism. And with good reason. "Turn the other cheek" suggests the passive, Christian doormat quality that has made so many Christians cowardly and complicit in the face of injustice. "Resist not evil" seems to break the back of all opposition to evil and counsel submission. "Going the second mile" has become a platitude meaning nothing more than "extend yourself." Rather than fostering structural change, such attitudes encourage collaboration with the oppressor.

Jesus never behaved in such ways. Whatever the source of the misunderstanding, it is neither Jesus nor his teaching, which, when given a fair hearing in its original social context, is arguably one of the most revolutionary political statements ever uttered.

> You have heard that it was said, "An eye for an eye and a tooth for a tooth." But I say to you, Do not resist one who is evil. But if anyone strikes you on the right cheek, turn to him the other also; and if anyone would sue you and take your coat, let him have your cloak as well; and if any one forces you to go one mile, go with him two miles. (Matt. 5:38-41, RSV)

When the court translators working in the hire of King James chose to translate *antistenai* as "*Resist* not evil," they were doing something more than rendering Greek into English. They were translating nonviolent resistance into docility. Jesus did *not* tell his oppressed hearers not to resist evil. That would have been absurd. His entire ministry is at odds with such a preposterous idea. The Greek word is made up of two parts:

anti, a word still used in English for "against," and *histemi*, a verb which in its noun form (*stasis*) means violent rebellion, armed revolt, sharp dissension. Thus Barabbas is described as a rebel "who had committed murder in the *insurrection*" (Mark 15:7; Luke 23:19, 25), and the townspeople in Ephesus "are in danger of being charged with *rioting*" (Acts 19:40). The term generally refers to a potentially lethal disturbance or armed revolution.[1]

A proper translation of Jesus' teaching would then be, "Do not strike back at evil (or one who has done you evil) in kind. Do not give blow for blow. Do not retaliate against violence with violence." Jesus was no less committed to opposing evil than the anti-Roman resistance fighters. The only difference was over the means to be used. The issue was *how*—not whether—one should fight evil.

There are three general responses to evil: (1) passivity, (2) violent opposition, and (3) the third way of militant nonviolence articulated by Jesus. Human evolution has conditioned us for only the first two of these responses: fight or flight.

Fight had been the cry of Galileans who had abortively rebelled against Rome only two decades before Jesus spoke. Jesus and many of his hearers would have seen some of the two thousand of their countrymen crucified by the Romans along the roadsides. They would have known some of the inhabitants of Sepphoris (a mere three miles north of Nazareth) who had been sold into slavery for aiding the insurrectionists' assault on the arsenal there. Some also would live to experience the horrors of the war against Rome in 66-70 C.E., one of the ghastliest in history. If the option *fight* had no appeal to them, their only alternative was *flight*: passivity, submission, or, at best, a passive-aggressive recalcitrance in obeying commands. For them no third way existed. Submission or revolt spelled out the entire vocabulary of their alternatives to oppression.

Now we are in a better position to see why King James' servants translated antistenai as "resist not." The king would not want people concluding they had any recourse against his or any other sovereign's unjust policies. Therefore the populace must be made to believe there were two and only two alternatives: flight or fight. Either we resist not, or we resist. And Jesus commands us, according to these king's men, to resist not. Jesus appears to authorize monarchical absolutism. Submission is the will of God. Most modern translations have meekly followed the King James path.

Neither of the invidious alternatives of flight/fight is what Jesus is proposing. It is important to be clear about this point before going on: *Jesus abhors both passivity and violence as responses to evil.* His is a third alternative not even touched by these options. Antistenai may be translated variously as "Do not take up arms against evil," "Do not react reflexively to evil," "Do not let evil dictate the terms of your opposition." The *Scholars Version* translates it brilliantly: "Don't react violently against someone who is evil." The word cannot be construed to mean submission.

Jesus clarifies his meaning by three brief examples. "If anyone strikes you on the right cheek, turn to him the other also." Why the *right* cheek? How does one strike another on the right cheek anyway? Try it. A blow by the right fist in that right-handed world would land on the *left* cheek of the opponent. To strike the right cheek with the fist would require using the left hand, but in that society the left hand was used only for unclean tasks. Even to gesture with the left hand at Qumran carried the penalty of ten days penance (*The Dead Sea Scrolls*, 1 QS 7). The only way one could strike the right cheek with the right hand would be with the *back of the hand*.

What we are dealing with here is unmistakably an insult, not a fistfight. The intention is not to injure but to humiliate, to put someone in his or her place. One normally did not strike a peer in this way, and if one did the fine was exorbitant (four *zuz* was the fine for a blow to a peer with a fist, 400 zuz for backhanding him; but to an underling, no penalty whatever; *Mishna, Baba Kamma* 8:1-6). A backhand slap was the normal way of admonishing inferiors. Masters backhanded slaves; husbands, wives; parents, children; men, women; Romans, Jews. One black South African told me that during his youth white farmers still gave the backhand to disobedient workers.

We have here a set of unequal relations, in each of which retaliation would be suicidal. The only normal response would be cowering submission. It is important to ask who Jesus' audience is. In every case, Jesus' listeners are not those who strike, initiate lawsuits, or impose forced labor. Rather, Jesus is speaking to their victims ("If anyone strikes *you* . . . would sue *you* . . . forces *you* to go one mile . . ."). There are among his hearers people who have been subjected to these very indignities. They have been forced to stifle their inner outrage at the dehumanizing treatment meted out to them by the hierarchical system of caste and class, race and gender, age and status, and by the guardians of imperial occupation.

Why then does Jesus counsel these already humiliated people to turn the other cheek? Because this action robs the oppressor of power to humiliate them. The person who turns the other cheek is saying, in effect, "Try again. Your first blow failed to achieve its intended effect. I deny you the power to humiliate me. I am a human being just like you.

Your status (gender, race, age, wealth) does not alter that. You cannot demean me."

Such a response would create enormous difficulties for the striker. Purely logistically, how can he now hit the other cheek? He cannot backhand it with his right hand. If he hits with a fist, he makes himself an equal, acknowledging the other as a peer. But the whole point of the back of the hand is to reinforce the caste system and its institutionalized inequality. Even if the master orders the person flogged, the point has irrevocably been made. He has been forced, against his will, to regard that person as an equal human being. He has been stripped of his power to dehumanize the other.

The second example Jesus gives is set in a court of law. Someone is being sued for his outer garment.[2] Who would do that and under what circumstances? The Old Testament provides the clues:

> If you lend money to any of my people with you *who is poor*, you shall not be to him as a creditor, and you shall not exact interest from him. If ever you take your neighbor's garment in pledge, you shall restore it to him before the sun goes down; for that is his only covering, it is his mantle for his body; in what else shall he sleep? And if he cries to me, I will hear, for I am compassionate. (Exod. 22:25-27, emphasis added)

> When you make your neighbor a loan of any sort, you shall not go into his house to fetch his pledge. You shall stand outside, and the man to whom you make the loan shall bring the pledge out to you. And *if he is a poor man*, you shall not sleep in his pledge; when the sun goes down, you shall restore to him the pledge that he may sleep in his cloak and bless you. . . . You shall not . . . take a widow's garment in pledge. (Deut. 24:10-13, 17, emphasis added)

> They that trample the head of the poor into the dust of the earth . . . lay themselves down beside every altar on garments taken in pledge. . . . (Amos 2:7-8)

Only the poorest of the poor would have nothing but an outer garment to give as collateral for a loan. Jewish law strictly required its return every evening at sunset, for that was all the poor had in which to sleep. The situation to which Jesus alludes is one with which his hearers would have been too familiar: the poor debtor has sunk ever deeper into poverty, the debt cannot be repaid, and his creditor has hauled him into court to wring out repayment.

Indebtedness was the most serious social problem in first-century Palestine. Jesus' parables are full of debtors struggling to salvage their lives. The situation was not, however, a natural calamity that had overtaken the incompetent. It was the direct consequence of Roman imperial policy. Emperors had taxed the wealthy so vigorously to fund their wars that the rich began seeking nonliquid investments to secure their wealth. Land was best, but there was a problem: it was not bought and sold on the open market as today but was ancestrally owned and passed down over generations. Little land was ever for sale, at least in Palestine. Exorbitant interest, however, could be used to drive landowners into ever deeper debt until they were forced to sell their land. By the time of Jesus we see this process already far advanced: large estates (*latifundia*) are owned by absentee landlords, managed by stewards, and worked by servants, sharecroppers, and day laborers. It is no accident that the first act of the Jewish revolutionaries in 66 C.E. was to burn the temple treasury, where the record of debts was kept.

It is in this context that Jesus speaks. His hearers are the poor ("if anyone would sue *you*"). They share a rankling hatred for a system that subjects them to humiliation by stripping them of their lands, their goods, finally even their outer garments.

Why then does Jesus counsel them to give over their inner garment as well? This would mean stripping off all their clothing and marching out of court stark naked! Put yourself in the debtor's place; imagine the chuckles this saying must have evoked. There stands the creditor, beet-red with embarrassment, your outer garment in one hand, your underwear in the other. You have suddenly turned the tables on him. You had no hope of winning the trial; the law was entirely in his favor. But you have refused to be humiliated. At the same time you have registered a stunning protest against a system that spawns such debt. You have said, in effect, "You want my robe? Here, take everything! Now you've got all I have except my body. Is that what you'll take next?"

Nakedness was taboo in Judaism. Shame fell not on the naked party but the person viewing or causing one's nakedness (Gen. 9:20-27). By stripping you have brought the creditor under the same prohibition that led to the curse of Canaan. As you parade into the street, your friends and neighbors, startled, aghast, inquire what happened. You explain. They join your growing procession, which now resembles a victory parade. The entire system by which debtors are oppressed has been publicly unmasked. The creditor is revealed to be not a "respectable" moneylender but a party in the reduction of an entire social class to landlessness and destitution. This unmasking is not simply punitive, however; it offers the creditor a chance to see, perhaps for the first time in his life, what his practices cause—and to repent.

Jesus in effect is sponsoring clowning. In so doing he shows himself to be thoroughly Jewish. A later saying of the Talmud runs, "If your neighbor calls you an ass, put a saddle on your back."[3]

The Powers That Be literally stand on their dignity. Nothing takes away their potency faster than deft lampooning. By refusing to be awed by their power, the powerless are emboldened to seize the initiative, even where structural change is not possible. This message, far from being a counsel of perfection unattainable in this life, is a practical, strategic measure for empowering the oppressed. It provides a hint of how to take on the entire system in a way that unmasks its essential cruelty and to burlesque its pretensions to justice, law, and order. Here is a poor man who will no longer be treated as a sponge to be squeezed dry by the rich. He accepts the laws as they stand, pushes them to the point of absurdity, and reveals them for what they really are. He strips nude and walks out before his compatriots, leaving stark naked the creditor and the whole economic edifice he represents.

Jesus' third example, the one about going the second mile, is drawn from the enlightened practice of limiting the amount of forced labor that Roman soldiers could levy on subject peoples. Jews would have seldom encountered legionnaires except in time of war or insurrection. They interacted primarily with auxiliaries headquartered in Judea who were paid at half the rate of legionnaires; they were rather a scruffy bunch.

In Galilee, Herod Antipas maintained an army patterned after Rome's; presumably it also had the right to impose labor. Mile markers were placed regularly beside the highways. A soldier could impress a civilian to carry his pack one mile only; to force the civilian to go further carried with it severe penalties under military law. In this way Rome tried to limit the anger of the occupied people and still keep its armies on the move. Nevertheless, this levy was a bitter reminder to the Jews that they were a subject people even in the Promised Land.

To this proud but subjugated people Jesus does not counsel revolt. One does not "befriend" the soldier, draw him aside, and drive a knife into his ribs. Jesus was keenly aware of the futility of armed revolt against Roman imperial might. He minced no words about it, though it must have cost him support from the revolutionary factions.

But why walk the second mile? Is this not to rebound to the opposite extreme: aiding and abetting the enemy? Not at all. The question here, as in the two previous instances, is how the oppressed can recover the initiative, how they can assert their human dignity in a situation that cannot for the time being be changed. The rules are Caesar's but not how one responds to the rules. The response is God's, and Caesar has no power over that.

Imagine then the soldier's surprise when, at the next mile marker, he reluctantly reaches to assume his pack (sixty-five to eighty-five pounds in full gear). You say, "Oh no, let me carry it another mile." Why would you do that? What are you up to? Normally he has to coerce your kinsmen to carry his pack; now you do it cheerfully and will not stop! Is this a provocation? Are you insulting his strength? Being kind? Trying to get him disciplined for seeming to make you go farther then you should? Are you planning to file a complaint? To create trouble?

From a situation of servile impressment, you have once more seized the initiative. You have taken back the power of choice. The soldier is thrown off-balance by being deprived of the predictability of your response. He has never dealt with such a problem before. Now you have forced him into making a decision for which nothing in his previous experience has prepared him. If he has enjoyed feeling superior to the vanquished, he will not enjoy it today.

Imagine the hilarious situation of a Roman infantryman pleading with a Jew, "Aw, come on, please give me back my pack!" The humor of this scene may escape those who picture it through sanctimonious eyes. It could scarcely, however, have been lost on Jesus' hearers, who must have delighted in the prospect of thus discomfiting their oppressors.

Some readers may object to the idea of discomfiting the soldier or embarrassing the creditor. But can people engaged in oppressive acts repent unless made uncomfortable with their actions? There is, admittedly, the danger of using nonviolence as a tactic of revenge and humiliation. There is also, at the opposite extreme, an equal danger of sentimentality and softness that confuses the uncompromising love of Jesus with being nice. Loving confrontation can free both the oppressed from docility and the oppressor from sin.

Even if nonviolent action does not immediately change the heart of the oppressor, it does affect those committed to it. As Martin Luther King, Jr. attested, it gives them new self-respect and calls on strength and courage they did not know they had. To those with power, Jesus' advice to the powerless may seem paltry. But to those whose lifelong pattern has been to cringe, bow, and scrape before their masters, to those who have internalized their role as inferiors, this small step is momentous.

These three examples amplify what Jesus means in his thesis statement: "Do not react violently against the one who is evil." Instead of the two options ingrained in us by millions of years of unreflective, brute response to biological threats from the environment, instead of flight or flight, Jesus offers a third way. This new way marks a historic mutation in human development: the revolt against the principle of natural selection.[4] With Jesus a way emerges by which evil can be opposed without being mirrored.

Jesus' Third Way

- Seize the moral initiative.
- Find a creative alternative to violence.
- Assert your own humanity and dignity as a person.
- Meet force with ridicule or humor.
- Break the cycle of humiliation.
- Refuse to submit or to accept the inferior position.
- Expose the injustice of the system.
- Take control of the power dynamic.
- Shame the oppressor into repentance.
- Stand your ground.
- Force the Powers into decisions for which they are not prepared.
- Recognize your own power.
- Be willing to suffer rather than retaliate.
- Force the oppressor to see you in a new light.
- Deprive the oppressor of a situation where force is effective.
- Be willing to undergo the penalty of breaking unjust laws.
- Die to fear of the old order and its rules.

Avoid	**Flight**	and	**Fight**
	submission		armed revolt
	passivity		violent rebellion
	withdrawal		direct retaliation
	surrender		revenge

It is too bad Jesus did not provide fifteen or twenty more examples since we do not tend toward this new response naturally. Some examples from political history might help engrave it more deeply in our minds.

In Alagamar, Brazil, a group of peasants organized a long-term struggle to preserve their lands against attempts at illegal expropriation by national and international firms (with the connivance of local politicians and the military). Some of the peasants were arrested and jailed in town. Their companions decided they were all equally responsible. Hundreds marched to town. They filled the house of the judge, demanding to be jailed with those who had been arrested. The judge was finally obliged to send them all home, including the prisoners.[5]

During the Vietnam War, one woman claimed seventy-nine dependents on her United States income tax, all Vietnamese orphans, so she owed no tax. They were not legal dependents, of course, so were disallowed. No, she insisted, these children have been orphaned by indiscriminate United States bombing; we are responsible for their lives.

She forced the Internal Revenue Service to take her to court. That gave her a larger forum for making her case. She used the system against itself to unmask the moral indefensibility of what the system was doing. Of course she "lost" the case, but she made her point.

Another story Jesus himself must have known and which may have served as a model for his examples: In 26 C.E., when Pontius Pilate brought the imperial standards into Jerusalem and displayed them at the Fortress Antonio overlooking the temple, all Jerusalem was thrown into a tumult. These "effigies of Caesar which are called standards" not only infringed on the commandment against images but were the particular gods of the legions. Jewish leaders requested their removal. When Pilate refused, a large crowd of Jews "fell prostrate around his house and for five whole days and nights remained motionless in that position." On the sixth day, Pilate assembled the multitude in the stadium with the apparent intention of answering them. Instead, his soldiers surrounded the Jews in a ring three deep. As Josephus tells it,

> Pilate, after threatening to cut them down, if they refused to admit Caesar's images, signaled to the soldiers to draw their swords. Thereon the Jews, as by concerted action, flung themselves in a body on the ground, extended their necks, and exclaimed that they were ready rather to die than to transgress the law. Overcome with astonishment at such intense religious zeal, Pilate gave orders for the immediate removal of the standards from Jerusalem.[6]

During World War II, when Nazi authorities in occupied Denmark promulgated an order that all Jews had to wear yellow armbands with the Star of David, the king made it a point to attend a celebration in the Copenhagen synagogue. He and most of the population of Copenhagen donned yellow armbands as well. His stand was affirmed by the Bishop of Sjaelland and other Lutheran clergy.[7] The Nazis eventually had to rescind the order.

It is important to repeat such stories to extend our imaginations for creative nonviolence. Since it is not a natural response, we need to be schooled in it. We need models, and we need to rehearse nonviolence in our daily lives if we ever hope to resort to it in crises.

Sadly, Jesus' three examples have been turned into laws, with no reference to the utterly changed contexts in which they were being applied. His attempt to nerve the powerless to assert their humanity under inhuman conditions has been turned into a legalistic prohibition on schoolyard fistfights between peers. Pacifists and those who reject pacifism alike have tended to regard Jesus' infinitely malleable insights as iron rules. The one group urges that they be observed inflexibly; the other treats them as impossible demands intended to break us and catapult us into the arms of grace. The creative, ironic, playful quality of Jesus' teaching has thus been buried under an avalanche of humorless commentary. And as always, the law kills.

How many a battered wife has been counseled, on the strength of a legalistic reading of this passage, to "turn the other cheek." This when what she needs, according to the spirit of Jesus' words, is to find a way to restore her own dignity and end the vicious circle of humiliation, guilt, and bruising. She needs to assert some sort of control in the situation and force her husband to regard her as an equal—or get out of the relationship altogether. The victim needs to recover her self-worth and seize the initiative from her oppressor. And he needs to be helped to overcome his violence. The most creative and loving thing she could do, at least in the American setting, might be to have him arrested.

As such an example suggests, "Turn the other cheek" is not intended as a legal requirement to be applied woodenly in every situation. Rather, it is the impetus for discovering creative alternatives that transcend the only two we are conditioned to perceive: submission or violence, flight or fight.

Shortly after I was promoted from the "B" team to the varsity basketball squad in high school, I noticed that Ernie, the captain, was missing shot after shot from the corner because he was firing the ball like a bullet. So—helpfully, I thought—I shouted, "Arch it, Ernie, arch it." His best friend Ham thought advice from a greenhorn impertinent. From that day on he sniped at me without letup. I had been raised a Christian, so I "turned the other cheek." To each sarcastic jibe I answered with a smile or soft words. This confused Ham somewhat; by the end of the season he lost his taste for taunts.

It was not until four years later that I suddenly woke to the realization that I had not loved Ham into changing. The fact was, *I hated his guts*. It might have been far more creative for me to have challenged him to a fistfight. Then he would have had to deal with me as an equal. But I was *afraid* to fight him, though the fight would probably have been a draw. I was scared I might get hurt. I was hiding behind the Christian "injunction" to "turn the other cheek." Instead I could have been asking, what is the most creative, transformative response to this situation? Perhaps I had done the right thing for the wrong reason, but I suspect that creative nonviolence can never be a genuinely moral response unless we are capable of first entertaining the possibility of violence and consciously saying no. Otherwise our nonviolence may actually be a mask for cowardice.

Oppressed people are justifiably suspicious that those with wealth or power are more concerned to avoid violence than bring about justice.

Nobel Peace Prize laureate Adolfo Perez Esquivel comments, "What has always caught my attention is the attitude of peace movements in Europe and the United States, where nonviolence is envisioned as the final objective. Nonviolence is a lifestyle. The final objective is humanity. It is life."[8]

Maybe it would help to juxtapose Jesus' teachings with Saul Alinsky's principles for nonviolent community action (in his *Rules for Radicals*[9]) to gain a clearer sense of their practicality and pertinence to the struggles of our time. Among rules Alinsky developed in his attempts to organize American workers and minority communities are these:

(1) Power is not only what you have but what your enemy thinks you have.

(2) Never go outside the experience of your people.

(3) Wherever possible go outside the experience of the enemy.

Jesus recommended using one's experience of being belittled, insulted, or dispossessed (Alinsky's rule 2) in such a way as to seize the initiative from the oppressor, who finds the reaction of the oppressed totally outside his experience (second mile, stripping naked, turning the other cheek—Alinsky's rule 3) and forces him or her to believe your power (Alinsky's 1) and perhaps even to recognize your humanity.

(4) Make your enemies live up to their own book of rules.

(5) Ridicule is your most potent weapon.

(6) A good tactic is one that your people enjoy.

(7) A tactic that drags on too long becomes a drag.

The debtor in Jesus' example turned the law against his creditor by obeying it (4)—and throwing in his underwear as well. The ruthlessness of the creditor is thus used as the momentum by which to expose his rapacity (5), and it is done quickly (7) and in a way that could only regale the debtor's sympathizers (6). All other such creditors are now put on notice and all other debtors armed with a new sense of possibilities.

(8) Keep the pressure on.

(9) The threat is usually more terrifying than the thing itself.

(10) The major premise for tactics is the development of operations that will maintain a constant pressure on the opposition.

Jesus, in the three brief examples he cites, does not lay out the basis of a sustained movement, but his ministry as a whole is a model of long-term social struggle (8, 10). Mark depicts Jesus' movements as a *blitzkrieg*. "Immediately" appears eleven times in chapter one alone. Jesus' teaching poses an immediate threat to the authorities. The good he brings is misperceived as evil, his following is overestimated, his militancy is misread as sedition, and his proclamation of the coming Reign of God is mistaken as a manifesto for military revolution (9).

Disavowing violence, Jesus wades into the hostility of Jerusalem openhanded, setting simple truth against force. Terrified by the threat of this man and his following, the authorities resort to their ultimate deterrent, death, only to discover it impotent and themselves unmasked. The cross, hideous and macabre, becomes the symbol of liberation. The movement that should have died becomes a world religion.

(11) If you push a negative hard and deep enough it will break through to its counterside.

(12) The price of a successful attack is a constructive alternative.

(13) Pick the target, freeze it, personalize it, polarize it.

Alinsky delighted in using the most vicious behavior of his opponents—burglaries of movement headquarters, attempted blackmail, and failed assassinations—to destroy their public credibility. Here were elected officials, respected corporations, and trusted police, engaging in patent illegalities to maintain privilege. In the same way, Jesus suggests amplifying an injustice (the other cheek, undergarment, second mile) to expose the fundamental wrongness of legalized oppression (11). The law is "compassionate" in requiring that the debtor's cloak be returned at sunset, yes; but Judaism in its most lucid moments knew that the whole system of usury and indebtedness was itself the root of injustice and should never have been condoned (Exod. 22:25). The restriction of enforced labor to carrying the soldier's pack a single mile was a great advance over unlimited impressment, but occupation troops had no right to be on Jewish soil in the first place.

Jesus' teaching is a kind of moral *jujitsu*, a martial art for using the momentum of evil to throw it, but it requires penetrating beneath the conventions of legality to issues of fundamental justice and hanging onto them with dogged persistence. As Gandhi put it, "We are sunk so low that we fancy that it is our duty and religion to do what the law lays down." If people will only realize that it is cowardly to obey laws that are unjust, he continued, no one's tyranny will enslave them.[10]

Picking the target, freezing it, personalizing it, and polarizing it are the means, then, by which intensity is focused and brought to bear (13). For example, infant formula merchants were discouraging breast feeding and promoting their product in countries where women could not afford the powder. Often the parents overdiluted the formula, causing malnutrition. Or they mixed it with unsanitary water, resulting in diarrhea and death.

But you cannot fight all the merchants of infant formula in the world at once; so you pick the biggest and most visible, Nestlé, even though doing so is technically unfair, since their competition gets off scot-free. The focus pays off, however. Nestlé's recalcitrance leads to worldwide outrage and an international boycott. To avoid similar treatment most of the infant formula manufacturers make some changes. Eventually the boycott leader, the Infant Formula Action Coalition (IN-FACT), in conjunction with the World Health Organization and the United Nations International Children's Fund, draws up a code regulating the marketing of infant formula. In 1984, after eight years of struggle, Nestlé finally signs an agreement promising to comply with the new standards. And the whole campaign has been instigated out of an office the size of a closet.[11]

Jesus' constructive alternative (12) was, of course, the reign of God. Turning the tables on one's oppressor may be fun now and then, but long-term structural and spiritual change requires an alternative vision. As the means of purveying that vision and living it in the midst of the old order, Jesus established a new counter-community that developed universalistic tendencies, erupting out of his own Jewish context and finally reaching beyond the Roman Empire.

Jesus was not content merely to empower the powerless, however. Here his teachings fundamentally transcend Alinsky's. Jesus' sayings about nonretaliation are of one piece with his challenge to love our enemies. Jesus did not advocate nonviolence merely as a technique for outwitting the enemy but as a just means of opposing the enemy in such a way as to hold open the possibility of the enemy's becoming just as well. Both sides must win. We are summoned to pray for our enemy's transformation and to respond to ill-treatment with a love which is not only godly but also, I am convinced, can only be found in God.

To Alinsky's list I would like to add another "rule" of my own: never adopt a strategy you would not want your opponents to use against you. I would not object to my opponents using nonviolent direct actions against me, since such a move would require them to be committed to suffer and even die rather than resort to violence against me. It would mean they would have to honor my humanity, believe God can transform me, and treat me with dignity and respect. One of the ironies of nonviolence, in fact, is that those who depend on violent repression to defend their privileges cannot resort to nonviolence. There is something essentially contradictory between crushing the dissent of a society's victims and being willing to give one's life for justice and the truth.

Today we can draw on the cumulative historical experience of nonviolent social struggle over the centuries and employ newer tools for political and social analysis. But the spirit, the thrust, the surge for creative transformation which is the ultimate principle of the universe—this is the same one we see incarnated in Jesus. Freed from literalistic legalism, his teaching reads like a practical manual for empowering the powerless to seize the initiative even in situations impervious to change. It seems almost as if his teaching has only now, in this generation, become an inescapable task and practical necessity.

To people dispirited by the enormity of the injustices which crush us and the intractability of those in positions of power, Jesus' words beam hope across the centuries. We need not be afraid. We can assert our human dignity. We can lay claim to the creative possibilities that are still ours, burlesque the injustice of unfair laws, and force evil out of hiding from behind the facade of legitimacy.

To risk confronting the Powers with such clown-like vulnerability, to affirm at the same time our own humanity and that of those we oppose, to dare to draw the sting of evil by absorbing it—such behavior is unlikely to attract the faint of heart. But I am convinced a host of people are waiting for the Christian message to challenge them, for once, to a heroism worthy of their lives. Has Jesus not given us that word?

3

Mysticism and Resistance

Dorothee Soelle

My personal experience of the relationship between mysticism and politics comes out of a dozen years' work with the peace movement in Europe and the United States. I do not wish to write off this experience, because I believe we still need it. In this movement, simple faith and worldly-wise skepticism battled against each other in each person. "Nothing ever changes," says the skeptic. "Have not wars always existed, and isn't the urge to make a profit the most natural thing in the world?" The reality of defeat was thus the most basic of our daily experiences.

How could that sense of defeat, of our own powerlessness, connect us to God? According to Jakob Boehme, God is "the Nothing that wishes to become Everything." Like the majority of mystics in the Western tradition, he thought of God as a movement, something flowing, growing, driving: a process.[1] If we participate in this process, we become a part of the God movement. We draw nearer to God as we take part in this movement.

God as the Nothing that wishes to become Everything means that we too must live with our own nothingness, that we must come to terms with our nothingness or be devastated by it. A Latin-American bishop, a mystic, described this as faith disrobing itself for him bit by bit. Faith must take off and lay down its garments one layer at a time. Without such undressing or destruction—Thomas Müntzer called it removing the coarseness (*Entgrobung*)—we cannot enter the process we call God. We must become the Nothing that wishes to become Everything.

The mystical cobbler, Jakob Boehme, became aware of the light that reflected off a metal pitcher in his workshop. This light changed his life; it started him down his path. We need to let such an experience make its way to us. We need to pay attention to it. Have we had similar experiences? Have we ever discovered something that we need in a splinter of wood or in a puddle at the edge of the street? The presence of God was there, in a poor cobbler's workshop.

Gegenwart, presence, is an interesting German word. It means literally that someone is across from me, present, paying attention and waiting for me. I am not alone; I am in the presence of another. If we say God is present, we are saying we are never alone. The strength of the Bible is that it speaks of this presence of God: a presence that calls out, promises, longs for, experiences, seeks, tells. The presence of God is the light of God.

In the classical definition, mysticism means experiencing the knowledge of God, *cognito Dei experimentalis*: the knowledge of God from experience as opposed to knowledge transmitted through books and doctrine or through tradition. There are two distinct paths to God: the normal, doctrinally buttressed, institutionalized path—and the unusual, experimental, and experiential, noninstitutional path.

I want to look at an example of the noninstitutional path. John Woolman was a North American Quaker who lived from 1720 to 1772.

> I was born in Northampton in Burlington County, West Jersey, in 1720. Before I was seven years old, I became acquainted with the workings of divine love. Through the care of my parents I learned to read as soon as I was able. I remember that one day after school I left my schoolmates and sat down to read the twenty-second chapter of Revelation: "Then the angel showed me the river of the water of life, bright as crystal, flowing from the throne of God and of the Lamb." As soon as I had read it, I felt a longing for the dwelling place that, according to my belief at the time, God had prepared for His servants. Even today I remember clearly the place where I sat and the blessed mood of that morning.[2]

I cannot do without the religious dimension of this way of thinking. For this I like to use the expression "the presence of God is present." That means first of all that I do not wish to speak of God as only in the past. God is indeed the greatest memory that we can remember. God hides God's self in the Bible and approaches us through tradition, but that is not enough. It is also not enough to speak of God as some kind of subjective past, as if God were a childhood memory. As soon as we become nostalgic when we talk about God, we have trivialized the here-and-now-ness of God; we have denied it, removed it.

I also do not wish to speak of God only in the future tense, in the hope of a world in which God will be more visible. This dimension of

God's time is necessary, and it should be stressed in contrast to those who still imagine the life to come as spatially separate. But the past and the future of God cannot satisfy us if we know nothing of the present presence of God: henceforth; now; here; amen, it is so; it was meant to be; behold!

I want to return to John Woolman, this eighteenth-century Quaker who left us his diaries. They offer a unique witness of the "and" in the title "Mysticism *and* Resistance." It was mystical piety and the certainty of the inner light that made him an activist for a radical change. Being one with God, in union with God, led him to a union with the conditions of all human beings alive, especially those most oppressed.

John Woolman grew up in a Quaker family near Philadelphia. He worked as a sales clerk, then a tailor. Occasionally he earned a little from teaching school and from farming. He also did drafting and preparing of contracts and legal documents. This latter occupation brought him into contact with slave owners who wanted to bequeath their slaves. Woolman's conscience would not allow him to write a will in which a slave was given to someone else. Thus he started to question those who asked him for this type of legal service, mostly wealthy, pious Quakers. Slowly he developed his personal position on the slavery question.

During his long and frequent travels he was dependent on the hospitality of the Friends, the Quakers. When, however, he noticed how the slaves of a co-religionist were dressed out in the fields—often, in the case of children, not at all—and their poor health, he preferred to sleep outdoors. The next day he would go to the owner in question and talk with him about slavery and the treatment of slaves. Woolman was convinced that greed led to destruction, for the rich as well as for the poor; that slavery destroyed the life God gave both those who owned slaves and made them work and those who were slaves; and that oppression was as deadly for the oppressor as for the oppressed.

After long conflicts the Quakers, influenced by Woolman among others, finally condemned slavery. Members were required to free their slaves, and slave owners were visited and monitored for compliance. Anyone involved in slave trading was banned from the fellowship of Friends. The Yearly Meeting of the Quakers in 1776 forbade Quakers to own slaves.[3]

I tell this story to demonstrate how a person may arrive at action from a deep mystical connection with God, and how mysticism and liberation—in this case of slaves and their owners—belong together. In addition, Woolman advocated a simple lifestyle. Slave holding corrupted the original simplicity of the settlers in the new land. It often led to the desire for luxury. Woolman thought about the clothing he wore and about what the departure from a certain simplicity meant for people's souls. He pondered how people either worked too much and ruined their health for the sake of false needs or exploited others for their own gain, behavior likewise driven by the dictatorship of false needs. The simplification of his lifestyle was for John Woolman the consequence of spiritual life, prayer, and the experience of the inner light. This simplification made possible a lifestyle not driven by concern with daily needs.

A third point at which Woolman as a Christian came into conflict with his times involved war. He refused to pay taxes during the wars against the Indians. He traveled to visit the Indians of Pennsylvania to attempt reconciliation. He encouraged all those who did not want to serve in the military. He said, "Luxury and oppression contain in them the seeds of war and destruction."[4]

Mysticism is not merely something for a few pardoned, elected individuals. The individual mystics did not think of their loneliness as confirmation of elite status; rather, they bemoaned their aloneness. So often they were not able to share the present presence of God with others. They could not impart God. They were mocked or persecuted for calling God present. I find a similar difficulty in the most important religious movement of our time, the one concerned with justice, peace, and the integrity of creation. We cannot impart God. Our political powerlessness is so vast that our language is not understood.

The unarmed God is ridiculous. He is slandered and mocked. When young people hold silent vigils for peace in the shopping malls of our cities—in the places where the golden calf is worshiped—the act of their standing there is a clear sign that God is present. In silence they speak of God's present presence. There is a mystical core in these new forms of piety that lives with one's own powerlessness and does not hide in churches. This core cannot be dampened by lack of response or rationalized away. God is there, even in the daily defeats each person must deal with in this struggle.

We know these defeats well. They are expressed in sentences such as "My family could care less"; "The newspaper didn't report on our action again"; "At work I'm ignored and mocked." Yet God *is* present. When the Present God is in my life and is not merely a tradition-laden memory and an eschatological future, this places me in a deep, unbridgeable conflict with the world in which I live. In our societies, God, his creation, and his favorite children are too often regarded as less than dirt.

When mystics speak of the experience of the presence of God, they do not primarily mean a God who protects and secures. In the language of mystics God is the light that shines for me, the water in which I can immerse myself, the fire that glows and warms. God is not the mighty fortress with thick walls that protects us from the evil enemy.

The experience of the God of the inner light, the birth of this spark in the soul, has radicalized humanity. Precisely because of the presence of God in humanity, humanity has become less and less tolerant of the exploitation and humiliation of its fellow creatures. In this manner, struggle and contemplation grow intertwined.

4

Just Peacemaking

Duane K. Friesen and Glen H. Stassen

How do we view our calling as Christians to be peacemakers in a world where injustice and conflict destroy life? More specifically, how can we as Christians work to build peace? Can we identify ethical guidelines that are faithful to a Christian vision of life and are both realistic and practical??

A group of twenty-three North American scholars, mostly Christian ethicists along with well-known international relations scholars, peace activists, and conflict resolution practitioners, worked at these questions for four years in a series of meetings and working conferences. Our beginning consensus was that the arguments which have long divided us, between Christian pacifists and those in the just war tradition, do not speak to the changing needs of our world and our time. We wanted to bridge these differences and find our areas of agreement.

At one of our meetings at the Abbey of Gethsemani (Kentucky, USA), we debated whether we should emphasize moral principles or political strategies. That discussion misled us to move toward abstract, historically disembodied ideals. It led us away from concreteness and historical actuality. It was ironical—or providential—that this struggle between empirical description and moral imperative took place at the Abbey of Gethsemani, where right before our eyes the monks were actually, empirically, engaging in the normative practice of prayer, beginning at 3:20 each morning. A few of us participated in those early morning prayers, and the monks' practice may have been what led us to a solution.

We found agreement by explicitly turning to the ethics of normative—ethically desirable—practices. The result is a list of ten actions which make up the Just Peacemaking Theory.[1] Casting the theory in the form of normative practices did several things for us. First, it brought together the empirical research of the international relations experts among us and the ethical arguments of the Christian ethicists and moral theologians.

Our approach also brought together the realists and the idealists among us. *Realists* say the world is characterized by power struggles and conflicts of interest. History does not take leaps, so we must learn to deal with the world as it is. *Idealists* say we should focus on ideals and imagine how we can move the world toward them. Bringing together these two often-polarized emphases, the realist-idealist practices of peacemaking we are pointing to do happen, empirically, in the real world, in the context of real threat, power struggle, and drive for security. They make power's expression in war less likely and peace more likely.

Describing just peacemaking in terms of normative practices also remedied the tension we experienced about the role of justice in peacemaking. When justice means historically actual practices that restore community, and we acknowledge our own complicity in injustice, then we can participate in modest and realistic ways that do lead to peace. This is in contrast to seeing justice as an absolute ideal, which can result in postponing peace until the kingdom arrives in its fullness.

The ten just peacemaking practices in our consensus model are not merely an ideal wish list. They are practices currently being carried out that are in fact spreading peace. Furthermore, they are engendering positive feedback loops, so they are growing in strength. They are pushing back the frontiers of war and spreading the zones of peace. We believe these emerging practices are also ethically normative; therefore, they can give realistic guidance to engagement by faith groups and other groups. We are saying that something intriguing is happening in our time. Understanding this can give us guidance and orient our participation in the peacemaking happening worldwide.

The Historical *Kairos*

Several historical forces have come together in our time to produce the Just Peacemaking Theory. Over fifty years ago the world was stunned by the horror of the devastation of World War II and the threat of atomic and nuclear weapons. The reality of that threat persuaded people and institutions to develop new networks and practices they hoped would prevent another world war and use of nuclear weapons.

Now over fifty years have passed, and so far we have avoided those two specters. New practices are actually getting results in ways many have not noticed. We believe we live in a moment of *kairos* when it is useful to name these practices, call attention to them, and support them ethically.

In this new era, after the Cold War and at the turn of the millennium, people lack a clear vision of what sort of peacemaking is effective and is in fact happening. Hence they do not know how they can contribute. The result is confusion, cognitive dissonance, apathy, and inward-turning—ironically just when the opportunity and need for spreading zones of peace is most at hand.

Just Peacemaking Theory is intended to give a road map to individual people, grassroots groups, voluntary associations, and groups in churches, synagogues, mosques, or meetings. The theory shows what people can do to fan the flames of peace.

As we experienced in our discussion at the Abbey, there is in our time a growing sense of the inadequacy of the debate between just war theory and pacifism. This has been the major division among Christians on the question of war. Debates dominated by these two paradigms inevitably focus on whether or not to make war.

That crucial question will not go away if the just peacemaking paradigm succeeds. However, in that two-sided debate another question regularly gets slighted: What essential steps should be taken to make peace? Have they been taken? Or should they yet be taken?

The just peacemaking question fills out the original intention of the other two paradigms. It encourages pacifists to be what their name, derived from the Latin, *pacem-facere,* means: peace-*makers.* And it calls just war theorists to fill in the contents of their underdeveloped principles of last resort and just intention. It invites them to spell out what resorts must be tried before moving to the last resort, what intention there is to restore a just and endurable peace—and then to act on the peace-promoting suggestions emerging from such discernment.

Ten Practices of Just Peacemaking

The ten practices of just peacemaking presented here are based on and grounded in the Christian faith. But we also offer them to others who can adapt them to their own faith perspectives. We divide the practices into three groups: *cooperative forces, justice,* and *peacemaking initiatives.* The first group, *cooperative forces,* may be seen as a dimension of love, realistically rather than sentimentally understood. A key dimension of love in scriptural teaching is breaking down barriers to community and participation in cooperative community.

Justice, the second grouping, is a central biblical theme. Third, growing numbers of us interpret grace-based peacemaking in terms of specific *peacemaking initiatives, or transforming initiatives.* The theological comments which follow our list of the ten just peacemaking practices show how these are grounded in Christian faith.

Strengthen Cooperative Forces

1. *Recognize emerging cooperative forces in the international system and work with them.* Historically, cooperative institutions like the League of Nations have broken down. But there are trends in today's world that make it much more possible to sustain voluntary associations for peace and other purposes.

The utility of war has declined, with trade and the economy taking priority over war. International exchanges, communications, transactions, and networks are growing stronger. There is a gradual ascendancy of liberal representative democracy and a mixture of welfare-state and laissez-faire market economy. We should act so as to strengthen these trends and the international associations they make possible,[2] insofar as they genuinely advance the common good and do not further hurt the poor and powerless.

When churches teach the wrongness and futility of war, send and receive missionaries, and welcome refugees, they are encouraging cooperative forces. Churches strengthen ties in this emerging international system by themselves becoming internationalized in their membership and leadership. They can work at this by sending members to international conferences, service projects, and work camps as well as learning from fellow Christians across international and especially North/South divisions. Churches were pioneering these practices long before international relations scholars were writing about them, and we need more of such activity.

2. *Strengthen the United Nations and international efforts for cooperation and human rights.* International relations increasingly involve not only the traditional military-diplomatic arena but also the modern arena of economic interdependence. Here governments are exposed to the forces of a global market they do not control. At the same time, the information revolution makes it harder for governments to control people's minds, and popular pressures can now set much of the agenda of foreign policies. States float in a sea of forces from outside their borders or from among their people. Acting alone, states cannot solve problems of trade, debt, interest rates; of pollution, ozone depletion, acid rain, global warming; of migrations and refugees seeking asylum; of military security when weapons rapidly penetrate borders.

As we approach the turning of the century, collective action is increasingly necessary. Citizens can encourage their governments to act in small and large crises in ways that strengthen the effectiveness of the United Nations and of regional organizations. We can include support for the United Nations as part of our church teaching and action or as an aspect of the strategy of peacemaking organizations in which we participate.

Many multilateral practices are building effectiveness to resolve conflicts; to monitor, nurture, and even enforce truces; and to replace violent conflict with the beginnings of cooperation. International cooperation is meeting human needs for food, hygiene, medicine, education, and economic interaction. Collective action sometimes includes UN-approved humanitarian intervention in cases like the former Yugoslavia, Haiti, Somalia, and Rwanda "when a state's condition or behavior results in . . . grave and massive violations of human rights."[3]

Advance Justice for All

3. *Promote democracy, human rights, and religious liberty. Spreading democracy and respect for human rights, including religious liberty, is widening the zones of peace.*[4] Democracies tend not to make war on each other. Established democracies fought *no wars* against one another during the entire twentieth century. And they generally devote lower shares of their gross national products (GNP) to military expenditures, which decreases threats to other countries. Influences that played significant parts in producing the recent extensive wave of transitions to democracy include church institutions that oppose governmental authoritarianism; citizens' groups and nongovernmental organizations dedicated to defending human rights; and states and international organizations more actively promoting human rights and democracy.

Powerful threats to democracy's spread exist. Among them are grim economic conditions in numerous struggling democracies; ethnic, racial, nationalistic, and religious conflict; instabilities during the transition to democracy; and external threats from nondemocratic neighbors.

The possibility of a widespread and growing zone of peace requires a network of persons who work together to gain public attention for those they are trying to protect from human rights violations.[5]

4. *Foster just and sustainable economic development.* Supporting human rights and democracy also requires sustainable development. The needs of today must be met without threatening the needs of tomorrow. Those who lack adequate material and economic resources need to gain access, and those who have such resources must learn to control their

use and prevent future exhaustion. Organizations like the Mennonite Central Committee and others have pioneered in fostering the development of appropriate technology. Sustainable development will require work on various levels. Access to resources such as water and land is a peace question in the Middle East, Latin America, and Asia.

Take Peacemaking Initiatives

5. *Reduce offensive weapons and weapons trade*. A key factor in the decrease of war between nations is that weapons have become so destructive that war is not worth the price. Offensive forces cannot destroy the enemy's defense before it does huge retaliatory damage. Further reduction of offensive weapons makes war even less likely. For example, President Gorbachev removed half the Soviet Union's tanks from Central Europe and all its river-crossing equipment. This freed NATO to agree to get rid of all medium-range and shorter-range nuclear weapons on both sides from Eastern and Western Europe—the first dramatic step in ending the Cold War peacefully.

As nations turn toward democracy and human rights, their governments no longer need large militaries to keep them in power. As the ten practices of peacemaking reduce the threat of war, nations feel less need for weapons. As they struggle with their deep indebtedness, they have less ability to buy weapons. The International Monetary Fund now requires big reductions in weapons expenditures before granting loans. Arms imports by developing nations in 1995 dropped to one-quarter of their 1988 peak.

6. *Support nonviolent direct action*. Nonviolent direct action, used effectively by Gandhi in India and the civil rights movement in the United States, is spreading widely. In recent decades it has ended dictatorship in the Philippines, terminated rule by the Shah in Iran, and brought about nonviolent revolutions in Poland, East Germany, and Central Europe. Nonviolent action has transformed injustice into democratic change in human rights movements in Guatemala, Argentina, and elsewhere in Latin America; in the nonviolent parts of the Intifadah campaign in Palestine; in the freedom campaign in South Africa; and in many other countries.[6] In contrast we can point to the failures of violent campaigns in Bosnia, Somalia, and Northern Ireland. Christian peacemakers are teaching the methods of nonviolence worldwide.

7. *Take independent initiatives to reduce hostility*. The recently developed strategy of independent initiatives successfully freed Austria from Soviet domination in the 1950s in exchange for Austrian neutrality and nonoffensive military. The Atmospheric Test Ban Treaty of 1963 was made possible after U.S. Presidents Eisenhower and Kennedy halted at-

mospheric nuclear testing unilaterally. Independent initiatives led to dramatic reductions in nuclear weapons via the series of initiatives by President Gorbachev plus the U.S. Congress and President Bush. Peacemaking breakthroughs have occurred through small initiatives taken by Israel and its Arab neighbors and by adversaries in Northern Ireland.

Independent initiatives have a number of characteristics. They are independent of the slow process of negotiation and designed to decrease distrust by the other side—but not leave the initiator weak. Such initiatives are visible and verifiable actions, have a timing announced in advance and carried out regardless of the other side's bluster, and include a clearly announced purpose—to shift toward de-escalation and to invite reciprocation. These initiatives need to come in a series. If the other side does not reciprocate, small initiatives should continue to keep inviting reciprocation.

The strategy of independent initiatives was advocated in various church peace statements in the 1980s. However, it needs to be understood more widely so it can be noticed when it causes breakthroughs and so citizens can press governments to take such initiatives.[7]

8. *Use partnership conflict resolution.* Conflict resolution is becoming a well-known practice at international as well as local levels. A key test of the seriousness of governments' claims to be seeking peace is whether they develop imaginative solutions that show they understand their adversary's perspectives and needs.

We prefer the term *partnership* conflict resolution. By this we mean active partnership in developing solutions, not merely passive cooperation. Adversaries need help to listen to each other and experience each others' perspectives. This multicultural literacy must go beyond the surface positions and interests of the adversaries to include aspects of their culture, spirituality, story, history, and emotion. We seek long-term solutions which help prevent future conflict, even as we work to heal and resolve immediate conflict. Justice is a core component for sustainable peace.

Martin Luther King Jr. said, "Peace is not the absence of tension, but the presence of justice."[8] John Howard Yoder describes the New Testament practice of fraternal admonition, long practiced (but not frequently and consistently enough) by churches, as a predecessor of conflict resolution.[9]

9. *Acknowledge responsibility for conflict and injustice; seek repentance and forgiveness.* The single most important initiative in German Chancellor Willy Brandt's *Ostpolitik* was the quest for reconciliation with then-Communist Poland. Poland, after all, was the first country to be blitzkrieged by the Nazi war machine and the country with the largest num-

ber of Holocaust victims (perhaps 3,000,000). In December 1970, Brandt courageously (with no sure guarantee of parliamentary approval) signed a treaty accepting the Oder-Neisse frontier and therewith the cession of 40,000 square miles of German territory (Silesia and parts of Pomerania and East Prussia). This decision he personally dramatized by kneeling silently at the Warsaw war memorial as an act of atonement for German offenses against the Polish people. That Brandt, of all people, should assume such a posture of repentance was especially remarkable in view of his own anti-Nazi credentials and his exile in Norway throughout the war. It was an extraordinarily winsome, powerful, long-lasting act of personal leadership. It made peace a human possibility.

Conflict is not really resolved nor the resolution really internalized until confession and forgiveness occur. This dimension of gospel grace also is deeply needed worldwide.

10. *Encourage grassroots peacemaking groups and voluntary associations.* Just peacemaking requires associations of citizens organized independently of governments, and linked together across boundaries of nation, class, and race, to learn peacemaking practices and press governments to employ these practices. Governments should protect such associations in law and give them accurate information.

The existence of a growing worldwide people's movement constitutes one more historical force that makes just peacemaking possible. A transnational network of groups, including faith groups, can partly transcend captivity by narrow national or ideological perspectives. Citizens' groups are not so committed to status-quo institutional maintenance as bureaucracies often are, nor are they so isolated and only temporarily engaged as individuals often are. Thus they can provide long-term perseverance in peacemaking. They can serve as voices for the voiceless, as they did in churches in East Germany and in women's groups in Guatemala.[10] They can help to initiate, foster, or support transforming initiatives where existing parties need support and courage to risk breaking out of cycles that perpetuate violence and injustice.

A citizens' network of NGOs (nongovernmental organizations) and INGOs (international nongovernmental organizations) can be a source of information which persons in positions of governmental authority may lack or resist acknowledging. NGO's can criticize injustice and initiate repentance and forgiveness. They can nurture a spirituality that sustains courage when peacemaking is unpopular, hope when despair or cynicism is tempting, and grace and forgiveness when peacemaking fails.

Toward a Theological Basis of Just Peacemaking

The practices of just peacemaking make pragmatic sense. We see historical evidence that these practices can accomplish the goals of peace and justice. However, we arrive at these normative practices of just peacemaking not only on pragmatic grounds but also from deeply held faith perspectives. With the eyes of faith we attribute the evidence that just peacemaking works to the "breaking in of God's reign" in history.

We two who have been involved in the process from the beginning (Duane Friesen, a Mennonite, and Glen Stassen, a Baptist) want to share the theological perspective that informs us. Our vision, shaped by our "believers church" tradition, is grounded in three theological convictions. First, we believe biblical discipleship is grounded in the life, teachings, death, and resurrection of Jesus Christ. Second, the church is the eschatological "sign" of God's reign in the world, embodied in a concrete gathering of persons who seek to discern together what just peacemaking means and to model peacemaking practices in our corporate and individual lives.

Third, the church must be committed to seek the peace of the city where she dwells (Jer. 29:7). The task of the church is to further God's reign not by withdrawal or quietism nor by uncritical support of or reliance on the government—but by engaging the issues of peace and justice actively in the brokenness of the world.

Discipleship

Discipleship is based in an "embodied," or incarnational, Christology. Christ is the servant Lord of the Gospels, who represents a specific and concrete way of life meant to be followed. This is an alternative to views of Christ which make "Godlike" claims for Christ but are divorced from Christ's way as a model for ethical practice. We resist Christologies that relegate Christ to a separate sphere of life (the spiritual), define the meaning of Christ primarily in terms of salvation for eternal life, or reduce Jesus' teaching to high, abstract ideals (like selfless, sacrificial love) unrelated to concrete practices able to guide us in the real world. We find inadequate a Christology (reflected in the orthodox creeds) preoccupied with the metaphysical relationship of the individual person of Jesus to an imperial God. Instead, we focus on the Lord who called his disciples humbly to follow his way of nonviolent love.

We can illustrate what an "embodied" Christology looks like by a brief examination of the classical text of Christian peacemaking, The

Sermon on the Mount (Matthew 5-7). In Matthew's portrayal of Jesus' teachings we see a vivid peacemaking model of a way to confront evil not through violent force but through transforming initiatives as an alternative to either passive withdrawal or violent confrontation.[11]

Most interpretations of the Sermon on the Mount view Jesus as teaching an impossible ideal that cannot be realized in a sinful world. The Sermon on the Mount is interpreted in dyads: (1) "You have heard of old, don't kill"; (2) "But I say, don't even be angry." In this interpretation the focus is on not being angry, which is easy to dismiss as impossible.

In fact, the Sermon is organized as triads: (1) traditional piety (i.e., "you shall not kill"); (2) the mechanism of bondage (nursing anger or saying, "you fool"); and (3) the transforming initiative ("Go, therefore, be reconciled"). There are fourteen such triads, from Matthew 5:21 through 7:1. In each, the second member of the triad, the mechanism of bondage or vicious cycle, does not use imperatives but continuing action verbs. It diagnoses the ongoing process of trouble we get ourselves into when we serve some other lord than God.

When, for instance, anger rules us, we often fail to take the steps necessary to act to correct a problem. If we recognize the triadic structure of the Sermon on the Mount, then we can see that the emphasis is on the concrete step we can take to deal with the conflict with a brother or sister. The third member of each triad names the imperatives, the transforming initiatives, the concrete commands of Jesus which are practical and doable (in this case, "go be reconciled"). This third element is always an initiative, not a prohibition.[12]

In preaching, teaching, and living this good news, Jesus modeled a way to confront evil to restore right relationships (righteousness or justice). We have vivid pictures in New Testament images, stories, sayings, accounts of Jesus' life, and ethical exhortations of how the followers of Jesus envisioned what it means to follow him in a life of discipleship. Not only the Gospels but also other writings (such as the ethical exhortations of Paul, for example, beginning in Romans 12), provide such pictures. The peacemaking practices of weapons reductions, nonviolent action, independent initiatives, conflict resolution, and repentance and forgiveness are public analogies, spillovers, or even sometimes expressions of obedience to these embodied actions and teachings of Jesus.

Jesus taught and practiced a total devotion to God's kingdom that called into question human devotion to less ultimate ends. This is particularly evident in Jesus' teaching on wealth and material well-being. Jesus is not ascetic in this teaching, not denying the importance of that which sustains bodily well-being. However, the stories and teachings of the gospel severely condemn those devoted to the accumulation of wealth and the goods of this world. The just peacemaking practice of sustainable economic development is an expression of Jesus' teachings about wealth, poverty, feeding the hungry, and covenant justice.

The Church as a Discerning Community

Discipleship is not primarily realized in the actions of heroic individuals. Rather, discipleship is actualized in the practices of a concrete community, in a social group which by its very existence as an alternative community in the world is a sign of God's reign, albeit in very earthen vessels.

The church has a variety of functions, only two of which we will elaborate here because of their direct implications for a theology of just peacemaking.

First, the church functions as a community of memory and hope to nurture the paradigmatic story that orients the community in time and sustains a vision of God's reign. The identification of the norms of just peacemaking by a group of persons from a wide diversity of backgrounds is not sufficient if we do not also nurture more intimate moral communities that can form people of character. The analysis of North American society reflected in *Habits of the Heart* has shown how this culture increasingly nurtures an individualism which damages commitment to the common good. Communities which nurture a commitment to a social vision are increasingly being eroded by an ethic of "self-interest" in which individual well-being is the ultimate value.[13]

We cannot take for granted the institutions of civil society (families, churches, synagogues, neighborhoods) that form people of character. Such communities can morally shape people willing to commit their energies to just peacemaking because they believe it is right in and of itself. The conditions of our world require that we be willing to embrace the stranger, those with no voice, if we are really serious about just peacemaking. A calculating self-interest will not sustain us. A deep commitment to the values of compassion and justice is essential for the costly and enduring commitment to just peacemaking required by the conditions in our world.

However, simply having a set of values is not enough to make someone an active peacemaker. Sociologist Robert Wuthnow suggests that the likelihood for compassionate behavior requires a combination of belief in these values and regular participation in an organized religious community.

> Religious inclinations make very little difference unless one becomes involved in some kind of organized religious community. Once you are in-

volved in such a community, then a higher level of piety may be associated with putting yourself out to help the needy. But if you are not involved in some kind of religious organization, then a higher level of piety seems unlikely to generate charitable efforts toward the poor or disadvantaged.[14]

Deliberate attention to nurture in the church, which keeps alive the memory of its paradigmatic stories (such as the Exodus or the "Good Samaritan"), is essential to the moral formation of people of character. Keeping alive such stories is important to the continued practice of a kind of compassion that reaches across barriers to generate reconciliation.

The church can serve a special role in nurturing a spirituality that sustains courage when just peacemaking is unpopular, hope when despair or cynicism is tempting, and a sense of grace and the possibility of forgiveness when just peacemaking fails. A church nurtured by an eschatological vision of God's reign, grounded in a vision that the slain lamb is the Lord of history (the book of Revelation) is particularly needed when popular culture fosters a mass spirit of hatred toward enemies that fan the flames of war.

Peacemakers then need to be sustained by a willingness to suffer if necessary, to endure abuse without retaliation, to overcome hatred of the enemy, and to keep hope and patience alive during a long period of struggle. The church can sustain trust in the possibility of the miracle of transformation when the evidence for change appears bleak, and joy even amid suffering and pain.

Just peacemaking will not long endure if its theological roots are based on the assurance of success, though we live at a moment when historical evidence of the promise of just peacemaking surrounds us. We need a realism about the depth of evil that can guard us from disillusionment. Aware of the limits of our own ability to predict and control the future, we can still, by the gracious power of God, embrace our common humanity through simple deeds of kindness and charity. In the context of hatred and violence, such acts may disarm an opponent and become the occasion for a transforming initiative for justice and peace.

When we emphasize the tenth practice of just peacemaking—encouraging grassroots peacemaking groups and voluntary associations—we most concretely have in mind those churches, church groups, and peacemaking groups that embody the peacemaking that the Jesus Christ of the New Testament taught and died for.

Second, the church structures a process of practical moral reasoning where the members of the community can both hear and speak to each other as they discern together what discipleship means. To be a member of a church means to commit oneself to a process of conversation. Commitment is not primarily to a fixed system of ethics. The church is a gathering of persons committed to speaking and listening to each other to discern what faithfulness means in the light of the vision of life revealed in Jesus Christ. This participatory model, when it functions well, can be a "school of learning" for the participatory democracy of the third practice of peacemaking. It has been so historically and can be so in our time.

Our emphasis on the church as community, over against individualism, also influences us to see the importance of the secular analogy. Here we mean those cooperative forces in the international system, the United Nations and regional organizations, that function as deliberative bodies but also encourage mutual admonition, mutual understanding, communication, common memories and narratives.

Seeking the Shalom of the City (Jer. 29:7)

The church is engaged in mission beyond its own borders. The church does not exist simply for itself but to participate in the liberating power of God's reign in the world. The Gospels portray Jesus as an agent of deliverance, God's anointed one (Messiah), who is commissioned to bring God's kingdom into the world. The kingdom of God represents the wholeness God intends for the entire cosmos. Jesus taught his disciples to pray that this kingdom come and to participate in the process through which deliverance comes about. The vision of God's kingdom is not a sectarian model for the church but a call to transform the world.

Though the kingdom is a reality which is still future in terms of its full manifestation, it is present already where God's reign is breaking into history. Jesus says, "If it is by the finger of God that I cast out the demons, then the kingdom of God has come to you" (Luke 11:20). The kingdom becomes present through Jesus when he gives sight to the blind, feeds the hungry, liberates people from demonic possession, and forgives sin so people can live a life of wholeness.

Compassionate presence is at the heart of the Christian faith. Jesus reveals a God who is not a detached sovereign ruling over the universe from a distance. The Greek word for compassion in the New Testament, *splagchoisomai*, means to let one's innards embrace the feeling or situation of another. Jesus is a compassionate presence with those who suffer in many of the stories of the gospels.

Jesus stands in solidarity with the marginalized. Those treated as outcasts in the social context of Jesus' time are just the ones on whom Jesus has compassion: the poor, widows, the sick, Samaritans, those labeled "sinners." We observe in particular Jesus' attitude and behavior toward women and toward children—a revolutionary stance in the cultural context of first-century Palestine.

Christ's call to discipleship means the church will frequently find itself at odds with the dominant culture in which it lives. In some sense, like the Hebrews in Babylon at the time of Jeremiah, the church is an "exile" community. But exile does not mean withdrawal into a special enclave separate from the world. Rather, like the Hebrews of Jeremiah's time, the church is called to "seek the shalom of the city where it dwells." The church exists not for itself but for the world, to be God's body in the world. The advice of Jeremiah to pray to God on behalf of the city in which we live is not a call for passivity—to let God act while the church watches and waits. To genuinely pray to God for the welfare of the city is to yearn with all one's heart for its well-being.

The classic study of Christ and culture by H. Richard Niebuhr develops a classification of types of responses of the church to culture.[15] Ethicists have debated at length the usefulness of Niebuhr's typology and the question of what the relationship should be of the church to culture.

In our development of just peacemaking norms, our response to culture varies. Sometimes we are sharply critical of the direction of our culture (i.e., practice five: opposition to the development of offensive weapons and the weapons trade; practice nine: the need for repentance and forgiveness). In other cases we affirm the positive directions in the larger culture (i.e., practice one: to strengthen the cooperative forces in the international system; or practice three: the spread of democracy and commitment to human rights).

When the church seeks the well-being of the city where it dwells, it will be drawn into participation with fellow citizens, from a variety of points of view, in the development of norms and practices that can contribute to the *shalom* of the city. The way in which this just peacemaking paradigm was developed is itself a model of the process of discernment, of citizens coming together even though they do not share all theological or philosophical assumptions.

Conclusion

The Just Peacemaking Theory suggests normative practices churches and peacemaking groups can use to build conditions that make peace more likely. In crisis situations, these are initiatives that should be tried before actors resort to war. Whether a government employs these practices is a test of the sincerity of its claims that it is trying to make peace.

Not all practices in our time are normative. There are powerful economic interests and natural drives for national security, that can work good or evil. There are interests that do not want to make peace— and interests that think they want to make peace but perceive things in such a way, and with such loyalties, that their actions work against peace. There are those who think the way to peace is to wipe out the enemy. There are enormous forces of evil. These include—

* nuclear weapons and their delivery systems as well as chemical and biological weapons;

* devastating poverty and its offspring, including population explosion;

* ecological devastation and nonrenewable energy consumption;

* ethnic and religious wars in nations like Cambodia, Bosnia, and the Congo.

Whatever peacemaking practices we may point to need to work their way into areas where they are still foreign. Each practice recognizes and seeks to resolve, lessen, or check one or more of these forces.

Our normative practices focus on peacemaking processes that are in fact taking place in our historical period and growing through positive feedback loops. If we begin to notice that these ten practices are already happening—resolving conflicts, proving useful and therefore spreading, and making reliance on war unlikely in many regions—then we *will* sense we may be able to encourage a transition from war as normal to war as abnormal.

We are not just expressing a wish. We are also calling those who have eyes to see to notice what new processes of deliverance are happening among us and spreading globally. We are urging not disembodied ideals to be imposed on history. Rather, we are advocating support for what serves functional needs in the midst of the power realities. These are the practices perceived by those who have eyes to see from the perspective of peace and justice and of faith and hope.

5

The Politics of Forgiveness

(In the name of God, the Magnificent, the Merciful)
Chaiwat Satha-Anand (Qader Muheideen)

Many people look forward to the rise of the twenty-first century with hope. There are good reasons for this. The world has changed so drastically in the last decade it is only vaguely recognizable if viewed from the perspective of the Cold War. Many rejoiced when the Berlin Wall collapsed and the Soviet Union dissolved, redrawing the world map both geographically and politically. Lester Brown, founder and director of Worldwatch Institute, delights that world leaders can now shift their focus from old agendas to the urgent new global challenges around resource and environmental policies.[1]

While there are signs of hope, signs of despair are not absent either. There are civil wars in the Sudan between Arab and black Africans, fighting in Chad between insurgents and government troops, tension between Orthodox Christians and Muslims in the Horn of Africa, and recurring rioting between Muslims and Christians in Nigeria.

In Asia, Buddhist Tibet and its Turkish-Muslim minority are oppressed by China. The December 1992 destruction of the Babri mosque in Ayodhya by militant Hindus and resulting communal violence mark a new intensity in India's long-standing conflict. These conflicts, and the carnage in Bosnia-Herzegovina, Rwanda, and Somalia, raise a disturbing point. Maybe the world *has* gone mad. Maybe novel thinking is needed to fight a new style of violent conflict plaguing humanity.

If the modern world is facing violent conflicts underscored by the "clash of civilizations,"[2] a politics of forgiveness is necessary. I use forgiveness not as a religious concept but from a political, conflict-oriented, nonviolent perspective. Yet I will discuss the idea of forgiveness in Christianity, from Jesus' teachings to Kenneth Kaunda's proposal, in Islamic teachings, and in Gandhi's thoughts. I will not so much compare as search for inspiration rooted in vital beliefs. I suggest nonviolence requires the politics of forgiveness·

Why Forgiveness Now?

Samuel P. Huntington proposes in a controversial article that "the fundamental source of conflict in this new world will not be primarily ideological or primarily economic. The great divisions among humankind and the dominating source of conflict will be cultural."[3]

Clashes of civilizations will occur because differences among civilizations are more fundamental than differences among political ideologies and political regimes.

Interactions between peoples of different civilizations are increasing. Meanwhile, the processes of economic modernization and social change throughout the world are both separating people from long-standing local identities and weakening the nation-state as a source of identity. Huntington believes cultural characteristics are less changeable. As a result cultural conflicts are less easily resolved than political and economic ones.[4]

Huntington's ideas are intriguing. If there is a new mode of violent conflict in the making, I see it captured by the kinds of questions participants in these conflicts raise. The basic question which characterized earlier modes of violent conflict was "Which side are you on?" But the question which characterizes the present mode of violent conflict is "What are you?"[5]

This question seems to seek an answer which strikes deep at the relationship between the problem of the self and its cultural world. It is the focus on culture (or culture's highest grouping—civilization) which is now responsible for the agonizing conflicts around the world.

I contend that the fundamental difference between the two questions does not depend on their dichotomizing worldview because both are similar in separating "us" from "them." The more dangerous quality of the second question lies in its rigidity and the almost unchangeable nature of answers it elicits. When asked the first question, people can choose—and could change sides. But it is much more difficult, if not impossible, to give up the faith, throw away the language of ancestors, or change skin color. A person can be half-American and half-Thai; it is more difficult to be half-black and half-white or half-Hindu and half-Muslim. This second question is more dangerous than the first because the answer has a sense of finality.

One of the clearest examples of a clash of civilizations is the case of ex-Yugoslavia. In her 1937 book, *Black Lamb and Grey Falcon*, historian Rebecca West imagines herself asking a Yugoslavian peasant, "In your lifetime have you ever known peace?" She shakes him, and he is transformed into his father, then his grandfather, then his great-grandfather. As she carries her questioning back in time for a thousand years, the answer remains the same: "No, there was fear, there were enemies without and in, there was prison, torture, and violent death." In the sixteenth century, the Croatian peasant uprising was suppressed with unimaginable cruelty by the Austrians. Later the Pope ordered thousands of Bosnian followers of a popular Christian sect killed. Then the Turkish *pasha* entered Sarajevo and began massive beheadings. The Sarajevans reconquered their city and began a bloody three-day massacre.[6]

Ex-Yugoslavia, like other countries, is a land steeped in history. A long, bitter tradition laced with direct violence and legitimized by cultural violence can easily become a repository of collective trauma. As new conflicts erupt, these traumatic experiences can be drawn on to fan the fires of hatred. Living with a surplus of traumas from the past can undermine any attempt, violent or nonviolent, to resolve the present violent conflict for a better tomorrow.

Ex-Yugoslavia is not the only place where collective traumas jeopardize efforts to construct a peaceful future. The same can be said about the Tamil-Sinhalese conflict in Sri Lanka, the Irish/Catholic-British conflict in Northern Ireland/England, the Hindu-Muslim conflict in India, and the militant Muslim versus the West conflict, spearheaded by Americans in violent encounters around the globe. With clashes of civilizations underlying violent conflicts, neither the brutality of violent means nor the power of nonviolent actions may be sufficient to meet the challenges. The concept of "forgiveness" can serve as a corrective device to enhance the effectiveness of nonviolence in coping with violent conflicts.

Analyzing Forgiveness

Since forgiveness is a concept underscored in Christianity, let me begin this discussion with the words of Jesus himself. The Gospel of

Luke states, "When they reached the place called the Skull, there they crucified him and the two criminals, one on his right, the other on his left. Jesus said, 'Father, forgive them; they do not know what they are doing.'"[7]

At least three points can be derived from this story of Jesus on the cross. First, the Jesus who asked God to forgive wrongdoers was the suffering Jesus who had been victimized. The request for forgiveness came from the victim himself. This is of utmost importance for the social-scientific understanding of forgiveness discussed below. Second, the sinners who tried to kill him did so out of ignorance and therefore deserved God's forgiveness. Third, from a theological perspective, the history of Christianity becomes a history of salvation once Jesus is accepted as the Redeemer. The meaning of Jesus as the Redeemer is realized when forgiveness is activated and sinners become Christians. In this sense, a human life is not a lost cause but a possibility for a better future.

Some may argue that forgiveness is important only in the religious realm. Yet in both Islamic teachings and Gandhi's thoughts, religious values and politics are inseparable.[8]

There are as well a number of modern politicians who regard forgiveness as crucial for their kind of politics. Dr. Martin Luther King Jr., for example, highlighted the significance of forgiveness in the context of love. He explained this as *agape*—an active seeking to preserve and create community. Agape love includes "a willingness to forgive, not seven times, but seventy times seven to restore community."[9]

No less instructive is the case of Kenneth David Kaunda of Zambia, a political leader who included the idea of forgiveness in his politics. Despite later political problems, Kaunda's life is particularly significant for those interested in nonviolence. As a former national movement leader, he advocated and practiced nonviolent action. Yet when he became president of Zambia, he changed and accepted violence as necessary for the conduct of politics.

Kaunda candidly voiced the existential tension he felt between his involvement in the use of force as president and his belief in the central importance of the cross as a Christian. He maintained that to rule out the use of force under the circumstances he faced in 1980 would have condemned millions of people to indefinite servitude. While he found no way of coming to terms with the cross as a political strategy, he claimed he rediscovered the power of forgiveness as a means of personal regeneration. He also argued that forgiveness corresponds well with the African temperament and has been exercised by other African political leaders, including Zimbabwe prime minister Robert Mugabe.

Kaunda highlights three points. First, forgiveness is not an isolated act and therefore is not the same as granting a pardon. On the contrary, forgiveness is "a constant willingness to live in a new day without looking back and ransacking the memory for occasions of bitterness and resentment." Second, forgiveness is not a substitute for justice. Kaunda reasoned that "To claim forgiveness whilst perpetuating injustice is to live a fiction; to fight for justice without also being prepared to offer forgiveness is to render your struggle null and void." Third, through the power of forgiveness people are freed from the burden of past guilt so that they can act boldly in the present. In this sense, to forgive one's enemies is not only a moral or religious matter. It is necessary for one's own sanity.[10]

I began this discussion through Jesus and Kaunda because the image of forgiveness resonates with a religious and especially Christian tone. These examples make the sociopolitical implications of forgiveness evident. Nevertheless, also needed is a critical analysis of the politics of forgiveness from a nonreligious perspective. I emphasize the secularized version of forgiveness because, to enhance its universal appeal for people of different persuasions, the concept needs to be freed from particular religious overtones. In addition, I believe that if the dynamics of forgiveness are critically analyzed, its power will be better understood and the concept may be taken more seriously by those engaged in present-day violent conflicts.

Forgiveness and Social Relations

Any violent situation includes victimizer and victim. The relationship between the two parties is that the former is more powerful while the latter is less so. If the victim remains passive, the power relationship remains unchanged. If the victim starts to fight back, the existing power relations become unstable: fighting back challenges and sometimes changes existing power relations.

This is the central point of Gene Sharp's nonviolence theory. Sharp urges that

> all responses to conflict situations be initially divided into those of *action* and those of *inaction*, and not divided according to their violence or lack of violence. In such a division nonviolent action assumes its correct place as *one type of active response.*[11]

Without nonviolent actions, or violent actions for those deeply trapped in the paradigm of violence, power relations remain unchallenged. When the former victim acts, for example, by engaging in nonviolent disobedience, he or she is no longer a victim but an equal of the former victimizer. In fighting back, the victim is able to free him or herself from the chain of passivity which successfully locked the social relations. Once freed and on equal footing with the former victimizer, the victim can contemplate forgiveness.

In this sense, forgiveness serves as a more radical alteration of social and power relations than revenge. During revenge, the avenger becomes a new victimizer and the foe is transformed into a victim. Some would call this situation "the paradox of opposites" when "we become what we hate."[12]

But the ones who forgive are superior to those forgiven. A person able to forgive rises above the memories of being victimized. Forgiveness restores wholeness, autonomy, and freedom to this person.[13]

Forgiveness and Time

In this process of restoration and change of social relations, time plays an important role. Politics are not shaped only by worldly concerns, such as "Who gets what? When? And how?" or "Who governs?" or "the political economy" of a given country. Politics are also profoundly influenced by the collective memories of people. These memories are both conscious and subconscious carriers of complex past experiences which, in turn, affect both perceptions and formations of future political options.[14]

Forgiveness is often mistakenly assumed to relate to forgetting. Kaunda's assertion is no different. But I believe the meaning of forgiveness cannot be realized unless those memories of past misery are retained. Forgiveness is not forgetting. An amnesiac loses the ability to forgive precisely because the person has lost memory. To forgive the victimizer in a conscious act full of intentionality, a clear memory is required.

The problem is how to face the bitter memory and then rise above it. This difficult task cannot be accomplished unless the former victims of violence also try to free themselves from being trapped by the memory of being victimized.

To free oneself from this invisible cage of memory, the nature of time as it affects the self must be understood. When a loved one dies, bereavement captures the imagination of those who remain and remember. Seeing the belongings of her dead husband, the wife's consciousness is caught in the past represented by his things. If both husband and wife were victims of violence, the traumatic experience returns. On a collective level, it is possible to institutionalize the retention of past misery. On May 20, 1984, an officially proclaimed "Day of Hatred," Cambodians were ordered to express their anger against the Khmer Rouge regime and its supporters.[15]

This memory trap makes genuine reconciliation among different Khmer factions difficult, despite the tremendous effort by the United Nations and other parties.

In bereavement, the past becomes fixed, because it acts as a wall preventing present reality from entering the individual's time consciousness. If the present does filter in, it is transformed immediately in terms of the past.[16] To free oneself from the wall of the past is not to undo the past. Murder or rape are irreversible. But those who survive can learn to accept these miseries as parts of life. They can learn to cross the wall and get on with newfound possibilities.

It is important not to forget the past; otherwise, forgiveness would be meaningless. But it is also necessary to not accept being trapped in the memory of that past, or former victims will be unable to find their place in the changing future.

Forgiveness and Justice

Kaunda asserts that forgiveness cannot coexist with injustice. In other words, forgiveness without justice is meaningless. But is forgiveness really impossible without justice? Can justice itself become a hindrance to forgiveness? To deal with these questions, we must raise a new question: "What kind of justice is at work in the process of forgiving?" This question allows us to approach forgiveness in a more dynamic way.

The Greek philosopher Aristotle understood justice to mean "a state of character which renders men disposed to act justly." Justice is also defined as that which is fair or equal; the just person is the one who takes his or her proper share. Aristotle used this concept of equality to categorize justice into distributive justice, corrective justice, and justice in exchange. Distributive justice focuses on equality between equals. Corrective justice is equality between crime and punishment. Justice in exchange, on the other hand, means equality between whatever goods are exchanged.[17]

In violent action and revenge, corrective justice is most relevant. The chain of violence, or the formula "violence begets violence," results mainly from retribution considered just because of its equalizing effect. This type of justice can easily become a hindrance to forgiveness because it perpetuates a cycle of violence which recreates traumatic memories again and again. The individual or group is trapped in the labyrinth of traumatic memory and the chances to forgive are gravely undermined.

The three types of justice suggested above are inadequate if we are properly to understand the dynamism of forgiveness. This is because in forgiving a new type of justice emerges. Justice in terms of Aristotle's equality may not present itself at the time forgiveness occurs. Yet when the victim forgives the victimizer, a radical alteration of power relations takes place which frees people from the memory cage of the past and allows a social space to come into being. This social space is both open-ended and future-oriented. While it does not immediately provide equality, it does create an opportunity for the parties involved to pursue justice as fairness in the future. Because of its transformative character, I call it *transformative justice*. It is at work in the process of forgiving.

Forgiveness: Islamic Teachings and Gandhi's Thoughts

Let me be up-front about choosing Islamic teachings and Gandhi's thoughts as my foci in exploring inspiration for the praxis of forgiveness. Islam is generally considered a potential actor in the clash of civilizations with the West. Evidence for this can be seen in the 1991 Gulf War and the 1993 World Trade Center incident in New York. Although the image of Islam is generally perceived to be closely related to violence, I suggest that Islam has a strong potential for nonviolent action.[18] If forgiveness can significantly contribute to nonviolence theory, then it certainly can benefit Muslim nonviolent actions as well. Finally, I am a Muslim who wishes to see the world transformed through nonviolent actions. I also include Gandhi's thinking because his perspective contains a wealth of wisdom badly needed in a world rich with ignorance.

I am not comparing Islamic thinking with Gandhi's thought. Instead I am using both as repositories of inspiration for the praxis of forgiveness. This is needed to link the above theoretical discussion with the living culture of Islam and the living thought of the Mahatma.

Muslim practice should be based on the Qu'ran and the traditions of the Prophet.[19] There are 12 verses dealing with forgiveness in the Holy Qu'ran that appear in the index at the end of the Yusuf Ali translation. Five verses deal with Allah's mercy to forgive (4:48, 116; 39:53; 53:32; and 57:21); one instructs believers to seek forgiveness from God (4:110); and one indicates that angels pray for forgiveness for all beings in the world (42:5).

The remaining verses teach Muslims to forgive other human beings. Muslims are instructed to "forgive and overlook" the People of the Book who wish to turn Muslims back to infidelity (2:109). More importantly, the Qu'ran commands Muslims to—

Hold to forgiveness;
Command what is right;
But turn away from the ignorant. (7:199)

Those who avoid the greater
Crimes and shameful deeds
And, when they are angry
Even then forgive; (42:37)

The recompense for injury
Is injury equal thereto
(In degree): but if a person
Forgives and makes reconciliation,
His reward is due
From God: for (God)
Loveth not those who
Do wrong. (42:40)

Tell those who believe
To forgive those who
Do not look forward
To the Days of God:
It is for Him to recompense
(For good or ill) each People
According to what
They have earned. (45:14)

These verses illustrate four basic points in relation to the Muslim tradition of forgiveness. First, forgiveness is a virtue commanded by Al-Qu'ran, which Muslims believe to be the Words of Allah. These Words must therefore be put into practice in daily life. Second, Muslims are asked to forgive even when angry. This shows that the force of human anger should be withheld and a space created to allow for the exercise and power of forgiveness. Third, although vengeance is allowed, forgiveness is a superior course of action. God considers forgiveness a good deed, and the one who forgives will reap rewards from the Almighty. In the language of my earlier analysis, while provisions for retributive justice do exist, forgiveness is clearly favored. Fourth, Muslims are told to forgive those who do not believe as they do. Forgiveness is not an injunction for practice only among Muslims. Tolerance of others outside their group becomes crucial for forgiveness.

Gandhi advocated the practice of nonviolence of the strong to liberate India from the colonial British. He maintained that compared to cowardice, violence is the preferred course of action.

> But I believe that nonviolence is superior to violence, forgiveness is more manly than punishment. Forgiveness adorns a soldier. But abstinence is forgiveness only when there is the power to punish; it is meaningless when it pretends to proceed from a helpless creature. A mouse hardly forgives a cat when it allows itself to be torn to pieces by her. . . . We in India may in a moment realize that one hundred thousand Englishmen need not frighten three hundred million human beings. A definite forgiveness would, therefore, mean a definite recognition of our strength. With enlightened forgiveness must come a mighty wave of strength in us. . . .[20]

Forgiveness does not figure prominently in Gandhi's thinking perhaps because it already exists as a part of *Ahimsa* and *Satya*. In the above passage, forgiveness seems to be conceived in the retributive mode and therefore considered "more manly than punishment." Moreover, the meaning of forgiveness will only be realized when the one who forgives has the power to punish and chooses not to. The moral choice assumes political significance. This is what Gandhi calls "enlightened forgiveness" which affirms a recognition of strength.

Gandhi's perspective is somewhat different from my earlier analysis. While he points out that one is able to forgive because one is *already* powerful, I have maintained that the nonviolent actions preceding the forgiving phase empower the victim. Forgiveness, once performed, helps transform power relations and in the process empowers the one who forgives while opening up opportunity for further future negotiation. The differences and/or similarities between Islamic teachings and Gandhi's thinking, and the rather abstract and theoretical discussion of forgiveness suggested above, should be considered in the context of the imminent threat of violent conflicts. Islamic teachings and Gandhi's thinking are fountains of cultural strength which can contribute much to the theory and politics of forgiveness, especially in the realm of praxis.

Conclusion: Forgiveness, Nonviolence Theory, and Sensitivity

Today the world is bursting with violent conflicts nurtured by hatreds which in some ways result from a clash of civilizations. It is no longer possible for those concerned with both the theory and practice of nonviolence to ignore the healing process without which direct violence will eventually reoccur. From a long-term strategic perspective, nonviolence theory needs to incorporate a crucial element which will alleviate, if not solve, this challenging problem. I have suggested here that forgiveness could be that crucial element. With this element added to nonviolence theory, a radical alteration of power relations will occur.

In addition, with proper understanding of the dynamism of forgiveness, the former victim may also find freedom from past traumatic experience and engage in constructive nonviolent actions for a better future. Contrary to retributive justice, the forgiving process will allow transformative justice to take place. This kind of politics of forgiveness can also find cultural nutrients in Islamic teachings and Gandhi's thinking.

I propose this modification of nonviolence theory because nonviolent actions will be badly needed in a fast-changing world. To accomplish this Herculean task, nonviolence theory needs to be critical, constructive, and strategic. In addition, sensitivity is also necessary so that we who cherish the ideal of nonviolence will not be blind to suffering and deaf to the cries of the oppressed.

Let me end with a prayer found on a piece of wrapping paper near the body of a child at Ravensbrück, a Nazi concentration camp where 92,000 women and children were killed during World War II.

> O Lord,
> Remember not only men and women of goodwill
> but also those of evil will.
> But do not remember all the suffering
> they have inflicted upon us;
> remember the fruits we have borne
> thanks to this suffering—
> our comradeship, our loyalty, our humility,
> our courage, our generosity,
> the greatness of heart
> which has grown out of all this;
> and when they come to the judgment,
> let all the fruits that we have borne
> be their forgiveness.[21]

6

Reconstruction: Healing a Nation's Soul

Gerald J. Pillay

Post-apartheid South Africa is a society emerging from decades of ideological conflict. After almost three hundred years of racial oppression, its indigenous peoples have for the first time the possibility of creating a democratic society. But change during these three hundred years has always been violent. How can South Africa establish a new pattern of transformation?

Much talk goes on in South Africa, and in Africa as a whole, about the need for a "theology of reconstruction." After the systematic political and economic subjugation of the indigenous peoples (and others who were not white) for almost three hundred and thirty years, the first priority was to empower those who had become marginalized. Now that political liberation has come at last, the obvious problems of making up for the social and educational backlog are formidable. Development and empowerment do not follow naturally from the vote. Amid the euphoria of political freedom lurk the dangers of exaggerated expectations, discontent, and disillusionment.

In the eighteenth and nineteenth centuries, the colonial subjugation of the local peoples in what was to become South Africa was often rationalized as an extension of Christian civilization. A particular reading of the Old Testament coupled with a newfound identity of *volk* or peoplehood created the possibilities of Afrikaner nationalism and the justification of this cause against both the Africans and the British. This dynamic formed the underpinning of the apartheid ideology. On the other hand, theology also provided the basis for the first dissenting voices (albeit few) within the Afrikaner volk.

Theology also was to provide the sustenance for the struggle against apartheid. The first voices of protest against the colonial excesses were those of church leaders. African church leaders were among founders of the African National Congress (ANC), one of the earliest political movements by Africans themselves on the African continent. The best-known Christian ANC leaders are Albert Luthuli, ANC president during the formative years of "passive resistance" in the 1950s, and Oliver Tambo, Nelson Mandela's predecessor.

During the 1960s, as black South Africans took greater interest in the emergence of black theology in the United States, the first tracts on African theology appeared in South Africa. Then a small but highly motivated group of writers produced the first writings of a South African liberation theology. By the 1980s the proclamation of Christian social witness drew on the theme of liberation for the poor and powerless in Scripture as well as social analysis, often referred to as "contextual theology." A key accomplishment of this theological movement was the formulation in the mid-eighties of the "Kairos Document," a statement outlining the theological justification for the struggle against apartheid.[1]

With the granting of the political franchise to all citizens in 1994, the first democratic elections were held and the first black majority government was inaugurated. Black South Africans are now in charge of their own destiny. Their own leaders in the cabinet must undo evils of the past and bring to completion what the new government has called the program of "Reconstruction and Development."

Already theologians are addressing this question of reconstruction. A monograph on *A Theology of Reconstruction* appeared in 1992 and deals with the role theology can play in nation-building and the extension of a human rights culture. The monograph is an exploration of the interface between theology and pertinent issues facing the fledgling South African democracy, such as cultural empowerment, democratization, lawmaking and nation-building, human rights, political economy, economic justice, and the political responsibility of religion.

Author Charles Villa-Vicencio defines a theology of reconstruction as "a corporate theology, given to democratic participation, expressive of interdisciplinary and inter-faith dialogue." It is "open-ended" and "driven by an eschatological vision." While offering "no final answer" it challenges society to "reach forward to the social goals which form part of the social vision incorporated in the biblical metaphor of the reign of God."[2]

In Villa-Vicencio's view, a theology of reconstruction is "theology committed to continuous social renewal and revolution." His book underscores some of the pressing social concerns in the rebuilding of the new democracy. In the context of South Africa, a theology of reconstruction seeks to give direction to the establishment of an equitable and just democracy where the historical divisions of race and class will be abolished and the bias toward the poor made explicit in both Christian witness and public policy.

The Deeper Problem

There is something incongruous about making theology the enterprise that follows in the wake of changed social and political circumstances: a kind of secondary activity that seeks perpetually to make sense of change. There is little evidence of how effective the theological critique of social systems has been. I do not seek to undervalue prophetic witness in a situation of injustice, but it is also true that the walls of apartheid only crumbled when it was no longer possible to support it financially or maintain it by force.

A theology of reconstruction at the level of social critique has still to show that its vision for society is valid. For many, the Christian vision is irrelevant or commands little respect. A situation of multiculturalism raises anew the question of the role for a Christian vision for society.

South Africa contains strong advocates of the view that the only valid reading of the Bible is the political reading of it. Liberation theology helped us focus on the social responsibility of the church and its imprisonment by unjust systems and provided a frame of reference for Christian activism. At the same time, by making political liberation paramount, this theology often paid scant respect to the life and spiritual integrity of worshiping Christian communities. A stark division occurred between spirituality and activism, despite some attempts to speak of the "spirituality of struggle."

In South Africa it is not yet clear what the influence of the work of protest theology was on the vast mass of the dispossessed. It is significant that the fastest growing churches in Africa are the African indigenous churches which did not embrace liberation theology. They flourish in their ability to speak authentically to the African soul in traditional cultural terms as part and parcel of their religious heritage, clothed in worship and liturgy.

A theology of reconstruction must, after "the struggle," reintegrate a generally fragmented theological vision. The struggle for justice and truth is part of the church's ongoing prophetic witness. But the lesson that the growth of these African indigenous churches has taught the established churches is that a theology that neglects the spiritual needs of people will have transient benefits. These churches demonstrate that mission, worship, and piety cannot be relegated to the periphery of any theology of reconstruction.

But there is also a prior question when we take up reconstruction. The question to be raised is what Christian theology can uniquely contribute to the healing of a society and nation. It seems trite to raise this question. So long as theology endorses what serves the common good, its validity is expected to be self-evident. However, it is not always clear why theology needs to be involved in what appears to be hard-nosed social reconstruction requiring the serious social and economic analysis the theologian is often not equipped to do. The problem is not solved by reducing all Christian theology to social ethics or, as some advocate, "an ideology of social transformation." If the question "What makes the contribution Christian?" cannot be unambiguously answered, the contribution of Christian theology is dispensable. How we perceive the nature of reconstruction is crucial to understanding the task of a theology of reconstruction.

There are at least two important questions such a theology must seriously address that are illustrated by the South African experience. The first question is how we overcome a deep historical pattern of relying on violence to bring about social change. The second question is how a society can heal entrenched divisions. We must resolve these two questions if we are to achieve a viable democracy, even if human rights are enshrined in the constitution. A theology of reconstruction has the indispensable responsibility to help in the formation of a humane society.

Exorcising Violence

What became the African National Congress began as a nonviolent movement in 1912. During the 1950s, the ANC organized the Passive Resistance movement by applying the methods of Gandhi to rouse the national conscience. Albert Luthuli, the ANC president, won the Nobel Peace Prize for his contribution to the nonviolent struggle to transform South African society.

The justification for the armed struggle was that African reasonableness had been answered only by violent government action. The Kairos Document, a statement which outlined the theological justification for the struggle against apartheid, has explained this option theologically. For good reasons the document called into question "state theology" which preserved the status quo and "church theology" concerned primarily with maintaining the integrity of the institutional church while posing no threat to an iniquitous system. Instead it called for a "prophetic theology" that prepared the way for the transformation of South African society. It made a distinction between the structural violence of apartheid and the violence of defenseless victims.[3]

Thus a variant of the "just war" position was being applied to the struggle against apartheid with the general endorsement of the churches. While leading churchpeople worked hard at preventing use of arms in the struggle, most Christians accepted that if all else failed there would be no compelling argument against violent resistance.

The nonviolence even of Luthuli was not a principled pacifist position. The Gandhian legacy had not put down strong roots in South Africa. On top of the violence in the South African history of colonial extension and subjugation, of rivalry between British and Boer fueled by the competition for economic control, of the application of apartheid ideology and the systematic and violent division of the country, came the violence of the freedom struggle.

Now the task facing the new democracy is how to quell the violence that has become endemic and threatens to destroy the newly acquired freedom of all. One attempt to address this problem was to set up a mechanism for a public atonement process. The former archbishop of the Anglican church, Desmond Tutu, chaired the Truth and Reconciliation Commission. Its task was to create the means and opportunity for those who committed human rights violations in service to the apartheid state to confess their complicity in the evils of the past system. The Commission gave opportunities equally for victims of such oppressors to tell their stories. The process, as traumatic as it has been for the nation, has in effect been a national catharsis. What will come of the revelations is yet to be assessed. Knowledge of the truth is necessary. Whether it leads to reconciliation is still to be seen.

The violence evident in society is not merely a political concern or a matter of criminality requiring more efficient policing. In cases of ethnic and racial violence, where violence is coupled with the motifs of revenge, ethnic cleansing or rivalry, intolerance for dissent, or oppression of minorities, it is vital to discern what the underlying motivations are. The spiral of violence during some three hundred years has become part of the South African social fabric.

Among the most threatening problems for the new democracy is uncontrollable levels of violence. The subjugation of the local people, rivalry between Boer and British, and imposition and maintenance of apartheid all evolved violently. A theology of reconstruction has to address this fundamental problem if there is to be lasting and meaningful reconciliation.

The reality of violence is fundamental to social existence. French anthropologist René Girard has done important work on the nature of violence and its outworking in a society. He analyzed primitive societies and the mechanisms for dealing with the problem of endemic violence embedded in their religious rites and views.

Girard shows that religious sacrifice actually is a means of containing violence. Religious practice contains what would otherwise be uncontrollable. In his writings he describes at length the mechanism of violence endemic within society, "continually functioning" but "perpetually misunderstood," which "assures the community's spontaneous and unanimous outburst of opposition to the surrogate victim."[4] His studies of sacrifice reveal that latent in society is a spiral of mimetic violence—violence in which victim and victimizer mirror or imitate each other. Sacrifice is then the mechanism that ritually curtails the explosion of violence. Such a view casts new light on many New Testament passages and especially on the meaning of the cross.

The problem of mimetic violence is how to break out of the vicious spiral, how to transcend what is so embedded in society. It is here that a Christian theology of reconstruction must make its unique contribution to the question of violence; it is at this point that the Christian understanding of the cross makes eminent sense. Violence is mimetic because the victim mirrors the victimizer and can easily become the victimizer. Christ, the innocent victim, willingly suffers the violence and forgives his persecutors. Mimesis is replaced by catharsis.

A theology of reconstruction is a theology of the cross unmasking the hidden and ritualized violence inherent in society, thereby exorcising it and bringing peace and healing.

Healing South Africa's Soul

After centuries of division based on race and culture, South African society now seeks a common nationhood. The rationale for apartheid was that, to prevent conflict and rivalry, different races needed self-determination and control over their own affairs. The imposition of racial divisions and the rigorous application of apartheid laws, a program of daring social engineering, was maintained on this logic. Such logic masked apartheid's real intent of ensuring white dominance and keeping white control of human and natural resources.

How can so fragmented a society be united? With a long historical view, the task is even more daunting. There never was a united black nation that may be recovered after colonialism or imperialism or Afrikaner nationalism or apartheid. South Africa as we know it is a relatively recent colonial creation: in 1910, the four provinces, two British colonies and two Boer republics, were brought together for the first time. The different African tribes shared no common culture or affiliation. Apartheid, and before it colonialism, exploited the traditional divisions to enhance the management and control of nonwhite peoples.

Now with democracy has come a desire to establish a nation. The implication is that within a nation there would be a place for everyone, both the different African peoples and the white and other minorities. But it is foolish to assume that after centuries of separation the vote can lead to the kind of transcendence that would allow groups to empty themselves of the drive for self-protection and control. The question of central importance then is how to heal the soul of a society conditioned by race and ethnicity.

To begin this healing, South Africa adopted a democratic constitution which has at its heart preservation of individual rights. Entrenching liberal values in the Constitution may achieve a great deal in breaking down intransigent tribalism. But can the attainment of nationhood against this history of separation be achieved only on the basis of protecting individuals? Haven't societies which have had the protection of these freedoms also become increasingly individualistic?

Individualism is counterproductive to achieving human or social solidarity. A society whose stability rests on a constitution depends entirely on the courts of law to keep the democracy intact. When the courts lose their ability to be effective arbitrators, then violence is the alternative.

Salvation in much of modern Western theology has been conceived as an individual matter. Nevertheless, there has also always been in Christian thinking the idea of the solidarity of the human race. "By one sin came into the world . . . in Adam all have sinned. In Christ (the 'last Adam') all may be restored" (Rom. 5).

This is an extremely difficult idea for modern Western society, an indication that a fundamental worldview change has taken place since Paul's age. Paul developed his Christology based on the idea of human solidarity without seeing any need to explain or justify it. The idea of human solidarity was an extension of Semitic social thinking and was familiar to his Greek readers as well. The Old Testament view that the whole nation is polluted by idolatry or disobedience and must as a nation atone had a counterpart in the idea of pollution in Greek culture. Paul universalizes what in traditional thinking had become tribal and national solidarity. The whole human race shares the potential to be the new Israel: "there is now neither Greek nor Jew; male nor female; free or bondman" (Gal. 3:28), a view of considerable sociological and historical significance.

In the seventeenth century, a noteworthy change occurred in the dichotomy between the individual and society. There were two markedly different notions of "the individual" alongside each other, largely linked to two different movements: Puritanism and science. The individualism of Puritanism was for human fellowship. The individualism of science fostered an atomistic view of society. A mixture of these two influences was the basis for Jeffersonian democracy in the U. S. and thus for the individualized emphasis on human rights.[5] In this mixture, accompanied by the secularization of the state, the Christian teleological frame of reference (priesthood of all believers and fellowship) was no longer a motivational factor. "Social contract" replaced the religious basis of human solidarity. Bills of rights and constitutions supplanted the role of tradition and social convention based on religious sanction.

Religion and other socially integrating forces (culture, education, subgroupings) remained and gave a semblance of social cementing, but the die was cast. The fracturing of social cohesiveness had tilted the scales to the side of individualism. The integrating religious rationale of society based on the solidarity of the human family was abandoned. In this regard, it is noteworthy that the phenomenon of human slavery accompanied the first democratic formations in the West. The period of the institution of slavery in the West coincided with the period of its Enlightenment. Slavery was formally abolished over half a century after the American and French Bills of Rights.

Furthermore, these so-called "rights" of individuals, for well over a century after their formulation, were in effect the rights of white landowning males. Even after the 1830 Revolution only about 200,000 out of the thirty million in France qualified to vote. The American constitutional affirmation that "all men are equal, and that they are endowed by their creator with certain inalienable rights" did not include white women until the suffragette struggles in the second decade of this century. Black folk in the 1960s still struggled for basic civil rights in the United States over 100 years after the abolition of slavery.

This antithesis between the individual and community reappeared in our time. The dialectical theologians formulated the crisis of human freedom in mainly individualistic terms. Liberation theology, on the other hand, addressed the human predicament not from the standpoint of the individual but from that of societal freedom.

The unresolved antithesis in theology between the individual and the community emerged again in the different emphases of these two theological schools of thought. Nevertheless, despite their different emphases on the individual and social structures and their divergent methodologies, the ultimate concerns of these two schools of theology are not all that disparate. Community is the condition for individual freedom. The encounter of an individual with God is mirrored in the encounter with other people and vice versa. There is in fact a trinitarian dimension to anthropology, person-God-neighbor, each dimension of which is indispensable.

The idea of community has been amply stated in church history, probably most consistently in the Eastern Orthodox tradition. The absence of true community is therefore not due to the absence of the idea, although there has been a tendency to stress *either* individuality *or* community, when even in divergent modern theological schools they are not mutually exclusive.

Yet the Christian claims about authentic community have increasingly become merely symbolic. The fact of institutional unity (Roman Catholic) or visible Eucharistic celebration and consistency with tradition (Eastern Orthodoxy) or active lay participation in ecclesiastical life and organization (Protestant) has not been a guarantee for real community in the world. Community is experienced as an absence. The idea is familiar but the manifestation rare.

The problem facing us in these last years of the millennium is probably more basic. A fundamental change has occurred in Western societies, and westernization with its technocratic acculturating media has transformed other cultures as well, most obviously the urban societies throughout the world. The change I refer to is the loss of a communal cementing force in society, the absence of a teleological frame of reference within which life may be lived. Religion has lost its traditional role. Along with the praiseworthy ideas of individual autonomy, progress, and democracy have come rank individualism bordering on narcissism, self-adulation, and moral licentiousness.

It appears that much of the theological enterprise and its precise formulations are done quite independently of the context of human loneliness and societal brokenness. Where there have been attempts to root the theological project in social analysis, these have either been relegated to a Third World concern or have themselves excluded authentic human fellowship.

Our thinking about being human must be recast in terms that seek to transcend the dichotomy between individualism and community. The task of a theology of reconstruction is to seek creative transcendence over the intellectual and social impasses that have come to be accepted as pervading the human predicament. It is one thing to value the human being, as traditional theology does. It is quite a different matter to create a meaningful context for being human. Both human creativity and love are transcendent acts that transform merely instinctual or conditioned behavior. Authentic fellowship is where individualism and selfishness are transcended and where human creativity is set loose. It is in the creative act of loving, an act of self-transcendence, that human beings find themselves. Community provides the wholeness that rescues individual striving from being empty action. There is a profound truth in the oft-quoted African proverb: "A person is only a person in the presence of other people."

Nicolai Berdyaev, whose thinking is both postexistentialist and post-Marxist, emphasized the need to transcend both the individual and the collective in the disclosure of personality. "Personality," he wrote, "is not a biological or psychological category but ethical and spiritual."[6] Personality consists of creative acts and is connected with freedom from the determinism of nature. Individualism, on the other hand, is a category of naturalism, biology, and sociology where the individual is seen in relation to the whole: an atom. The realization of personality is the continuous self-transcending creative act, not egoistic affirmation; it bears "witness to the fact that man is the point of intersection of two worlds; that in him takes place the conflict between Spirit and nature; freedom and necessity; independence and dependence." In this view, "Transcendental man does not evolve, he creates."[7]

Here is the first aspect of the reformulation of the anthropological question: being a human being must be stated in terms that surpass the traditional view of the individual and take as primary human creativity and human transcendence. The transformation from being merely an *individual* to being a *person* is the transformation into an "ek-static being" that can be looked upon "not from the angle of his limits but of his *overcoming his selfhood* and becoming a *related* person."[8] In *relation* the individual becomes a person.

The second aspect of reformulating the anthropological question is recasting of the idea of society into the terms of community and authentic fellowship, for it is only in this context that personality can be formed. Where a society is anti-individual or where it is merely a conglomeration of individuals thrown together by common needs (a society based on necessity, not freedom) then such a society is merely a collective (a herd). The collective is a distorted form of community which suppresses personality and gives the illusion of belonging. Collectives hold up such values as the survival of volk, class, race, or social system.

The Russian idea of *sobornost* is helpful here. The word is extremely difficult to translate. "Altogetherness" comes close. Sobornost is the dynamic of life in community. Berdyaev defines it as "the interior concrete universalism of personality."[9] Jaroslav Pelikan points out that the great virtue of this idea is that it "transcends the antitheses that are regarded in Western thought as mutually exclusive."[10] Non-Western cultures, which have maintained a sense of interconnectedness longer, are more likely to provide apt cultural metaphors to explain this Christian view of society.

Authentic community nurtures human freedom and is the necessary and sufficient condition for personality. A theology of reconstruction faces several decisive anthropological tasks. First, it must articulate what may perhaps best be described as a "trinitarian" model of personality that goes beyond the traditional and contemporary preoccupation with the individual and makes sense of both human freedom and creativity.

Second, a theology of reconstruction must develop a view of community (as illustrated in the idea of sobornost) that transcends the traditional antithesis of individualism and communalism. Until now "the neighbor" has been a category in theological ethics. It belongs to the heart of Christian anthropology. We may have to mine African or oriental thought for new ways to express this transcendence without which true society or even a democracy will become impossible in spite of its technological and scientific advancement and the redistributions of power.

Finally, such a theology must translate personality-in-community into practice. A theology of reconstruction must help make theological claims real in the world. In a socially arid realm the church must be authentic community. But how can we restore or implant a teleology in a broken world and within a fractured social consciousness? This third task is probably the most crucial and difficult and will remain a formidable challenge in this decade and beyond.

Theology and the Vision of God

A great dilemma of much of theology today is that it is undertaken without directly informing worshiping communities. It hardly ever enriches the churches' dogma and thus at best can too easily be merely an informed background to the churches' lives. Its immediate preoccupation is the guild, that relatively small band of subject specialists who have a vested interest in supporting the specialist academic journals. A prior challenge in formulating a theology of reconstruction must surely be the restoration of wholeness to theological purpose that still existed in early Christianity: a "catholic" wholeness.

In referring to catholic wholeness, I mean the period of early Christianity during which an interconnectedness existed between life and thought, reflection and spirituality, and theology and worship. It was a time when theology was steeped not merely in reflection but also in awareness of participating in the mystery of salvation. Rational reflection in theology (the attempt to speak appropriately about God) was grounded in "life in God." Knowledge arose out of contemplation and required self-discipline and watchfulness.[11]

A theology which heals the soul of a nation begins with this restoration of purpose and vision. A theology of reconstruction is fundamentally a theology of healing society by restoring living community and exorcizing violence. Such theology promotes the renewing of the earth and the evolution of a humane society and lives out the Christian understanding of salvation.

A Local
Culture of Peace

A Local Culture of Peace

Introduction by Judy Zimmerman Herr

"All politics is local," is a saying attributed to former U.S. national political figure Thomas P. ("Tip") O'Neill. O'Neill was suggesting that even on a national or international level, we make decisions and act based on our local perceptions and interests.

A corollary statement in the context of this volume might be, "All peacemaking is local." We may make broad statements about the need for peace in the world, but we work at making peace in local contexts. Elise Boulding suggests that peacemakers in the international arena have credibility to the extent that they have worked at peacemaking in their home communities. When forces of international capital and economic self-interest drive national governments, citizens should see the local community as the base from which a renewed sense of civic life can grow.

But to do this requires some intentionality. In describing the need for local peacemaking teams to help build new societal patterns in South Africa, Andries Odendaal and Chris Spies offer an illustration of this kind of local peacemaking. In yet another community context, the Wajir Peace Group works amid a minor internal war to bring peace through local structures and a fruitful mix of cooperative ventures between ordinary people, local government, and military.

The local context is usually defined geographically. Elise Boulding draws our attention to the "locality" offered by communities of faith, which preserve a particular identity even as they span the globe. This community of faith can be a site of peacemaking as well, as Doug Hostetter shows in his description of the Bosnian Student Project. Here a very local activity also reaches around the world and links local sites in response to a situation of need.

No book would be comprehensive enough to document all the many ways in which people around the world are busy building a culture of peace in their specific localities. These representative examples point toward the need continually to look for spaces in which peace may be nurtured and encouraged to grow.

7

Cultures of Peace and Communities of Faith

Elise Boulding

Religions play a crucial role in building a culture of peace. This role always begins locally, in the settings in which members of each community of faith find themselves. Such local influences account for the great diversity of ways in which the peace witness of each faith is practiced. However, these local communities are also part of their particular global network, so there is constant interplay between the local and global faces of each set of religious practices.

When we are thinking in terms of peace culture, many other elements come into play as well. It helps to think of peace culture as a mosaic, made up of varied ingredients: historical memories of peaceful peoplehood; teachings and practices of communities of faith on gentleness, compassion, forgiveness, and the inward disciplines of reflection and prayer; ways families care for one another and nurture the next generation; economic behavior that deals carefully with earth's resources and is oriented to human need and human sharing; forms of governance that ensure justice for all; and means of dealing with conflicts, differences, strangers—with those who are "other"—in a problem-solving, reconciling manner.

An important part of this mosaic is expressing love of creation and the Creator through ritual, celebration, music, dance, the arts. The symbol of the Tree of Life appears frequently in religious imagery to bind together the elements of a universally intuited culture of peace.

It is important to reflect on the special role communities of faith have in creating and sustaining a culture of peace at a time when a culture of violence and war threatens to overwhelm many societies.

Two Contrasting Cultures

A particular challenge we must face and deal with is that most if not all our communities of faith have—through the vicissitudes of human history—generated two conflicting images of how to practice that faith. One image is of an embattled community of believers surrounded by enemies with evil ways. This is a community called to holy war by divine command, by a God who will lead his people to victory over evildoers. The three peoples of the Book—Jews, Christians and Muslims—share a history of call to violent struggle, as do other communities whose call to battle comes with different yet recognizably similar imagery.

The second image is of a community of believers living at peace with neighbors, called by a loving God to deal nonviolently with other peoples when conflicts arise, prepared to practice forgiveness and reconciliation and to leave room for other ways of thinking, believing, and acting. The component of struggle in this image is the inward struggle to achieve goodness, virtue, compassion.

We may be entering the third *axial age* in history. The first age represented the rise of universal religions. The second is the age of unprecedented contact between cultures and civilizations across all the five continents. This age is marred by premature declarations of a universal culture, particularly from the West. The third axial age holds the promise of bringing these cultures and civilizations into a creative, mutually respectful relationship of interactive development and growth that enhances the uniqueness of each while enriching the lifeways of all.

Each culture, each civilization, each community of faith has a rich heritage of peaceful ways of resolving conflicts to bring to this new axial age. The tragedy, however, is that this precious heritage of peace culture belonging to all peoples is to a great extent a hidden one. The cultures of the historical record are overwhelmingly warrior societies. They are defined by stories of battles won and lost, nations and states conquered or conquering. Yet the cultures of everyday life are largely peaceful. In families, neighborhoods, schools, workplaces, organs of governance—in the entire daily conduct of what we tellingly call the civil society—when differences arise, we negotiate.

Interpersonal and intergroup differences pervade the core of social life, because no two human beings are alike. Each of us sees, hears, thinks, and feels in ways unique to our own individuality, yet most of our activities involve others. Therefore, to accomplish even the simplest social task requires some negotiation across differences. Some of us are better negotiators than others, but we all do it!

One major task is to recover and make visible the actually existing peace culture which makes our ways of life sustainable in every society. This claiming of our own skills of peacemaking and reconciliation must involve a major effort to change the practices of media coverage of news, practices which highlight violence and give little space to creative conflict resolution. This is becoming an increasingly important field of research in peace studies.

A second major effort, to which peace research historians are already committed, is to correct the war-biased historical record by documenting all the ignored peacemaking activity that has gone on in and between states. This means also chronicling the lives of the peace heroes and heroines. It means showing how inventive humans have been through time in resolving serious differences without violence. Since much of this inventive peacemaking came about through the creative intervention of church, temple, synagogue, and mosque, this becomes an opportunity to honor that historical role of religious institutions. It becomes an occasion to counterbalance the easy emphasis in the historical record on holy wars backed by religious as well as state authorities, such as the Crusades of the late Middle Ages.

Balance or Cultural Transformation?

The task is partly righting the balance in the historical records and in present-day media between violent aspects of human activities and peaceful ones. However, we can hardly be satisfied with simply achieving balanced reporting on violent versus peaceful behavior! There is a far greater challenge facing us at a time when to continue traditional habits of warfare means to threaten the very survival of life on the planet. That challenge is to undertake deep reflection on the meaning in today's world of the warrior-hero model.

Moving beyond reflection, the challenge is to undertake a reworking of the inner dynamics of fighting behavior, even while honoring the courage and dedication of the fighter, so the tremendous cultural energy that has gone into fighting for one's people can be transformed into nonviolent energy for righting of the many wrongs that feed violence and counterviolence. The Seville Statement on Violence (UNESCO 1989) gives us the basis for a transformation of warrior cultures into cultures of peace, since it records the findings of the scientific community that war is a social invention, not an urge biologically determined in the human species.

Every community of faith has examples of inspiring women and men whose basic life energies have been transformed into a heroic practice of nonviolent rebuilding of a peace culture in shattered societies. Gandhi, one of the better-known nonviolent heroes of our century, is in fact but one of many. What is most important about such figures is not their exceptionality but that they become teachers for their society and enable others to rechannel energies into what Pannalal Dasgupta calls "the nonviolence of the brave."[1]

That same rebuilding of a peace culture is evident in the work of Sulak Savaraksa and his many colleagues in the Network of Engaged Buddhists, as exemplified by the peace march they organized in Cambodia during 1994 national elections. Such rebuilding is inherent in the nonviolence movement Servicio Paz y Justicia (SERPAJ, meaning "service of peace and justice"). Founded by Adolfo Perez Esquivel of Argentina and fellow activists, SERPAJ is an eleven-country network that reaches from Central America to Chile.

Ibrahim Rugova is the rebuilding Muslim leader who has brought the Albanian population of Kosova into peaceful, nonviolent witness to the integrity of their society in the face of attempts at ethnic cleansing by a neighboring ethnic group. Another rebuilder is Wangari Maathai, the Kenyan biologist and university professor who helped rural women form the Greenbelt movement—an effort to transform deteriorating communities and the decaying ecosystems they inhabited into revitalized social bodies through the communal planting of trees.

Kenneth Boulding used to say that "what exists is possible." Since major nonviolent public activity is taking place amid violence on every continent, rebuilding and making visible the hidden cultures of peace, then the transformation of military cultures into nonviolent cultures of peace at societal and intersocietal levels is possible.

Allies in the Work of Transformation

The image of the international system as consisting of 185 states all armed (with few exceptions) for military defense and capable of military aggression makes the cultural transformation I speak of seem almost impossible. Yet states themselves, apparently so basic to the structure of the international system, are becoming obsolete as guarantors of human security for the peoples within their borders. Highly technologized weapon systems aimed at potential enemies outside state borders are increasingly irrelevant to the problems of resource scarcity and historical traumas that set states against one another. They are even more useless for addressing the diversity of needs and interests of peoples within their borders.

The concept of the modern state as a melting pot for constituent nationalities turns out to be a myth as we become increasingly aware that there are thousands of ethnic groupings (anthropologists sometimes speak of "the 10,000 societies") spread across the borders of these 185 states. There are also 20,000 nongovernmental organizations, or NGOs, which are peoples' associations forming the core of the global civil society, crisscrossing all national and ethnic boundaries, as well as countless local grassroots associations. These phenomena have arisen from the inadequacy of the state system to provide peace, justice, and security for the world's peoples. The need for new arrangements that will allow cultural autonomy, religious freedom, and economic well-being for the peoples now denied them is increasingly evident.

The United Nations system with its many agencies and growing partnerships with NGOs and NGO-organized entities may be thought of as a transitional structure, badly hampered by the preoccupation with sovereignty of its member states. At the same time, by creating new nonterritorial space for action on conflicts that overwhelm those states, it carries the promise of new sociopolitical arrangements for the future.

At present ethnicity appears to be a source of violence and terror in the world, yet each people has its own traditions of peaceful conflict resolution, traditions hidden during prolonged periods of different colonialisms and social displacements and by exploitative practices of economic development. It is the global civil society that is and will be uncovering these hidden traditions of peace culture, through the work of the many NGOs committed to peace, justice, and social well-being for the oppressed. Ethnic transnational peoples' associations, which incorporate ethnic diaspora and have positive social goals of bettering the life of their people in the context of a commitment to a peaceful world order, also have a role. Ethnic NGOs have grown more than fivefold 1970-1994, to a total of 574 now registered with the Union of International Associations. While not all are equally peace-oriented, on the whole this is a positive sign of the growing capability for peaceful problem solving of ethnic transnationals.[2]

One special category of NGOs should concern us here: transnational networks of communities of faith. If we count all the transnational associations oriented toward religion and theology and include religious orders, as of 1997 there are 3,320 listed in the database of the Union of International Associations. This is more than double the number in 1970, when there were 1,581. These include both associations related to specific communities of faith and such interfaith organizations as the World Conference of Religion and Peace and the World Parliament of Religions.[3]

Faith-based organizations tend to be qualitatively different from secular NGOs in members' commitment to the goals of the NGO, in continuity of membership over time, and in the amount of resources and volunteer time available. In other words, faith-based NGOs can contribute out of proportion to the members they represent and to the achievement of significant goals relating to rebuilding and strengthening peace culture. We should be alert to occasions for both ethnic and religious NGOs to develop new ways to work together across the many differences that divide them so as to speed the decline of the war culture and the flowering of a culture of creative peacemaking in the new axial age.

Rebuilding a Culture of Peace

The introductory statement in the program for the 1994 UNESCO Conference on "The Contribution by Religions to the Culture of Peace" held in Barcelona stated that religions could always take the side of justice, nonviolence, and peace because they love truth, are free, and have great spiritual strength. But how? Communities of faith will need to do better in the future than they have in the past. A statement issued recently by the Kholoq-e-Azeem Society of Islamabad, Pakistan, could as well speak for every one of our communities of faith. The society says that "there is abundance of natural wealth and also human resources which ensure a bright future for the world of Islam. But the spiritual, cultural and humanitarian values which form the very basis of Islamic teachings are sadly lacking everywhere."[4] No religious community lives up to the potential of its teachings.

As a sociologist and peace researcher, I will address one set of challenges in relation to this fulfillment of potential: developing specific peacemaking skills, identifying and training for new peacebuilding roles and strategies, and providing the infrastructure to carry them out. Resources will need to be drawn on that have not been adequately used in the past—including the skills and creativity of women. Let us look at a few examples of strategies underused by communities of faith that could make them more effective peacemakers.

Training in Conflict Resolution

Some religious bodies are now encouraging training in conflict resolution and the skills of listening and nurturing at the level of the local worshiping community. Such training can help parents meet the needs of their children more fully and prepare children to behave non-violently in environments where there may be considerable violence. Such training can also help local worshipers be peacemakers in their own city, town, or village, and can even help worshipers settle differences among themselves in mosque, temple, or church. Seventeenth-century English Quaker William Penn, when asked by a fellow believer if he should give up wearing a sword, said, "Wear thy sword as long as thou canst." Persons who have no other skills to deal with violence feel the need of weapons. If they are to give up weapons they must have other means of dealing with conflict and aggression. These skills at the local level contribute to a strong and viable peace culture that can produce skilled problem-solvers for larger conflicts.

Recognizing Women as Partners in Peacemaking

Taking women into full partnership in public peacemaking is a step still to be taken by many communities of faith. Women are expected to be peacemakers in the home and local community, but the imagination and inventiveness they have developed through centuries of practice in these settings is rarely used in larger conflicts. The story of women's peacemaking inventions in settings of war and communal violence is part of the hidden history of peace culture. The nineteenth and twentieth centuries include particularly noteworthy but largely unrecorded examples of such peacemaking.

Global Peace Services

Gandhi's vision of locally based *shanti sena* or "peace armies" acting as unarmed, nonviolent peacemakers in conflict settings around the world has borne fruit in a number of faith-based peace team projects. Here members are trained to serve where violence has gotten out of hand. Peace teams, both secular and faith-based, place themselves between parties in combat and provide protective accompaniment for endangered persons in high-violence situations. They help create safe spaces for normal activities like farming, education, and care of children; for refugees; and for humanitarian provision of health and food services amid war.

Expansion of these presently widely scattered groups through a coalition of religious NGOs on all continents who would coordinate peacebuilding partnerships between outside helpers and local men and women in conflict areas is a concept emerging from faith-based groups in Sweden. The vision has so far been referred to as Global Peace Services.

The coalition process is slow and the need great, but peace services are growing in two parallel and intertwining trends. One trend is the development of peace services and training centers in local communities torn by violence, entirely by local initiative and with local leadership, though with some support from outside. The examples are legion. Almost unknown to the outside world is the Center for Peace, Nonviolence, and Human Rights in Osijek, Croatia, close to the Serbian border. This Center was begun by a local doctor and concerned citizens. They protect the human rights of Serbs and Croats, Christians and Muslims, work with the displaced and the injured, and carry out community-wide peace education to empower children and adults with the skills of nonviolent conflict resolution. They have received support from British Quakers and both religious and secular groups in Germany, Sweden, and Spain.[5]

In Chiapas, Mexico, indigenous Christian and secular groups empower victims of violence to rebuild their communities, with Servicio Internacional para la Paz (SIPAZ, meaning "international service for peace") and other international groups providing a supportive network of nonviolence trainers to help them. In Africa, the Nairobi Peace Initiative based in Kenya networks with other centers in Africa with support from the Mennonite Central Committee, the International Fellowship of Reconciliation, and other peace groups in Europe and the Americas to provide local nonviolence training in regions of civil war.

The Buddhist Dammayietra Center in Phnom Penh, Cambodia, trains monks, nuns, and laypersons for annual interfaith pilgrimages to end violence in Cambodia, with help from trainers in Asia and Europe. In the United States, inner-city neighborhoods struggling with violence form their own community centers, supported by local interfaith groups, to rebuild peaceful relations and end the poverty that spawns violence. Contrary to the general view, most of the peace work today on every continent is being done through local initiatives.

The parallel trend at the global level is for Peace Service groups to train nonviolent peace teams for work in any part of the world. Peace Brigades International, Christian Peacemaker Teams, World Peacemakers, and Witness for Peace are among the dozen or so groups training and fielding such teams. The two trends are intertwined because it is generally agreed that no one should be part of an international team who has not first worked in areas of conflict and violence in their own country. The *Peace Teams/Peace Services Newsletter* initiated by Elise

Boulding in 1993 and now edited by Yeshua Moser in Bangkok, Thailand, reports on these types of activities in an effort to strengthen the networking and collaboration among growing numbers of peace service centers and teams. The development of training manuals such as the new publication from the Christian Council of Sweden brings together the best of knowledge and skill in the field in a way that can be adapted for local use and encourages local initiatives.[6]

Healing the Victims and Perpetrators of Violence and War

Once an individual or a community has experienced severe violence, time alone cannot bring healing and the capacity for peaceful social relationships. Traditional societies know this and provide healing rituals for those who have experienced war and for other kinds of hurts. The needs of the many victims of intergroup violence and war in this decade and the decades preceding it—men, women, children, the elderly—will require the establishment of posttrauma healing centers wherever the culture of peace needs rebuilding. Such centers must also address the traumas of the perpetrators of violence—soldiers, guerrillas, gangs, and individual abusers. Both types of groups need healing, though of different kinds. Women who have faced mass rape, and adults and children who have witnessed genocidal killing, urgently need group therapy to come to terms with what they have experienced and to be able to reestablish trusting relationships with others.

This need is especially great among children who have grown up knowing nothing but constant warfare and have never had systematic schooling or even opportunities for productive work. They require staggering amounts of rehabilitative work to enter socially responsible adulthood. That hundreds of thousands of such children and youth are spread over several continents is a matter deserving serious reflection.

Adults who have become used to killing and maiming others will have to be helped to develop a new level of self-understanding and rebuild their identities as human beings capable of engaging in normal everyday activities in families, as workers, and as citizens. The kind of healing needed has a deeply spiritual base, and every religious body of every faith will have an important part to play in this healing work.

Zones of Peace

Every temple, church, mosque, and synagogue is in a profound sense a zone of peace, a special type of space dedicated to the embodiment of a culture of peace in human togetherness. Developing a deeper awareness of this aspect of peacebuilding is important for every local place of worship. The extension of the concept into civic life, so that spiritual energy is available for the creation of zones of peace in widening circles of public space, is a challenge for communities of faith. Zone of peace treaties, creating nuclear-free zones or completely weapon-free zones, are a significant political aspect of the zone of peace movement which needs the support of religious bodies since states find it so hard to give up weapons. Local declarations of a community as a zone of peace have the greatest potential for actually creating local peace cultures.

Once a community has made such a declaration, it immediately becomes possible to develop a wide range of peacebuilding activities in the community: sister city projects between continents, conflict resolution curriculum in the schools, public peace gardens, economic conversion projects that wean local manufacturers from military contracts to civilian types of production.

Envisioning a Future Culture of Peace

Given the levels of violence in the world today, it is hard to imagine a world in which the energies fueling militarism have been transformed into peacebuilding energies. Yet it is also true that it is impossible to work for something one can't even imagine. That is why the prophetic voice proclaiming the earthly peaceable kingdom is so important in each religious tradition, even though the details of the prophecy may vary. The religious imagination has suffered in the secular atmosphere of the twentieth century. Even the basic hope for a better future is jeered at as being "unrealistic."

Yet that prophecy and that hope are the most precious resource of humankind, and the very capacity to imagine the other and better is, as Fred Polak so eloquently put it in his 1953 *Image of the Future*, our most completely human capacity. The envisioned future draws us toward it by helping us organize our thinking and behavior to bring it about. That is why it is so important to put much energy into imagining, envisioning, dreaming about, meditating about—and yes, praying about—a future culture of peace. The elements of the peace culture that already exist, hidden from the unobservant eye, provide the materials for our spiritual imagination to work with. They inspire us as we look through the violent present to the possible human futures that lie on the far side of that violence, and they provide the social energy for transformative action in the present.

Neighbors in the Bosnian Tragedy

Doug Hostetter

Just then a lawyer stood up to test Jesus. "Teacher," he said, "what must I do to inherit eternal life?" He said to him, "What is written in the law? What do you read there?" He answered, "You shall love the Lord your God with all your heart, and with all your soul, and with all your strength, and with all your mind; and your neighbor as yourself." And he said to him, "You have given the right answer; do this, and you will live." But wanting to justify himself, he asked Jesus, "And who is my neighbor?" Luke 10:25-29 NRSV

"After my parents were sent off to the concentration camp, it was the neighbor with whom my father had coffee every afternoon who stole everything from our house before burning it to the ground." —Damir

"My next-door neighbor, who took care of me while Mother was working as I was growing up, now lives in our home. They took everything that once belonged to us."—Dalila

"It was three days before my best friend could finally speak. She had returned after being yanked from my side as we slept in the women and girls' section of the concentration camp. She said she had been raped all night by seven Serbian soldiers. One of them was a classmate from our high school."—Alisa

During the war in Bosnia the United States branch of the Fellowship of Reconciliation (FOR) tried to answer that question posed to Jesus almost 2,000 years ago. We did so by asking our members and friends to open their homes to students who had been driven from their homes in Bosnia by ethnic/religious hatred and war. The Bosnian Student Project of the FOR helped more than 150 Bosnian students of all backgrounds to escape from the war zone and continue their education in the U.S. Students who had been hated because of their religious background in Bosnia were welcomed into the homes of Americans of all ethnic and religious backgrounds.

The project not only saved the lives of scores of excellent students, it also gave Americans something positive to do in the face of an overwhelming tragedy. The project enabled its American participants to affirm their commitment to pluralism and tolerance by working together with people of other religious traditions to love and accept students who were victims of war and genocide.

One day one of Mohammed's disciples asked, "What should one do when confronted by evil in the world?" Mohammed responded, "You should change it with your bare hands." He paused for a moment and continued, "If you discover that you are not able to change it with your bare hands, you must tell your friends and neighbors about this evil." He paused again, and continued, "And if you find that you are too shy or embarrassed to speak about this evil, you must take this evil and hold it in your heart."

I repeated this story from the Hadith (part of Islamic sacred writing) to a Christian monk friend of mine.

He responded, "In the Christian tradition the taking of an evil, about which you do not know how to respond, into your heart is called *prayer.*"

What this monk knew and the story from the Hadith hints at is this: if you prayerfully take an evil into your heart, God will give you the courage to speak out and eventually show you the way to change that evil with your bare hands.

When war broke out in Bosnia in spring 1992, and stories of rape, murder, and concentration camps began to emerge, the Fellowship of Reconciliation in the United States began to search for ways that U.S. citizens could respond to this enormous tragedy. In early 1993 a retired professor from Fairleigh Dickinson University who lives near FOR headquarters organized a small delegation of American Muslims to visit Bosnian refugee camps in Croatia. During the visit they discovered that there were thousands of Bosnian students who had been attending universities in Croatia when Croatia and Bosnia were both parts of Yugoslavia.

When Croatia became an independent state in 1991, it also declared itself a Catholic nation. To make matters worse, in 1993 Croat

(Roman Catholic) and Bosnian armies were fighting each other in Bosnia. Muslim and mixed-family students from Bosnia were no longer welcome in Croatian universities, but because of the fighting most of these students were also unable to return to their families in Bosnia. Most Bosnian students were completely without funds, and male students especially were vulnerable to being beaten up by other students or arrested by Croatian military police. Despite their desperate situation, the students had organized themselves into an Association of Students of Bosnia and Herzegovina to try to find a way to continue their education.

When the delegation of American Muslims came to visit the Association of Students, they discovered a small office teeming with Bosnian students without so much as a single chair in the entire room. The professor, also Imam (leader) of a Sufi Muslim community in New York, decided to seek scholarships for some of the students in this desperate and dangerous situation. Once back in the United States he sent letters on mosque stationery to over 300 colleges and universities requesting scholarships for some of these excellent students who were unable to continue their education because of their religious background. Only one college responded, stipulating readiness to offer a scholarship to a talented Bosnian student so long as the student was Christian.

The Imam quickly agreed and referred to the school two Bosnian Croat sisters who were refugees from Sarajevo. The U.S. Embassy in Croatia, however, refused to grant student visas to the sisters. As Bosnian Croats (Roman Catholics), the embassy pointed out, the sisters would have no difficulty attending the university in Croatia. In desperation, the Imam looked for friends who might help. He remembered that during the Persian Gulf War the Fellowship of Reconciliation had sent twenty tons of medicine to help the mostly Muslim civilian victims of that war.

He called FOR and asked for a meeting. After giving his report on the desperate situation of Bosnian refugees and students, he asked about FOR plans for work related to Bosnia. I reported that FOR would likely put together a delegation of U.S. Christians, Muslims, and Jews to visit Bosnia and speak out against using religion to divide people and nations or as a tool of genocide. The Imam agreed that sounded like important work but asked, "Is there anything FOR could do to help the thousands of Bosnian students who are unable to continue their education simply because of their religious background? Could FOR help to find scholarships and homes for some of these students?"

For a year I had agonized over what a pacifist organization could do in response to the enormous evils of war and genocide in Bosnia. Suddenly, as if in answer to prayer, this project was placed in our hands.

The FOR's work started with university students from Bosnia who were trapped in Croatia, but it soon expanded to include Bosnian students—high school or college, inside or outside of Bosnia—who were unable to continue their education due to "ethnic cleansing" or the war. We had to find talented students in refugee camps and inside Bosnia who could also be successful in U.S. schools. After finding the students we had to search for a way to get them out of the war zone and to the U.S. We had to develop a network of friends in high and low places, inside and outside governments.

We needed friends in several countries of the former Yugoslavia who could help the students get passports, visas, and transportation across national borders and sometimes through battle lines. These friends had to be people who, in the middle of a war, would be willing to help young people who had no money and were often of a different religious or ethnic background than their own.

We also had to locate U.S. schools which would grant full scholarships to academically excellent students who had no money and often lacked official transcripts and other documentation usually required for school admission. Many of our students came from schools destroyed by the war or located in parts of Bosnia held by armies of an opposing ethnic group. Transcripts, diplomas, and other documents for some of our students were destroyed when these young people were forced into concentration camps or were stopped at Serb checkpoints as they tried to escape Bosnia.

We had to find families who, based on a one-page faxed biography, would open their homes to a young person they had never met. In a capitalist, predominantly Christian country (with strong Jewish and smaller Muslim minorities), we had to find homes for children who had grown up in a socialist state in families which were primarily Muslim or inter-ethnic. We searched for families able to love and care for students traumatized by personal experience with the horrors and tragedies of an unspeakable war. We needed individuals or congregations who would contribute the funds for passport, visa, and airfare for each student.

The task initially seemed overwhelming. We had no money, but the FOR could offer a large office, some administrative support, a small computer, two phones, a portion of my staff time and access to the network of FOR local chapters and religious peace fellowships across the U.S. If we were going to "change this evil with our bare hands," we were going to need help from many people!

The project had a number of strengths which aided its success.

1. *It was elegantly simple.* We proposed to find homes and schools for Bosnian students who had lost homes and schools due to religious

intolerance and war. This was easy to communicate and simple to understand.

2. *It empowered individuals.* Individuals or congregations anywhere in the country could offer housing, raise funds for transportation, or encourage a school to offer a scholarship to a talented Bosnian student.

3. *It offered a positive statement of faith.* "You are my neighbor, a friend, and a child of God. I will open my home, my school, and my congregation to you," such an action said. There was also an implicit corollary: "I will not be complicit with war and genocide."

4. *It offered a participatory model of interfaith cooperation.* The FOR staff volunteers at the national office included people from a number of different faith backgrounds. Local organizers were encouraged to use the project as an opportunity for interfaith cooperation.

The interfaith aspect of the project had profound implications in Bosnia, in the U.S., and for numerous students. Many of the Bosnian students had been driven from their homes and deprived of the ability to continue their education by "Christian" armies or governments which, in the tradition of the Crusades, had slaughtered or expelled from their area all people of other religious traditions. The Bosnian Student Project offered American Christians an opportunity to distance themselves from the triumphalist, sectarian tradition of the "Christian" armies of the Middle Ages and enabled them to identify with a much older Judeo-Christian tradition of hospitality, compassion, and love as practiced by the Patriarchs, Christ, and the apostolic church. It was a great shock to many students who had been driven from their homes by "Christian" armies in Bosnia to see that the families and schools that gave them love, shelter, and education in the U.S. were also Christian.

Lejla, a Bosnian Muslim student from Mostar, was a freshman at the University of Sarajevo in 1992. When war broke out, she quickly returned to be with her family in Mostar. Mostar was first shelled by the Serb (Orthodox Christian) army for several months until a combination of the Bosnian Army and a separate Bosnian Croat (Roman Catholic) army was finally able to drive the Serb artillery from the mountains surrounding Mostar. After the Serb army had retreated, however, the Bosnian Croat army turned on the Bosnian army and the Muslim civilians living in the city and drove them across the Neretva River into the older, smaller part of the city called East Mostar.

In East Mostar, Lejla and her family took refuge in the basement of an old apartment building that was disintegrating under the daily shelling of the Croat army. After six months Lejla's parents were able to help her and her younger sister escape East Mostar and travel to stay with friends of the family who lived in Croatia.

Lejla enrolled at the University of Zagreb and continued her studies for several months. Then Croatia passed laws which granted full rights for Croats (Roman Catholics) from Bosnia to attend Croatian universities—but determined that Muslims from Bosnia would be foreign students. Bosnian Muslim students suddenly were not allowed in student dorms or cafeterias and were required to pay high foreign student university fees.

Once again Lejla was unable to continue her education. Happily, the Bosnian Student Project found a full tuition scholarship for her at Iona College, a Catholic school in New Rochelle, New York, as well as a home with an African-American Catholic family who lived near the college. Lejla's friend and mentor at Iona College was Sister Kathleen, who had worked hard to secure the scholarship for Lejla.

Some Christians saw it as their special responsibility to demonstrate a faith distinct from that of the people slaughtering in the name of Christ in Bosnia. One evangelical Methodist layman heard about a Mennonite school in his area that had offered scholarships to two Bosnian Muslim students. He brought the issue of Bosnian students to his prayer group. After prayer and discussion they decided they had a Christian responsibility to help rescue Bosnian Muslim students.

So they approached a local evangelical Christian college and asked if the college would give a scholarship to a qualified Bosnian Muslim student. After some consideration, the president of the college authorized a scholarship for Dino, a young man from Sarajevo and the first Muslim student ever admitted to that Christian school. The Bosnian Student Project forwarded the papers by fax to Sarajevo. Because Dino was of military age and Sarajevo at the time was under heavy military siege, the Bosnian government refused to grant papers for Dino to leave.

After several months of unsuccessful attempts to get the papers, we suggested to the sponsor that he select another student, perhaps a female or a student who lived in some less threatened location. The sponsor brought the matter to his prayer group. After prayerful consideration, members of the group reported being convinced that they should bring Dino. They would pray that Dino be granted his papers.

On July 4, 1995, the apartment where Dino and his family lived in Sarajevo was hit by a Serb artillery shell. The apartment was completely destroyed, but miraculously no one was killed. The following week Dino's papers were approved. A few days later, on a moonless night, Dino passed through the tunnel under the Sarajevo airport and crossed the no-man's land at the other end to reach a Bosnian village a few miles away. He slept the night in the village and the next day caught a ride to safety in a Bosnian tank traveling over Mt. Igman.

Although the majority of the families who took in Bosnian students were Christian, Americans of other religious traditions also participated in this project. The Bosnian Student Project sought to find and unite people of all ethnic and religious traditions in a common effort to help the students from Bosnia.

The program had special appeal to American Muslims because most of the students who had been driven from their homes by ethnic cleansing in Bosnia were Muslim. This project offered a concrete way to help Muslim students from Bosnia who were in desperate need. The Jerrahi Order of America is a Sufi Muslim religious order with a congregation in Spring Valley, New York. The leader of this congregation, Tosun Bayrak, had initially discovered the plight of the Bosnian Muslim students in Croatia and asked the FOR to help them. The Imam and his congregation were perhaps the strongest supporters of this project. Families of the congregation hosted over a dozen Bosnian students, and the Imam, his wife, and many members of the congregation gave innumerable hours of volunteer work to the project.

The program also had strong appeal to many Jewish Americans. The genocide of Muslims in Bosnia had many similarities to the Nazi genocide of Jews fifty years earlier. Many of the Jewish host families were survivors, or relatives of survivors, of the Holocaust. For Jews who had lived through that terrible period through the kindness of a Christian, this project offered an opportunity to return the favor to a Muslim who was also in desperate need of protection. Bryna and Harvey Fireside, who later wrote *Young People from Bosnia Talk about War* (a book which interviewed our students, discussed genocide, and described the Bosnian Student Project), were particularly sensitive to genocide. As a young boy, Harvey and his family were forced by the Nazis to flee their home in Vienna because they were Jewish.

Maja was a freshman at the University of Sarajevo when the war broke out. Her father was Muslim and her mother Serb (Orthodox Christian). The family had lived comfortably in a suburb of Sarajevo populated by people of many ethnic groups. The area where Maja's family lived was captured by the Serb army in the early days of the war. Maja's parents felt it would be safer for her and her sister to travel to Belgrade, Serbia, to stay with their aunt.

Soon after the girls had gone to Belgrade, Maja's father was captured and taken to a Serb prison camp where he was brutally tortured. He was eventually rescued by a Serb family friend who, because of his military rank, was able to take her father from the prison camp and bring him to a hospital outside the country. After his recovery he and his daughters moved to Turkey. Maja's mother, who was Serb, was humiliated by the Serb soldiers for being married to a Muslim and expelled across the battle front into the area of Sarajevo controlled by the Bosnian Government. She escaped Sarajevo on a Red Cross convoy to Croatia and eventually joined the rest of the family in Turkey.

With the family finally together again, Maja turned her attention once more to education. She enrolled in an English school run by a Muslim voluntary agency helping Bosnian refugees in Turkey. The classes went well until the agency learned that Maja's mother was Serb (Orthodox Christian). It seems the school was for *Muslim* refugees from Bosnia; since Maja was only half-Muslim, she was ineligible to attend, and Maja and her sister were asked to leave. When the Bosnian Student Project called Maja to inform her we had found a home and a scholarship for her to attend college in the U.S., Maja's first question was, "Do you know that my father is Muslim and my mother is Christian?" Maja was assured that the Bosnian Student Project was open to all Bosnian students who were unable to continue their studies, regardless of race, religion, or ethnicity.

Bryna and Harvey Fireside, who were acutely aware of the horrors of religious prejudice, were the key organizers in finding the scholarship for Maja and a year later for her sister as well. The committee they put together to find homes and scholarships for Bosnian students included the Protestant chaplain from Ithaca College, the Jewish chaplain from Cornell University, and Muslim, Christian, and Jewish members of the faculty and the wider community. This committee also included Serbs and Croats from the academic community who wished to contribute to the effort to help victims of ethnic nationalism in Bosnia. The committee met every three weeks to hear from the students, to receive updates on the situation in Bosnia, and to distribute responsibilities related to the project.

The interfaith nature of the project was important not only to the U.S. participants but also to the students and their families. Every Bosnian student in this project knows that his or her scholarship to a U.S. school would have been impossible without the collaboration of people of many faith traditions in several different countries.

Because of the religious sectarian overtones of the war in Bosnia, the FOR felt that the programmatic response to that war should be strongly interfaith. In the former Yugoslavia we worked with the World University Service (WUS), which helped us locate needy students, secure necessary papers, and arrange transportation.

The director of the WUS office in Sarajevo was a Serb (Orthodox) and the director of the Zagreb office was a Croat (Roman Catholic). Most of the students were Muslim or of mixed family. In the Bosnian Student

Project office in the U.S., the director was Mennonite and the office manager American Muslim. Christian, Muslim, and Jewish volunteers helped the national office during the project.

The project encouraged all organizers to use this opportunity to include people from other religious traditions. A number of FOR local chapters were surprised to discover mosques in or near their communities and were even more surprised to learn that many of these Muslim congregations welcomed the opportunity to cooperate with Christian and Jewish neighbors to help students from Bosnia. This was the first project in the history of the FOR-USA in which Christians, Jews, and Muslims actively worked together on the same project at a community level. The project offered a chance for Americans of many faith traditions to affirm their commitment to tolerance and pluralism through concrete action.

The project tried to be sensitive to the currents of the war and respond to the needs of the victims. Initially we helped Bosnian students who were no longer able to attend the universities in Croatia. Later we expanded to help college-age Bosnian refugees anywhere in the world who could not continue their education, as well as students inside Bosnia who could no longer attend school because of the war.

When we learned that armies in many areas of Bosnia were killing captured Muslim civilian males as young as age fifteen, we expanded our program to include high school students as well. With the inclusion of high school students, the range of U.S. participants broadened significantly. One no longer needed to live in a university town to become involved; an individual or parish anywhere in the country could sponsor a student.

The project worked through people. Our first task was to find those who cared and were willing to try to make it possible for a student to come to their community. We developed a brochure and two packets related to the project. In developing our materials we tried to be interfaith so our project would model our belief in tolerance and be accessible to Americans of all faith traditions. The central slogan of the project is a quote from the Talmud, "To save one life, it is as if you had saved the world." It seemed somehow appropriate to use a quote from Jewish sacred literature to inspire Christians (and others) to help rescue Muslims (and others) who were victims of religious intolerance.

I wrote articles about the project for many publications and offered to speak about Bosnia to any church, synagogue, mosque, or school who would invite me. Whenever I spoke I also took at least one Bosnian student with me and sometimes more. I introduced the FOR as a community of people of faith from all nations and races committed to using the power of love and truth to resolve conflict and help the victims of oppression. I spoke briefly about the war in Bosnia and asked the accompanying students to tell the story of what happened to them, their families, and their communities. It was painful for the students and their audiences to relive the tragedies of war. But the telling of these stories had a cathartic and empowering effect on them. They became participants, not helpless victims. It allowed the students to validate the tragedy of their past, help in their own healing, and educate their audiences about the dangers of religious and ethnic bigotry.

Americans are used to hearing stories of genocide or wars of racial hatred coming out of developing countries. U.S. audiences assume that these tragedies happen due to lack of education, poverty, or religions which tend toward violence. The stories these young people told broke American stereotypes of societies which succumb to ethnic violence and genocide. These students had grown up in a European country, gone to excellent schools, played basketball, watched MTV and American sitcoms, and loved U.S. popular music. The stereotypes of Muslims as religious fanatics out to create a fundamentalist Islamic state evaporated as soon as the students opened their mouths. To bring matters even closer home, the political and military leaders in Bosnia who had organized the soldiers to drive these young people from their homes were themselves university-educated Christians.

People were deeply moved by the tragic stories of young people who were so much like their own children and had grown up in a society not very dissimilar from their own. Many wanted to help, but most felt incapable of doing anything in the face of such enormous violence and suffering. I explained that while it was true we had no control over the actions of any of the governments or armies in Bosnia and little influence over the actions of the U.S. government or NATO, we could always control our own actions. The Bosnian Student Project could use any person who wanted to get involved to save the life of one Bosnian student and help her or him continue school.

The FOR encouraged U.S. participants in this project to recognize the profound religious implications of their action. We also asked participants to respect the religious backgrounds of the students and the other religious groups with whom they cooperated. We expected host families to welcome students into their homes and places of worship—but also to look for a house of worship consistent with the religious upbringing of the student if the student wished. We asked host families and schools to love and accept the students as they were, regardless of ethnicity or religion, and requested that there be no attempt to convert the students to another religion.

How could a Christian school or congregation welcome Muslim or mixed-family students into their midst and still accept the students as they were? Several of our Bosnian Muslim students received scholarships to Christian colleges which required attendance at chapel services. A Christian organizer who had found a scholarship at one of these colleges wrote about this problem to a Muslim Imam who worked with the project. The Imam responded, "I would like to emphasize our point of view with regard to religion. As Muslims we believe that there is one God, one religion and one race; we are all children of Adam and Eve. We would prefer to place Bosnian Muslim children in parochial colleges, as we hope the atmosphere and conditions would be moral. In the absence of mosques, we would be favorable towards the children going to chapel and, in a serene atmosphere, to meditate, say their own prayers, and participate."

The First Baptist Church of Granville, Ohio, came up with an innovative solution to the question of how to be welcoming and inclusive without pressuring the Bosnian Muslim student whom they sponsored to convert. The pastor reported, "The congregation has accepted Sanela as a Muslim member of our Baptist church. I introduced her the first Sunday as our Bosnian Muslim sister. We feel so privileged to have her with us. Being a friend of Sanela, holding her as she cries and we cry with her, has helped our congregation to move beyond the limits of religious separation.

"We couldn't have had a more meaningful gift to our congregation. Everyone in the congregation feels helpless at the enormity of what she represents, and we are privileged to stand with her in this suffering. At an Advent service we invited her to light one of the advent candles and say a prayer with us."

For the student who had fled the religious intolerance of Bosnia, the experience was healing and transforming. Sanela wrote, "This church is just like my mosque back home. They are my family. Did you know that Baptists and Muslims pray to the same God?"

In Oakland, California, a Serbian-American woman, member of the Society of Friends (Quakers), opened her home to a Bosnian Muslim art student. The host mother had been born in Belgrade, Serbia. Although she had come to the U.S. as a child, she had returned to Belgrade every summer while growing up and still spoke fluent Serbo-Croatian, the common language of Bosnia, Serbia, and Croatia. When she opened her home to a Bosnian student, her own mother, also a U.S. citizen, warned against allowing a "Muslim fundamentalist" into her home. Still she welcomed a Muslim student whose doctor father had been killed in Sarajevo by Serb artillery the previous year.

By all accounts, everyone has enjoyed and learned through the new relationship. The mothers of both the host and the student agreed that it was a wonderful placement and that the "enemy," when viewed up close, looks a lot like oneself.

In much of the world Muslims and Jews are considered antagonists. The Bosnian Student Project learned that this did not need to be the relationship between these two faith traditions. Two Bosnian Muslim students in this program were hosted by the families of rabbis. The family of a Jewish doctor from the Boston area contacted our program to offer to host a Bosnian high school student. The host mother explained that while the family observed the strict Kosher Jewish dietary laws, they would welcome a Bosnian Muslim high school student who needed a home.

A year and a half later, after the high school student had graduated and moved on to a university in a nearby city, I called the host mother to see how things had gone. "Mirza has become like another one of our children. Even now that he is off to college, he returns home to be with our family every other weekend. A month ago was our twenty-fifth wedding anniversary. The children decided to organize a big party to celebrate with our family and friends. Mirza came and spoke about how important we had been in his life. He couldn't finish his speech because he broke down crying. He has really become part of our family."

A Jewish family in North Carolina who had hosted a Bosnian high-school student from Sarajevo called me one day to report that their student's father had been killed as the result of a sniping incident. The death had occurred during the middle of the siege of Sarajevo; there was no possibility the student could return for her father's funeral. "How can we help Maja mourn the tragic loss of her father?" the host mother asked. In the end this Jewish-American host mother worked with a Lebanese Muslim Imam who lived in North Carolina and her own rabbi to find suitable rituals and prayers to help this young student survive and recover from the tragic loss of her father. Unfortunately, many of our host families needed to provide this kind of support. In the same year that Maja's father was killed, two other students lost their fathers and one student his mother.

Communication with the parents of Bosnian students was often difficult because none of our host families spoke Bosnian and very few of our students' families spoke English, but many of them tried to communicate. One Bosnian mother struggled to tell us what had happened to her family and how this project looked to her. She and her husband had sent their two sons to Croatia shortly before the war started, but the parents had chosen to stay in their town to save their house. Because they were Muslims, both she and her husband had been incarcerated in a concentration camp.

They were fortunate. With the help of several Serb friends they escaped shortly before her husband was scheduled to be killed, and after months of hiding made it safely to Croatia. They lost everything but their lives and their two sons. It appeared that the entire world was willing to look the other direction as genocide progressed against them. "You are more than friends for us. You are second parents for our children. We are so conscious how much you sacrifice that our sons not suffer with us in the war which continues in our country. Our children are safe and going to school. Thank God."

In the last year of the war I was able to travel to Bosnia to visit some of the families of students. I came with photos of children who had not been seen by their parents for almost four years and photographed parents for homesick children in our project. It felt like a sacred obligation to be a bridge between members of a family separated by war. The tears of joy and pain on both sides of the Atlantic were almost too much to absorb. One mother explained, "You have been the face of God to us at a time when the whole world seems to have turned its back on the Bosnian people."

The Bosnian Student Project's principle weapon in its struggle against genocide was love and inclusion. Purveyors of genocide always try to destroy the human link between their victims and "the rest of us." The very students whom others were trying to kill, destroy, or drive out were welcomed into our homes and schools. In our own small way, we helped to rebuild the human community which others were determined to destroy. We did not stop the war or end the genocide—but did give witness to our belief that these students of a different ethnicity, religion, and nationality than our own are our neighbors. They are part of our human family—children of God.

We also saved the lives and secured an education for scores of Bosnian students. Each student knows that it was only through the cooperation of people of many faiths in the U.S. and the former Yugoslavia that they were able to continue their education. Perhaps it is in the investment in life and hope for these students that the true value of the project can be seen. Alma, a Bosnian Muslim student who was in Bihac during the four years of the war, wrote, "I got the opportunity to come to the United States and finish my high school education. I wanted to expand my views about the world and people, and I wanted to convince myself that all people are not capable of the hatred that I saw during my war experience. I came to the United States because I also wanted to receive a wide range of education, so I could return to my country and contribute to its reconstruction. I don't want history to be repeated one more time, and I don't want to carry revenge in me. I came to the United States for education that will open my eyes and in that way help me to open the eyes of others."

After her first day in college in the U.S., Bojana, a Bosnian Serb student who spent two years of the war in Gorazde and two years of the war in Pale, wrote this letter to fellow students killed in the war: "Today was my first day in the college! I enjoy seeing young people and being surrounded by natural freedom and their voices and laughter. I don't feel very much as an artificial part of them. Something assimilates, and something remains apart. I feel very blessed to have found the happy problems of peace. Things to do. . . .

"This is the first day I was thinking of you so deeply. This is the first sense of getting into a normalcy, and in a completeness it is easier to notice that you are missing. I cannot resist the thought that you are absent. It drags me to a loneliness. You were supposed to be in your classes too.

"Many of us went on. Many of us will work for peace to prevent new empty places in the world. There's nothing to justify, but there's a lot to be changed. I don't have any comforting explanation for what happened, but I hope that it is a strong reason for the world to care for their children by taking care of each other."

Building Community
Peace in South Africa

Andries Odendaal, Chris Spies

Democracy came to South Africa like manna in the desert—unimaginable and unexpected. For many decades the prospect of "one person, one vote" had hovered over the country, filling some with desperate hope and others with abhorrence. When it became a reality, people of all sorts stood in lines kilometers long, baked for hours in the sun, and filled the moment with quiet dignity, pride, and gratitude. It was a moment of eschatological proportions.

Yet realized eschatology is not the same as heaven. The end to apartheid and colonialism in South Africa did not wipe out the history of the previous 500 years. Free access to the ballot box for everyone did not obliterate the economic, demographic, and historic realities of the country. Peace was made, but it still needs to be built.

The key question is this: will a democratic South Africa be a peaceful and stable South Africa? The role of democratization in conflict resolution and peacebuilding is a topic of discussion and research among conflict resolution scholars lately. There is a growing consensus that democratization is a vital precondition for peace; democratic states rarely go to war with each other.[1]

For South Africans a more relevant question is whether democracy is also a safeguard against internal ethnic or racial conflict and civil war. Can democracy protect a country from implosion? Does universal and free access to the ballot box guarantee that historic animosities between different groups will be sufficiently contained? Diamond, for one, believes this is the case. He writes that democratic governments do not "ethnically cleanse" their own populations and "are much less likely to face ethnic insurgency." The respect for competition, civil liberties, property rights, and the rule of law are to be the safeguards for a stable internal and external social order.[2]

Democratization is indeed a necessary condition for peace, but it is not a sufficient condition. Democratization creates a legitimate framework which makes peace possible, but the content of that framework has to be created. The grassroots or local level is particularly important in making democracy work, as this is the arena in which democracy becomes real to people. At the local level democracy is raw with intensity and often lacks sophistication.

At this level problems like racial prejudice or ethnic intolerance become persons. They have faces and addresses. If democratization or peacebuilding is to have any effect, the local level is a crucial testing ground. What follows is a look at the perceptions and experiences of people at this level, at the way these perceptions contribute to conflict, and at suggestions for local-level peacebuilding. Our comments come from observations of communities in the Western Cape, one of South Africa's nine provinces.

Local Perceptions of Community

The Western Cape is unique in South Africa for more than one reason. First, the Black population group forms a minority in this province. According to the 1991 government census, the Coloured population, a community of mixed-race origin, comprises 58.3 percent of the province, the White population makes up 24.5 percent and the Black population 16.4 percent. The primary language is Afrikaans, the first language of the majority of Whites and Coloureds. Second, the Western Cape is the only province under the rule of the National Party (NP), previously the Whites-only ruling party of apartheid, because a majority of Coloureds voted for this party in the national elections of 1994.[3]

During the local government elections of 1995, however, the Coloured vote shifted to the African National Congress (ANC), South Africa's current ruling party. All the towns of the Southern Cape, for example, are now under ANC rule at the local level. So on the one hand, Coloured and White interests seem to be merging. On the other hand, there is evidence of deep divisions and high levels of distrust. The Black population is in the ambiguous situation of being outnumbered at the local level, yet at the level of national government they are in the majority. In some towns the ANC rules locally, but provincial NP executives may overrule them, to be in turn overruled by the central (ANC) government. In the struggle for resources and positions, strings can be pulled in all directions, creating a complicated cross-stitching effect.

Conflict resolution and peacebuilding are the arts of dealing with perceptions and identity. In each of the three population groups at the local level, perceptions are developing which will severely test the ability of the democratic framework to deal with the resulting tensions and conflict. We will take a brief look at these perceptions to understand the continuing need for deliberate peacebuilding. Obviously what follows is a generalized and simplified version of the much more complicated and nuanced discourse in each group. Our goal is to describe a developing pattern, to draw a picture with broad strokes.

The Black Community

The Black community is the most disadvantaged of all the communities of the Western Cape when judged by such socioeconomic indicators as income, employment, housing, and availability of facilities such as schools and clinics. In the Western Cape they are regarded by the other groups as "inkommers" (immigrants). Historically there has not been a large presence of Black people in the Western Cape and during the apartheid years the Coloured Labour Preference Act restricted them from gaining permanent employment. Following the repeal of this law, a large influx took place during the late 1980s, especially to towns that offered a distinct possibility of employment.

The very state of being disadvantaged dominates the discourse of this community and influences its members' perceptions of issues like racism and justice. They believe they have the moral right to be first in line for developmental opportunities and allocation of resources and jobs because they are most disadvantaged. They argue that the Reconstruction and Development Programme (RDP), the government's plan to address poverty and the lack of infrastructure in disadvantaged communities, should benefit their communities first and foremost—even to the exclusion of less disadvantaged communities.

They believe racism is the attitude of those who deny the obviousness of this right or who make this right conditional on the more mundane laws of the land. In one town, for example, informal taxi operators, those operating without legal registration and licensing, argue passionately that they have a right to operate as taxis without valid permits because they are poor and because the RDP is "for them."

Another aspect of this community is the intense pressure on its leaders. Not many people have leadership experience on a Town Council or other such representative structures. Those who do have the requisite skills serve on many committees. There is enormous expectation for them to perform well and deliver their communities from poverty. All this causes intense pressure, exacerbated by an uphill battle to come to grips with the new situation and its demands.

Township communities and those of squatter camps often exhibit remarkable dignity and staying power considering their conditions. At the same time, however, one cannot escape the impression that these are battered communities. Their leaders, as much victims of the battering as the rest, now find their hands on the levers of power. They are expected by the wider community to exercise that power with fairness, empathy, and concern for the interests of other groups as well. The fact that there are some who succeed is remarkable. Others, however, show signs of stress-related behavior, such as alcohol abuse and avoidance of responsibilities.

The Coloured Community

The Coloured community is in the grip of a severe crisis of identity. The race classification system of apartheid used the concept *Coloured* as a catchall for those neither White nor Black. This group is thus diverse. According to skin color—that all-important badge of power and privilege of the old South Africa—the members range from almost black to almost white. Some trace their lineage to the Khoi-San people, who have probably the greatest claim to being aboriginal South Africans. There is currently a revival of Khoi-San nationalism led by the Griqua people, who are pressing hard to be recognized as an aboriginal minority group distinct from Coloured.

The majority of Coloureds, however, do not have a strong sense of cultural identity apart from being South Africans. A high level of consciousness of color prevails. Identity and status are still attached to skin color (the lighter the better).

At a secondary school for Coloureds in one rural town, the appointment of a deputy principal was criticized by some of his colleagues because he is too dark-skinned. The school reported low levels of cooperation among staff and serious demoralization. Further investigation revealed that consciousness of status among the staff contributed significantly to the problem. In another town a Coloured farm manager complained about his lack of power. Though he enjoys all the power of a manager on paper, his subordinates refuse to accept his authority because he is not the White boss.

For a community that has internalized the message that Whites provide the norm, the new South Africa has brought significant internal turmoil.[4] Coloureds see themselves as "sandwich people" squeezed between White and Black power blocs. The sandwich has now been turned around, but they remain the middle being squeezed. For them the dawn of liberation was therefore an ambiguous experience. Some have embraced the new democracy with enthusiasm. For others, however, democracy intensified fears of being a neglected minority. They were used to thinking of the Western Cape as their territory. Now they have to share scarce resources like land, houses, and jobs with the recent (Black) immigrants, who are socioeconomically more deprived than they are, but who now hold the levers of national power. This insecurity and resentment is an important contributor to conflict in communities.

The White Community

The mood among Whites can be described as indignation. The indignation relates to perceived lowering of standards in public life and perceived incompetence of the new bureaucracy. It is probably part of a process of mourning; it is natural that Whites would mourn the loss of power and control. For centuries the belief was instilled in them and reinforced through practical experiences that the only way to survive on this harsh continent was through firm control. This paradigm has been dramatically overturned. The new paradigm says survival will be guaranteed through democratic behavior, the quality of their cooperation with Africa's people, and the indispensability of their contribution.

But mourning the death of the old paradigm has to be a discreet affair. It is not acceptable to long for the old South Africa from public platforms. Some still wave the old flag at sport events, but few would call for a return to the days of former President P.W. Botha, with its human rights abuses and international isolation. There is a mixture of accepting the moral superiority of the current democracy while resenting and fearing the insecurities and loss of control that go with it. The consequence is indignation.

Indignation is a fairly useless emotion. It undermines the cooperation with others which is vital to the new paradigm. It is not helpful in dealing with the legitimate aspects of the mourning process. Indignation causes people to withdraw from public life, to withhold their contribution, and to find comfort in a collective gloating over the failures of the newly empowered.

Acting on Perceptions

The interaction of these perceptions creates conflict. The perceptions derive in part from the material conditions attached to racial identity which is the legacy of the colonial and apartheid past. In part they also stem from the nonmaterial sphere of insecurity, fear, and resentment. As a consequence, there is a clear tendency for people on the local level to mobilize along ethnic or racial lines. Each town and village is ethnically and racially diverse. Each town has an ethnic majority and one or more minorities. The competition for resources and job opportunities is highly influenced by this demographic reality. The following two case histories highlight this dynamic.

The Housing Crisis at Grabouw

"Melrose Place" is the name given a forty-six-hectare piece of land in Grabouw, where hundreds of homeless Coloureds and Blacks want to live. They impatiently watched in 1994 as bulldozers cleared the land where 1,300 plots for low-cost housing would soon make a dream come true. People talked about Melrose Place as if they would soon live in the TV soap opera setting itself. The "new" South Africa looked promising. Little did they realize that Melrose Place would turn out to be as plagued with backstabbing and conflict as the soap opera.

Two years and twenty-two million Rand later, shrubs and trees are growing on the land. No houses have been built. Only streets, hundreds of electricity poles, a new squatter camp called "Snake Park" on the edge of Melrose Place, and damages and legal costs to the local municipality can be pointed to.

Not only did the bulldozers level the terrain for development, they also cleared out more than 200 illegal shacks erected by Coloured people. The trucks dumped damaged corrugated iron, poles, and meager personal belongings in the adjacent bushes. This "transit area" was soon known as Snake Park, named after the many snakes the evicted people had to deal with. During protest actions, police and residents of Snake Park shot at one another. The police used rubber bullets, and the residents employed catapults (slingshots).

This scenario is not uncommon in present-day South Africa. As in many other deprived areas created by apartheid, the previous local (White) councils had not built enough houses for the poor. In Grabouw no new state-owned houses were built for twenty-six years in Coloured townships. New families and grown children had to live in backyard shacks and overcrowded homes.

No provision was made for Black housing either, because Blacks were required by the Group Areas Act and the Coloured Labour Preference Act to leave the area after 1955. After the lifting of the apartheid laws in the late 1980s, the Black men working as seasonal or migrant farm workers and living in single quarters on the farms brought their families to live with them. In a few months thousands of Black people moved into the village. Having no place to stay, they erected shacks on an open public space where the White, Coloured, and industrial areas intersected.

The then-White-controlled municipality refused to provide services for "squatter areas." The farmers were indifferent ("It's not our problem—it's a problem for the town"); the Coloureds were getting apprehensive ("We were here first"); the Whites were alarmed at the prospect of having Black squatters a stone's throw away ("Our house prices will fall"); the churches did not respond to the needs of the poor at all; and the business sector had mixed feelings ("More people mean more customers, but what about the crime rate?").

A Coloured residents' organization, GRACO, associated themselves with the Pan Africanist Congress (PAC), a minority national political party, because "the PAC takes land issues seriously." Their leader, a middle-class school teacher, mobilized support around bread-and-butter issues like the need for proper housing, jobs, and fighting crime, but also around the issue of identity.

It soon became apparent that the fear of having to live among Black people was probably the main force behind the illegal occupation of Melrose Place. GRACO was adamant that Coloureds had the first right to choose where to live and who they wanted to live with. "We believe that nobody has the right to force people simply because they have no other choice. We are not prepared to be abused as guinea pigs," they wrote in a memorandum to the municipality in January 1996. Though nationally the PAC supports a nonracial society with an Africanist ethos, the Grabouw PAC branch was rallying around the land issue as an exclusively Coloured party, pushing a policy of "Coloureds first."

The ANC, the majority party in the local council since 1995, were adamant that they would never accept the re-introduction of "apartheid." The slogan capturing their position is "One person, one plot." Every person on the waiting list would have to qualify according to prescribed criteria and would receive equal treatment. Among Black people the irritation with GRACO grew. In their view, these leaders were ignoring the desperate plight of Blacks and were seeking to promote their own sectional interests. More and more letters attacking the leaders of GRACO and PAC appeared in the press. Among Whites, however, the dominant feeling was that "they" (meaning the Blacks and Coloureds) should sort out their own problems. They denied having any responsibility for this conflict.

During the first half of 1995, one of us attended as impartial observer forty-three different negotiation meetings between the major players. Each time the negotiations deadlocked because neither the ANC nor the PAC members moved beyond stated positions. They were trying to win the moral high ground and positioning themselves through threats to use power and legal action. It soon became clear that hidden agendas, negotiating in bad faith, uncontrolled and unverified information-spreading, political power struggles and opportunism, internalized oppression, pending and potential legal actions, and the prospect of winning the upcoming local government elections were factors which formed the hidden part of the iceberg.

Currently about 200 of the plots have been allocated by the local council. But GRACO supporters who do not meet the criteria to qualify for a plot have erected shacks on some of those plots in defiance of the council. Rejecting the allocation process, their leader allegedly stated, "This time we will fight to the death."

The Transport Crisis at Mossel Bay

Fynbos refers to the indigenous shrubs and flowers of the Western Cape. This ecosystem enjoys worldwide recognition for its uniqueness and beauty. Many areas of fynbos, however, are threatened by invading plant species, especially in the water catchment areas of the mountains. This negatively affects the ability of the soil to retain water.

The Department of Forestry and Water Affairs developed a plan to deal with this problem and at the same time address the serious problem of unemployment. Using RDP funds (money donated to the government with the specific aim of addressing the poverty and infrastructural needs of disadvantaged communities), they would hire unemployed people to remove the invader plants by hand. In this way jobs would be created, the fynbos would be protected, and the steady flow of rivers and streams would be enhanced. The value of the water saved in this way would be higher than the cost of the project. It appeared to be a clear win-win situation.

When the project was implemented in Mossel Bay, however, it created serious conflict. Part of the plan was to use local transportation to take workers to fynbos areas. People in the Black community jumped at the opportunity and used almost anything that moved to transport workers. It became a lucrative business. The official taxi association, however, felt aggrieved that the government used vehicles which did not meet official requirements for public transport. They felt the right to transport people belonged to them since they had legal transport permits. The legal taxi owners were, with some exceptions, Coloureds.

The conflict between legal and informal transporters became so intense that, despite efforts to negotiate deals that would accommodate

ments are sometimes involved in dealing with conflict relevant to their departments, but increasingly the government is seen as party to the conflict. The consequence is a catch-22: development is hampered because of conflict, but because of frustration at the slow pace of development, conflict escalates.[6]

The quest is to transform the conflict at the local level into sustainable, peaceful relationships and outcomes. An additional reason for taking this quest very seriously *at the local level* is to inoculate the country against the pest of "ethnic entrepreneurs." South Africa has in the past suffered deeply from ethnic nationalism. The potential for future ethnic or racial conflict will always be there. Current consensus holds that democracy and a culture of human rights on a national level are the best safeguards against violent ethnic conflict.[7] South Africa today enjoys one of the most human rights-friendly constitutions in the world.

However, at the local level, where people through the power of their perceptions find themselves pitted against others in their struggle for survival, violent conflict continues to happen along ethnic or racial lines. The inoculation of the country against the instinct to deal destructively with other identity groups has to happen at the local as well as national level. This inoculation will happen, we believe, when communities undergo successful conflict resolution processes and are allowed to learn from and be empowered by those experiences.

Components for Building Peace

Many local conflict resolution efforts continue across the country. The culture of talking to opposing groups or parties to find common ground has been firmly established in South Africa in a remarkably short period.[8] The implementation of the National Peace Accord has contributed to this new culture, specifically by involving local communities in the process.[9] If it were not for a general willingness to deal with conflict in this way, much higher levels of violence and ungovernability would exist. Often such efforts at conflict resolution involve negotiations between the parties without third-party help. When such help *is* used, it usually involves professional mediators or facilitators.

It is important to find a form of third-party intervention that looks beyond merely defusing the tension and reaching compromises around a specific issue. Conflict resolution should be not an ad hoc event but a process which, to meet the needs of all, ultimately aims to transform social institutions, relationships, and procedures for allocating resources. It should empower the whole community to deal constructively with future conflict, thus creating the inoculation effect.

This will happen, we believe, when careful attention has been paid to the roots of the conflict and to the frustration of basic human needs that supply the energy for the conflict. Important theoretical work has already been done in this respect.[10] But empowerment will also happen when the local peacebuilders' own understanding of the conflict and their capacity to deal with it have been enhanced. It is this last aspect that we wish to draw attention to by suggesting four central components to a foundation for local peacemaking.

Team Building

A successful conflict resolution process at the local level should not be a process managed by a professional third party without the involvement and empowerment of local peacebuilders. Each community has its own natural peacebuilders. These are the people who can establish relationships of trust and respect beyond the borders of their own group. Though none are neutral or completely impartial amid conflicts in their community, they are perceived to be especially capable of an objective opinion, self-criticism, and empathy for people of other groups. None may have sufficient credibility as individuals to be a neutral third party, but if a team of such people is assembled representing the different groups, the team may enjoy such credibility.

The tasks of such a team are to take ownership of the peace process; to establish a mandate for themselves in the community and, if applicable, for skilled conflict resolution practitioner(s) from outside; to analyze the conflict;[11] to design and implement a peace process; and to oversee and monitor agreements reached. The team should create a safe space where members can talk about their deeper concerns and feelings and where options can be investigated in a nonbargaining atmosphere.

The facilitation of the team meetings should be done by skilled person(s) due to the sensitive nature of these meetings. The team is therefore not the place where negotiations or bargaining should be allowed to happen. A culture or atmosphere should rather be fostered which will enhance constructive conflict resolution by breaking down stereotypes and establishing relationships of trust.

Establishing a Mandate

An important aspect of empowerment is to establish some form of implicit or explicit mandate for local peacebuilders. The experience of peacemaking during South Africa's transitional period shows that the credibility of the peacemaker is an all-important ingredient in the process. Once a mandate has been established, local peacemakers can act with great effect.

Building such a mandate is no easy task because these efforts may easily be interpreted as signifying lack of confidence in the abilities of the legitimate rulers. There is, however, an emerging distinction between the role of policy and decision makers and the role of peacebuilders in a highly complex and diversified community. The first role has been institutionalized, while the second has not. Government is the institutionalized decision maker in the field. It will always be tainted by controversy and seen as partial by one or another of the minorities. Peacebuilders, though, have to look at process and ensure sufficient communication between role-players and adequate understanding of the different perceptions. Peacebuilders should not be involved in the power struggle. Their challenge is to negotiate and establish a mandate for their role in the community.

Training

A serious obstacle to peacebuilding efforts is lack of interest in the ongoing process. Often after a conflict has been defused and some agreement reached, those involved lose interest and do not attend follow-up meetings. Thus conflicts are defused but not solved. It is important to realize that while a conflict is "hot," a high level of interest and energy exists and should be exploited. This is when the most effective opportunity for training and skills development exists.

Training should have two legs to stand on. On the one hand there is a need for directive training, including the sharing of information concerning the theory of conflict resolution and training in basic mediation skills. Adults, however, learn best when reflecting on their own actions. Thus a vital part of the training process should be to create opportunities for those dealing with a specific conflict to step back and reflect on what has happened. These reflections should then be captured in a number of learnings that can help plan the next step of the process. After implementation, the cycle of *action-reflection-learning-planning-action* should be repeated and become part of the "toolkit" of the peacebuilders.[12]

Involvement in such a process is long-term. South Africa has become a happy hunting ground for institutions or individuals presenting quick-solve two-or-three-day workshops on conflict resolution and related topics, or for facilitation or mediation sessions for a few hours at a time. The value of these interventions is not disputed; they contribute to creating a culture of tolerance and greater mutual understanding. Yet the greater need at this stage is for the design and implementation of long-term processes and strategies to resolve conflict. The touchstone of these interventions should at all times be whether local peacebuilders have been empowered.

Creating Self-awareness

The effectiveness of peacebuilding ultimately depends more on the person of the peacebuilder than on acquired techniques. In South Africa, as in all traumatized countries, all citizens have been affected to some extent by the violence of the conflict, by the injustice of oppression, and by the reigning prejudices. It is not productive to develop conflict resolution skills without at the same time helping participants come to grips with their own pain, anger, fear, and prejudice. Peacebuilding has to start with a process of making peace with one's own individual and collective past. The context of a team is ideal for this process. It creates a safe space to talk about one's hurt or fear in the presence of representatives of those identity groups associated with that hurt or fear. Such a process promotes the self-awareness and healing without which it will be virtually impossible to play an effective role as peacebuilder.

Conclusion

The framework for peace has been established in South Africa. However, local communities are still being ripped apart by the force of their divergent perceptions and the frustration of their basic human needs. The need for concerted efforts at peacebuilding through empowering local peacebuilders is clear. As suggested above, this can best be done through a team-building approach. While this methodology still needs refinement, there can be no doubt about the urgency of the task.

10

Breaking the Cycle of Violence in Wajir

Dekha Ibrahim, Janice Jenner

A virtually unknown war was fought among Somali clans in Wajir District of Northeastern Kenya between 1992 and 1995. Eclipsed by bigger wars in Somalia, Ethiopia, the Sudan, and elsewhere in Kenya, this fighting was little recognized even in Kenya, let alone by the international community. However, for the 275,000 mostly nomadic Somali herders living in Wajir District in northeastern Kenya, the results of the fighting were devastating. This is the story of that war and the remarkable community-based initiatives that brought an end to the violence. It is the story of courageous, creative people who took on the responsibility of bringing peace to their land and their community.

"If members of your clan are killed by a person from the clan of another in the peace group, will you continue to be part of this group and continue to work to bring an end to the violence in Wajir? If not, now is the time to leave the peace group." This was the challenge that Oray and other men and women in the newly forming Wajir Peace Group heard and adopted in mid-1993. Oray, a mother of three young children, was ready to do anything to stop the violence that was destroying her people. She, along with others, made the commitment to work toward a peaceful society regardless of what happened.

Soon Oray's commitment was tested, and then tested again, and then yet again. Raiders killed two children in her extended family, and Oray's family was bitter, angry, and ready to avenge the deaths. They urged Oray to stop working with those belonging to the killers' clan. Oray replied, "But we have to do anything and everything to stop this violence so that everyone will feel secure."

Then 500 goats were stolen from Oray's uncle. Again her family urged her to stop her work with people of the enemy clan, and again she refused and kept up her work aimed at stopping the violence. "We must work for peace, to preserve the little we have left," Oray insisted, and continued her work with the peace group.

After that, ten people in her family were killed in one raid, and then three more in a later raid. Altogether, Oray had lost fifteen people in her family. Still she continued her work for peace. Her family distrusted her, calling her stupid, mad, and arrogant. The other clans also distrusted her, wondering what her motivations really were. Still she persisted, in spite of her personal tragedies, and she continues today as a vital worker for peace in Wajir District.

The Roots of the Conflict

Wajir District lies in the extremely arid Northeastern Province of Kenya. Wajir borders both Ethiopia and Somalia and is one of the most sparsely populated and least developed areas in Kenya. Its 275,000 people are almost entirely ethnic Somali. Over eighty percent are nomadic pastoralists, moving with their herds of camels, cattle, and goats in search of pasture and water. The extreme dryness and unpredictability of rainfall means the people require free movement over large areas to sustain themselves and their herds. Traditionally, the Somali clan system provided organizational structure and conflict-resolution strategies that assured the survival of the people in these harsh climatic conditions. Today collision between the modern nation-state and traditional systems has led to problems of control and conflict.

The roots of the Wajir conflict that occurred 1992-1995 are tangled and unclear. The traditional systems used for centuries to regulate Somali society were disrupted by British colonial administration. Following Kenya's independence in 1963, the Somalis of northeastern Kenya fought an unsuccessful war for independence from the new government. The new government continued the British policy of isolating and marginalizing its Somali citizens.

Northeastern Province, including Wajir District, remained under a State of Emergency from 1963 until 1992. Following independence, a series of interclan conflicts occurred, some based on clan boundary disputes, some on political leadership issues, some simply over the scarcity of resources. Most of the clan fighting since Kenyan independence has pitted the Degodia camel-keeping pastoralists against the cattle-keeping Ajuran and Ogaden clans.

Conflicts in neighboring countries have had a severe effect on Wajir District. Wars in Ethiopia and Somalia had significant impacts on Wajir, chiefly in the flow of refugees, weapons, and mercenary soldiers into the District as well as the realignment of clan alliances in Wajir which further eroded clan stability.

A series of severe droughts over the past twenty years led to massive livestock death and subsequent impoverishment and displacement of large numbers of people. This, coupled with chronic underdevelopment and unemployment, led to a community which was vulnerable, desperate, and easily manipulated into violence.

Most top District government officials, as well as members of the security forces, were Kenyans from elsewhere in the country. Their culture, religion, and worldview differed greatly from those of local people. These differences caused misunderstandings and distrust, and many locals tended to view the government administration with suspicion.

Also during this time, in December 1992, Kenya held its first multi-party elections. The vote, conducted in parliamentary districts based on colonial boundaries, led to the Ajuran clan being without a voice in Parliament. This imbalance in perceived political power exacerbated problems already existing among the three major clans in Wajir District.

For all these reasons, the situation in Wajir by 1992 was quite unstable. Large populations of people were destitute and on famine relief. There was a buildup of tension between the various clans, distrust between the government administration and the local population, and a huge influx of refugees and weapons from Ethiopia and Somalia.

Conflict in Wajir, 1992-1995

The conflict in Wajir during 1992-1995 included both interclan conflict and general lawlessness and banditry. While there is no doubt that some of the general lawlessness was caused by the large numbers of refugees, the major impetus to the violence was the local interclan conflict. Elders and chiefs of the three major clans directed their own local militias, consisting of youth from their own clans as well as hired mercenaries from Somalia and Ethiopia. At the height of the fighting in 1993-1994, local people were openly recruiting, arming, and transporting fighters in the trading centers and Wajir town, asserting that this was for their own safety.

The fighting actually began with incidents between the Ogaden and Degodia clans as the Ogaden perceived the Degodia to be encroaching on their land and political base. Violence erupted with clashes and livestock raids in southern Wajir District. The incidents continued without any attempt by the District Administration to stop them.

The Degodia forged an alliance with neighboring people from the Borana ethnic group, ending a long-standing Ajuran-Boran alliance. This prevented the Ajuran from migrating west into Boran territory to escape the worst effects of the drought. Following the election of a Degodia MP in Wajir West constituency in December 1992, the Ajuran and Ogaden allied themselves against the Degodia. Fierce fighting erupted in several areas in Wajir District. Again there was no government intervention to halt the violence.

After June 1993 the situation worsened, with clashes in Wajir town and surrounding areas continuing well into 1994. The violence included stock theft, highway robbery and hijacking of vehicles, looting and arson of homesteads, looting and destruction of businesses, rape, injury, and murder. By late 1993, almost no part of Wajir District was safe; insecurity brought the normal activities of the District to a halt.

The results of the conflict were numerous. The loss of animals greatly worsened an economic and food situation already made serious by the drought and influx of refugees. During "normal" livestock raids, livestock are often simply redistributed among populations in a given area, without great loss of animals to the area as a whole. However, in this case huge numbers of animals left the district. The Ogaden and Ajuran formed alliances with clans in Somalia, and the animals they stole went directly into Somalia; the Degodia formed an alliance with the Borana, and the animals they raided went west and north into Ethiopia.

With roads unsafe, buses stopped running; the only road transportation to and from the District was on large trucks. Trucks were frequently attacked, robbed, and hijacked. This increased both the risk and the cost of transporting people and goods, including relief food, throughout the district. Schools in many areas closed, and teachers, civil servants, and business people left the district.

After an attack on the UNICEF compound and the murder of a UN pilot in 1994 in Wajir town, UNICEF and NGOs pulled out of the district, greatly affecting the drought relief work. Business and economic activity came to a near halt, and feelings of mistrust and fear pervaded all levels of society. People refused to buy or sell to anyone who was not of the same clan, and it became unsafe to venture into other clans' areas, whether in Wajir town, the trading centers, or the pastoralist areas. The government was seen as unconcerned and unable to enforce security, and traditional systems of clan-based justice resulted in escalating violence.

Because of the remoteness and the nature of the conflict, exact figures of the destruction caused by the violence are difficult to obtain. The best estimates available are as follows:

(1) About 1,213 people were killed.

(2) An estimated 2,000 people were injured and/or raped.

(3) The number of livestock stolen is estimated to be 1,000 camels, 2,500 cattle, 15,000 sheep and goats. The economic loss of these thefts is $900,000 (U.S.). Again, most of these stolen animals were taken from the District; they were not simply redistributed among the District's population.

(4) The number of homesteads raided, looted, and burned is estimated at around 1,500, both in pastoralist areas and in trading centers and Wajir town.

(5) About 500 businesses were looted and/or destroyed.

(6) About 30 vehicles (including buses, trucks, and smaller vehicles) were robbed and/or hijacked. Five vehicles were stolen and never recovered.

(7) Forty-five primary schools and five secondary schools with 15,000 students were affected by the violence. Ten primary schools were closed completely, disrupting education for 2,500 students. It is estimated that 50,000 children were traumatized by violence and/or displacement during that time.

(8) About 165 civil servants, including teachers, either left the District or refused to accept their posting there, severely affecting the provision of government services.

(9) About 1,000 guns have been turned over to the government. It is estimated that 1,000-1,500 guns remain in the hands of the people of Wajir. With each gun costing about $200-300 (U.S.), the amount of money used to purchase guns and thus not available to the people for other purposes was $500,000-600,000. This figure does not include costs of ammunition or of hiring the mercenary fighters from outside the District.

It must be remembered that these losses occurred among a population of 275,000 already impoverished people. Multiplying the effects of the violence in Wajir by 1,000 would give an estimate of the disruption caused by violence if similar fighting had occurred in the U.S.

Community Efforts Toward Peacemaking

Throughout 1992 and 1993, the violence in Wajir District continued to escalate. People in Wajir now say, "We were living in hell during that time. Wajir was like a mini-Mogadishu." Violence and insecurity were prevalent throughout the district; shooting occurred even during the day. In the trading centers and Wajir town, it was unsafe for people to be outside after dark or to visit areas not controlled by their own clan.

In June 1993, fighting broke out between women traders at the Wajir market. The market stall owners refused to sell to members of other clans, saying these products would be used by the other clans to kill their relatives. Since Somali women retain their own clans after marriage, this sometimes resulted in the refusal to sell to their husbands' relatives. An appeal by local women to the District Administration to intervene and restore security to the market was dismissed because the fighting was "a women's problem."

Also in June 1993, a wedding was held in Wajir town attended by many of the educated, elite Somalis of all clans. A discussion ensued at the wedding about the fact that they could all attend this celebration together but could not visit each other's homes because of clan problems. Two educated Somali women attending the wedding, one of whom was Dekha Ibrahim, decided it was necessary to get involved with solving the problems of violence in Wajir themselves. The next day they began meeting with the women of the market to discuss what was happening and the causes and results of the fighting. The two women were soon joined by an older, traditional woman leader, and the three of them met every afternoon with the market women throughout June and July.

Slowly they convinced the market women that the fighting at the market was not helping anyone, it was not restoring peace to the area, and it was continuing the cycle of violence. The market women began to express the opinion that although it was the men who had started and were continuing the violence, it was the women and children who suffered the most. From this group of market women, Wajir Women for Peace was born. The group gradually expanded to include other women in Wajir town and also women from the rural areas.

Women are crucial in the process of peace and conflict in Somali society. When fighting is occurring, they sing "songs of war," taunting their men to continue the conflict. Likewise their singing "songs of peace" can shame the men into stopping the fighting. The efforts of the Women for Peace group throughout Wajir District have been catalysts in bringing the violence to an end.

In August the women approached other educated Somalis in Wajir town, both men and women, and convened a meeting to discuss the situation in Wajir and what could be done to restore peace. These educated professionals met and decided to form what came to be known as the Wajir Peace Group (WPG). As one later said, "It was the first time we elite entered into the situation at all."

Representing all clans in the District, these professionals developed severe guidelines for the group and for themselves. Early discussion established that if people wanted to be part of the group, they would have to commit themselves to continuing the peace work, "no matter what happens: If my clan were to kill your relatives, would you still work with me for peace? If you can't say yes, don't join the group now." Some people left, but the core group that remained was—and is—strongly committed to peace in Wajir District. One woman in the group subsequently lost fifteen family members in the fighting; she remains an active member and a strong voice for peace in Wajir.

The first task the Wajir Peace Group took on itself was talking with the major clan elders, whom they saw as responsible for the violence and who would also be responsible for bringing peace. The members of the WPG each went to elders of their own clans and talked about their desire for the restoration of peace and security in the area. These talks met with limited success but did begin the process of debate between the traditional elders and the educated younger people.

The WPG then approached elders of minority clans not directly involved in Wajir conflicts. These elders were asked to act as mediators between the warring elders. After lengthy discussion, they agreed to do this and convened a meeting of elders representing all the clans.

The first meetings were stormy and difficult. Some elders resented "these children" (as they called the members of the WPG) questioning their actions and usurping their roles. A breakthrough finally came when a very old elder gave a lengthy speech saying, "All these children want is peace. We have failed as elders because we have not protected our people. Our children want peace. Will we give them war?"

A series of meetings between the clan elders finally led to a several-day meeting of elders in late 1993. Under the leadership of Mr. Hamad Khalif, then Member of Parliament for the Wajir West constituency, the elders agreed to a code of conduct, the "Al Fatah Declaration," which established guidelines for the return of peace to the District. The elders also formed an "Elders for Peace" group at this meeting.

The WPG also began working with other groups in Wajir. The youth were seen as a major target, and a Youth for Peace group was soon started. The youth began to realize that although the old men controlled the violence, it was the young men who did the fighting and died. Youth for Peace, which started in Wajir town, soon began sending delegations throughout the district, talking to the youth about their roles in either promoting or stopping the violence.

Similar work was done with the business community in Wajir. Approached with the idea that "peace is good for business," many business people joined the peace work, and from the beginning supported the work of the groups financially. The work of the religious leaders was also key. Sheiks (Islamic leaders) from other areas of Kenya, including Mandera, Garissa, and Nairobi, traveled to Wajir and spent a month on preaching tours to call the people back to the Qu'ran's message of peace. These sheiks traveled to all the outlying parts of the district, sometimes in dangerous conditions, to call their people back to peace and the rejection of violence.

Many members of the WPG were civil servants. Thus from the beginning there was concern to integrate the work of civilian groups and the government in restoring peace and security. However, until April 1994 the District Administration was weak and/or uninterested, and cooperation was difficult.

In April 1994 a new District Commissioner (DC) was appointed to Wajir District. This DC has been central in the work of restoring peace to Wajir. He has been actively involved in the entire peace process and has made government resources available to restore security to the district. It is clear that without a strong, committed, interested administration, the peace process in Wajir would not have been possible. In addition, the DC clamped down hard on corruption and bribery and worked to ensure that the administration was responsive to needs of the people.

A major problem during the war was vehicle hijackings. Lack of government response had led to clan-based retaliation and escalating violence. Within a few weeks of the arrival of the new DC, a truck was hijacked on a major road and thirty-five people riding in it were murdered. Immediately on hearing this, the DC personally went to the scene of the hijacking along with army and other security personnel. The security forces were able to track down and arrest the perpetrators. They were dealt with promptly under Kenyan law, and the elders from the various tribes agreed that no traditional revenge was necessary since the perpetrators had been arrested and jailed. This was the first major indication that the government was taking its responsibility for security seriously and that a return to security and a breaking of the cycle of escalating violence was possible.

A Rapid Response Team was set up to deal with problems occurring around the District. This team consisted of members of the District Security Committee, elders, women, and youth. When problems started in a certain area, the Rapid Response Team would travel to the area, meet with various people involved, and usually convene a meeting of elders and others to work on resolving the problem.

One example of the success of the Rapid Response Team occurred in Batalu. Two young men of different clans were fighting over a gun;

one killed the other. The murdered man's clan took revenge by killing some of the murderer's clan, and the cycle continued. By the time the Rapid Response Team arrived, seventeen people from both clans had been killed and the situation was escalating. A series of meetings with elders and others led to the conclusion that the first death was a murder and the perpetrator should be dealt with by Kenyan law. However, the other deaths were attributable to traditional Somali practices and would be dealt with by traditional Somali justice, which would involve the payments of large fines of camels. The District Administration agreed to this. The first murderer was arrested, and the other deaths were dealt with by traditional methods. The cycle of violence was stopped.

The WPG held workshops for many groups in the District, including elders, women, youth, chiefs, administration, security forces, and religious leaders. There were also Training of Trainers workshops so the workshops could spread to more District areas. All the workshops focused on ways of restoring peace and security to the District.

The chiefs were seen as vital to the process of continuing the violence or of restoring peace. Chiefs in Kenya have great powers and often receive little training in their roles and responsibilities. The workshops for chiefs focused on training in these roles as defined by the Chiefs' Act and introduced to the chiefs their vital role in providing security for their people.

Also important were the training sessions held for the District security forces, especially the army and the police. Most members of the security forces are from other parts of Kenya, with deep prejudices and suspicions about Somali people. Training sessions were held which explained Somali culture and ways of interacting with Somali people. Members of the security forces were then asked to provide training to Somali people on "how to interact with the police and the army." The training sessions for the security forces as well as for the civilian population built trust between the people and the government.

One important part of this trust building was the army commander's commitment to stop the looting, rape, and other abuses by army personnel when they were out on missions. His success at stopping these actions, as well as curtailing public intoxication by his soldiers, improved relations between the people and the army.

A program for the return of guns was initiated. Chiefs were given the responsibility of collecting weapons from their locations, and an amnesty was granted to those people returning weapons to the government. As peace and security slowly returned to various parts of the district, guns and other weapons were turned in to the government. To date, over 1,000 guns have been turned in to the government; it is estimated that 1,000-1,500 guns remain in the district, "but most are buried in the sand" (hidden).

A number of innovative methods cemented steps taken to ensure peace. For example, in October 1993 the Degodia and the Ogaden clans reached an important agreement over the return of stolen livestock. This agreement was one of the first activities of the Elders for Peace group and included a ceremony in which stolen camels were returned to the Ogaden and stolen cattle to the Degodia. An attempt to get this agreement reported in the Kenyan media was unsuccessful, but the WPG then called the BBC Somali Service in London. The BBC broadcast an interview of the chairman and secretary of the Elders for Peace group who had negotiated the agreement. The BBC Somali Service is widely listened to all over Northeastern Kenya; hearing their own elders talk of the peace agreement was important in convincing the people to respect this agreement.

By late 1994 it became evident to members of the Wajir Peace Group that some formalization and integration of the various types of peace work going on in the District was necessary. There was concern that the individual peace groups would be unable to continue effectively without some coordination of efforts. In addition, leaders of the peace groups wanted to assure that the peace efforts had some formalized organization in the District so peace work could continue even if the Administration changed to one indifferent or even hostile to the work of the peace groups.

The WPG leaders explored a number of options for this formalization. One option seriously considered was registering as an NGO. They rejected this because of concerns that it might become difficult for government departments to work within an NGO structure. Similarly, they rejected the option of formalizing the peace groups as a direct structure in one of the government departments because of the difficulty NGOs and citizen groups would have in being a full part of the process.

The one structure in district administration in Kenya that brings together government, NGO, and citizen groups is the District Development Committee, which coordinates development activities in each district. It had become evident to the leaders of the peace groups that peace is a vital and necessary part of development, and they eventually decided to unite the peace groups as a subcommittee of the District Development Committee. This was done in May 1995, with all peace groups represented under a united group now known as the "Wajir Peace and Development Committee" (WP&DC). The chair of the WP&DC is the District Commissioner; members include the heads of all government departments, representatives of the various peace groups, religious leaders (both Muslim and Christian), NGO representatives, and District officers and chiefs. The meetings of the WP&DC were closed at first but are now open for any citizen of the District to attend.

An important WP&DC activity has been sponsoring two districtwide peace festivals, first in July 1995, then June 1996. The first festival was a one-day event in Wajir town, with the theme "Peace is a Collective Responsibility." It included presentations by schools, community groups, and peace groups. Presentations included songs, dramas, poems about peace and peacemaking, and speeches by local dignitaries.

In addition, a Peace Prize was given to the chief who had done the most to promote peace in his location. The prize was a large trophy and about $200 for use by the location's peace committee to continue their efforts towards restoring peace. The winning chief was chosen by a committee of elders representing all clans in the District. The peace prize was such an honor that it was necessary to hold an unplanned workshop for chiefs the following day to instruct them in what they needed to do during the following year to win the prize at a subsequent peace festival.

The second festival was expanded to an entire week of activities in each of the twelve divisions of Wajir District. Local activities and presentations took place in each division. Members of the WP&DC spent the week visiting each of the divisions to provide help and support to the division festivals. The theme of the 1996 Peace Festival was "Amani ni maziwa; amani ni maendeleo; amani ni maisha" (peace is milk; peace is development; peace is life).

Following the Divisional Peace Week, a one-day festival was held in Wajir town. The winners from each division came to town to perform their winning presentations. Many presentations focused on the relationship between peace, food, development, and life, with school children giving quite dramatic renditions of the suffering caused by war and the happiness that comes from peace.

Certificates were given to the performing groups. Certificates were also presented to the chief or subchief in each division who had done the most to promote peace. Again a trophy and cash prize were presented to the best chief in the District and again choices were made by a committee of elders. The criteria for selecting the chiefs for the peace prizes were that the chief needed to have stopped livestock theft in his location, to have resolved problems quickly when they occurred, and to have had guns turned in to him by the people of that location.

All festival money was raised locally. In 1996 this amount was around $4,600. The WP&DC believes if peace is to be sustained in Wajir District, it must be owned by the people of Wajir; a too-heavy reliance on outside money will doom the peace efforts of the community groups.

Local contributions to peace have been crucial from the beginning. The activities mentioned above have occurred with remarkably small amounts of money, which again underlines the unique cooperation between the community and the government in working at restoration of peace and security. Government departments, in the face of inadequate funding, supplies, and personnel, have contributed fuel, personnel, vehicles, and other items for the work of the peace groups. The army and police have also often supplied fuel, logistical help, vehicles, and personnel to help with the work of the groups. Business people have contributed both cash and materials for help, and individuals in the community have also donated.

In the early days of the Wajir Peace Group, each member gave an individual contribution of $20 (equivalent to one week's wage), and contributed $4 monthly to keep the group going. In addition, the WPG rented and furnished an office for the use of the Elders for Peace group. This commitment by the local community to the work of peace is indicative of the continuing success of the peace efforts.

However, the role of NGOs and donors has also been important in the work of the peace groups in Wajir District. Special mention should be made of Oxfam (United Kingdom and Ireland), which from the beginning has been intimately involved in the work of the peace groups. In addition to providing funding for various activities, Oxfam has been generous in the use of their vehicles, personnel, and logistics (fax, photocopying, and so forth) for the work of the peace groups. Other funding has been provided by Quaker Peace and Service and the Mennonite Central Committee. Donors have provided about half the funds used by the peace groups, with the other half coming from local sources.

The international community has also had some involvement. UNICEF provided help before its pullout from the District in mid-1994. Currently World Bank-funded projects are providing badly needed infrastructure to the District through construction of roads and a commercial airport to help in the export of livestock and other products.

The Fruits of Peace

The people of Wajir are now enjoying some positive effects of the cessation of violence and restoration of District peace and security. Individual investment is increasing, and many new shops and services are opening in the District. A large new commercial building is currently under construction in Wajir town.

The local peace groups were able to restore or compensate much of the property which had been stolen during the fighting. According to a diary kept during that time by Mzee Dubow Yusuf, a member of the Elders for Peace group, three stolen vehicles were recovered; 7,057 sheep and goats, 706 camels, and 1,722 cattle were returned to their rightful owners; and approximately $10,000 (U.S.) was raised to enable business people to restock their looted shops.

With the return of peace, local fundraising is now possible. Since 1994 local citizens have contributed $225,000 to development in Wajir, including the construction of three secondary schools, bursaries for students going to higher education, support of sports clubs, and construction of mosques. In June 1996 elders and chiefs working for peace in the Rift Valley Province of Kenya visited Wajir to attend a workshop led by Wajir's elders and chiefs on the peace process in Wajir. The visitors were surprised and impressed by the work done by the Wajir groups, and the sharing of information was valuable for both groups.

In August 1996 a group of nineteen American university students visited Wajir District for two weeks as part of a semester foreign study program in Kenya. The students traveled through several areas of the District, stayed with nomadic families, viewed development work, learned from sheiks about Islam, and generally experienced life in Wajir. They traveled to and from Wajir by road, something only possible because of the return of peace and security to the District. Two years previously, neither the District Commissioner, the peace groups, nor the American university would have approved such a visit because of the insecurity in the District. Buses are now operating in Wajir, making travel possible again for Wajir's citizens. Scheduled bus service is now available from Wajir to Mandera, Moyale, and Garissa.

The confidence of NGOs and donors to invest in Wajir District is returning. Oxfam committed $1,500,000 to development assistance in the District during 1995-1997. This did not include relief help also being provided by Oxfam. Mennonite Central Committee and Quaker Peace and Service are continuing to assist the WP&DC. The Kenyan Government Arid Lands Program, funded by the World Bank, is working in pastoralist development and in providing infrastructure, including a new road. Kenya government is funding a new commercial airport .

Assumptions Underlying
Conflict Resolution in Wajir

The peacemaking efforts of the community and government groups in Wajir grew out of desperation at a situation that was causing local people untold hardships. There was no articulation beforehand of theories of conflict. However, some values and assumptions with which the peace groups operated can be identified.

The peace groups operated with the assumption that the conflict in Wajir District is multifaceted. The conflict stemmed from historical contexts, including the colonial legacy, previous interclan conflicts, the conflict between traditions and the modern state, conflicts in neighboring countries, chronic underdevelopment and marginalization, national and local leadership crises, and environmental factors.

However, the peace groups also recognized that although the Wajir violence included significant national and international components, the primary cause was local and involved interclan problems in the District. The groups recognized that there were many players or interest groups in the District who were responsible for starting, escalating, and generating the violence for their own ends. Traditional Somali systems of justice, while able under the best of circumstances to control and regulate disputes, can also be used to quickly escalate individual disputes to clan levels. Access to modern weapons greatly exacerbates problems of violence within a traditional society like Northeastern Kenya.

There has never been a clear articulation of the peacemaking process. Most of what was accomplished was done by people with "a heart for peace" rather than training in conflict resolution. Only one person has received extensive training in peacemaking, at a three-month program at Selly Oaks College in the United Kingdom on "Responding to Conflict." Therefore, as with the assumptions about the conflict itself, the values and assumptions on which the peacemaking efforts were based can only be seen in hindsight.

The various peace groups in Wajir operated on the assumption that everyone has a stake in peace; thus all groups must be included in working toward peace. Peace cannot be restored without involvement from all significant sectors of society, both civil and government. All clans must be involved in bringing about peace. Also required is involvement of all sections of society, including elders, women, youth, business people, religious leaders, civil servants, and security personnel.

The peace efforts in Wajir District recognized that Kenyan constitutional law and traditional Somali systems of justice are both legitimate ways of solving conflicts in the Somali community. It is possible to use the systems either against or in support of each other. The peace groups and the District Administration struggled to find the proper balance between the two quite different systems of administering justice and restoring peace and security. The groups recognized that peace efforts must be legitimized by existing community and government structures.

Peace groups could not remain free-floating but needed to be attached to something which legitimized them. For this reason, the peace groups formalized themselves under the District Development Committee.

The peace groups have seen peace as the responsibility of local communities. The leaders (chiefs and elders) and the citizens of each location are who will bring peace or war to their location. Outside organizations can help but not direct the peace process. The main efforts must come from the local population. As a part of this, the peace groups recognized that peace is important enough to pay for locally. While there has been some help with outside funds, the leaders of the peace movement in Wajir have believed strongly that major funding for peace work must come from the local community. Overreliance on outside funds will lead to the collapse of the peace efforts by the local people.

The peace groups recognized that when people feel secure, they will turn in their illegal weapons to the government. In Wajir, guns were often not owned by individuals but by clans. As peace returned to various areas, people came to feel that the dangers of retaining the guns outweighed their worth, and more of them turned in weapons.

The Wajir Peace and Development Committee made the celebration of peace an important part of their work. They operated on the principle that peace festivals, songs, dramas, and other ways of celebrating their success are vital parts of maintaining the peace. Similarly the peace groups realized that recognizing peace workers is important. This is seen in the awarding of chiefs' prizes at the festivals, as well as communication to the national government about government employees who have done significant work for peace. One Kenyan army major was promoted because of letters of commendation from the Wajir community for his work for peace during his time in Wajir.

The peace groups recognized that development cannot occur without peace, and that peace cannot be sustained without development. Now that there is a cessation of violence in Wajir District, greater effort is being placed on development that will allow the peace to continue. Those working for peace in Wajir have recognized the fruits of peace. These include the revitalization of economic activity in the District, the hosting of a workshop for chiefs and elders from the Rift Valley, the two-week visit by American university students in late 1996, and the return of public transport to the District.

Conclusion

There are far too few success stories in Africa's search for peace. The Wajir experience should serve as an example to other community groups in Kenya, around Africa, and elsewhere in the world that peace is possible and that citizens' groups, working with the local government, can bring about peace instead of violence. We hope the Wajir peace story can be shared, discussed, and replicated in many communities throughout the world. And we hope Oray's children will never need to hide from gunfire in Wajir.

A Global Culture of Peace

A Global Culture of Peace

Introduction by Robert Herr

We have all heard the expression "think globally, act locally." It's a shorthand way to help us remember to connect grand theories to every-day life. However, too often we see this turned on its head. Programs aimed first of all at global problems are not easily applied at the local level. Trickle-down peacemaking provokes as many questions as trickle-down economics. Today there is growing appreciation that local realities need to inform global understandings. And if global events rest firmly on life in local communities, transcultural work in peacemaking should start with this orientation.

But the struggles we face cannot be worked at only through local programs and activities. Everything will not somehow work out if we all just take care of our own backyards. The struggles we confront tran-scend local contexts. What is crucial is that we reflect on the linkage be-tween these two. We need to make clear, conceptual links between ordi-nary people living and working together on the one hand and global peacemaking on the other.

This section draws attention to the link between local contexts and global realities. At its best the Christian church physically embodies this single unity, from locally-gathered congregation to worldwide fellow-ship. These chapters look at both theoretical descriptions for this unity and practical examples of Christian work undertaken on a global scale.

David Jackman's account of Quaker work relating to the United Nations presents a picture of the connection between local communities, where peace must become apparent, and national and international are-nas, where its impact is so needed. Peace teams, international conflict mediation, and human rights are each addressed from this perspective.

To "seek the peace of the city where you dwell" (Jer. 29:7) has been a biblical theme through the ages, calling people to work for the well-being of neighbors regardless of national orientation. These chapters re-mind us again of this and provide examples of its application.

11

Churches in a Planet-Sized Peacemaking System

David Jackman

This seems to be a time in world affairs for sober second thoughts. Recently I attended a breakfast presentation at the midtown New York headquarters of a prominent philanthropic organization. The speaker was Marrack Goulding, then chief of the United Nations Department of Political Affairs and its former head of peacekeeping. Goulding's topic was "What's Gone Wrong with Peacekeeping?"

Not surprisingly, Goulding held that, contrary to popular opinion, much had gone right in the scores of UN peacekeeping operations during the last decade. Unfortunately, these successes were deemed uninteresting by the news media and therefore often did not attract much public attention. The large, complicated, and troubled missions in Yugoslavia and Somalia, on the other hand, received lots of attention. For Goulding and for the UN these have been, if not outright failures, at least difficult learning experiences.

When Goulding listed the reasons for the UN's peacekeeping difficulties, he headed the list with the word *euphoria*. In the early 1990s the UN had just completed a number of important peacemaking negotiations that ended seemingly intractable conflicts in several parts of the world, such as the well-run and successful peacekeeping mission in Namibia. These missions represented a whole new order of complexity and importance. "We thought we were invincible," Goulding explained, somewhat ruefully.

Consequently, when the public demanded action to curb the genocidal war in Yugoslavia and the even more devastating chaos in Somalia, the UN Security Council ordered a peacekeeping response. The UN Secretariat put the operations together but did not include a long-term peacemaking strategy, an assured centralized command, or adequate resources. The resulting mess, which, to be fair, was not entirely the fault of the UN, has tarred the credibility of the whole organization. In this atmosphere, the subsequent statements on peacekeeping by both Secretary-General Boutros-Ghali and his successor Kofi Annan have emphasized a back-to-basics theme.

I have described all this at length because I think it mirrors the confusion many Christians feel when they address the question "What is our peace witness today?" In the vast political opening after the end of the Cold War we were excited, had great hopes, and felt that some of our vision might actually come to pass. Now it all looks worse than before. The world situation is complicated with new players, proliferating tensions, and a kind of warfare that seems frighteningly old and distinctly irrational.

But before we sink into despair, it would be good to take a second look at the UN experience. The peacemaking record is really not so bleak; in fact it is marked by many significant, new, positive developments. While the press and public were focused on Bosnia and Somalia, the UN and its agencies, national governments, and a large number of nongovernmental groups have been slowly assembling the framework for a comprehensive, planet-sized peacemaking system.

No, it isn't yet complete, nor is it entirely understood and supported by all participants. Nevertheless the system is being assembled, its parts elaborated, assessed, and, most important, connected. These developments are relevant to Christian peacemakers in several ways.

First, as individuals, groups, and formal agencies, we are involved already in creating parts of the system. For example, Mennonites are involved in international conflict prevention. European churches have sent observers to peace operations in Namibia and South Africa. Church relief organizations participated in refugee aid programs in Rwanda, Burundi, and Congo. Earlier other churches organized solidarity programs with groups in Central America. Canadian churches help to fund professional research into peacekeeping, arms trading, and other security policy questions. All these activities are related to UN programs in war prevention, emergency peace operations, and postwar peacebuilding.

Second, the ongoing elaboration and success of such a system will depend on our encouragement of public support, and we can't speak for its promise if we do not understand its scale and nature. Too often we take our understanding of UN peace actions from the news media, which frequently ignore the wide range of ongoing peace-related activities organized by the world community.

For example, the media have judged the UN efforts in the former Yugoslavia a failure. But actually this UN peace operation and its humanitarian mandate were remarkably successful. The UN goal of preserving a civilian population amid modern warfare was unprecedented. That the UN mandate was too narrow to end the war was not the fault of the UN peacekeepers but rather the responsibility of the major powers. These countries could not agree on a common peacemaking strategy. They attempted to fill the gap with a humanitarian operation. The resulting public protest, which focused on UN peacekeepers' apparent failure to end the war, missed the point and allowed the most culpable actors, the permanent five members of the Security Council, off the hook.

Third, we aren't going to be effective and ultimately confident peacemakers unless our efforts fit sensibly into a wider structure. Church-based peace efforts will always be small in scale when compared to the overwhelming devastation of war. Inevitably these efforts will only address some parts of the complex structure that war prevention and postwar recovery require. This apparent gulf may occasionally slow the responses of Christian peacemakers and will certainly dishearten rank-and-file church members and the general public. If peacemakers describe their work as part of a larger coherent system, it will instill more confidence in participants and supporters alike. More practically, awareness of the wider peace system will allow church-based peace workers to design projects that explicitly build on, or open the way for, the efforts of a wide range of other actors.

Let me sketch in outline what is coming into place. Some of what I present can be found in the UN Secretary-General's "Agenda for Peace 1995" and in a growing set of more specialized publications. Increasingly, peacemaking work is being seen as a cycle of overlapping and interrelated programs that begin with conflict preventive actions, move to more crisis-oriented steps if events spiral toward violence, and finally result during postviolence stages in peacekeeping, humanitarian actions, and long-term development programs.

The overall aim is not to suppress societal conflict, which can be positive, but to "inoculate" societies against using violence as a means of conflict management. This means that the UN system consciously recasts long-term effort in economic or social development, human rights, and education work into a conflict-sensitive framework. UN agencies, national governments, and many international nongovernmental organizations (NGOs) are already reassessing their programs in light of the need to see themselves as conflict managers.

Inevitably there will still be states that threaten violence to achieve their aims. These developments are monitored and responded to under "preventive diplomacy." In this there is an official "track one" dimension which includes multilateral groups and state actors. There is as well a growing unofficial dimension called "track two" which is made up of NGO conflict interveners. While much of this work is diplomatic in nature, involving fact-finding, negotiation, mediation, and official agreements, it also entails efforts to defuse violence with community-level communication, training, and empowerment programs, often conducted by NGOs.

It is important to note that these developments are reflected in the work of larger humanitarian agencies, such as the International Red Cross and the United Nations High Commission for Refugees (UNHCR). Such groups see the need to stem the threat of disaster by engaging in conflict-oriented work.

The determining factor in whether or not a conflict spirals into large-scale violence may well be the stabilizing influence of a peacekeeping force. These operations are likely to include military forces because they require some of the capabilities that, at present, only the military is organized to provide. But peacekeeping operations already include many civilians who organize and administer the nonmilitary aspects of peace plans, such as elections, refugee repatriation, policing, demobilization of combatants, and provision of humanitarian aid. In the future, partly due to the great expense of using military units and partly due to the widening scope of peace agreements, the proportion of civilians engaged in peacekeeping missions is likely to increase.

The need to link peacekeeping to longer-term postwar peacebuilding programs will also lead to greater use of civilians for clearing landmines, restructuring governments, building infrastructure, demilitarizing economic life, and an almost endless list of other tasks needed to move a nation beyond war-time destruction. It may be that for church agencies the greatest scope for action will be in the violence-prevention and postviolence rebuilding stages of the peacemaking structure. These are the places where our capacities for disarmament, economic conversion advocacy, humanitarian aid, grassroots training, conflict resolution intervention, and emphasis on a long-term vision for a nonviolent society have a clear place.

This is not to say that we do not have a contribution to make during war-time. However, there are major obstacles to our working alongside (let alone with or under) military forces. There are perhaps even larger obstacles to our providing large-scale help during the extreme environment of wartime programs. But even with these limitations, there is ample scope for our participation in the emerging international peace structure.

For example, the work churches are doing in culturally sensitive conflict resolution training can be applied to preventing violence long before it erupts. Equally useful is the application of these systems to help inoculate postwar societies against a return to fighting. Church agency work in victim support and reconciliation could have an important role to play in postwar healing. Church positions on economic justice, social services, and community organizing could provide a useful basis for helping to rebuild countries after war. Even the traditional church experience with emergency relief work, if linked more consciously to an awareness of conflict dynamics, could play a useful role in the emerging peace system.

Before we ride off in all directions, however, there are four lessons we need to learn from experiences of the past decade. Such lessons are taught as much by failure as by success. We are living at a historically distinct moment, and we need to respond to new factors. While none of the following lessons are utterly new, their combination is. Certainly, the need to heed them is more crucial than ever.

Learning New Lessons

Lesson 1: Peace starts at home

This lesson seems familiar, but it has a new wrinkle that applies to our current difficulty in feeling confident of choosing the right responses. We are continually pulled by the media and by our own personal experiences to react both to the big stories of large-scale violence and to the very real and vivid needs of our own communities.

Is there a dichotomy between these global and local levels? Interestingly, when one looks at the lists of international postwar peacebuilding programs, many of the projects are desperately needed in all communities. Whether the topic is building community-centered economics, disarming civilians, shrinking dependence on the military, or looking at long-term reconciliation among groups (racial, ethnic, or class), it looks as appropriate in Toronto, Des Moines, or Los Angeles as in Nairobi, Lima, or Bangkok.

More crucially, by working on a local manifestation of a world problem we are going to have an effect on the larger situation. This is true because some of these problems have their roots in local situations. For example, the arms production and trade policies of countries in one area quickly become a significant component of conflict in distant places. Sometimes our inability to act beyond our communities is fed by failures at home. When we do not confront racial, ethnic, and religious intolerance at home, we are diminished in our ability to understand or act in more distant places. Finally, we all need practice if we are to be useful. And practice comes by developing alternatives at home.

This doesn't mean we should stop supporting or being involved in international work. It does mean we should look closely at how involved we are in righting the parallel problems at home.

Lesson 2: We only have to do a small part

If the world is developing a clear, comprehensive, well-articulated peace structure, then we can use that fact to combat the inevitable worry that we have to fix everything. We can choose what is appropriate or crucial for us to do and know that others will do likewise. Too often nothing gets done when we treat peace work as a huge, amorphous cloud of needy symptoms. We need to explore situations, identify what our best contribution can be, then stick to it.

This isn't a recipe to limit the whole range of actions by churches. It is a suggestion that each church grouping should stick to what it recognizes as its own areas of expertise and assume others will do the same. If there is anything one can notice from events around the UN, it is that the world is not lacking in thoughtful, capable, active social change groups. It is in sore need of groups willing to focus and cooperate.

Lesson 3: Alliance is essential

We are no longer working alone—if we ever were—on building peace. Many of the principles, structures, and techniques that the historic peace churches have brought to the world have been internalized and re-expressed by others. This allows us the opportunity to work on aspects that are new and at the growing edge, or to work on smaller, more defined areas in larger efforts. It also brings the realization that there are large programs in which we can be one of many actors.

Some analysts have wondered if the emerging peace structure can be centrally coordinated by the UN or some other body. Increasingly, the answer is that alliance, not central coordination, is the most likely organizing principle. We are realizing that groups will cooperate by consensus, under agreed principles, but without one all-powerful chief. Agreeable as this notion is to many of us, it also requires us to be more ready than ever to participate responsibly in more diverse groupings.

In our work of relating to the UN we are often called to listen to and act in concert with governmental officials, military experts, NGO specialists, activists, and many others. At our best we recognize that new circumstances are drawing together new allies and that we can play an important part by offering contributions that flow directly from our deepest spiritual roots and traditional concerns. It is a real challenge to work closely with those with whom we share some but not all values and where we no longer have the comfort of being righteously in opposition.

Lesson 4: What we do and how is most important

Perhaps this lesson is easier to see at the UN, where we are inundated daily by waves of paper, oceans of opinion, charges, statements, and reports. The world is not lacking in words, and it should be no surprise that merely sharing our opinions, however well stated or illustrated, seems to have little effect on national or international peacemaking.

Too often we become dispirited because the world doesn't seem to be listening. It is my experience that there is nothing more powerful than new information. Our goal should be to bring new perspectives to real problems. In fact, many professional peacemakers are hungry for such input. The more we can share of our practical experiences and our distinctive way of acting, the more likely it is that we will be heard.

Moving Ahead

If asked to put some of these lessons into operation, I would suggest the following priorities for church peace programs. First, we have to do a better job of describing the outlines of the new, comprehensive peacemaking system. We must emphasize the many interrelated parts and our involvement in them. Some of our activity is not directly linked to peacemaking, but all of our efforts, from development projects to relief work to solidarity and fellowship programs, have important roles to play in peacemaking. It is important that we make this clear as we talk about church programs.

Second, we should take a critical look at the peace programs we are currently operating or supporting. How do these relate to other groups now working in the field? Do we have areas of special competence? Are we supporting these adequately and making them known to others? At the same time, are we encumbered with projects that duplicate the work of others? If there is reason to continue these, could they be better linked to, or coordinated with, those of other groups?

Third, the effort by church programs to enable host communities to recognize their own value and take care of themselves is an important direction to maintain. Too often the one-way, top-down, quick-fix solutions that peace emergencies seem to call for can leave the recipient communities helpless when the interveners leave. The basic principle of any conflict resolution process is that the people involved are the experts and are responsible for their own settlement. This is equally valid for relief or development work conducted in a conflict setting. Official, governmental, "track one" peacemakers can lose sight of this in the rush to get quick results. It is often left to unofficial, church or nongovernmental "track two" groups to hold out for approaches that empower host communities to participate in building peace.

The emerging peace system definitely has a place for religious organizations. It is likely an even larger role than we realize. I was reminded of this in my first year of work at the Quaker United Nations Office in New York. Our office invited a number of diplomats, including military officers, to a discussion on UN peacekeeping. The presenter, a Quaker overseas worker, presented her arguments effectively, and the participants left the meeting amid animated conversation. At the door I overheard one officer telling another, "You know, maybe we should let the Quakers run the world for a while!" Let's hope all our organizations can work in a way that continues to inspire such confidence in us.

Exploring
Civilian Peace Teams

Lisa Schirch

The cry "Something must be done!" is heard around the world in reference to any number of violent conflicts. The call for intervention is complex: interventions may take many shapes. The United Nations, regional organizations, or powerful countries such as the United States are usually charged with the responsibility to "do something" in destructive conflicts. Civilian interventions model an alternative to these increasingly unpopular military peacekeeping interventions.

Four ongoing nongovernmental organizations are involved in civilian intervention projects. Peace Brigades International (PBI) has responded to invitations to intervene from grassroots groups in Guatemala, El Salvador, Sri Lanka, Colombia, Chiapas, the Balkans, and among Native Americans in the United States. Witness for Peace (WFP) is an ecumenical organization formed in the early 1980s to challenge U.S. policy and provide a nonviolent presence in Nicaragua and later Guatemala, the Middle East, South Africa, and Haiti. Christian Peacemaker Teams (CPT), a religious organization sponsored by the historic peace churches, has intervened in Haiti, Israel/Palestine, and urban areas in the U.S. The newly formed Balkan Peace Team (BPT) documents human rights violations, accompanies peace and human rights activists, and is a protective presence in the former Yugoslavia. A variety of short-term coalitions and ad hoc groups have also intervened in conflicts.[1]

Johan Galtung distinguishes between two types of interventions:

dissociative efforts to separate the parties and *associative* efforts to bring parties together to address issues.[2] In crisis situations, peacekeeping interventions are increasingly popular. Peacekeeping is a dissociative approach to peace: it keeps the parties to conflict apart from each other to prevent, reduce, or stop violence, and may provide space for both parties to cool off and negotiate. Most civilian groups are involved primarily in dissociative peacekeeping activities but may also engage in a number of other associative or activist projects.

Peacekeeping

There are a number of types of peacekeeping. Two do not involve peacekeepers. Buffer Zones separate the parties with unoccupied demilitarized areas. Peace Zones are civilian-occupied spaces where no fighting takes place. Nurtured in such zones are dialogue and negotiations over the rules of war and peace as well as development projects.

Traditional peacekeeping is based on the idea of peacekeepers who place themselves between parties. Such *interpositioning* is commonly thought to deter violence since a party who harms a peacekeeper may suffer political and economic punishment from the world community. Civilian peacekeepers have interposed themselves in conflicts in Nicaragua and the Philippines as well as during the Gulf War.

When the parties in conflict are not easily separated or the violence is primarily one-way, interpositioning may be inappropriate or impossible. Intercessionary peacekeepers then hope to deter violence by interceding on behalf of particular communities or principles, such as human rights. *Accompaniment* is a type of intercessionary peacekeeping which aims to deter violence by having interveners live with particular individuals or groups such as activists, refugees, and communities threatened with violence because of their involvement in certain types of work or activities. It helps create and protect space for the parties to work for nonviolent social change.

With its formation in 1982, Peace Brigades International popularized the idea of accompaniment in Guatemala and later in El Salvador, Sri Lanka, and other conflicts. Balkan Peace Team members began to accompany and escort threatened individuals or groups in the former Yugoslavia in 1994. During the Gulf War, the Gulf Peace Team accompanied convoys of relief supplies into Iraq.

Other civilian groups provide a *presence* with groups or communities. Presence is focused on reducing the risk of violence to a community. In Nicaragua, Witness for Peace pioneered this new form of intercessionary peacekeeping by being a protective presence in Nicaraguan towns beginning in 1983. To deter "contra" attacks, WFP volunteers lived with Nicaraguan families in areas where contra forces were active. Since the early 1990s, Christian Peacemaker Teams has conducted presence projects in the Palestinian West Bank city of Hebron and in Haiti. The Cry For Justice coalition also provided a continuous nonviolent presence in Haiti during the fall of 1993, when Haiti's ousted President Aristide was expected to return to power.

In addition to these primary dissociative methods of separating the parties, peacekeepers may undertake other activities. Peacekeepers may observe, investigate, supervise, and document many types of conflict-related activities. These may include military actions, infringement on agreements or ceasefire lines, elections, refugee camps, or attacks on civilians. Reports from these observations are sometimes funneled through emergency response networks, which are composed of thousands of people ready to send faxes, telexes, and letters or to make phone calls, protest human rights violations, and press for change.

Civilian peacekeepers are often explicit and intentional about their desire for media attention to educate others about the conflict. Witness for Peace volunteers have conducted hundreds of popular education seminars when they return to their home countries. Such efforts, for example, helped educate and inform both U.S. citizens and government officials about the role of the U.S. military in Nicaragua.

Above all, many civilian peacekeeping groups intervene to show solidarity with the people in conflict. During the war in Nicaragua, some Witness for Peace volunteers saw their presence as more than an effort to deter violence. It was an opportunity for Americans to share in the pain of the war their government was waging, to stand with the grieving, attend funerals, harvest coffee and beans, and engage in other acts of solidarity with the victims of violence. Many long-term volunteers in peace teams, as well as short-term symbolic civilian interventions in the former Yugoslavia, the Middle East, and Cambodia, name solidarity as one of their primary objectives.

Peacemaking

Peacemaking, in contrast to peacekeeping, takes an associative road to peace. Bringing the parties together in a conflict resolution process, such as mediation or facilitation, enables them to settle, manage, transform, or resolve their conflict. A number of civilian groups have combined peacekeeping activities with peacemaking activities. The Balkan Peace Team brings parties together for dialogue. Christian Peacemaker Teams has also tried to combine mediation and reconciliation efforts with its intercessionary peacekeeping work in Washington, D.C., Los Angeles, and Haiti.

Peacebuilding

Peacebuilding activities include social, political, and economic development projects that bring the groups together to prevent destructive conflicts from occurring or recurring. These are often associated with a stage of conflict in which there is no direct violence. In the former Yugoslavia, the Italian-French coalition Mir Sada/We Share One Peace and the U.S.-based Sjema Mira, both civilian interventions, brought relief supplies as part of their hope to provide an overall peacebuilding presence.

Activism

If the parties to a conflict have radically different levels of power, awareness of the conflict is low, or use of violence is one-sided, some civilian interveners use activism or nonviolent direct action to raise awareness of the conflict and increase the negotiating power of one or more of the parties. Christian Peacemaker Teams has held demonstrations in front of the U.S. embassy in Haiti and engaged in nonviolent sit-ins in Israel/Palestine to raise awareness and resist military presence.

Combining dissociative, associative, and activist activities in one civilian intervention project is controversial. Whereas some point to the need to address all these areas in order for an intervention to succeed, others maintain that success requires more limited, realistic goals and activities, given limited human and material resources of most civilian interveners.

Combining peacebuilding and activism is particularly controversial. Some civilian peacekeeping groups avoid undertaking development projects. They are concerned that development aid to one side may be seen as solidarity work, damaging their impartiality; that it may provoke material expectations that conflict with their primary mandate; that it may overlap with work being done by many development organizations; or that it may be interpreted as neocolonialism. Other civilian interveners feel peacebuilding activities provide entry into a conflict and may increase the credibility of the interveners if done in culturally sensitive and appropriate ways.

Some also see activism as inappropriate because it sides with one of the parties and decreases the impartiality of the intervention. Others point to the need both to confront the power structures which perpetuate the violence and protect those victimized by the violence.

The Future of Civilian Peace Team Interventions

Ongoing violence in Rwanda, Sudan, East Timor, Colombia, and dozens of other violent conflicts raging around the world call for a response. Delicate political situations in South Africa, Congo, and Bosnia also deserve attention. Civilian peace teams have a successful history of preventing or reducing violence, providing space for and contributing to peacemaking and peacebuilding activities, documenting conflict-related activities, and educating others about the conflict. Due to the failure of many official, military-based interventions, and the compelling promise held forth by civilian interventions, the possibility of expanded use of civilian peace teams is receiving increasing attention. However, difficulties and complexities will need to be addressed if this young but growing peace activity is to produce the fruit it promises.

Civilian interveners usually intervene because they are invited, extensive human rights violations are apparent, or a nonviolent mandate compels them to do something to stop the violence. Yet without clear criteria for responding to conflicts, and given a history of ad hoc intervention choices, we are left with questions about why some conflicts are chosen and others not. Is intervention appropriate where there is no direct violence, where the violence is "structural," causing poverty? The existence of urban crime and violence in many of the home countries where peace teams are based also suggests the need for further analysis of the motives and choices peace teams use to determine where they intervene.

The role of "outsiders" in a conflict also raises difficult questions. Many civilian conflict interveners are from Western countries and assume their international presence deters violence. This may be so, but their effectiveness is lessened if aggressors do not fear international condemnation. In Haiti, for example, UN observers were routinely treated with disrespect by a military that did not respond to international political or economic pressure. On the other hand, a Filipino civilian intervener in Haiti noted that he could relate to the Haitians better than his American counterparts because he had personally struggled against military repression in his country.

While Westerners are often skeptical of the credibility of insider or partisan third party interventions, local groups of elders, women's groups, and religious organizations have proven to be effective interveners in some conflicts. Some of the earliest civilian interventions were conducted in India by Gandhi's followers, the Shanti Sena. Long-term commitment, clear moral principles, experience, and wisdom brought the Shanti Sena credibility to interpose themselves in conflict situations. Interveners from inside the conflict have been incorporated into the work of PBI and other foreign-based civilian interventions as well. Who the most effective interveners are in different contexts remains a question needing more thought.

Most of the civilian peace team interventions have been composed of less than a dozen individuals. Some propose forming larger teams which may interposition more effectively between warring parties or conduct other peacekeeping intervention activities on a much larger basis.

What changes would increasing the size and scope of peace teams bring? Official interventions are often criticized for self-interested motives and violations of state sovereignty. While unarmed civilian interventions may pose less of a threat to governments than their official counterparts, larger or more active civilian peacekeeping teams will likely draw critical attention. More carefully soliciting governmental and military responses to civilian peace teams may give civilian interveners a better sense of their effectiveness in deterring or stopping violence and may also increase officials' understanding of the purpose and activities of civilian peacekeepers.

An increasing number of UN staff and government officials are interested in the idea of employing civilian peacekeepers. However, is it helpful to have both armed and unarmed peacekeepers involved in the same project? As some veteran peace team volunteers point out, the nonviolent principles which guide their work, such as being willing to confront violence of any type, may be sacrificed if they are included in structures that include a military component. How these two may cooperate is not immediately apparent, but research focusing on how civilian peacekeeping may fit into official UN structures, or how UN forces may be able to learn from and use the theory and practice developed by civilian conflict interveners, may inspire more creative collaboration.

Finally, too often a Western mold of intervention is fitted over a new cultural context with little regard for the indigenous resources which may help transform the conflict. Civilian peace teams will need to focus more on the perspectives of the people in the conflict who interact with or observe civilian interveners. This may shed light on the assumptions civilian interveners bring to the conflict and help refine methods of engaging and drawing on local cultural resources for conflict resolution.

Most interventions take place under crisis conditions that prohibit reflective analysis. While quick-fix solutions are attempted, the roots of the conflict and the aftermath of war require long-term, coordinated, culturally tuned interventions. While lessons learned by peace teams in one conflict may not transfer directly to other contexts, we can learn from past experiences and shape future civilian interventions in an on-going effort to reflect on and improve the practice of promoting peace. The energy and resources for looking carefully at civilian interventions are gaining momentum. Time and effort spent examining and developing solid theories and practices regarding interventions are well worth the effort, so that when crises arise, we can say more than "Something must be done!"

13

Applying
Civilian Peace Teams

Kathleen Kern

In 1986 a group of Mennonite church leaders from the United States and Canada founded Christian Peacemaker Teams (CPT) to support nonviolent forms of struggle, activism, and public witness. Shortly after this founding, the Church of the Brethren and Friends Meetings (Quakers) joined in support of CPT. In 1990 CPT sent its first delegations to Iraq in response to the growing threat of war and to the Oka Indian reservation in Quebec to intervene in the standoff between the Mohawks and Quebec provincial police.

In April 1992, as the sentencing for the Rodney King trial approached, Mennonite churches in the Los Angeles area called CPT and requested that it send a delegation to south Los Angeles because the situation there was about to "explode." Gene Stoltzfus, director of CPT, explained that it took nearly two months to put a delegation together. After the Los Angeles riots, members of the CPT Steering Committee decided CPT needed to have a full-time Christian Peacemaker Corps ready to move immediately into conflict situations.

Since its founding in October 1993, the Christian Peacemaker Corps has responded to invitations in Haiti, the West Bank city of Hebron, the Columbia Heights neighborhood of Washington, D.C., Bosnia, Chechnya, and Chiapas. The CPT steering committee considers the following questions when individuals or organizations from situations of conflict extend invitations:

(1) Is the proposed action one our constituency can support? Is there a critical mass of supporters?

(2) Is there a trusted welcoming body in the crisis setting with whom we connect? Is the area one in which CPT or its supporting denominations have experience and relationships of trust?

(3) Is the action explainable as Christian witness?

(4) Can we talk freely and with integrity in our constituency about what we do?

(5) Is there enough stability in the area that sending people is not negligent? Is it a situation in which there is time for love and nonviolent engagement to work?

(6) Do our governments contribute to the problems in the given location?

(7) Is the mission one for which we have people available who can imagine new ways of living nonviolently and develop actions that bring hope to situations of stalemate and hopelessness?

(8) Can provision be made for coping with language barriers?

(9) Is the time frame of the mission clear for the benefit of staff, volunteers, and the hosting body?[1]

CPT's longest-term involvements have been in Haiti, Hebron, and Washington, D.C. Accounts of these experiences help to illustrate the kind of work such peace teams engage in.

Haiti

In 1990, in closely monitored elections, an overwhelming majority of the Haitian people chose Jean Bertrand Aristide to be their president. After serving in office for seven months, he was overthrown in a coup d'etat led by the man he appointed to head the Haitian military, Raoul Cedras. In July 1993, the U.S.-brokered Governors Island accords signed by both Aristide and Cedras specified that Cedras would step down at the end of October 1993. In return, Aristide agreed to refrain from criticizing U.S. policy and to encourage Haitians not to flee the country.

In the period between July and October, CPT had joined with a coalition of organizations that operated under the name Cry for Justice.[2] The coalition's purpose was sending teams to different areas in Haiti to provide a violence-deterring and human rights-monitoring presence. In September 1993, when the Organization of American States (OAS) human rights monitors left Haiti because the situation was too dangerous for them, the need for international teams became even more desperate. At the invitation of Father Samedi and the parish of St. Helene in the western seaport town of Jeremie, CPT stayed on.

On October 25, U.S. President Clinton ordered the warship Harlan County with hundreds of military and technical advisers on board to enter Port au Prince harbor and set the stage for Aristide to return. Hundreds of armed paramilitary opposed the Harlan County when it attempted to dock, and Clinton ordered the ship to pull away—to the astonishment of almost everyone. For nearly a year, while the embargo tightened and Aristide remained in exile, the CPT team maintained a presence in Jeremie.

Serving as a presence included a variety of activities. Following daily worship, the team visited people throughout the community of St. Helene and in this way accumulated a great deal of information about military and paramilitary activity. When the team heard reports of human rights abuses, they reported them to contacts in Port au Prince, who in turn disseminated them to various human rights agencies. Eventually people began coming to the team with stories of human rights abuses they wanted documented.

Jeremie was not a place where dramatic things happened, but as the United States tightened the embargo on Haiti, CPT members saw the slow starvation of the people they worked among. Two highlights of the CPT experience in Jeremie were the Bat Teneb and a community demonstration after the United States military arrived in Haiti in September 1994.

At noon on February 7, 1994, the bells of the downtown cathedral in Jeremie began to chime as usual, but they were soon drowned out by the noise of dozens of people banging on pots, pans, and the tin roofs of their houses. That morning, CPT's interpreter told the team that people would be participating in a Bat Teneb ("beating away the shadows") all across Haiti that day. Bat Teneb has a long tradition in Haiti as a sign of social protest; this February 7 marked the third anniversary of Aristide's inauguration. Because of the coup d'etat, he had spent the previous two Februaries in exile.

The team walked through the neighborhood at noon to see how many people would pick up their pots. The entire action lasted a minute or less, and members of the team assumed it would not make much impression. But two hours later, ten heavily armed Haitian soldiers gathered outside the rectory compound. Haitians living in the rectory encouraged the four team members to go down to the heavy metal gate and talk to the soldiers. The soldier in charge said that someone had reported several Haitians standing on the roof of the rectory, banging drums, and generally disturbing the peace. He asked about the purpose of the people making that noise. A team member said no one in the neighborhood seemed disturbed by the noise. After further dialogue, the soldier said, "Give a message to the people who made this noise. If they do this again, they will be arrested, and you will be arrested too."

United States forces arrived in mid-September 1994 to return President Aristide and supervise a peaceful handover of power. On September 30, Haitians organized nationwide demonstrations to commemorate the 5,000 people killed for political reasons since the 1991 coup. Several days before September 30, patrols of soldiers from the U.S. Special Forces began to come up to the rectory several times a day, asking for Father Samedi, the parish priest. When the team finally learned that they wanted to talk to Father Samedi about the demonstration, they told the soldiers he was not in charge of organizing it, but they could introduce them to the people who were.

The team helped set up the meeting between the demonstration's organizers and the American Special Forces officers. The American officers reported that the Haitian military personnel had told them that the people of St. Helene were planning to engage in indiscriminate killing and looting during the demonstration. One organizer said, "Well, we want to dump the cement slab [on which the army and paramilitary units had performed ritual sacrifices to prevent Aristide's return] into the ocean. Is that looting? And we want to do the same to the one in the FRAPH compound."[3]

Finally the organizers from St. Helene and the officers agreed that they could throw the wharf slab into the ocean but not the one in the FRAPH compound. Largely because of this open communication, of all the major population centers in Haiti, Jeremie alone had a demonstration in which no one got hurt.

The project in Jeremie did not represent the totality of CPT's Haitian experience. Contacts in Port au Prince forwarded CPT reports to the press and connected these reports to the larger picture of what was happening in Haiti. CPT also sent short-term delegations of North Americans to Haiti to learn about the situation, engage in public witness, and report to their home congregations. When the Jeremie project closed in the winter of 1995, CPT kept a three-person team in Haiti to monitor election campaigns and investigate paramilitary violence. Members of the team served as election monitors in the December 1995 elections. During 1996 the work included training people in dispute resolution, reporting on disarmament procedures, working for judicial change, providing a presence for communities in central Haiti during periods of civilian police absence, and working with Haitian legislators on human rights and security.

Hebron

Hebron is a city of 120,000 Palestinians and 450 Israelis. It is also home to the Il-Ibrahimi mosque, where legend has it that Abraham, Sarah, Rebekah, Isaac, Jacob, and Leah are buried. The site is called the Cave of Machpelah by the Israelis (see Gen. 23) and is a holy site for Muslims, Christians, and Jews.

In 1929 an Arab mob attacked the Jewish Quarter established in the sixteenth century by Jews fleeing the inquisition in Spain. At least sixty-seven men, women, and children were hacked to death and many more wounded. Over 400 were saved by their Muslim neighbors, but the massacre still looms large in the collective memories of both Jews and Muslims in Hebron. Because the biblical patriarchs and matriarchs are purportedly buried in Hebron and because there had once been a thriving Jewish Quarter there, the Hebron area became a special target for the right-wing religious adherents of Gush Emunim ("Bloc of the Faithful") when Israel's settlement policy began to take root in the 1970s.

Kiryat Arba, the oldest settlement in the West Bank, was founded in 1970 by Rabbi Moshe Levinger. He and a group of supporters took over the only hotel in Hebron. To get them to move out, the army gave them an old soldiers' camp on the outskirts of Hebron. Gradually, however, they moved inside the city center under protection of the Israeli military despite protests from local Palestinian inhabitants. In 1980 six yeshiva students in Hebron were killed by a militant offshoot of the Palestinian Liberation Organization (PLO). The Israeli military response was swift. Two more settlements appeared in the center city.

Relations between the settlers and Palestinians continued to deteriorate throughout the period of the *intifada*, the popular Palestinian uprising of the late 1980s and early 1990s. The tensions culminated in the February 1994 massacre in the Il-Ibrahimi mosque. Official reports of the massacre stated that settler Baruch Goldstein, a medical doctor from Brooklyn, New York, began spraying Muslim men and boys with bullets at 5:30 a.m. According to the Israeli government, twenty-nine worshipers died in the mosque. Palestinian sources put the figure higher. A curfew imposed on Palestinian Hebronites lasted for two months, but the settlers were excluded and allowed to roam the streets freely. By the time a CPT delegation arrived in Hebron a year later as part of a fact-finding tour, people expressed as much bitterness about the collective punishment imposed on them as they did about the massacre.

CPT was initially invited to the West Bank to help document settlement expansion. When CPT members explained to personnel in the mayor's office what they had done in Haiti, they invited CPT to maintain a presence in Hebron. A four-person team was sent to Hebron in June 1995.

Team members began every morning with worship in the park in front of the mosque. Following this members would pick up trash, fix broken benches in the park, play with local children, or visit journalist friends to pick up news. Twice a week, two members of the team taught English classes to Palestinian high school students. These classes often turned into discussions on nonviolence. Every Saturday the team spent the afternoon and early evening hours on Dubboya Street to serve as a violence-deterring presence when hundreds of Israelis from settlements throughout the West Bank and Israel converged on Hebron to demonstrate support for the settlers. Dubboya Street connects the Jewish settlements of Tel Rumeida and Beit Hadassah. There is a history of violent encounters on this street between settlers and the street's Palestinian residents and shopkeepers.

Visiting families who lived near settlements was another important aspect of the team's work. One day the team stopped to visit a family who lived between the settlement of Tel Rumeida and an Israeli soldier camp. They were told the family's cistern had run dry. In the summer, the Israeli settlements between Bethlehem and Hebron consume most of the water. Consequently, people in Hebron who live on the high ground, as this family does, do not get running water due to low pressure in the pipes. They must buy their water from the municipality of Hebron or from private sources.

However, the municipality had decided to stop delivering water to people who lived near settlements because of settlers' rock throwing. The team contacted the municipality to say they would accompany any water trucks it might send out. A few days later a call came that a water truck was ready to go. Two team members walked with the water truck through the settlement of Tel Rumeida. But though they were told they could accompany the truck, soldiers detained them both.

Despite what seemed at the time a setback, the water truck incident produced three positive outcomes. First, a lawyer for the Society of St. Yves volunteered to represent the two CPT team members. She and her legal staff also eventually provided free legal help to several of the families in Hebron.

Second, a *Washington Post* reporter came to spend a day with the team, which resulted in an article highlighting CPT's experience in Hebron.[4] While talking to a settler in Tel Rumeida, the reporter dispelled some rumors that had been circulating about one CPT-er being a supporter of the more militant Palestinian organization, Hamas. Sporadic death threats that the team had been receiving stopped.

Third, the subsequent publicity drew both Israeli and international attention to the water shortage in Hebron. The Israeli public expressed outrage when they saw footage of the settlements in the West Bank with swimming pools and well-watered lawns, then learned that Palestinians in Hebron did not have enough water for drinking and washing. Prime Minister Rabin sent a fact-finding mission to Hebron to determine the extent of the water shortage—even though the West Bank cities had been complaining for years of water shortages.

On July 22, 1995, CPT and members of the Jerusalem-based Hebron Solidarity Committee (HSC) responded to an invitation to open the gates of Hebron University. The military had kept them closed since the beginning of the intifada, even though the University does not stand near a settlement, checkpoint, or road the military uses. Students either had to climb the front gate or walk nearly ten minutes out of their way to come in through the service entrance.

Using sledgehammers, the CPT team and members of the Hebron Solidarity Committee attempted to open the gates, to the applause of students and faculty. After about an hour, the Israeli military appeared and arrested team members and an HSC member for refusing to leave a closed military zone.

In spring 1996 the focus of the team in Hebron shifted outside the town, where almost sixty houses came under threat of demolition, ostensibly because the Palestinian families there had built homes without a permit. In reality, they were not granted permits to build on their own land because it lay between the settlements of Givat Ha Harsina and Kiryat Arba. CPT began supplying information to the Israeli organization Peace Now and the Meretz party in Israel and helped bring about meetings between members of these groups and the families from the threatened houses.

CPT also became involved around this time with a professor from Hebron University who owned land next to the Susia settlement south of Hebron. The settlers from Susia had tried at various times to take the land away, but the professor had won his case in the Israeli courts. He asked for CPT's assistance when the settlers put a fence around part of his land and planted olive trees in the middle of his wheatfield. The team helped take down the fence on one occasion and harvest the wheat on another. When the team tried to transplant the olive trees from the wheatfield back to settler property, they were arrested.

Several suicide bombings in Jerusalem, Ashkelon, and Tel Aviv occurred in February and March of 1995. After the number 18 bus had been bombed at about the same time and place in Jerusalem on two consecutive Sundays, the team decided to ride the bus on the third Sunday as a public witness against violence. The team sent out releases to all the Arab, Israeli, and international news media in the area, explaining CPT's commitment to confront violence in any form against any group of threatened people.

Washington

Between May and July 1994, three CPT members investigated the possibility of setting up a project in Washington, D.C. CPT's steering committee had expressed a need to address the issue of violence in North America as well as overseas. Since one member lived in Washington, D.C., and since the murder rate in D.C. was at that time the highest in the nation, the capital city seemed an appropriate location. CPT received an invitation from the Sojourners Neighborhood Center to establish a "violence-free zone" embracing a single neighborhood in which all residents were invited to help eliminate violence.

The D.C. project officially began in September 1994. The first team began by instituting a Listening Project in the Columbia Heights neighborhood. Discussions with residents soon identified a local crack house as the locus for much of the violence in the neighborhood. The team's focus became closing down the crack house.

Team members soon discovered that many of the neighbors had attempted to do this before but were unaware of the efforts of their fellow neighbors. CPT invited all the residents of the area to the Sojourners Neighborhood Center to begin strategizing. They invited a resident of the crack house to come to one of the neighborhood meetings. She told the neighbors about the substandard living conditions under which she and her fellow residents had to live, including the lack of heat and hot water. The Columbia Heights neighbors subsequently helped the crack house residents by looking for housing for them and storing the belongings of those people who wanted to look for their own housing

On December 7, 1994, the Columbia Heights Community held a candlelight vigil in front of the crack house. Initially planned to call the city's attention to its negligence in allowing the house to remain open, the vigil turned into a celebration. Six days earlier, the city government had sent two people to close down the house and brick it up.

In October 1994, CPT helped provide a safe Halloween for Columbia Heights children after listening to neighbors lament that their children had not been able to participate in trick-or-treating for the past ten years. They handed out fluorescent green signs for neighbors to put in windows to indicate that their houses were safe places for children to come and ask for treats. The October 1994 Halloween was such a success that the area for the October 1995 Halloween was doubled. Over twenty-five Orange Hat citizen patrollers in four squads kept watch on every block and helped trick-or-treaters cross dangerous intersections.

On Halloween night 1995, over 350 children enjoyed safe trick-or-treating throughout the South Columbia Heights neighborhood thanks to the combined efforts of area residents and Christian Peacemaker Teams. While some residents patrolled the streets with flashlights and whistles to ensure a violence-free environment, families sat on their porches to greet the excited children dressed in colorful costumes.

The event also spread to other communities. A member of Sojourners Neighborhood Center got her own community in Northeast Columbia Heights to put out flyers as well. By encouraging people to come out for Halloween, her neighbors enjoyed the largest trick-or-treating in years. "We stole your idea," she said, "and we are glad we did!"

Although CPT borrows from decades of Mennonite, Brethren, and Quaker volunteer experiences around the world and from the experiences of activists of many religious backgrounds, it is still a relatively new phenomenon. Traditionally, people from Anabaptist backgrounds have been "the quiet in the land," and committing civil disobedience— even to the point of getting arrested—is a concept with which many members of Mennonite and Church of the Brethren congregations are not comfortable.

Because of its newness, there are many dilemmas Christian Peacemaker Teams has not fully sorted out. Like Peace Brigades International, CPT has a policy against giving monetary or material aid. This places teams in difficult situations when their hosts live in extreme poverty. CPT is still working to develop appropriate relationships with the military and paramilitary people that teams encounter in the course of their work. Most of the people who have invited CPT to serve as a violence-deterring presence are not pacifists, and CPT will continue to struggle with the issue of what it means to stand in solidarity with people and still remain true to its own pacifist convictions.

Despite these struggles, CPT is establishing a unique niche in peacemaking. Because it is rooted in the congregations of the Mennonite and Brethren churches and Friends Meetings, it offers a venue for these Christians to participate in peace teams. CPT's religious base has also helped it communicate more effectively with the Catholics of St. Helene and the Muslims and Jews of Hebron. Members of CPT understand what it means to act out of religious conviction, which provides an opening to dialogue with religious peoples involved in conflict.

14

Remember and Change

John Paul Lederach

I carry with me the words I once read on a wall of West Belfast, "While Ireland holds these graves, Ireland unfree shall never be at peace." Of interest here is not so much the partisan view the phrase expresses as the metaphor it weaves about conflict. Across the forty-five or so armed conflicts in our world, the graves are held present in peoples' minds because they represent the sacrifice, the loss, the trauma, the deep pain of years and generations of conflict. More often than not the pain is submerged from years of needing to survive without thinking about it.

Ironically peace opens a space where we think about it. And it places before us a "remembrance" dilemma. As the possibilities for peace emerge, the graves and great-grandchildren meet. How can we change for the good of our children yet not forget the sacrifices of our parents? How can we remember and honor, with all the pain that may represent, yet at the same time live in relationship with those we feel helped create the pain?

As is the case with most dilemmas, we must not permit ourselves the luxury of choosing one over the other. We cannot afford to pursue a simplistic "forgive and forget" approach nor to stagnate in a "remember and refuse to change" cycle. The challenge of postconflict peacebuilding lies in creating the individual and collective mechanisms that provide us the space to remember and step toward change.

Recently I conducted training workshops or helped with team meetings for peacebuilding initiatives with colleagues from Northern Ireland, Somalia, Sudan, Colombia, and Guatemala. Most of these events and meetings represent another step in a longer journey we have traveled over the years. Each takes place in a context of long-standing violent conflict and a deeply divided society. Sudan and Colombia suffer the distinction of being the locations of the longest standing wars on their respective continents. In both cases the wars have gone on for more than forty years.

At least two generations of children have grown up in these realities. When we seek ways to take up and sustain the journey toward reconciliation in these societies we must face the challenges and dilemmas they pose. There are no quick fixes or magic wands we can wave that will make everything better. There is no Holy Grail of conflict resolution. Reconciliation is hard, tedious, slow work. And, solutions cannot be imported from outside. They have to emerge from the soil where the conflict is rooted.

In working with deep-seated and violent conflict it is important to start by sensing the bigger and longer-term picture. We need a way to think about the context, history, people, and process of peacebuilding. First, we need a set of lenses to look at the peacebuilding process that can help us identify the problems and dilemmas posed by any particular moment in the process. Second, we must approach peacebuilding like a system, a system with a design and architecture.

We use the lenses, then, to look at this system. To draw a metaphor, we can approach peacebuilding somewhat like a building inspector might approach a house. An inspector whose job it is to discover the heating patterns in the building wants to know where the heat is going, whether it is sufficient, and whether the system is efficient. In our case, the lenses are focused on where energy in the peacebuilding system is being used up. Is it spread evenly? Is it "overheating" some places and "underheating" others?

With these energy-seeking lenses on, we can make three initial observations about peacebuilding. First, we tend to focus enormous energy on *immediate tasks*, too often decoupled from *longer-range design* of social change necessary for creating and sustaining a comprehensive approach. Here we must talk further about peacebuilding and time.

Second, we are driven too often by a *hierarchical* instead of an *organic* focus on political process. Here we must talk about the levels of activity needed to sustain peacebuilding.

Third, we tend to approach conflict and peacebuilding with increasing narrowness, at times almost myopic focus, on the *technical tasks of political transition* over the social, economic, psychological, and spiritual *processes of transformation*. Here we must talk about the nature of change.

Time Frame: Immediate and Long-Range

Peacebuilding is a complex endeavor due to three phenomena: simultaneity of activities, gravity of issues, and pressure for rapid response. Everything is happening at once. Everything is of critical importance. And everything is urgent. This is further exacerbated by the "CNN effect." As described by Ernie Regehr, "problems not in the headlines should be ignored, but once they have the attention of CNN they should have been addressed yesterday."[1] These characteristics point us toward the question of time and more specifically how we think about time and our actions.

It is useful to have a conceptual framework for thinking about time and action, to develop a mechanism that permits us to look at immediate needs as embedded in a longer-ranging design. I propose a nested paradigm as illustrated in Figure 1.

The immediate, often crisis-driven component, is represented here by the word "action." It refers to the need we feel to respond to evolving events. In the international NGO community, recent crises like those of Bosnia, Somalia, or Rwanda have made popular the term *disaster management*. In peacebuilding we are often driven by the emerging crises that put the peace process in jeopardy and call for crisis negotiation or mediation. The time frame of the "action" component is short-term, a matter of months. The question that seems to preoccupy our minds is this: How do we respond to these immediate needs to keep the process alive? The dilemma, however, is that we never leave the crisis. In most of these situations we live in what we could define as a permanently emerging crisis.

We need a way to see beyond the crisis. This leads logically to the notion of *preparation*, of equipping people to undertake better action. In peacebuilding endeavors this includes training and preparing the way. Preparation evolves in a more extended unit of time than action, often conceived in terms of projects that lay out plans for one to three years. However, preparation often relates back to responding more effectively to the crisis. We need something much more extended.

At the far end of the paradigm is *outcome*. Outcome is a way of talking about vision and wanted change. This refers both to structural and to social change. What visions do people have for a given setting? For example, in a peaceful situation how are political, economic, and social systems constructed? How do people relate? What characterizes their relationships? As the African American poet Langston Hughes once put it, we need "dreamkeepers," people who keep alive a vision of what could be or of what should be. What is particularly challenging about this is that we must be able to think in terms of generational change. This

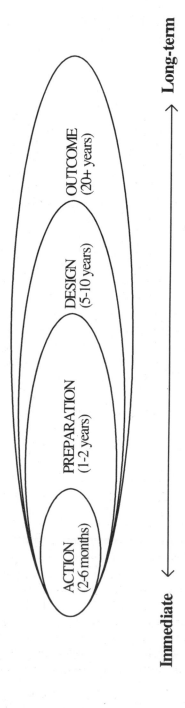

Figure 1. Time Frame for Peacebuilding
Copyright © 1998 by John Paul Lederach

suggests a simple idea: if we do not know where we are going it will be difficult to get there. We must create the space to dream and provide vision.

Between the two extreme ends of crisis and vision we find the idea of *design*. This component of peacebuilding has the operational function of linking immediate action and long-term goals. Its primary task is to develop a conceptual plan, a peacebuilding architectural *design for social change*. It compels us to think in decades. Decade thinking is not easy but is critical for peacebuilding. The design component pushes us to grapple with tough questions. How is our immediate action linked to wanted social change? What are the steps we follow to move from where we are to where we want to be?

This paradigm suggests that different activities related to peacebuilding require distinct units of time in which we reflect and act. The units are related to each other and must be seen as connected rather than isolated. It is vital that we develop the capacity to think operationally in decades and generations to link immediate action and shorter-term preparation with longer-ranging wanted changes.

Taking this a step further, Figure 2 suggests a scheme based on a set of questions I find helpful in thinking about specific pieces of work. The scheme is built as a matrix that cross references time with the outcome of the activity. There are four basic questions. What are we trying to accomplish? What is the nature of our relationship? What is the unit of time in which we can think and plan? How much do we know about the context?

In response to the first question I suggest three categories that form one side of the matrix. *Purpose* refers to the bigger picture of what we are attempting to accomplish in the context or setting. *Goals* relate to narrower aspect of what a particular event is attempting to achieve. *Objectives* refer to the more specific activities in the event. These three categories can be cross-referenced with perspectives emerging from the nature of the relationship and the unit of time in which we plan. An event is a one-time activity which may be conducted for a few hours to a few days. A project refers to a series of events taking place across a year or two. A program connects the projects into a longer-term, decade-length effort.

We can now return to our original point. If we overlay our two schemes we can describe what typically happens in peacebuilding and suggest a possible alternative. Typically the process of peacebuilding is driven by a crisis orientation. This tends to produce response to immediate needs through narrowly defined and short-term objectives. Projects and programs that relate to the longer-term agenda for social change are defined by what is necessary and possible emerging from the crisis.

OUTCOME

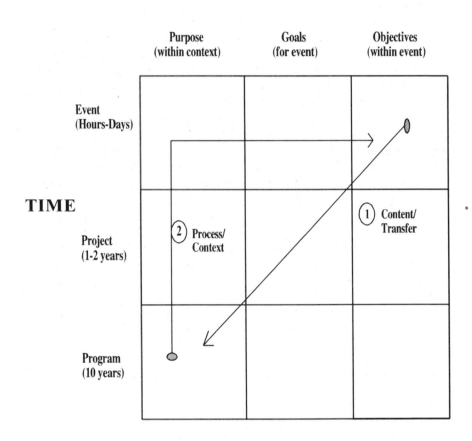

1. Content/transfer relies on delivering a package of preconceived models and skills assumed to be relevant for the context.

2. Process/context initiates with assessment of needs in context and devises specific training activities that respond to those needs.

Figure 2. Approaches to Training

Copyright © 1998 by John Paul Lederach

Peacebuilding needs a social architectural design that thinks in decades and in which specific events and responses are defined by a measured understanding of the context, purpose, and program.

Think of this in relationship to a context of conflict and rapid change. The entire social, political, and economic system is changing. New realities and newly defined shared futures seem almost in reach. Yet the context is that of people emerging from years of stagnated cycles of violence, who by basic human nature may find more security in clinging to what is known and understood than in moving toward the unknown, even if it promises to be qualitatively better. In this context, peacebuilders feel overly responsible to take care of every detail, lest the process fail. While vigilance is necessary, it is far more important to develop the capacity to think about immediate action as embedded in broader context and program developments.

In sum, let me make three points about time frame. First, we must respond to but not be driven by a crisis mentality. Second, we must create the space for long-term vision but not be isolated from practical steps that root the vision in the realities of day-to-day life. Third, we must explicitly think about and develop the capacity of social change design as a discipline and responsibility that links crisis and vision.

Levels: Hierarchical and Organic

Peacebuilding needs to happen on a variety of levels at the same time. Figure 3 presents a conceptual framework that outlines three levels of peacebuilding activity: top, middle, and grassroots.[2] The top level of peacebuilding is official "table talks." During the postconflict phase the peacebuilding system is driven by a hierarchical instead of an organic focus on political process. In other words, the approach to peacebuilding is top-down and energy is centered on top-level leaders and activities. This is taking place at a time and in a context of significant and far-reaching change. But this evolving contextual change poses some dilemmas for those involved.

People experience contradiction in terms of the pace of change. Peace can be experienced as simultaneously moving too slowly and too rapidly: too slowly because expectations have been raised by the possibility of peace; too rapidly because the reformulation of perspectives and concessions offered to create movement can generate a feeling of having given away too much and received too little. We may feel swept along by the rapid pace of events.

Everyone feels an identity dilemma, but it may be especially critical for leaders caught in the public limelight. Those involved struggle with

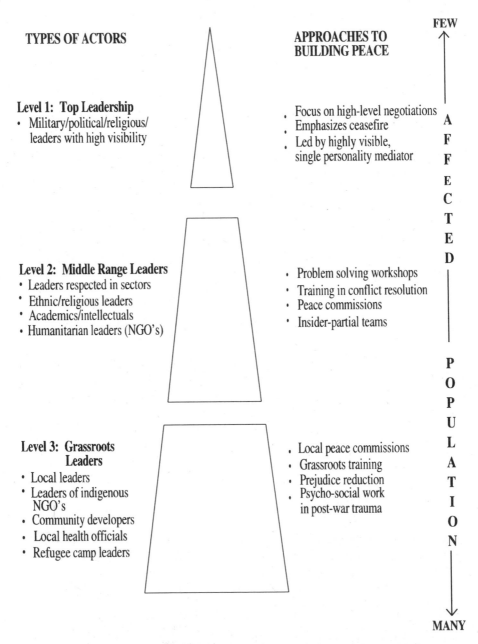

TYPES OF ACTORS

Level 1: Top Leadership
• Military/political/religious/
  leaders with high visibility

Level 2: Middle Range Leaders
• Leaders respected in sectors
• Ethnic/religious leaders
• Academics/intellectuals
• Humanitarian leaders (NGO's)

Level 3: Grassroots
        Leaders
• Local leaders
• Leaders of indigenous
  NGO's
• Community developers
• Local health officials
• Refugee camp leaders

APPROACHES TO BUILDING PEACE

• Focus on high-level negotiations
• Emphasizes ceasefire
• Led by highly visible,
  single personality mediator

• Problem solving workshops
• Training in conflict resolution
• Peace commissions
• Insider-partial teams

• Local peace commissions
• Grassroots training
• Prejudice reduction
• Psycho-social work
  in post-war trauma

FEW

AFFECTED

POPULATION

MANY

Figure 3: Actors and Peacebuilding Foci

Copyright © 1998 by John Paul Lederach

how to change yet hold onto the core of who we are. In settings of deep-rooted conflict, identity is shaped mainly by defining ourselves against the enemy. There is little room for ambiguity or gray areas. Moving from deep and violent conflict toward reconciliation changes this. Old answers no longer explain. We find ourselves caught in a classic struggle: how do we create the space for remolding and shaping our identity so it is not based exclusively on the enemy—yet clearly articulate the core purpose of who we are and are about? What do we hold onto amid such change?

People across the population, particularly at the grassroots level, not only feel an identity dilemma but also are caught in a process paradox. They pay enormous attention to the official negotiating table as the measuring stick of personal and group validation. Their identity, sacrifice, and years of struggle are validated or invalidated by what happens at the "table." But at the same time, they feel marginalized because they do not have direct access to the process.

Enormous pressure is brought to bear on the official, top-level process to bear the fruit it is incapable of delivering on its own. Expectations may be nearly impossible to fulfill. This is the weakness of the hierarchical approach to politics in the postconflict phase. In the worst case postconflict scenario, the leadership is able to manipulate the context for personal gain because there is little or no accountability—in other words, "power corrupts, and absolute power corrupts absolutely." At the same time, the people may feel lack of genuine access, participation, responsibility, and ownership in the process. In this case, on the other side of the coin, powerlessness is the seedbed of violence. Both possibilities are forerunners to the collapse of peace.

We need to conceptualize and develop an organic rather than a hierarchical approach to politics. An organic view of political process, or what Harold Saunders calls "whole body politic,"[3] envisions peacebuilding as a web of interdependent activities and people. The web links and cuts across levels, types of activity, and time. It creates a binding effect, holding people and processes together. It is systemic in orientation, understanding that changes in one component of the system affect the whole system, but no one component controls the process of change in the whole. This calls for building an infrastructure for peace, particularly at the middle and grassroots levels. It is this foundation that will ultimately hold up the house. At the end of the day the roof is sustained by the infrastructure.

The single most important aspect of encouraging an organic perspective of peacebuilding politics is creating a genuine sense of participation, responsibility, and ownership in the process across a broad spectrum of the population. People must move from sitting back and reacting toward a proactive engagement that helps shape and define the process. In other words, a key task is to seek ways to engage and inspire others to a sense of their own responsibility and validation, rather than relying on a process that is too often remote, rife with pitfalls, and incapable of meeting their needs. Peacebuilding and politics in the postconflict phase must be seen as an open, accessible system that rests on a broad base of participation rather than the narrowness of the official talks.

Processes of Transition and Transformation

Finally, in postconflict peacebuilding there is a tendency to focus energy on technical tasks of transition rather than broader processes of transformation. A visualization of a postconflict paradigm can be seen in Figure 4. Again this is best depicted as a web, consisting of a nested paradigm involving four related peacebuilding activities. Consider for a moment each of the four.

At its most immediate level, defining the agenda of peacebuilding involves identifying the various tasks that need to be addressed. These include dealing with people, structures, and processes. Tasks may involve everything from demobilization and disarmament to governance and employment, as they relate to movement from destructive conflict toward redefinition of relationships.

The second circle, transition, suggests that each of the identified agenda tasks will move through a technical, logistical component of implementation. The technical aspect of repatriating refugees, for example, is the transport, location, and aid provided to them as they return to their country of origin. This transition is embedded, however, in the third circle, the transformative processes that go beyond the technical aspect and reach toward the deeper questions. The technical side of disarmament, for example, is to remove the guns. The transformative side raises the question of the role and place of the military in a new context, under a newly formed structure of governance.

Finally, all of this takes place in the broadest circle, the search for relational reconciliation. This is a search because reconciliation represents a dialectic. It is both a place toward which we journey and the journey which, once initiated, opens a social space. In both instances reconciliation is about relationships. Reconciliation is not primarily about ending something, it is about building something.

To this paradigm we can add four distinct and necessary dimensions in postconflict peacebuilding: the sociopolitical, socioeconomic, social-psychological, and spiritual. Many postconflict peacebuilding

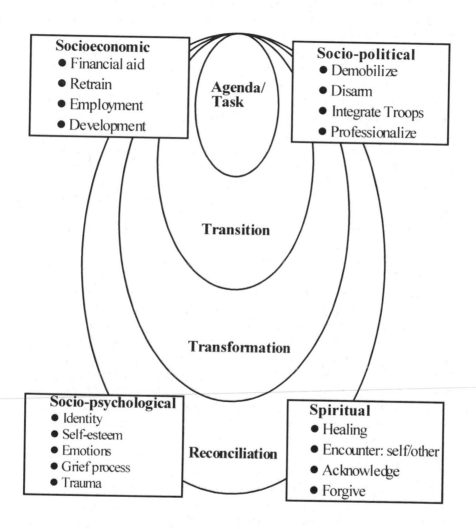

Figure 4. The Web of Reconciliation

Copyright © 1998 by John Paul Lederach

systems focus their energy too narrowly on political transition—or the top part of the paradigm. The focus is reduced to the technical tasks of transition related to sociopolitical concerns, and at times crosses over into socioeconomic issues. As such, the system rarely moves to encompass the transformative and relational concerns or the social-psychological and spiritual dimensions of human experience.

An example comes from work with ex-soldiers and their families in Nicaragua. When the war ended, the peace accords mandated that armies be reduced. From a sociopolitical perspective, this is referred to as the process of demobilization, disarmament, and reintegration. The technical side involved the logistics of keeping troops encamped and separated, and simultaneously disarming them. The socioeconomic aspect of the process involved providing the demobilized soldiers with a fresh start, often in the form of financial aid or training for new vocations. The transformative aspect of the process is how a postconflict economy should be conceived, how to deal with unemployment, and how to pursue development and distribution of resources in ways that support the peacebuilding effort.

The social-psychological dimension was not officially dealt with. These are a different set of concerns, aimed more at transformation and reconciliation. Here the demobilized soldier is seen as a person dealing with accumulated emotions and intense trauma. For this soldier, there are significant personal questions of identity and self-worth. The person may be resented by others for his or her actions and likely carries deep feelings of anger, resentment, and loss attributed to others. There is need to mourn loss of family, friends, youth, and time. In other words, this phase represents more than the transition of social roles. It involves the transformation of persons and the social networks in which they live and move.

This is coupled with the spiritual dimension. *Spiritual* here signifies moving beyond the issues and toward an encounter. Conflict and reconciliation always involve a journey toward an encounter with self and the other. The purpose of the reconciliation journey is healing. Healing is found in constant movement between self and the other, or in many settings, between myself and my former enemy. This involves a willingness to acknowledge the truth and the pain of injustices experienced, and an openness to offer and accept forgiveness, to start a new relationship.

But these encounters pose deep questions. The encounter with self raises the difficult question "What have I done?" The encounter with the enemy raises the equally complicated question "What have they done to me?" Both are necessary questions on the road to healing. In our example, the spiritual dimension suggests that we see the demobilized individual not merely as a soldier to be disarmed or retrained, not as a person with psychological needs, but as a human being on a journey toward restoration and healing within a society seeking the same.

The challenge of reconciliation is how to open the social space that permits and encourages individuals and societies to acknowledge the past, mourn the losses, validate the pain experienced, confess the wrongs, and reach toward the next steps of restoring the broken relationship. This is not forgive and forget. This is not remember, justify, and repeat. True reconciliation is to remember and change. *Spiritual* is the best term to describe this search that goes beyond the political, economic, and psychological. From a personal faith viewpoint, the journey toward reconciliation is necessarily a journey toward self, enemy, and God. We must extend our focus on peacebuilding to include the possibility of such transformation and the restoration of relationship.

Conclusion

As we think about reconciliation in deeply divided societies, we need a sustainable approach to peacebuilding that moves beyond a number of frontiers. We must move beyond a short-term, crisis orientation and toward development of our capacity to think about social change design in terms of decades. We must move beyond a hierarchical focus on politics and toward the construction of an organic, broad-based approach that creates space for genuine responsibility, ownership, and participation in peacebuilding. We must move beyond a narrow view of postconflict peacebuilding as a political transition and toward the formation of a web that envisions a whole body politic, whole persons seeking change in a radically changing environment.

To do this we must face the challenges of fear and hope. We need vision and hope to orient our steps and sustain our action. Yet hope must be linked to the realities of the context and provide us with a way forward. We must recognize the presence of fear all around us—fear of what is to come, fear of the unknown, fear of losing something important to us. Yet we must not succumb to nor be paralyzed by fear. Despite our fear, we act on hope because we believe reconciliation can take place. In this journey of reconciliation we believe it is possible to remember the past and at the same time choose to respond to the present based on a vision of the future.

15

Providing Space for Change in Mozambique

Andrea Bartoli

M ozambique is a peaceful country experiencing amazing recent economic growth. These developments have occurred in the past
three years and are results of a long process which brought peace for the
first time after 400 years of colonization, an independence war, and more
than fifteen years of internal struggle. Although Mozambique is still
considered one of the poorest countries in the world, the last three years
mark an economic and social upswing for a population badly wounded
by long wars. Mozambicans are now enjoying the country's first period
of peace and working together no longer for survival but to assure future generations a higher standard of living.

First credit for this success story must go to the Mozambicans
themselves and their leaders. But the Mozambique peace process contains elements that make it a unique success story. For the first time a
major conflict ended using the good offices of a nongovernmental organization which not only facilitated communication, offering informal
diplomatic services and allowing positions to be clarified, but also participated informally in the track-one diplomatic effort with governments and international organizations.

The Community of St. Egidio, the international Catholic organization which played this role, has since been involved in other conflict
resolution activities. Since 1992, five more agreements have been signed
by factions involved in internationally relevant conflicts in Guatemala,

Algeria, Kosovo, Albania, and Burundi. Not all of these conflicts have been resolved, but in all five cases the communities and their representatives have been able to negotiate partial agreements, creating formalized documents signed by the armed parties involved in the conflict.

How was it possible for an organization that did not have conflict resolution as its mission to perform such an impressive sequence of successful activities? How was it possible in the first place that an NGO like St. Egidio participated first as observer and later as mediator in the Mozambican peace process? And how did religious motivation help support and strengthen this newly developed role?

The History of Mozambique's Conflict

Located in the Southern region of Africa, bordered by Malawi, Zambia, Zimbabwe, and South Africa, flanked to the east by an incredibly beautiful and long Indian Ocean shoreline, Mozambique gained independence from Portugal in 1975. This independence was a sudden development, the result of the change of government in Portugal, which had been a presence in Mozambique since 1498. For centuries, Portuguese settlers and traders concentrated along the coast, trading ivory and gold internally. In the nineteenth century, slaves were the country's main commodity.[1]

Despite similarities to many European colonizations, that of Portugal in Mozambique did not completely disrupt local structure and authority. The interior of Mozambique was never colonized in the totalitarian way that many European settlers in North America and South Africa transformed the entire cultural, economic, political, and social landscapes of their conquered territories. Many ethnic groups have lived for centuries in what we now call Mozambique.

During this century, Portuguese control of Mozambique increased administratively, politically, and militarily. Mozambique remained under colonial control longer than many other countries as Portugal did not participate in the de-colonization process that peaked in the 1960s. On the contrary, Portugal not only denied the legitimacy of Mozambique and its demands for independence but continued to encourage settlement of Europeans on what it continued to deem Portuguese territory. Human rights abuses were widespread, and the Portuguese confrontation with the nationalist forces was militarily aggressive.

In June 1963, three major groups of the nationalist forces of the independence movement formed the *Frente da Libertaçao de Moçambique* (FRELIMO). The President was Eduardo Mondlane, an anthropologist with a Ph.D. from an American university. In 1964 the armed struggle against Portuguese colonial power officially started, but internal tension in FRELIMO's leadership itself marked the first years of the movement. The killing of Mondlane by a parcel bomb brought to power Samora Machel, who favored a radical policy aiming not only to challenge the Portuguese but also to liberate people from traditional authorities. Under Machel's leadership and with the support of China and the Soviet Union, FRELIMO expanded its presence into the north of the country. By 1973, they had reached the central area of the country, and the Portuguese could not confront them effectively, despite their superior military capabilities.

In September 1974, after a brief negotiation following the April coup in Lisbon, Portugal relinquished power to FRELIMO without obtaining assurance of free and fair elections as a prerequisite. FRELIMO was recognized as the "sole legitimate representative of the Mozambique people" and immediately asserted its mission to create a socialist country. The task was immense: to create a new state—a new nation—from an area that had never before had such a unified identity, did not have a strong local administrative structure, and did not share much common cultural history. Adding to the difficulty, the Portuguese left the country completely deprived of a functional infrastructure, taking away most capital and human resources of significance.

The priorities of the new government were in the sectors of education, health, and institution building. To make sure that tribal, regional, racial, or religious identities were not emphasized by Mozambicans, a new nationalist, socialist identity was promoted. The government was particularly harsh toward traditional local authorities in place since colonial times. The government nationalized much of the economy and directly controlled property and many of the country's functions.

Unfortunately, the same government lacked trained and experienced personnel. Although technicians from the Soviet bloc arrived, they were ill-prepared to cope with the impossible task of turning the country around. While the FRELIMO government was able to set the tone for a liberated Mozambique, it was also forced, by lack of resources and ideological rigidity, into an impasse. The assertion of the legitimacy of a new nationalist socialist authority over traditional ones created dissatisfaction and tension among the people. This dissatisfaction was exploited by neighbor Rhodesia and its military intelligence to fuel their opposition to the FRELIMO government.

The nucleus of military resistance to FRELIMO was first called Mozambique Military Resistance (MMR), later changed to Resistencia Nacional Mozambique, or RENAMO. Rhodesia initially supported this opposition to FRELIMO because of Machel's decision to close Beira's rail and road corridors, which cut off Rhodesian access to the sea. At the time, Mozambique was providing support in western Mozambique for the bases of Robert Mugabe's ZANU troops, who were fighting the Rhodesian government.

Mozambique was damaged by this confrontation with Rhodesia. Its involvement in the war on the side of Mugabe's ZANU troops came at a high price. RENAMO started as a small movement supported by Rhodesia and continued as a much stronger military threat to the well-being of the entire country. Supported later by South Africa, RENAMO was able to force the government onto the defensive.[2]

During the 1980s, RENAMO gained a terrible reputation as the "Khmer Rouge" of Africa, a notion formally articulated in Robert Gersony's report to the U.S. State Department in 1988. On that occasion all of RENAMO's violent practices against civilians were so vividly described that it was impossible for the U.S. government to support RENAMO as it had supported UNITA in Angola. Anticommunist rhetoric was not enough to overcome the concern about widespread human rights abuses. RENAMO did not have an articulated ideology or an organizational structure to present goals and a political platform. More a military insurgent movement, RENAMO was unable to envisage much of any political strategy.

The Community of St. Egidio

The Community of St. Egidio is an international Catholic association founded in Rome in 1968 to live the gospel while serving the poor in friendship. Born out of the initiative of an eighteen-year-old Italian youth, the Community did not make conflict resolution part of its original mission. The main purpose of the Community has been to serve the poor through forming small communities of laypeople. The majority of the current 15,000 members of the Community of St. Egidio are women and men with families and working obligations.[3]

The Community gathers regularly for prayer and meetings, always serving the poor in their local area. This service ranges widely and includes teaching children, helping the ill and dying, teaching foreigners, working in soup kitchens, and offering services to the handicapped. Tending to local needs and service to the poor constitute the priorities of the Community and are at the very core of its experience. While the Community does not require any vows of its members, it nevertheless fosters stability. The experience of the Community is strongly relational and assumes that it is crucial in both human and spiritual terms for people to connect to and be supported in their own environment.

The first five years of the Community were characterized by strong creative initiatives toward the establishment of better service to the poor, together with being a fellowship of disciples trying to live the gospel together. It was a time in which the Community did not have a name and was externally perceived as a group of young adults who formed to maintain friendship after they had finished university. In 1973 the Community was given a church in Trastevere, a central quarter of Rome. The church was dedicated to St. Giles (in Italian, *Egidio*). There was no connection between the Community and this Greek nobleman who traveled to Southern France in the seventh century to found a monastery and become famous as a protector of the poor. The name *Community of St. Egidio* was chosen based on the name of the church.

Since then, every evening the Community of St. Egidio holds an open prayer service in that church. This open prayer has been an occasion to welcome people from all over the world with their sorrow, difficulties, and requests. St. Egidio has transformed itself from a small community of young adults in Rome to an international association which follows closely many conflicts around the world.

The Peace Process

The connection of the Community of St. Egidio with Mozambique was from the beginning personal. In the early 1970s a young priest from Beira, Jaime Gonçalves, was studying in Rome and participating in the life of the Community. When in 1974 it was clear that the new Portuguese government wanted to change its colonial policy and allow the independence of Mozambique and Angola, the Holy See decided to change the Bishops in Mozambique from white Portuguese to native African. Father Gonçalves became Bishop of Beira and was sent immediately to his new diocese.

Due to its strong ideological commitments, the FRELIMO government was not eager at that time to establish cooperative links with churches and religious leaders. There were especially strong tensions between FRELIMO and Catholics, who were perceived to be too closely linked to the former colonial power. Religious activities and education were restricted and properties were confiscated. When Bishop Gonçalves came back to Rome and participated in prayer with the Community a few years later, he made everyone aware of the difficulties in his country faced by his people and church.

Gonçalves was certainly no supporter of former colonial power. A fervent nationalist, he wanted to encourage a better relationship between church and state in Mozambique. The Community offered to help, using not its own strength (at that time membership in the Community was around 500 people, almost all under twenty-five) but its Italian connections.

The members of the Community hoped for a positive intervention of the Italian Communist Party with FRELIMO to foster broader religious freedom in Mozambique. The Italian Communists supported Mozambique's freedom movement substantially and established themselves as a crucial point of reference in Europe for the newly independent government. Moreover, companies close to the Italian Communist Party were interested in investing in Mozambique through various forms of economic cooperation. Because the Italian communists were committed to democratic values and procedures, it was possible they would support a more inclusive approach towards religious leaders and people. For these reasons, the Community, previously lacking direct contact with Italian communist leaders, made a telephone call to the office of Enrico Berlinguer, at that time Secretary General of the Italian Communist Party. He agreed to come to St. Egidio to meet Bishop Gonçalves.

The meeting between Gonçalves and Berlinguer was extremely positive and opened the door to further cooperation between Italian Communists, Mozambican Catholics, and the Community of St. Egidio to remove restrictions against the practice of religion in Mozambique. Through these channels, official contact between the Community of St. Egidio and the Mozambican government was established, and strong relationships developed with many members of the government. The relationships were nourished by mutual activity. These included delivery of food and medicine through two solidarity shipments in 1985 and 1988, organizing an exhibition of Mozambique artists in Italy to portray the country as not only a recipient of help from a European country rich in resources and culture but also as a proud contributor to the global community, and fostering a better relationship between Mozambique and the Vatican.

Connections with RENAMO were established by the Community in the late 1980s. In February 1988, through a representative of RENAMO in Germany, the Community requested RENAMO to demonstrate its interest in negotiation by liberating a Portuguese Sister who had been kidnapped by the group. The Sister was released by RENAMO on April 25, 1988, exactly at the time and in the manner requested by the Community. The Community then established direct contacts with RENAMO leaders, who expressed the desire for peace negotiations. With the help of Kenya, RENAMO attempted to organize a meeting between delegations from the two parties, possibly in Kenya itself. Kenya was at that time perceived to be a country willing to relate to RENAMO, providing support via the Moi regime with lodging, transportation, and passports. The new role of Kenya demonstrated the diminishing role of South Africa in relation to RENAMO.

Immediately the problem of future negotiations emerged. On the one hand, RENAMO wanted a formal negotiation in a third country with strong international involvement and explicit recognition of its role. On the other hand, the government was not interested in even recognizing RENAMO and wanted to avoid as much as possible the involvement of international actors. At the same time, the desire for peace and the necessity of pragmatic steps caused President Chissano to encourage the Community of St. Egidio and Bishop Gonçalves to pursue the established contact in such as way as to open the possibility of serious negotiation. The FRELIMO leadership was at this stage vacillating between an inflexible hard-line approach and a more open one of dialogue and negotiation.

In spring and summer 1989, RENAMO and FRELIMO had contacts in Nairobi with the help of Kenya and Zimbabwe. The two sides never met directly but only participated in a dialogue through facilitators, members of the Christian Council of Mozambique. The talks, however, never progressed past the preliminary phase and closed on August 14, 1989, with no resolution. After the failure of another attempt, this time American, to resume talks between the two sides, RENAMO leader Alfonso Dhlakama decided to visit Rome for the first time in February 1990. Well-received by the Italian Foreign Ministry's representative through the services of the Community, Dhlakama reconfirmed RENAMO's interest in dialogue.

A few months later, through the initiative of Aguiar Mazula, a creative Minister of Labor in the FRELIMO government, the possibility of direct, secret talks without precondition between FRELIMO and RENAMO was reaffirmed. During a visit of Minister Mazula to the Vatican, he requested the Holy See to support those talks being held in St. Egidio. The same request was given to the Italian authorities. The FRELIMO government made clear its readiness to send a delegation of officials led by Minister Armando Guebuza, a man high in the ranks of FRELIMO. After the visit of Dhlakama, RENAMO confirmed its preference for Rome as the venue for direct talks and agreed to hold the talks under auspices of the Community of St. Egidio.

The first session of talks took place July 8, 1990, at the Community's headquarters in Rome. The talks were secret and the delegations highly qualified. There were four observers: two representatives of the Community of St. Egidio (Andrea Riccardi and Matteo Zuppi), Bishop

Jaime Gonçalves, and Mario Raffaeli representing the Italian government. A document was signed at the end of the session which read, "The two delegations, acknowledging themselves to be compatriots and members of the great Mozambican family, expressed satisfaction and pleasure at this direct, open and frank meeting, the first to take place between the two parties." This was a remarkable statement for representatives of two sides of a fourteen-year armed conflict that caused thousands of deaths, refugees and displaced people, and extensive infrastructure damage.

In July 1990 the parties agreed simply to "dedicate themselves fully, in a spirit of mutual respect and understanding, to the search for a working basis from economic and social conditions for building a lasting peace and normalizing the life of all Mozambican citizens." The framework was established, and they agreed to meet again in Rome in the presence of the same observers.[4]

The significance of this first joint communiqué can hardly be underestimated. It was clear from the beginning of the talks that there was no interest in dividing the country or in a secession movement; nor was there interest in exploiting ethnic, tribal, and religious differences. On the contrary, the Mozambican identity was perceived by both as the framework for further negotiation. A crucial element was added to the talks by the representatives of the Community, who not only acted as hosts of the talks but also invited the parties to focus on what united them while putting aside what divided them. This approach can be found in the document and is probably the most striking, if brief, example of the spirit of Rome that was conducive to the final agreement signed in Rome on October 4, 1992.

The entire process was based on the assumption that it was up to the parties involved in the armed conflict to stop it. The Community of St. Egidio had never had the force to impose a solution of its own. The only role it could play was to facilitate contacts among the parties themselves while keeping the hope for peace alive in times of difficulty. Certainly most of the credit must be given to the parties themselves and to the Mozambican people, who were able widely and openly to support the transformation of Mozambique into a democratic, pluralist society. Support for the peace process was strong and significant and involved civil society at large and especially the churches.

Religious Community as Mediator

The Community of St. Egidio nurtured contact between the two sides for a long time before being asked to be observer in the mediation process. It was in this period that many elements of its future success were laid down. The Community of St. Egidio was able, before the talks themselves, to establish channels of communication sufficiently strong and reliable to endure the mistrust and the miscommunication that necessarily arose from the process. These channels were generally based on long-lasting personal relationships and relied on a crucial common perception that St. Egidio was interested in the process per se and not driven by special interests or any particular political agenda.

A volunteer organization that strictly requires every member to work to participate in its activities, the Community was putting its scarce resources to the benefit of the process in a clearly disinterested way. The fact that nobody was paid by anyone for this service was probably part of the appeal to both parties, who recognized the value of commitment and personal sacrifice. It was also evident that the commitment of the Community of St. Egidio preceded its involvement as observer in the talks. It was not an ad hoc solution but the result of a long-standing friendship with a country and its representatives.

The impartial commitment of the Community was crucial in attempting to resolve a conflict in which the two sides were completely disconnected, with no ties between the FRELIMO and RENAMO leaders. The two parties did not know each other, came from different regions of the country, belonged to different tribes, and had very different experiences, all of which contributed to great mistrust. It is hard to imagine a more thorny relationship, considering the atrocity of the war and the fact that the two sides were supported by ideological enemies, the Soviet bloc on one side and South Africa on the other.

Significantly, while the fall of the Soviet bloc helped the conflict lose any ideological, anticommunist rhetoric, the change of South Africa made possible an equilibrium that would have been unthinkable in previous years. Nevertheless, the absence of contact between the two parties constituted what was probably the most relevant obstacle to the negotiations themselves. All other attempts to induce direct talks between the parties had failed because of lack of communication and understanding. In so delicate a negotiation, the possibility of relying on trustworthy interlocutors was an essential element in fostering trust between the two sides themselves.

The setting of the first meeting and of all the subsequent negotiations was also an expression of the particular character of St. Egidio. Located in a beautifully restored little convent, the Community offered its assembly room for the talks, and simply and elegantly created an environment that was conducive to exchange. Far from the conflict, not pressured by the everyday sequence of military attacks and dangers, the negotiators in Rome were able creatively to explore new possibilities for solving the problems on the agenda.

All needs of both sides were cared for, from communication to lodging, from transportation to translation systems. A team of volunteers supported the work of the two main litigators from the Community, making sure that the entire experience of the delegation in Rome was pleasant and conducive to dialogue. Before and after formal meetings, members of the community held extensive talks to explore and redefine positions. No meeting was ever allowed to occur formally unless positive conclusions were foreseen.

As we all know, the precondition for successful human communication is a positive psychological space. In a tense situation determined by years of war and political opposition, that space was simply nonexistent, created only as a result of the process itself. The strategy of the Community in that respect was to help all participants in the talks associate their experience with success, thus creating the psychological space previously missing.

The whole Community, while delegating the burden of direct talks to Andrea Riccardi and Matteo Zuppi, participated as much as possible, providing services of all kinds (secretarial help, translation, communication, food, transportation). While lowering the costs that were covered (especially in the beginning) by the Community itself and later by the Italian government, the presence of many members of the Community helped dramatically to set the tone of the whole experience for more than two years. Members of the delegations were welcomed and treated graciously during their presence in Rome, experiencing a level of care highly unusual in the more formal, traditional diplomatic setting. Dental care and special tours and meetings were among the many aspects of an all-encompassing courtesy. This atmosphere was crucial to the creation of the space necessary for dialogue.

The Community members involved in the actual talks did not have training as conflict resolvers, nor were they diplomats in a traditional sense. But the strength of the Community role has to be found in the perception of both sides that while the Community was disinterested regarding any particular political agenda, it was deeply committed to peace itself. That perception allowed the Community to play a role on several occasions as a nonthreatening representative of peace, and its strength came not from the possibility of imposing its own solution to the problem discussed but from the continuous re-addressing of the talks with peace as the final goal.

The Community also provided channels of communication to the international community at large while at the same time keeping peace efforts discreet. This discretion was an essential element of the talks and crucial in earning the trust of both parties, who were enabled to talk directly while external influences were minimized. The delicate equilibrium was preserved. The Community continued to defend the agreed-on setting of direct talks during the whole negotiation process while constantly informing the international community of progress.

The professional help of the Italian government and American diplomats was especially important. While direct talks were indispensable to any serious attempt to end war in Mozambique, it was necessary to nourish the talks with ideas and suggestions that were not expressions of any given side, articulating issues in the debate in a richer way. Even in this case, the lack of training and experience by the observers was transformed into a positive factor; instead of relying on a self-centered approach, the team decided to use professional expertise from different sources when available and acceptable to both sides. Through this mechanism, military experts joined the mediation team to discuss the specificity of a cease-fire, while government officials helped to define electoral law and other crucial elements of the agreement. The international community was brought officially into the process when the signing of the first set of protocols made such an action necessary.

The entire process was based on the will of the parties, coordinated by the primary actors, and supported by the international community. These characteristics continued even after the final signature of the agreement itself. The process which started in Rome continued in Mozambique through the United Nations' ONUMOZ (United Nations Observor Mission to Mozambique) intervention and created the possibility for a peaceful solution of the Mozambique crisis. The process relied heavily on the parties themselves, who started talking to each other directly for the first time in July of 1990 and, step by step, were brought together in a relationship still in place today.

FRELIMO is in power after a free and fair election (held in 1994), and RENAMO is represented in Parliament as an opposition party. The transformation of both sides is remarkable, but the change of RENAMO from an insurgent military group to a politically active party is especially striking. Without RENAMO's abandonment of the military armed struggle and its acceptance of the political arena as the appropriate realm of action, no peace would have ensued. FRELIMO, on the other hand, agreed to share political space with other interlocutors, transforming the political system to a multiparty democracy where power is distributed between legislative, executive, and judicial branches.

The strength of the agreement has been stressed many times by Aldo Ajello, Special Representative of United Nations Secretary General

1992-1994. Ajello was able to continue the peace process in a different way and on a larger scale beginning in October 1992, when the UN took the lead as coordinator of the resolution process. The implementation of the agreement by the international community was slow: the first military contingent supposed to arrive in Mozambique a few days after the signing of the agreement arrived instead six months later, and the money necessary to support the whole process was slow in being collected. The parties themselves were reluctant to proceed in demobilizing their own forces rapidly. Nevertheless, the agreement was flexible enough to allow renegotiation of terms of implementation. A new timetable was negotiated, and finally free and fair elections were held in autumn 1994. Joaquim Chissano was elected, and the new democratic and peaceful phase of Mozambique's history began.[5]

St. Egidio continued to play a role during these two years, facilitating contacts, addressing hot political issues, and lobbying in the international community for implementation of the agreement. The Community opened an office in New York, still operating today, to follow this and the many other dossiers in which the Community has been involved since. The Community remains active in Mozambique with humanitarian projects but also through a network of small communities of young Mozambicans who share the vision of St. Egidio to live the gospel and serve the poor in friendship.

The Community usually does not send missionaries anywhere, preferring to support local initiatives of individuals and groups who want to join their way of life. This is why Communities of St. Egidio around the world are not formed or led by Italians who migrate abroad but by natives. Of the 15,000 members, more than 10,000 are still in Italy, and half of the entire body of members is in Rome. Linked to all the other communities of the world by bonds of friendship and other personal relations, all Communities of St. Egidio around the world share not only a generic reference to the poor but also a commitment to direct, personal, faithful service to them.

The Community discovered Mozambique out of this love for the poor and recognizes that this link to the poor has been transformed into a true friendship, faithful and passionate. This is why, beyond the political reasoning that made it possible for St. Egidio to be involved in Mozambique in the first place, its relationship with the country is complex and rich and continues beyond the political face of the relationships.

The Community believes deeply that one of the most dramatic elements of our contemporary experience is the lack of communication between the rich North and poor South of the planet. Indifference is the most common attitude of representatives of the North toward the sorrow, need, and requests of the South. The Community believes a reason for its successful involvement in the Mozambique peace process is found in this passionate, unwavering alliance with the South. This has also meant openness on the Community's part to new requests for help by other representatives around the world in conflict situations.

A question which often arises is this: how does the Community decide to become involved in a particular conflict? Just as often, there is an underlying assumption that there is some kind of selection strategy based on a set of criteria and a political framework intrinsically linked to the Community. This assumed paradigm, that the Community's strategy in choosing the targets of its activities is to carefully contemplate and rationalize their selections, does not describe the reality of these decisions. On the contrary, the Community operates under a spiritual framework in which the pastoral care of others overshadows political factors and influences; the concern for the poor is a strong enough reason for spending time and energy in listening and intervening in situations of conflict.

The first and most important action of the Community's members involved in a situation of conflict is to develop personal relationships with the main actors in the conflict itself, exploring ways in which empathy can make its way and create the common space of communication that was not there previously. The work, then, has less to do with ordinary political activities—especially of traditional diplomats—than with the experience of personal friendship.

The human quality of all the conflict resolution exercises in which the Community has been involved is also shown by the continuity of the relationships that has usually preceded talks and continued afterwards. In the case of Mozambique, it is clear that the bonds of the Community with the country dated from sixteen years before the beginning of the negotiations and remain in place after peace has been achieved.

Such continuity is lacking in many official diplomatic attempts and brings to the process a genuine, personal dimension and strength. Such involvement is not ephemeral, occasional, or uprooted. This commitment, which has over almost two decades manifested itself in the form of sincere friendship, remains the Community's priority for the people and country of Mozambique. When the time for the role of mediator was finished, the Community was happy to oblige by discarding it. What the Community will not abandon, however, is the well-rooted friendship with Mozambique, established along the country's path to peace.

Human Rights: Dignity, Community, Freedom

Martin Shupack and Rachel Brett

Human rights is the common language of international morality and popular aspiration today. Oppressive governments are denounced as human rights violators. Political leaders contemplating new trade relations feel obligated to give at least minimal consideration to human rights. Community organizations, laborers, and other ordinary citizens throughout the world appeal to universal human rights to call for fair treatment, democracy, and social justice.

Christian churches have for decades promoted human rights. The Bible speaks eloquently about God's concern for people's rights.[1] Believers are instructed to "defend the rights of the poor and needy" (Prov. 31:8, 9). Yet Christians recognize that the deepest human needs—for grace, forgiveness, and fellowship with God and others—must be received as gifts, not demanded as rights.

In relationship to God, human rights too are gifts. But in relationship to organized society, the essential requirements for safeguarding dignity and justice must not be viewed as gifts. They are rights of persons that the state is bound to respect and ensure. Within the civil, political, economic, social, and cultural arenas, human rights identify the prerequisites for a life of dignity, community participation, and freedom.

The first part of this chapter discusses human rights in international law, articulates a Christian understanding of human rights shared by Catholics and Protestants, and offers convictions about human rights rooted in the beliefs and practices of the historic peace churches.[2] Part two describes a practical example of the human rights work of one peace church agency.

What Are Human Rights?

Human rights are fundamental claims or entitlements acknowledged to be morally justified and to take precedence over other societal interests. Each person possesses a full range of human rights simply by being human. Grounded in a belief in human dignity, human rights express the minimal requirements for human well-being.

Human rights are usually divided into two categories. *Civil and political rights* protect personal liberty and physical security. Among these are the rights to life, liberty, and security; the rights not to be enslaved or tortured; the rights to recognition as a person before the law and to equality before the law; protections against arbitrary arrest, detention, and *ex post facto* laws; the right not to be imprisoned for nonfulfillment of a contractual obligation; the right to privacy; freedom of thought, conscience, religion, expression, movement, assembly, and association; protection for marriage and the family; the rights to participate in government and vote in periodic genuine elections that freely express the will of the people; and the rights of members of ethnic, religious, or linguistic minorities to enjoy their own culture, practice their religion, and use their own language.

Economic, social, and cultural rights protect people's material sufficiency and community participation. These include the rights to work, to fair wages and just and favorable working conditions, to form trade unions and engage in lawful strikes, to job security, and to rest and leisure; the rights to an adequate standard of living for self and family, to sufficient food, clothing, housing, health services, and medical care; the right to social security in the event of unemployment, sickness, disability, widowhood, and old age; the right to education; and the right to take part in the cultural life of the community and share in the benefits of scientific advancement.

In addition to these two categories, some advocates propose recognizing a third set of human rights. These rights belong not so much to individuals as to "peoples." Rights to development, peace, and a healthy environment are often mentioned. The right of peoples to self-determination and to freely dispose of their own natural wealth and resources is one collective human right well-established in international law. This, however, is usually viewed narrowly as an anticolonial and anti-imperial provision and not as related to the aspirations for autonomy of ethnic minorities or indigenous communities.

The equal validity and importance of all human rights was reaffirmed in the Vienna Declaration and Program of Action of the 1993 UN World Conference on Human Rights as "indivisible and interdependent and interrelated."[3] Human rights are codified as international law in a series of treaties that legally bind the states party to them. At the same time, all states are bound through customary international law to observe the mostly widely accepted human rights standards. The most prominent human rights instruments are the Universal Declaration of Human Rights, the International Covenant on Civil and Political Rights, and the International Covenant on Economic, Social, and Cultural Rights. Each of these instruments requires the implementation of the enumerated rights without discrimination or distinction of any kind, such as those of "race, color, sex, language, religion, political or other opinion, national or social origin, property, birth or other status."[4]

Human rights are often viewed as the rights of individuals. However, thematic human rights treaties and declarations provide some specific protection for persons who are members of vulnerable groups, including workers; racial, ethnic and religious minorities; women; indigenous peoples; and children.[5]

How Are Human Rights Christian?

Christians have been human rights advocates since before the adoption of the Universal Declaration in 1948. The Catholic Church emphasized the primacy of rights inherent in human nature in the first modern Catholic social encyclical *Rerum Novarum* in 1891. *Pacem in Terris*, issued by Pope John XXIII in 1963, placed human rights at the center of Catholic social teaching.

The World Council of Churches at its first assembly in 1948 proclaimed the responsibility of churches to "take a firm and vigorous stand" against "flagrant violations of human rights."[6] International bodies of Reformed, Lutheran, and Baptist churches, as well as regional and national church bodies, have issued studies and statements on international human rights. The historic peace churches have been human rights advocates throughout the world on behalf of child soldiers, conscientious objection to military service, indigenous communities, and other concerns.[7]

Christians in general have affirmed the same catalogue of rights codified in the Universal Declaration and the Covenants. Yet they have articulated a moral vision of human rights in distinctively Christian ways, shaping the essential meaning of human rights on the basis of the key Christian narratives and convictions. We can see this by examining three fundamental values universal to human rights discourse: dignity, community, and freedom.

Dignity

International human rights legal instruments recognize the inherent dignity of the human person as the basis of human rights. Christians view this dignity as given by God, locating its ground in the biblical story. Christian teaching affirms that all human beings possess inviolable sanctity and immeasurable worth because they are created in God's image. The divine image precedes all national, ethnic, socioeconomic, and personal differences. Human rights flow from this transcendent dignity. Since human beings are created in God's image as male and female, men and women are equal in dignity and rights.

As a bearer of God's image, each person must be respected as a creative, self-determining subject, with the right to participate in the decisions that shape society. Also God has charged humankind with the care and keeping of the earth. This implies ecological duties and means that every person possesses economic rights to a just share of the earth's goods. Oppression, impoverishment, slavery, torture, and killing desecrate this image of God.

God's redemptive acts in Jesus Christ provide an even stronger ground for human rights. Jesus' life, death, and resurrection demonstrate God's immeasurable love for each person and the supreme value God places on human well-being. Every man, woman, and child is a person for whom Christ died. Because redemption is an undeserved gift of God's grace, not something earned or achieved, all persons are equal in dignity and rights. In Jesus, God has established sovereign claim to humankind, buying women and men back from sin, death, and oppression. Human rights are therefore anchored in "God's right to—i.e., God's claim on—human beings."[8]

Human rights identify the conditions of life required for the concrete realization in organized society of this exalted human dignity. In contrast to views that recognize only selected civil and political rights, but not social and economic rights, Christian faith respects the equal validity and indivisibility of all human rights. This is because a human being is created in God's image and loved by Christ as a spiritual and physical whole. Whatever is required for the protection of this God-given dignity, whether freedom of worship or an adequate wage, must be recognized as a human right. Whatever violates this dignity, whether torture or the denial of sufficient food, violates human rights.

Christian accounts of human rights, therefore, recognize not only "negative" rights that protect individuals from government abuse, but also "positive" human rights mandating government action on behalf of sufficiency and dignity for all. In the Christian view, government has a vital role as protector of ordinary people from the powerful, self-serving individuals and destructive social and economic forces that would abuse and exploit them.[9]

A peace church conviction is that *dignity is servanthood*. For Christians who identify with the historic peace churches, human dignity is most fully expressed in the nonviolent servanthood of Jesus Christ. True dignity rejects a self-centered misuse of rights language and focuses compassionate concern on the rights of others—especially impoverished and marginalized people. Nonviolent servanthood embraces the Christian spirit of love for enemies and a commitment to protect the enemies' human rights.

Human rights are often appealed to as an educational and mobilization tool to empower disenfranchised communities. In this context, the spirit of nonviolence, exhibited, for example, in the civil rights movement in the United States, is more faithful to Christ than are purely power-based strategies that seek to advance ideological or narrowly partisan agendas and that depersonalize adversaries and treat them as expendable.

When engaging policy makers, advocates for human rights can take the form of a servant by speaking to "that of God" in those whom we address. Providing reliable information and firsthand accounts, we tell our stories of the human reality we encounter. This can be done without moralizing or self-righteousness, by treating respectfully and hearing the concerns of those who do not share our views. Telling the truth in love, as we have experienced it, we can invite a compassionate, just response by those in power.

Community

In a Christian account of human rights, community is as important an underlying value as dignity. Neglecting the importance of community plays into the excessive individualism that mars Western society. Human beings are created to reflect the divine fellowship within the Trinity. Through Christ, women and men are called to unity in one body and one new humanity. Thus it is only through mutual interdependence that human beings can fully reflect God's image. God's image is seen neither in disassociated individuals nor in collectives which require a loss of individual identities, but in persons-in-community. Human rights should be seen as building blocks of a just and moral social order.

Because the Christian story emphasizes community, it affirms the equal importance of human duties. Each person has a duty to seek the common good and contribute to the emancipation of an oppressed neighbor. All persons should exercise their rights in an ethical manner and refrain from violating rights of others.

Emphasis on rights without equal recognition of responsibilities breeds a conflictual social environment in which all claim their rights but no one accepts responsibility for ensuring their enjoyment by others. On the other hand, an emphasis on responsibility without an equal stress on rights can lead to charity but not justice.

Recognizing the importance of community leads to a new appreciation for the norm of equality—beyond the traditional Western notion that government must extend equal respect and concern to all citizens. In the Christian story, the norm of equality applies to actual life conditions. This equality is not mathematical equivalence, but a principle of the distribution of wealth which ensures that everyone has the resources sufficient for life, dignity, and participation in community.[10]

Among members of one human family called to unity as brothers and sisters by Jesus' death and resurrection, vast disparities of wealth should be unthinkable. Authentic community does not permit some people to live in luxury while others lack food, shelter, or medical care. This means people have a responsibility to work together through churches, voluntary associations, and government policies and laws to develop societies where everyone truly has enough. Indifference to the economic afflictions of others violates the commandment to love our neighbors as ourselves.

The call to community and the duty to defend the rights of others transcend all boundaries. The "debt of love" owed to neighbors and enemies mandates compassionate solidarity across all the hostile barriers of nationality, ethnicity, class, and culture.

A peace church conviction is that *restoring community is vital.* Peace churches emphasize that human rights flourish in the context of relationships. Nurturing community, healing broken relationships, and seeking the common good are seen as foundational to realizing human rights. Based on this conviction, some members of peace churches are involved in articulating restorative justice approaches in the aftermath of civil wars and genocidal violence.

Restorative justice processes recognize that violence and crime represent a profound violation of people and their relationships. The just and appropriate response by society is to provide mechanisms for healing and wholeness: for the victims and offenders, for their families, and for the community as a whole. This is the approach of Jesus in Matthew 18, and it resonates with the history and practice of peoples throughout the world, including in the West. Mechanisms and opportunities for restorative justice could provide more profound satisfaction for persons devastated by violence and do more to bring an authentic and lasting peace to torn communities than the retributive notions embodied in modern Western legal systems.

Freedom

Christian discussions of human rights affirm the Western notion of freedom as an inviolable realm of personal choice and group autonomy protected from arbitrary state encroachment. The human vocation to respond to God in faith and represent God's character in the world can only be carried out in freedom. From Adam and Eve's freedom to choose—and to reap the consequences—in Eden, to the absence of coercion in the spread of the gospel in the New Testament, God reveals a radical respect for personal choice. Protecting this freedom requires limits to the power of government, which must not usurp the claim on allegiance that belongs only to God. The state has legitimate coercive functions, but within important limits.

The Jesus story, however, complements these traditional elements of individual and associational autonomy with a dynamic vision of freedom as emancipation. In his death and resurrection, Jesus defeated and disarmed the fallen "powers and authorities" that structure societies in oppressive ways. Christ's resurrection opens new historical possibilities for human liberation. Viewed in light of the good news of God's emancipatory work in Christ, human rights express the just claims of human beings to be set free from the demonic and dehumanizing forces of violence, political oppression, economic exploitation, and cultural alienation.

In this Jesus story, freedom must be regulated by love, by solidarity with the neighbor in need. The norm of love can resolve serious conflicts among rights. The rights to be free from hunger and joblessness take precedence over some traditional autonomy rights. For example, any rights to property and free commerce must be subordinated to everyone's right to a life of sufficiency and dignity.[11] This means that governments have an obligation to regulate the global market and provide a social safety net so that the basic needs of all people can be satisfied.

Freedom is not an end in itself. True liberty involves release *from* individual and social sin and bondage, but also freedom *for* communion with God and other human beings. Here again, the Christian story expresses a substantive goal for human rights. Rights do not exist simply to restrain government abuse and ensure minimal material welfare.

Rather, freedom should enable people to orient their lives toward God in faith and their fellow human beings in love and justice.

A peace church conviction is that *freedom of conscience is crucial.* For the peace churches, as historically oppressed minority religious movements, the freedom to worship God according to conscience has been of primary importance. Because Christians in the peace church tradition believe that war is sin and that following Christ requires rejection of any participation in killing, the right of conscientious objection to military service is also a central concern.

The historic peace churches were among the first to assert in word and deed that "no government has the authority to abrogate the right of individual conscience."[12] According to *A Declaration on Peace*, jointly published by Mennonites, Quakers, and the Church of the Brethren, the body of Christ (the church) must never lend its members to the enterprise of defending and preparing to defend the nation-state against its real or merely putative enemies by means of organized military force and violence.[13]

The first conscientious objection laws, implemented during the American colonial period, exempted Mennonites, Brethren, Quakers, and members of other religious bodies whose teachings rejected participation in war.[14] Since then, in the face of persecution and suffering, pacifist Christians have worked with others to establish in the laws of nations the right of conscientious objection to military service not only for themselves but for all.

In the United States, for example, advocacy efforts by the historic peace churches, joined by other denominations, succeeded in having alternative service under civilian direction provided by law during the Second World War. In recent years, peace church members in Honduras and Colombia have led national movements for the legal recognition of conscientious objection. By 1995, twenty-six countries had recognized conscientious objection to military service. International human rights bodies have indicated that conscientious objection can be a legitimate expression of the right of freedom of thought, conscience, and religion.

The first part of this chapter reviewed why human rights should occupy a central position in the practical expression of the divine message by all Christian churches, including the historic peace churches. The second part will illustrate the distinctive features the peace churches can bring to human rights work with international organizations, with specific reference to the activities of the Quaker United Nations Office in Geneva.

Distinctives of Peace Church Work for Human Rights

How does the fact that we are a peace church affect the way in which Quakers approach human rights issues at the international level? The answer comes essentially in two parts. It affects the way in which the Quaker United Nations Office actually works, and it affects the issues we choose as our priorities. More broadly, though, it should also be said that Quakers give high priority to critically supporting the United Nations. We believe it is essential to complement our involvement on the ground and lobbying national governments with working for change on a global level. Quakers have been involved with the UN from the beginning. Indeed, the Quaker office in Geneva was established during the time of the League of Nations.

How We Work

When most people think about human rights work at the international level, they think of Amnesty International—researching and publishing reports on specific countries, denouncing human rights violations at the UN, sponsoring letterwriting campaigns, using the media, and so on. Although Quakers share the same concerns (and indeed Quakers have and continue to be both international secretariat staff and local members of Amnesty), as an organization this is not our approach.

For the most part we work on issues rather than countries. In part, this approach is pragmatic. Because we are both a field work agency and a church, we may have people—expatriate workers or local church members—on the ground. To publicly accuse a government of human rights violations may have severe repercussions for our people in that country. However, it is not only pragmatic. This approach also reflects the way we approach people.

In one of the earliest Quaker writings, George Fox called on Friends to "walk cheerfully over the world, answering that of God in everyone," and the conviction that there is something of God in everyone and that we should be appealing to it has been prominent in Quaker thinking ever since. Even if people are representatives of their governments, even if we identify as wrong some deeds they may have committed, condoned, or diplomatically covered up, we should not forget that they too are human beings created in God's image. Because there is something of God in them, they are capable of change and repentance.

We are convinced that working together through education and persuasion produces more enduring effects than trying to force changes merely by creating new rules or bad publicity. At the same time, we recognize that the two types of activities may complement each other and be more effective than either on its own.

This does not mean we evade addressing real situations. In general, however, we address them thematically rather than on a country-by-country basis. This tends to be quiet, low-profile work, whittling away at attitudes, moving forward incrementally, collecting and analyzing the information to show what happens, why it happens, and why and how it should be changed.

At times such work may become high profile, as with our study on child soldiers which created considerable media interest because of its breadth and the way in which the analysis showed the issue in a new light. However, even here, in what many people consider to be a particularly sensitive area politically, we sought to defuse confrontation and not to point the finger at particular governments or armed opposition groups. Instead we tried to show why children are forced or drawn into conflict, which children are affected, what happens to them, and how to approach demobilization, rehabilitation, and reintegration. We addressed specific recommendations not only to the drafters of international agreements, but also to military authorities in countries which use child soldiers and to the leaders of armed opposition groups. Our aim was to show those who make the decisions on the ground that using children may not be in their own best interests and to point toward steps they could take to avoid the practice.

A similar convergence of interests can be seen in our work on conscientious objection to military service. Again rather than campaigning publicly about the lack of proper recognition of conscientious objection to military service in, say, the Russian Federation, we have promoted standards at the UN recognizing the right of conscientious objection and the conditions which alternative service must meet. We have ensured that Quakers and others working on this issue in the Russian Federation receive copies of these standards so they can take them up within the country.

In the wider acceptance of conscientious objection and the movement away from systems of conscription, our allies have included those military commands who realize that an efficient force cannot be composed of unwilling recruits. It might seem strange that as a peace church we should be involved in this sort of dialogue with military authorities about minimum ages for recruitment, the treatment of recruits, and so on. Should we not hold firm to our conviction that all war and all preparation for war is contrary to the will of God? Should we not refuse to engage in any discussion about measures short of the abolition of all armed forces everywhere?

That our ultimate goal is to establish a peaceful and just world where armed forces are no longer necessary or acceptable is never in doubt. The question is the means we use in our efforts to achieve that end. Some take the role of prophets, speaking and living out the ultimate vision. Others use the step-by-step approach which engages those in a position to make decisions, recognizing that we need to start from where they, and the world, actually are and move things along in the right direction.

The work of the Quaker UN Offices inevitably falls into the latter category. This does not necessarily mean that we avoid articulating our vision of the way things should be. There are many opportunities to explain who we are and why we do what we do since those we work with are often meeting Quakers and Quakerism for the first time and want to know what motivates us. Paradoxically, our "abnormal" views, once understood, often lead to greater trust because people realize we have no vested interest but are truly impartial. We are not seeking benefits for Quakers nor publicity or self-advancement for Quaker work.

One of the peculiarities of international human rights work is that many of the government representatives are not specialists. Many foreign services work on the basis of employing generalists who move to a new post every three or four years, often dealing with a completely different subject. Our educational and persuasive approach, together with our reputation for both expertise and fairness, mean that we are often looked to as a source of information as well as for interpretation and understanding of what is happening both on issues and at UN meetings more generally. This has resulted in a considerable demand from government representatives as well as others for the briefing papers and analytical reports we produce on our priority areas of work or more generally on key UN meetings.

There is a distinction between public accusation and the provision of information about the human rights situation in a particular country to UN bodies or the governments represented in them which may be achieved quietly and even on occasion confidentially. During the recent conflict in Chechnya, Quakers were one of the few outside groups with firsthand information about what was happening in the region. Because of the nature and extent of the human rights violations and the lack of other sources of information, the authorized Quaker bodies made a policy decision that we should publicize our information. In fact, the Quaker UN Office was the channel for much of the information from both Quaker and other sources for the UN Secretary General's Report to the 1996 Commission on Human Rights, as well as for routinely (quietly) informing representatives of governments we judged most likely to influence the behavior of the Russian government and its armed forces.

Along with work on issues, there is another way we seek to promote human rights: by encouraging and facilitating dialogue and discussion across the different regions, cultures, and religions of the world. For several decades Quakers in Geneva and elsewhere have organized off-the-record meetings where diplomats can meet and explore issues in an informal but completely confidential way. In the past these have included crossing the East-West and Arab-Israeli divides. Recently in Geneva we have focused specifically on drawing in diplomats from all five of the UN's geopolitical groups since, at the time we started them, no such discussions across the regional groups were taking place.

We do not expect everyone to agree on substance, but too often disagreements occur because of misunderstandings and lack of trust. If we can help reduce these, it becomes possible to address areas of substantive disagreement. It may even be possible to clarify areas of and reasons for disagreement. To play this role requires that we approach people in a nonconfrontational way and that our trustworthiness be taken for granted, so people know that what is said in confidence will not be revealed or exploited.

What We Work On

We see all human rights as important. However, to maximize the effectiveness of our interventions we must focus on areas not being addressed adequately by others and in which our insight or knowledge allows us to make distinctive contributions. Any nongovernmental organization (NGO) which lacks a specific focus and the ability to establish priorities in its work is likely to find its effectiveness diffused and its interventions ignored as mere rhetoric. What makes people—government representatives or not—take notice is receiving new information or insights from what they consider a reliable source.

Since we are a small movement (there are only about 300,000 Quakers worldwide), it is vital to focus on areas in which we can make the greatest and most unique contribution. It is not surprising that, as a peace church, our contributions in the human rights field at the UN all center around the interface between human rights and armed conflict.

The seeds of armed conflict are sown where there is oppression, exploitation, discrimination, and disparities of wealth and power. These factors build on themselves, leading to increasing tension, suppression, and violence until, if nothing is done, armed conflict erupts. Armed conflicts themselves are a frequent source of human rights violations. Even when the conflict ends, if the underlying causes and the additional problems created by the fighting (including the situation of refugees and internally displaced persons) are not addressed, seeds of the next conflict are already being sown.

The human rights issues which take priority in the work of the Quaker UN Office in Geneva are, on the one hand, those which deal with countering the militarization of society, and on the other, those which address the protection of human rights in armed conflict situations. The first category includes our work on conscientious objection to military service, child soldiers, and most recently, the inhuman, degrading, and brutalizing treatment of recruits in many armed forces. In the second category, we work on the protection of human rights in civil wars and situations of internal violence characteristic of recent years. To our long-standing work for refugees, we have added concern for the even larger number of "internally displaced persons" who are not technically refugees because they have not crossed an international border but remain within their own country.

In relation to conscientious objection, our principal aim has been to have the international community, and through it all states, recognize a right to refuse to perform military service on grounds of conscience. We have worked to ensure that where military service is compulsory a suitable civilian alternative is available for conscientious objectors.

The work has gone through a number of phases. First we worked at getting the issue on the UN agenda at all. The second stage has involved gaining recognition of the basic right of conscientious objection, followed by developing the grounds for recognition and the criteria to be met by alternative service. Finally we have worked to bring national practices to the attention of appropriate UN bodies to improve compliance with the standards now agreed to by the UN. This has taken many years of steady, persistent work with other NGOs and supportive governments, at times without evidence of progress or apparent prospects of success. In the end, it was the geopolitical changes of 1989 which enabled the Commission on Human Rights to recognize conscientious objection as a right. However, without the groundwork done over the previous years, the opportunity could easily have been missed.

Similarly, the Quaker UN Office in Geneva was in 1979 asked by the Friends World Committee for Consultation (FWCC) to take up the issue of child soldiers. Between 1979 and 1989, our focus was on raising international awareness about what was initially a little-recognized phenomenon. We sought to ensure that the Convention on the Rights of the Child (being drafted during this period) protected children from recruitment and use in warfare. Unfortunately, the latter effort failed. Since 1989, the work has focused on building momentum for a new effort at standard-setting in this area. This has led to drafting of an optional protocol (still in progress) to the Convention on the Rights of the Child.

At the same time, the Quaker work on child soldiers led the UN Committee on the Rights of the Child to hold a discussion on children in armed conflict. As a result, they recommended drafting an optional protocol to raise the age of recruitment and requested that the UN Secretary General appoint an expert to study the impact of armed conflict on children. In 1993 the UN General Assembly endorsed that request, and Graça Machel of Mozambique was appointed. She presented her study to the General Assembly in 1996.

Because of its known involvement with the issue, the Quaker UN Office in Geneva was commissioned to undertake the research on child soldiers for the study. Although the Quaker UN Office had overall responsibility, this became a collaborative project with the International Catholic Child Bureau and a steering group of other interested international NGOs. They commissioned country case studies, wherever possible from local organizations, covering all regions of the world.

For What Reward?

Because we only work on those issues which we see as essential and our work on them is based on faith rather than results, we are prepared to keep working on them over many years even when there is no evidence of results. Furthermore, at the end of the day, if results are achieved, we do not find it essential or even useful to claim credit. It may be equally desirable for governments with which we have worked to take the credit. For our work to gain too high a profile might make similar work harder another time. And a government which gets credit for our work is usually favorably disposed toward working with us again! For us the reward is the achievements themselves. Our work is a small attempt, growing out of our faith, to contribute to the growth and strengthening of community, dignity, and freedom.

Peacemaking in Ecumenical Perspective

17

Theology for a Just Peace

Lauree Hersch Meyer

Concluding the volume, this essay reviews the contemporary land-scape and addresses some theological implications for peacemakers in our violence-fraught world. I suggest no solution to war and violence; peacemakers rarely suppose they have that power. I do inquire into the significance and scope of what peacemakers do and why, in our various contexts, we work for peace in the widest possible ecumenical dialogue.

After the Cold War

Using the words *Cold War* indicates my location in Western civili-zation.[1] The collapse of East-West ideological conflict ended the hegem-ony of discourse rooted in European ideologies and set the stage for new dynamics to shape political, economic, cultural, and religious conversa-tion and reflection. The end of the Cold War coincided with, perhaps catalyzed, and brought to Western awareness a paradigm shift—a change in how people see things—in international affairs.

The changes open the way for more serious ecumenical and inter-national discourse among people of faith in different nations and cul-tures. The end of the Cold War brought less change in the perception and work of peaceworkers in Eastern and Southern cultures than of Western nations. Several dimensions of the new reality are of particular concern to peaceworkers.

First, Western civilization now knows it no longer sets the terms for much of the international conversation and action. The contexts, thought, and perspectives of peoples from many cultures and ethnic groups are audibly present and visibly central in international interactions. This change was particularly notable in the participant composition and agenda of recent World Council of Churches' Faith and Order conferences and commission meetings. The center of religious vitality is shifting to Southern and Eastern countries as church life diminishes in Europe and North America and blossoms in Latin America, Africa, Korea, and elsewhere. There is a new awareness among Western Christians of the growing presence of Muslim, Buddhist, and other faiths in countries that traditionally viewed themselves as Christian cultures.

Second, the decline of Western hegemony brings a new appreciation that each people's cultural particularities include values and practices essential to that people's identity. What is at home in one context is often alien to or an irritant in other contexts. For example, the United States' stress on individual responsibility and the Chinese emphasis on collective responsibility are in tension with one another as each recognizes and resists the other's values.

Even when people understand or can function in another culture's terms and values, cultural and contextual differences *make* a difference. Where differences are manifest in tension, hostility, or war, it is difficult to achieve agreement on general goals and guidelines like justice, social cohesiveness, self-determination, and human rights. Since specific realities basic to one people often trouble those at home in another context, peacemakers seek to meet all people on their own terms and work inductively. All peaceworkers consciously live and work amid these tensions.

Third, the post-Cold War landscape opens the way to strong, broad ecumenical dialogue. Christians learn to recognize peacemakers in all traditions as God-given kinfolk. Reference to the world as a "global village," commonly used to refer to closely linked communications technologies, or transnational corporations, is spoken of by Christian peacemakers as God's *oikumene*, God's whole created household, all who are our kin in Christ Jesus.[2] Christian theology and ethics often embody only fragments of our faith, which holds that because God created and loves all persons and all creation, all people who love God are fulfilled when they love what God loves. The historic peace churches, made up of Mennonites, Church of the Brethren, Friends/Quakers, and Fellowship of Reconciliation (HPC/FOR), understand that we are called to be peacemakers. We see in Jesus' life and work how God works in human lives to bless and restore creation.

Today most of the more overtly violent conflicts take place among peoples in a single state, in much of Eastern Europe, for example, or in the Sudan. Though these peoples share many cultural values, they are more concerned with asserting their separate identities than any commonality. In the absence of any universally binding criteria for what counts as a single culture, peace negotiations take place among people with very different presuppositions about what it means to be *this* people.

Contemporary peacemaking efforts must accept the lesson taught by Somalia and Bosnia that no nation-state or set of nation-states can create, keep, make, or build lasting and genuine peace for someone else. The active, voluntary participation of the peoples in conflict and the creation of trusted local institutions is essential if hostility, mistrust, and differences are to be settled.

As peacemakers from Southern and Eastern countries have long known, the world is inhabited by peoples of diverse identities who are informed by many visions; live by different values, traditions, and aspirations; and express themselves through many perspectives in many voices.[3] When violent conflict erupts, internationally imposed cessation of active combat may be a necessary condition for peace, but it is inadequate to support and nurture the trust or build the community needed for lasting peace. Nor, as seen in Cambodia, is an imposed but alien political system an adequate basis for building a communal life able to nurture members into self-respecting, trustful, compassionate, mature persons.

Peacemakers throughout the world know that no one or several nations can create, keep, make, or build peace. Where the force of domination is used to "pacify" amid violence, the other's integrity is disregarded, resulting less in peace than in an absence of armed conflict. Peaceworkers recognize that neither they nor those with whom they work are value-free; all partake of and express particular (political and religious) values, perspectives, presuppositions, and traditions. Ending conflict among peoples with different values and presuppositions can begin as a conversation in which participants hear and honor the other's sense of history and identity.

Peaceworkers from Western traditions among the HPC/FOR until perhaps the 1960s often assumed that their kind of pacifism was the only way to live faithfully. By living among, working with, and learning to honor peacemakers from Eastern Europe, Latin America, South Africa, and Israel-Palestine, whose citizens had no wish to be culturally Western, Western peacemakers learned that peacemaking sometimes looks different in different contexts. Learning from the contextual life-experiences of others, HPC/FOR peaceworkers became more pragmatic, practical, realistic, generous, and openhearted. Their conviction that God is present in all peoples came alive as they recognized spiritual kin among peacemakers who held different cultural, class, or power assumptions from theirs.

Writers of the preceding chapters, all committed to peacemaking, are at home in several contexts. Each writes from practical experience, discussing matters with which they are familiar and about which they care deeply. They offer no general blueprint or "peace solution" to a violence "problem."[4] Rather, they offer their life experiences and commitments, inviting believers into a bouquet of specific ways people of faith live and work as peacemakers in local communities and on the international level.

Peacemaking in Theological Context

The theological context of peacemaking asks questions about what it means to be human, how to live well in community, how to respond to and engage life amid violence and war, and how to live as a peacemaker, whatever one's life situation. These practical matters elicit inductive (thinking from specifics to principles) theological reflection. While in recent centuries Western culture has come to associate inductive thought more with the arts than with theology, Christian theology arose as inductive reflection on concrete experiences that were irrefutably different from what believers had been taught. When a leader like Jesus arises who embodies change, the parent community is sometimes polarized.

Similarly, leaders in the Protestant Reformation refuted the parent community's authority in ways that led to distinctly diverse Christian identities. Changes constantly appear in religious communities, often not related to polarized positions over issues, but arising from pragmatic, inductive adjustments to daily life. Challenge to an implicit or explicit communal position, usually projected by its deductive (from principles to application) reasoning, is normally met with resistance. It rarely seems "reasonable" to affirm what implies one's demise. Cultural change seems more readily absorbed and diversity more quickly tolerated when issues are not challenged and polarized but are absorbed as adaptions to living in this particular age and place.

The Bible is full of stories about people transformed by experiences that contradicted initially held beliefs. While it takes time to learn to talk clearly *about* experiences that have been life-changing, talk disconnected from real life generates inner tension. Theological reflection that becomes cerebral and deductive lends itself to contradictions between rhetoric and reality. Contradictions in dogmatic teachings are especially costly where power discrepancies exist: when, for example, more powerful persons (bishops, bosses, pastors, parents) are held less accountable for behavior that less powerful folks (employees, parishioners, children) are punished for.

When cultural changes enhance class or identity differences, claims to trust in "one true way" are invalidated as people sense the dissonance of leaders whose actions betray their words. When such contradictions become great enough, new ways of viewing reality arise. As people of faith, peacemakers who think practically, inductively, and contextually work to embody the rhetoric of faith in the practices of life.

It is significant that how people see things changes. Whether people welcome or resist those changes, they are real. They also offer a chance for genuine ecumenical conversation, for today virtually all dynamics involve both intranational and international communities. Partaking in such conversations, people of faith cross religious and/or national borders to offer support. Such peacemakers are loyal citizens of their own countries. At the same time, they have a deep loyalty to all people: to all God created and loves, to the whole inhabited universe. Perhaps the Church's oldest legacy, visible in early New Testament writings as in its mystical, radical, and peace traditions, is the conviction that citizenship in God's realm or kindom[5] is basic and has priority over national claims for loyalty, especially in times of political conflict and hostility.

Many peoples of faith enjoy the protection of the nations in which they live and work, fully participating in life as citizens of their countries, while others experience repression or prejudice. In all situations, peacemakers aim to understand and contribute to the wholeness of both their own and of other peoples. Seeking to act on the basis of reality, peacemakers often plan actions pragmatically, motivated by love. Peacemakers know local groups must be involved for communal well-being to be achieved. They are committed to living out their rhetoric in daily practice.[6]

Peaceworkers know that national and international peacekeeping, however valuable and necessary, is insufficient for peacemaking and peacebuilding.[7] They honor history, often re-interpreting old stories (as did Jesus, Gandhi, Martin Luther King), recognizing that the chaotic or undesirable fragments of preceding politico-socio-religious structures are the building blocks of any new creation.

The cacophony of newly audible and articulate voices can be confusing. But it is also a divine blessing, however startling or hard to hear. Though few of us likes engaging our limits, accepting limits is one rendering of the Genesis 11 story. It goes like this:

Once there was a community of people who were very alike. Having learned to think and act very similarly, they believed they could, with effort, reach to and know God's mind. God saw it coming and responded first by limiting their (perhaps unintended) idolatry and then imagining a new way for blessing to occur. God limited their idolatry by "confusing their tongues." As a result, they experienced the dissonance of being different peoples, each with their own tongue, stories, and identity. Then the God who had made humankind "in God's own image" and completed creation with blessing,[8] blessed each people particularly. Now peoples would come to know God in their particular situation and culture, in the anguish and hope, the burden and joy, of their specific daily way of life. The fulfillment of each people's promised inheritance, as to the descendants of Abraham and Hagar, was to "be a blessing to all peoples." In this changed situation, each was still called to live as "image-of-God" people able to bless one another and all creation as God blessed them. But now blessing was offered and received in each people's particularity.

When we bless one another in God's image, we seek to embody God's reign, God's kindom. Peacemakers do not control what our nations, communities, friends, or others do. But we can control our commitment; we can seek to live out our vision of God's kindom. Peacemakers believe God blesses each person in their age and place. They believe blessing and life for all is more abundant in as much as they honor and bless all whom God loves. They see in Jesus another way to respond to injustice than by passivity or violence.[9] Jesus' "third way" shows how downtrodden people may assert their dignity with generosity and an open heart, denying the powerful the ability to humiliate them.[10]

Citizens in God's kindom do not dominate or subjugate their kin. Peacemakers are citizens of God's cosmic community, committed to forgiving and blessing others as God forgives and blesses all humankind as far back as memory and story reach. Another story informs that commitment:[11]

God completed creation with blessing (Gen. 1:28), a blessing that contained no guarantee of peace though it did empower humans with the ability to choose and act. Genesis 3 tells how, when humans began to choose and act, they became self-aware and self-protective. When God then approached them, they first tried to hide to evade the results of their actions. Later they denied their responsibility by blaming the other. Nothing indicates that they wished to bring suffering, violence or evil on themselves and the other. The story indicates that having the *power* to bless does not assure that actions will result in blessing, or that the freedom to act will gain the wanted results. Even so, when man and woman blamed and betrayed the other, God remained actively present without controlling them. God heard the stories of each, identified the results of their actions, *then* named what was now life-giving and capable of providing blessing in this new situation.

People who live in God's image pay attention to the results that come from the actions of people, communities, and nations. In-God's-image people seek to identify what is life-giving in each new situation when a loved and familiar world collapses, often while experiencing the pain of betrayal.[12] Being in community with one's kin in God helps keep one's spirit and energy focused and a sense of self-worth and direction intact. Peacemakers keep learning that the "Body of Christ" is Christian language for all one's known and yet-unknown kin whom God loves and in whom God's presence is alive and well, daily renewing and restoring creation.

Whatever the narrative, storied legacy of a people is, it holds great religious and cultural power. Local leaders' initiative draws on it, and all who are heirs to its inheritance are nurtured to be self-reliant, to rely on its imagery for guidance about what is good and true. Peoples the world over are returning to their more ancient, storied life- and community-building legacies. From those diverse and particular social contexts, thought about what should be done differs, mirroring the incarnate and life-giving shapes of that particular people at this time and in this unique place.[13] *Incarnation* was a word early Christians began using to identify God's very presence at work in Jesus Christ in material reality. Its meaning continues to refer specifically to God's action in Jesus Christ, in the Church as Christ's Living Body, and more generally to God's presence working in reality, as "enfleshed."

Peacemaking in the Post-Cold War Landscape

My identity as a radical Western Christian churchwoman, rooted in a peace church tradition, is audible in this essay and remains evident as I reflect on contemporary peacemaking. Geographical bonds that artificially had held together Eastern European peoples for less than a century have today been dissolved. Ancient identities are activated and hostilities erupt along older faultlines of tribe, culture, religion, and civilization. Much of the world seems to have been unprepared for the ethnic and religious clashes that agonize contemporary life in Eastern Europe and parts of Africa and Asia. Any Western notion that some battle was won after the Soviet Union collapsed has itself collapsed. The collapse of Soviet communism did not give birth to a new era of peace and prosperity, let alone one made in the image of Western democratic ideology; it did offer some peoples new possibilities for autonomous identity.

Throughout the former Soviet Union, as in Asia, Africa, and Latin America, religious cultures are being reclaimed. Western nations' responses to such initiatives indicate that identity is becoming a crucial question. Western nations tend to identify modernization with Western civilization, but other nations distinguish them, largely embracing modernization while rejecting Western culture and values. However much nations today function as a "global village" in technology, communications, and economics, the world is by no means a community. Violent regional wars devastate entire cultures in Bosnia and the Sudan while Western nations hardly notice, except as their own interests are involved.

The Cold War ideological question "Whose side am I on?" no longer sets the international political agenda. Questions about loyalty permitted nations to change their minds when it seemed prudent to do so. "Who am I?" is a less flexible contemporary identity question. Only with difficulty can Serbs or Muslims or Chinese or Koreans change their minds about who they are, though inner conviction does result in identity change. Even so, while ideology provides individuals and nations with permeable boundaries, identity is deeply etched in peoples' formation and civilizational context. Those presuppositions and values are not readily relinquished, even by intent, though perhaps persons growing up with multiple cultural legacies, like children of mixed cultural parentage, may choose with which culture(s) to identify.

Helpful understandings of peacemaking touch people where they live: they are personal, pragmatic, practical. For peace to arise in conflict-ridden situations, leaders are required who are trusted by all in the conflict. Likewise, national governments, regional officials, and local leaders are all needed for different peacemaking tasks. As the South African case indicated, conflict itself may be grounded in and justified by different understandings of democracy in action.

Peacemakers of all faiths and in all nations will be increasingly challenged as identity questions become more central, old alliances fragment and new relationships emerge, shifting the global balance of power.[14] Peacemakers will be challenged to distinguish between the technological assets of modernity, various ideological and cultural presuppositions, and the community with which they identify and which they serve.

No matter with whom peacemakers' sympathies lie, all who seek to be peacemakers partake of and understand the cultural thought patterns, political structures, and interpersonal dynamics of the identity groups that formed them better than those of other peoples and groups. As a result, peacemakers increasingly work with local leaders and as part of multicultural teams.[15] In a world riddled by violent conflicts and a "clash of civilizations,"[16] the power of nonviolence is not enough; something like a politics of forgiveness is needed if people are to be(come) sane, whole, blessed.

What's Next?

Through long years of peace efforts, the HPC/FOR has learned that peaceworkers do not control what other people or nations do. As "servant leaders" they work for peace in a variety of ways matching their contexts and understandings. They seek to bless one another from their particular worldviews, perspectives, and angles of vision. However excellent, this incarnate behavior is confusing when they seek one-size-fits-all answers to questions of peacemaking.

One blessing the post-Cold War era offers is being disillusioned of the hope of achieving peace by thinking, living, working in one agreed-on way (building a single "tower" of Babel). All peoples rightly celebrate what has been given them, yet none has the ability to make peace in *their* image. Living as in-God's-image peacemakers, a different though modest learning HPC/FOR members have gained is not to insist on having things as we wish. That is a power even God relinquishes.

This by no means implies having no values, stance, or position. To the contrary, as is visible in Jesus' life, it means clearly articulating and living one's values and engaging others' perspectives and values, yet not equating their value with mutual agreement. God blesses all peoples with the ability to be peacemakers in their age, place, and context, and all peoples may be fulfilled by blessing one another, using their energies to imaginatively bring forth new life amid the real configurations of changing reality.

The foregoing reflections about things that make for peace highlight the centrality of context and identity as effective forces in reconciliation. Despite a human inclination to "fight or flight" in the face of violence, fear, humiliation, mistrust, hostility, and suffering, peacemakers are called to receive God's life-giving presence from one another. However understandable our efforts to control or evade conflict are, peacemakers know that violence simply goes underground when people seek to deny, evade, or contain it. Even when the lamb and lion lie down together, the lion does not become another lamb.

Peacemakers who work without force in communities subjected to violence are regularly challenged with the words, "But nonviolence doesn't work!" There are indeed many examples where nonviolence (like violence) fails to bring the wanted results. Nonviolence is not an effective way of imposing one's will on others without regard to their interests, though nonviolent strategies like those of Gandhi, King, and Romero can be effective means of social change and of empowering socially marginalized people. Nonviolence offers no guarantee that people will not suffer, but it does demonstrate that people who lack the clout of class or political and socioeconomic power can effectively exercise the power of shared identity.

The post-Cold War era's peacemaking dynamics can be dangerous. It is often lonely, difficult, and intimidating to be a peacemaker. It is lonely, as friends whose primary identity and loyalty is ordered by national priorities or ideologies are apt to have something of a "tower view" of God's kingdom rather than a from-the-margins view of God's kindom. It is difficult, because there is no sure recipe or formula, no reliable set of rules, no guarantee for success or of being understood or appreciated, and it is rarely clear whether one's efforts will take root and live. It is intimidating, since those in power are free to choose and are often deaf to requests for mercy or justice.

Perhaps the finest legacy of the historic peace churches is that they do not see peace as a pragmatic necessity calculated on the basis of need. The gift the HPC/FOR offers the wider church, and for which we often have been called irrelevant or naive, is the intent we live by. We understand peacemakers' fundamental identity and action to revolve less around concerns for security, risk, or loyalty to one's nation or religion and more around their commitment to love, to live as a member of God's kindom. Like healthy parents, teachers, ministers, lovers,[17] our peacemaking actions are a labor of love, a gift freely given.

A gift truly given is released. The desire to know how it is used or valued enmeshes and makes captive one's spirit much the same way as seeking vengeance when one is wronged. We believe peacemakers are less helped by asking, "Will this work?" or "Is peace possible?" than by asking, "How can I best live in (or as) God's image here and now?" or "Do I follow Jesus when I act this way?"—knowing that peacemakers in other traditions refer to the Divine Presence with other language.

Citizens of God's kindom are called simply to live God's presence where and as we/they are. Dispirited people who experience community after having been isolated or separated, and who find the strength to relinquish fear to act on their own behalf, experience empowerment and self-confidence. So peacemakers reconstruct and recreate the situations in and with which they live, always with an aim to strengthening the self-confidence of any who were violated, giving first priority to empowering all who are marginalized. Reconstruction imaginatively heals society by the restoration of living community and the exorcism of violence.[18] Here we call to mind the Genesis 1 story of God's creation of the world we know from "chaos."

Forgiveness, like reconstruction, is a spiritual work of peacemaking directly connected with and necessary for enduring social identity and nation building. When the one violated forgives a violator, it does not mean they are saying everything is now all right. Nor is forgiveness all that is needed, for it does not change material reality or restore justice. But forgiveness does break the cycle of vengeance and helps transform power relationships. A spiritual act that recalls one's power, forgiveness frees the one forgiving from the bondage of hostility toward the other. Thus the one violated is free *from* fear, anger, hostility, and desire for revenge, and free *for* creative, constructive work. Through a "politics of forgiveness," those materially victimized act as spiritual equals, thus restoring their sense of wholeness, autonomy, and freedom. When victims remain passive, by contrast, the victim-victimizing power relations are reinforced.

Christians tell how God's Divine Words gave birth to material reality, and how God's same creative Word became human in Jesus, a Palestinian Jew. Stories that people of faith tell and retell are a legacy to each generation to support and guide us, our children, and our children's children. A "politics of peacemaking," however global its vision, is grounded in practices that are local, in actions that are understood by, done with, and related to particular peoples, places, and situations. Shared actions build community and create a safe place to deliberate about further actions and needed change.

Like God's creation words, human words manifest in material reality what lies hidden in the heart. Like God's Jesus Word, human words take up residence and life in others' hearts and lives. People "do" theology by manifesting what is in their heart. The incarnate, actual, living power of behavior cannot be matched by faith words. Yet faith words witness to how people understand God present in each age and place, in each culture and situation. Throughout life, ears to hear and eyes to see may become more acute, finding God's presence moving among people, many of whose teachings we reject. Or we may see God's compassion in the actions of people we mistrust. Or hear God's Spirit amid questions, reflections, witness that trouble us.

Through our peacemaking work, members of the HPC/FOR know God works to renew all creation through people and in situations we find as surprising as Jesus' contemporaries found his actions. The blessing we offer from our legacy is that peacemakers find signs of God's creative work throughout God's whole household and creation, God's whole *oikos*.

Peacemakers will always be surprised by how God is present in places and cultures and situations they earlier resisted. Clinging to what we know about God's presence and action as if those signs themselves were sacred, people easily confuse their identity as members of God's kindom with their national or religious identity. So let us celebrate others' ways of being faithful as a God-given blessing. Let us rejoice that God prepares a table where all peoples and all creation are kin. Let us be open to the blessings of change, to being transformed by God's divine presence active in peacemakers of all nations and faiths.

Notes

Dedication

1. Quotes from M. R. Zigler are found in Donald F. Durnbaugh, *Pragmatic Prophet: The Life of Michael Robert Zigler* (Elgin, Ill.: Brethren Press, 1989), 191-192.

Chapter One

1. Contra Celsum. VIII, 55.

2. Justin, 1 Apol., XXXIX.

3. Bishop Nicolai Velimirovic, *The Prologue: Lives of the Saints*, vol. 3, entry for September 16 (Birmingham, England: Lazarica Press, 1986).

4. For an extensive review of primary church texts concerning war and military service, see Jean-Michel Hornus, *It Is Not Lawful for Me to Fight* (Scottdale, Pa.: Herald Press, 1980).

5. Ibid.

6. Ibid.

7. Butler, *Lives of the Saints*, vol. 3, entry for March 12. See also Robert Ellsberg, *All Saints* (New York: Crossroad Publishing Company, 1997), p. 112.

8. Ellsberg, p. 288.

9. Donald Attwater, *St. John Chrysostum* (London: Havrill Press, 1959), p. 72.

10. Father Stanley Harakas, *In Communion*, Orthodox Peace Fellowship Occasional Paper (May 1992).

11. For a thorough study of the life of St. Silouan and his writings, many of which concern the love of enemies, see Archimandrite Sophrony Sakharov, *St. Seraphim of Sarov* (Crestwood, N.Y.: St. Vladimir's Seminary Press, 1975).

12. Among various collections of Desert Father stories, a good beginning is Thomas Merton, *Wisdom of the Desert* (New York: New Directions, 1960).

13. *Communion and Otherness*, Orthodox Peace Fellowship Occasional Paper No. 19 (Summer 1994), pp. 1-4.

14. The most complete biography of Mother Maria in English is Serge Hackel, *Pearl of Great Price* (Crestwood, N.Y.: St. Vladimir's Seminary Press, 1981). An essay about her is in Ellsberg.

15. Valentine Sander, *St. Seraphim of Sarov* (Crestwood, N.Y.: St. Vladimir's Seminary Press), 1975.

16. Hackel.

Chapter Two

1. *Anthistemi* is the Greek word most frequently used in the Septuagint to translate the Hebrew *qum* and often carries the sense of "to rise up" against someone in revolt or war (Gen. 4:8; Num. 16:2; Judg. 9:35; 43; 20:33; 2 Chron. 13:6; Ps. 94:16 [93:16 LXX]; Isa. 14:22; Amos 7:9; Obad. 1; Hab. 2:7). *Epanistemi* is used synonymously: Deut. 19:11; 22:26; 33:11; Judg. 9:18; Job 20:27; 27:7; 30:12; Ps. 27:3; Isa. 31:2; Mic. 7:6. So also *katephistamai* (Acts 18:12—"made insurrection," KJV; "made a united attack," RSV); and *akatastasia* (Luke 21:9—"revolutions," JB; "insurrections," KJV, NEB). *Anthistemi* is also used of armed, violent warfare in 3 Macc. 6:19; Rom. 13:2; and Eph. 6:13. Liddell/Scott define it as "to set against, especially in battle." We can be virtually assured that it is used in Matt. 5:39 in the sense of "to resist forcibly" because the Jesus tradition elsewhere cites Mic. 7:6—"For the son treats the father with contempt, the daughter *rises up* against her mother, the daughter-in-law against her mother-in-law; a man's enemies are the men of his own house" (see Matt. 10:34-36; Luke 12:53). And Jesus may have formulated the statement about debtors giving their clothing to creditors in contrast to Hab. 2:7, where the wealthy are threatened with visions of debtors suddenly *rising up* in bloody revolt. Both passages use a form of *qum*.

2. Matthew and Luke are at odds on whether the outer garment (Luke) or the inner garment (Matthew) is being taken. But the Jewish practice of giving the outer garment as collateral for a loan makes it clear that Luke is correct.

3. *Babylonian Talmud, Babba Kamma* 92b.

4. Gerd Thiessen, *Biblical Faith: An Evolutionary Approach* (Philadelphia: Fortress Press, 1985), p. 122.

5. Therese de Coninck, ed., *Essays on Nonviolence* (Nyack, N.Y.: Fellowship of Reconciliation, n.d.), p. 38.

6. Josephus, *War* 2.172-74; *Antiquities* 18.55-59. Despite the similarity to a wolf's baring his throat to show he is overmastered, the two acts are polar opposites. The wolf is surrendering; these Jews were being defiant. The wolf seeks to save its life; these Jews were prepared to die for their faith. The Jews later tried the same tactic against the Emperor Gaius (Caligula) and again prevailed, aided by the providential death of the emperor (*Ant.* 18.257-309).

7. William Robert Miller, *Nonviolence* (New York: Schocken Books, 1966), p. 252.

8. "An Interview with Adolfo Perez Esquivel," *Fellowship* 51 (July/August 1985): 10.

9. Saul Alinsky, *Rules for Radicals* (New York: Random House, 1971).

10. Gandhi, *The Science of Satyagraha*, ed. Anand T. Hingorani (Bombay: Bharatiya Vidya Bhanan, 1970), p. 67.

11. Conversations with Doug Johnson and Elaine Lamay of INFACT.

Chapter Three

1. Jacob Boehme, "The Signature of All Things," in *The Signature of All Things, With Other Writings of Jacob Boehme* (London and Toronto: J. M. Dent and Sons Ltd.; New York: E. P. Dutton and Co., 1926), p. 22. Boehme was a German mystic who lived 1575-1624. For his early experiences, see also his *Aurora*.

2. John Woolman, *The Journal of John Woolman*, ed. Thomas S. Kepler (Cleveland and New York: The World Publishing Co., 1954), p. 1. The *Journal* has been published numerous times and is considered a classic in American Quaker history.

3. Woolman, *Journal*. Throughout his writing, Woolman repeatedly expresses his concern about Quakers who own slaves; see, for example, pp. 38-40.

4. John Woolman, "Considerations of the True Harmony of Mankind, and How It Is to Be Maintained," first printed 1770, in *A Journal of Life, Gospel Labours and Christian Experiences, of the Faithful Minister of Jesus Christ, John Woolman, to which are added His Last Epistle and Other Writings* (Philadelphia: Friends' Bookstore, 1876), p. 297.

Chapter Four

1. Set out in more detail in the book *Just Peacemaking*, ed. Glen Stossen (Cleveland, Ohio: Pilgrim Press, 1998).

2. Paper for the project by Paul Schroeder.

3. Paper by Michael J. Smith.

4. Paper by Bruce Russett, with some material from John Langan, S.J., on human rights and religious liberty. For some of the extensive empirical evidence, see Russett, *Grasping the Democratic Peace: Principles for a Post-Cold War World* (Princeton, N.J.: Princeton University Press, 1993); Spencer Weart, *Never at War: Why Democracies Will Never Fight Each Other* (New Haven, Conn.: Yale University Press, 1997); Bruce Russett, "Counterfactuals about War and Its Absence," in *Counterfactual Thought Experiments in World Politics: Logical, Methodological, and Psychological Perspectives*, ed. Philip Tetlock and Aaron Belkin (Princeton, N.J.: Princeton University Press, 1996).

5. Michelle Tooley, in *Voices of the Voiceless: Women Struggling for Human Rights in Guatemala* (Scottdale, Pa.: Herald Press, 1997), tells this story in a way that is both ethically informed and readably accessible for church members.

6. Paper by Susan Thistlethwaite, John Cartwright, and Gary Gunderson. For more extensive examples and engaging narrative, see Daniel Buttry, *Christian Peacemaking* (Valley Forge, Pa.: Judson Press, 1994).

7. Paper for the project by Glen Stassen.

8. Steven Brion-Meisels, David Steele, and Edward L. Long Jr.

9. See, for example, Yoder's "Sacrament as Social Process" in *The Royal Priesthood* (Grand Rapids, Mich.: Wm. B. Eerdmans, 1994).

10. Paper by Duane Friesen. For the work of groups in churches to bring about the East German nonviolent revolution, see Jörg Swoboda, *Revolution of the Candles*, trans. Richard Pierard (Atlanta: Mercer University Press, 1997); on Guatemala, see Tooley, *Voices of the Voiceless*.

11. John H. Yoder, *The Politics of Jesus* (Grand Rapids, Mich.: Wm. B. Eerdmanns, 1972); Walter Wink, *Engaging the Powers* (Minneapolis: Fortress Press, 1992); Glen H. Stassen, *Just Peacemaking: Transforming Initiatives for Justice and Peace* (Louisville, Ky.: Westminster/John Knox Press, 1992).

12. Stassen, *Just Peacemaking*, p. 46.

13. *Habits of the Heart*, ed. Robert Bellah, Richard Madsen, William M. Sullivan, Ann Swidler, and Steven M. Tipton (Berkeley, Los Angeles, and London: University of California Press, 1985).

14. Robert Wuthnow, *Acts of Compassion: Caring for Others and Helping Ourselves* (Princeton, N.J.: Princeton University Press, 1991), p. 156.

15. H. Richard Niebuhr, *Christ and Culture* (New York: Harper & Row, 1951).

Chapter Five

1. Quoted in Richard Falk, "Challenges of a Changing Global Order," *Peace Research* 24, no. 4 (November 1992): 18-19.

2. Samuel P. Huntington, "The Clash of Civilizations?" *Foreign Affairs* 72, no. 3 (Summer 1993): 22-49.

3. Ibid., p. 22.

4. Ibid., pp. 25-29.

5. Ibid., p. 27.

6. Dick Dougherty, "Yugoslavs: Scores to Settle," *The Honolulu Advertiser*, Sunday, March 7, 1993.

7. Luke 23:33-34, *The New Jerusalem Bible*. It is interesting to observe the NJB note that "some good and diverse ancient authorities" omit this verse.

8. For Islam, see Seyyed Hossein Nasr, *Ideals and Realities of Islam* (London, Sydney, Wellington: Unwin Hyman, 1988), p. 95; John L. Esposito, *Islam and Politics*, rev. 2nd ed. (Syracuse: Syracuse University Press, 1987). For Gandhi, see Gopinath Dhawan, *The Political Philosophy of Mahatma Gandhi* (Ahmedabad: Navajivan Publishing House, 1962).

9. Martin Luther King Jr., *Stride Toward Freedom* (New York: Harper and Row, 1958), p. 87.

10. The account of Kaunda's forgiveness is from Kenneth David Kaunda, *Kaunda of Violence*, ed. Colin Morris (St. James Place, London: Collins, 1980), pp. 178-184. The quotations are from pp. 180, 181, 182, respectively. See my discussion of Kaunda's change in Chaiwat Satha-Anand, "Exploring Myths on Nonviolence," *Gandhi Marg* 11, no. 3 (Oct.-Dec. 1989): 286-302.

11. Gene Sharp, *The Politics of Nonviolent Action, Part One: Power and Struggle* (Boston: Porter Sargent Publishers, 1973), p. 65. Emphasis in the original.

12. William Irwin Thompson, *Evil and World Order* (New York: Harper Colophon Books, 1977), p. 19.

13. Geiko Müller-Fahrenholtz, "Is Forgiveness in Politics Possible?" Paper given at International Peace Research Association Conference, Gronigen, Netherlands, July 3-7, 1990.

14. Ibid.

15. Bangkok *Post*, May 18, 1985.

16. John Berger and Jean Mohr, *A Seventh Man: A Book of Images and Words about the Experience of Migrant Workers in Europe* (London and New York: Writers and Readers, 1982), p. 178.

17. Aristotle, "The Varieties of Justice," in *Justice: Alternative Political Perspectives*, ed. James Sterba (Belmont, Calif.: Wadsworth Publishing Company, 1980), pp. 14-25.

18. See Glen D. Paige, Chaiwat Satha-Anand, and Sarah Gilliat, eds., *Islam and Nonviolence* (Honolulu, Hawaii: Center for Global Nonviolence Project, Matsunaga Institute for Peace, University of Hawaii, 1993); and Chaiwat Satha-Anand, *Islam e Nonviolenza* (Torino: Edizioni Gruppo Abele, 1997).

19. The Qu'ran used throughout this paper is *The Glorious Qu'ran*. Translation and commentary by A. Yusuf Ali (USA: The Muslim Students' Association of the United States and Canada, 1977). It should be noted that Yusuf Ali cautions that three words are used in the Qu'ran with a meaning close to "forgiveness." They are '*Afa*, which connotes forgetting; *Safaha*, which means to turn away or to treat a matter as if it did not affect one; and *Gafara*, which is an attribute of God (p. 47, note 110). I have touched upon the idea of forgiveness in relation to peacemaking relying on the life of Prophet Muhammad (*pbuh*) elsewhere. See Chaiwat Satha-Anand, "Core Values for Peacemaking in Islam: The Prophet's Practice as a Paradigm," in *Building Peace in the Middle East: Challenges for States and Civil Society*, ed. Elise Boulding (Boulder, Colo. and London: Lynne Rienner Publishers, 1994), pp. 295-302.

20. M. K. Gandhi, *Nonviolence in Peace and War*, vol. 1 (Ahmedabad: Navajivan Publishing House, 1948), pp. 1-2.

21. This prayer appeared in *Reconciliation International* (Fall 1991): 23.

Chapter Six

1. *The Kairos Document: Challenge to the Churches, A Theological Comment on the Political Crisis in South Africa* (Braamfontein, South Africa: Institute for Contextual Theology, 1985).

2. Charles Villa-Vicencio, *A Theology of Reconstruction: Nation-Building and Human Rights* (Cambridge: Cambridge University Press, 1992), p. 280.

3. *The Kairos Document*.

4. René Girard, *Things Hidden Since the Foundation of the World* (Stanford, Calif.: Stanford University Press, 1987), pp. 299-300.

5. See A. D. Lindsay, *The Churches and Democracy* (London: Epworth Press, 1934), p. 12ff.

6. Nicolai Berdyaev, *Slavery and Freedom* (London: Geoffrey Bles, 1943), p.

25.

7. Nicolai Berdyaev, *Truth and Revolution* (London: Geoffrey Bles, 1953), p. 18; see also Berdyaev, *The Meaning of the Creative Act* (London: Victor Gollancz, 1955), p. 156.

8. See J. D. Zizioulas, *Being as Communion* (Crestwood, N.Y.: SVS Press, 1985), p. 226, and Martin Buber, *I and Thou* (New York: Scribner, 1958), p. 62.

9. Berdyaev, *Slavery and Freedom*, p. 68.

10. Jaroslav Pelikan, "Orthodox Theology in the West: The Reformation," *The Legacy of Saint Uldimir: Byzantium, Russia, America*, ed. John Meyendorff (Crestwood, N.Y.: St. Vladimir's Seminary Press, 1990), pp. 164-165.

11. G. L. Frank, "Only the Saint is Truly Rational," unpublished paper, Pretoria, South Africa, 1996.

Chapter Seven

1. Pannalal Dasgupta, "A Minimum Programme of Action," *Gandhi Marg* 15, no. 3 (October-December 1993). Gandhian workers in today's India have probably given as much thought to the dynamics of this transformation from violence to nonviolence as any nonviolent activists today. M. L. Sharma's analysis of "People's Participation in Nonviolence" deals in depth with issues addressed here and follows Dasgupta's article in the same issue of *Gandhi Marg*.

2. The Union of International Associations (Brussels, Belgium) publishes the *Yearbook of International Organizations* biennually and has a computerized database available to scholars. I thank Anthony Judge and Jacqueline Nebel of UIA for providing me the above information from their database.

3. Figures updated 1997, courtesy Union of International Associations.

4. *The Muslim World, A Weekly Review of the Motamar* 32, nos. 3 & 4 (5-12 Safar 1415 AH): 6.

5. Sr. Mary Evelyn Jegen, *Sign of Hope: the Center for Peace, Nonviolence and Human Rights in Osijek* (Uppsala, Sweden: Life and Peace Institute, 1996).

6. Yeshua Moser edits the *Peace Teams/Peace Services Newsletter* from Nonviolence S.E. Asia, 495144 Soi yoo-omsin, Jaransanitwong 40 Rd, Bangkok 10700, Siam-Thailand. For a recent training manual, see *Empowerment for Peace Service: A Curriculum for Education and Training in Violence Prevention, Nonviolent Conflict Transformation and Peacebuilding* (Stockholm, Sweden: Unit for Justice, Peace and Creation of Christian Council of Sweden, 1996).

Chapter Nine

1. See, for example, Bruce Russett and William Antholis, "Do democracies fight each other? Evidence from the Peloponnesian War," *Journal of Peace Research* 29, no. 4 (1992): 415-435; Hazel M. McFerson, "Democracy and Development in Africa," *Journal of Peace Research* 29, no. 3 (1992): 241-248; and S. Gates, T. L. Knutsen, and J. W. Moses, "Democracy and peace: a more skeptical view," *Journal of Peace Research* 33, no. 1 (1996): 1-10.

2. Larry Diamond, *Promoting Democracy in the 1990's: Actors and instru-*

ments, issues and imperatives. A report to the Carnegie Commission on Preventing Deadly Conflict (New York: Carnegie Corporation, 1995), pp. 6-7.

3. Wilmot James, Daria Caliguire, and Kerry Cullinan, *Now That We Are Free: Coloured communities in a democratic South Africa* (Cape Town: IDASA), 1996.

4. Julian Sonn, "Breaking down the Borders," in James, Caliguire, and Cullinan.

5. African National Congress, *Reconstruction and Development Programme* (Johannesburg: Umanyano), 1994.

6. Davin Bremner, "Development's Catch-22," *Track Two* 3, no. 1 (1994): 1-5.

7. Hurst Hannum, "Minority Rights: Introduction," *The Fletcher Forum of World Affairs* 19, no. 1 (1995): 1-4.

8. Cyril Ramaphosa, "Power Sharing and Constitution Making," *Track Two* 5, no. 3 (1996): 12-14.

9. Andries Odendaal and Chris Spies, *Local Peace Committees in the Rural Areas of the Western Cape: Their Significance for South Africa's Transition to Democracy.* Occasional Paper, a *Track Two* Publication (1996).

10. See J. W. Burton, *Resolving Deep-Rooted Conflict: A Handbook* (New York: United Nations), 1987; Manfred Max-Neef, Antonio Elizialde, and Martin Hopenhayn, *Human Scale Development: Conception, Application and Further Reflections* (New York: Apex), 1991.

11. Burton.

12. A. Kaplan, J. Taylor, D. Marais, and S. Heyns, *Action Learning: Building Capacity for Development* (Cape Town: Juta), 1997.

Chapter Twelve

1. This chapter is based on two dozen interviews of people involved in civilian peace teams, in research funded and directed by the Life and Peace Institute of Sweden. The research is reported on more extensively in Lisa Schirch, *Keeping the Peace: Exploring Civilian Alternatives in Conflict Prevention* (Uppsala, Sweden: Life and Peace Institute, 1995).

2. See Johan Galtung, "Three Approaches to Peace: Peacekeeping, Peacemaking and Peacebuilding," and Johan Galtung and Helge Hveem, "Participants in Peacekeeping Forces," both in *Peace, War, and Defense: Essays in Peace Research,* ed. Christian Ejlers, vol. 2 (Copenhagen: PRIO, 1976).

Chapter Thirteen

1. Christian Peacemaker Teams Steering Committee minutes, October 10, 1993, revised April 16, 1994.

2. Other participating groups included Pax Christi, Peace Brigades International, Witness for Peace, and the Washington Office on Haiti.

3. FRAPH, the Front for Haitian Resistance and Progress (pronounced as *frappe,* French for "to hit"), was ostensibly the political wing of the Haitian military. Most of the violent attacks the team witnessed or heard about in Jeremie

were perpetrated by FRAPH members.

4. John Lancaster, "Hebron Daunting for Ex-D.C. Activist: Advocate's Efforts Result in Israeli Detention," *Washington Post*, Saturday, July 15, 1995, p. A16.

Chapter Fourteen

1. Ernie Regehr, "War After the Cold War: Shaping a Canadian Response," in *Ploughshares Working Paper 93-3* (Waterloo: Project Ploughshares, 1993).

2. This is articulated in John Paul Lederach, *Building Peace: Sustainable Reconciliation in Divided Societies* (Washington, D.C.: United States Institute of Peace, 1997).

3. Harold Saunders, *The Concept of Relationship* (Columbus, Ohio: Mershon Center, 1993).

Chapter Fifteen

1. For more details on the history of Mozambique, see Malyn Newitt, *A History of Mozambique* (Bloomington, Ind.: Indiana University Press, 1995). On the resistance struggle, see Eduardo Mondlane, *The Struggle for Mozambique* (New York: Penguin Books, 1996); H. Abrahamson and A. Nilsson, *Mozambique: The Troubled Transition from Socialist Construction to Free Market Capitalism* (London: Zed Books, 1995).

2. Much has been written about the war and the role of Rhodesia and South Africa. See, for example, Africa Watch, *Conspicuous Destruction: War, Famine, and the Reform Process in Mozambique* (New York: Human Rights Watch, 1992); H. Andersson, *Mozambique: A War Against the People* (London: Macmillan, 1992); M. Chincongo, *The State, Violence, and Development: The Political Economy of War in Mozambique—1975-1992* (London: Catholic Institute for International Relations, 1994); William Finnegan, *A Complicated War: The Harrowing of Mozambique* (Berkeley: University of California Press, 1992); D. Hoile, *Mozambique: A Nation in Crisis* (London: Claridge Press, 1989); D. Hoile, *Mozambique Resistance and Freedom: A Case for Reassessment* (London: Mozambique Institute, 1994); Lina Magaia, *Dumba Nengue: Run For Your Life, Peasant Tales of Tragedy in Mozambique* (Trenton, N.J.: Africa World Press, 1988).

3. See Andrea Ricardi, *Sant'Edgidio: Roma e il Mondo* (Paris: Beauchesne Editeur, 1996).

4. For accounts of the peace process, see C. Aldin and M. Simpson, "Mozambique: A Delicate Peace," *The Journal of Modern African Studies* 31, no. 1 (1993); Andrea Bartoli, "Somalia and Rwanda vs. Mozambique: Notes for Comparison on Peace Processes," in *Somalia, Rwanda and Beyond: The Role of the International Media in Wars and Humanitarian Crises*, ed. Edward Girardet (Geneva: Crosslines, 1995); Catholic Institute for International Relations, *The Road to Peace in Mozambique 1982-1992* (London: CIIR, 1994); Cameron Hume, *Ending Mozambique's War: The Role of Mediation and Good Offices* (Washington, D.C.: United

States Institute of Peace Press, 1994); Roberto Morozzo della Rocca, *Mozambico, dalla Guerra all Pace: Storia di una Mediazione Insolita* (Milan: Edizioni San Paolo, 1994); M. Vanancio, "Mediation by the Roman Catholic Church in Mozambique, 1988-1991," in *Mediation in Southern Africa* (London: Macmillan, 1993); Alex Vines and K. Wilson, "The Churches and the Peace Process in Mozambique," in *The Christian Churches and Africa's Democratization*, ed. P. Gifford (Leiden: Brill, 1995).

5. On the ONUMOZ process and elections, see L. Bowen, "Beyond Reform: Adjustment and Political Power in Contemporary Mozambique," *The Journal of Modern African Studies* 30, no. 2 (1992); Robert Lloyd, "Mozambique: The Terrors of War, the Tensions of Peace," *Current History* (April 1995); Richard Synge, *Mozambique: UN Peacekeeping in Action, 1992-1994* (Washington, D.C.: United States Institute of Peace Press, 1997); Alex Vines, *Angola and Mozambique: The Aftermath of Conflict* (Washington, D.C.: Research Institute for the Study of Conflict and Terrorism, 1995); UN Department of Public Information, *The United Nations and Mozambique: 1992-1995* (New York: United Nations Blue Book Series, 1995).

Chapter Sixteen

1. Biblical references to rights include, among others, Job 36:5-6; Ps. 82:3-4; Prov. 31:4-5, 8-9; Eccl. 5:8; Isa. 10:1-2; Jer. 5:27-28; Lam. 3:35; and Exod. 21:9-10.

2. Historic peace churches is a designation commonly applied to Mennonites, Friends (Quakers), and Church of the Brethren because of their rejection of war and official adherence to the teaching of biblical pacifism.

3. United Nations World Conference on Human Rights, Vienna Declaration and Program of Action, 1993, par. 5.

4. See Article 2 in each of the three instruments.

5. Treaties protecting members of vulnerable groups include, among others: the International Labor Organization (ILO) conventions on workers' rights; the Genocide Convention (1948); the Race Convention (1965); the Declaration of the Rights of Disabled Persons (1975); the Women's Convention (1979); the Declaration of the Elimination of All Forms of Intolerance and of Discrimination Based on Religion or Belief (1981); ILO Convention No. 169 Concerning Indigenous and Tribal Peoples in Independent Countries (1989); the Convention on the Rights of the Child (1989); the Declaration on the Rights of Persons belonging to National or Ethnic, Religious, or Linguistic Minorities (1992); the International Convention on the Protection of the Rights of All Migrant Workers and Members of Their Families (1990).

6. World Council of Churches First Assembly, Amsterdam, Report of the Church and the Disorder of Society (1948), quoted in Robert Traer, *Faith in Human Rights: Support in Religious Traditions for a Global Struggle* (Washington, D.C.: Georgetown University Press, 1991), p. 21.

7. On a global level, the major Catholic Church papal social encyclicals from *Rerum Novarum* in 1891 through *Centesimus Annus* in 1991 make language of natural and human rights integral to Catholic social theory. Key studies and

statements by global mainline Protestant church organizations include Lutheran World Federation, *Theological Perspectives on Human Rights*, 2 vols. (1977); World Alliance of Reformed Churches, Allen O. Miller, ed., *A Christian Declaration on Human Rights: Theological Studies of the World Alliance of Reformed Churches* (Grand Rapids, Mich.: Wm. B. Eerdmans, 1977); and the Baptist World Alliance, "Declaration on Human Rights," in *Celebrating Christ's Presence Through the Spirit: Official Report of the Fourteenth Congress* (1980), pp. 246ff.

Regional and national churches and ecumenical organizations have also produced numerous important human rights statements and studies. For references to Mennonite human rights views and activity, see Mennonite Central Committee, *Peace Office Newsletter* 25, no. 3 (July-September 1995). These official church statements provide the basis for the Christian views on human rights expressed here. More complete reference may be found in Martin Shupack, "The Demands of Dignity and Community: An Ecumenical and Mennonite Account of Human Rights," *Conrad Grebel Review* 14, no. 3 (Fall 1996): 241-258, which forms the basis for the first part of the present chapter.

8. World Alliance of Reformed Churches, *A Christian Declaration*, 144.

9. Recognition of this role of government recurs throughout the papal social encyclicals from *Rerum Novarum* to *Centesimus Annus*. It is also emphasized in Protestant documents, e.g., the statement "Toward a Just, Caring, and Dynamic Political Economy," adopted at the 197th General Assembly of the Presbyterian Church (USA) in 1985, printed in *Minutes of the General Assembly* Presbyterian Church (USA), 1985. See also the following Scripture texts addressed to rulers: Jer. 22:11-17; Prov. 31:8-9; Ps. 82:1-4.

10. See, for example, 2 Corinthians 8:13-15.

11. The right to own property is included in the Universal Declaration of Human Rights but not in the Covenants. International law does not recognize "free commerce" or the "the right to economic initiative" as a human right; though Catholic social teaching does acknowledge it, along with the right to hold property, as a right subordinate to the principle of the "universal destination of earth's goods," i.e., to the common benefit of all. See John Paul II, *On Social Concert*, par. 15; John Paul II, *Centessimus Annus*, par. 30, 31, 35; Paul VI, *Populorum Pogressio*, par. 22.

12. "Reaffirmation of the Opposition to War and Conscription for Military Training," Church of the Brethren Annual Conference, 1968, in *Words of Conscience*, ed. Beth Ellen Boyle, 10th ed. (Washington, D.C.: NISBCO, 1983), p. 70.

13. Douglas Gwyn, George Hunsinger, Eugene Roop, and John Howard Yoder, *A Declaration on Peace* (Scottdale, Pa.: Herald Press, 1991), pp. 86-87.

14. See L. William Yolton, "Conscientious Objection"(paper pub. Washington D.C. : NIBSCO, 1996) for a short history of conscientious objection.

Chapter Seventeen

1. Throughout this chapter, the words *Western civilization* or *Western nations* refer to the countries and culture of Western Europe and North America. Despite great diversity among these cultures, their shared history and world-

view is recognizably distinct from the history and culture of Asian, African, Latin American, Middle Eastern, and/or Eastern European countries.

2. Ecumenical/*oikumene* meaning "the whole household of God" and coming from the Greek root *oikos*, house. In this chapter, the word *ecumenical* is used in a global, not intra-Christian sense.

3. Persons and groups on the margins of power must understand both their own identity and culture and that of the more dominant power(s) around them. Western peoples may learn the value of diversity and the importance of other peoples values and perspectives (long known to Eastern and Southern countries) if they recognize and accept the decline of their hegemony.

4. See Dorothy Sayers' "Problem Picture" in *The Mind of the Maker* (San Francisco: Harper Collins, 1997); originally published 1941.

5. Kin-dom, in contrast to king-dom, indicates the kin-ship of all human-kind.

6. See especially ch. 4.

7. See especially chs. 5, 7.

8. Gen. 1:28.

9. See especially chs. 5, 8.

10. See ch. 2. Wink's thought is practical, pragmatic, and not ideological. He presupposes that in Jesus' context there would have been public knowledge of such incidents. Wink is clear that the abused must know and use the prevailing legal provisions. And he is aware that Jesus' teachings are less readily applicable to systemic violence than to individuals responding to their oppressors.

11. See especially Gen. 1, 3.

12. One reading of the Genesis 1–11 stories notes the escalations of violence throughout. See Ulrich Duchrow and Gerhard Liedke, *Shalom: Biblical Perspectives on Creation, Justice and Peace* (Geneva, Switzerland: WCC Publications, 1998), especially pp. 47ff.

13. See "Fencerow Theology: Spiritual Openness to the Cosmic God," in Stephen L. Longenecker, ed., *The Dilemma of Anabaptist Piety: Strengthening or Straining the Bonds of Community?* (Forum for Religious Studies, Bridgewater College, Bridgewater, Va.: Penobscot Press, 1997). See also chs. 7, 9, 10.

14. See ch. 4. As other civilizations come into more power, Western nations will be challenged to relinquish the dependence on exercising force and learn to achieve their ends by other means. Also, in his *The Clash of Civilizations and the Remaking of the World Order* (New York: Simon and Schuster, 1996), Samuel P. Huntington observes that the West separated the functions of "God and Caesar" and gained dominance less through "ideas or values or religion [than] by its superiority in applying organized violence. Westerners often forget this fact; non-Westerners never do," p.51.

15. These chapters (see esp. ch. 10) have consistently emphasized the need for local initiative. In addition, inasmuch as peacemakers often understand themselves as counter-cultural because of deep ideological or ethical dissent from the public policies of their own nations, their self-identity may be organized around global rather than national identity questions. If identity concerns be-

come more important in conflicted situations, peacemakers' identity and self-understanding (as global citizens) may strongly differ from others' perception of them (as disloyal to us).

16. Satha-Anand's reference to Huntington (ch. 5, n. 4) was expanded in Huntington's book cited in note 14.

17. For example, mystics, who hardly expect God to protect or secure their life.

18. See especially ch. 6.

Bibliography for Further Reading

BIBLICAL/THEOLOGICAL

Bailie, Gil. *Violence Unveiled: Humanity at the Crossroads*. New York: Crossroad Publishing Company, 1997.

Friesen, Duane K. *Christian Peacemaking and International Conflict: A Realist Pacifist Perspective*. Scottdale, Pa.: Herald Press, 1986.

Gwyn, Douglas, George Hunsinger, Eugene F. Roop, and John Howard Yoder. *A Declaration on Peace: In God's People the World's Renewal Has Begun*. Scottdale, Pa.: Herald Press, 1991.

Hauerwas, Stanley. *The Peaceable Kingdom: A Primer in Christian Ethics*. Notre Dame, Ind.: University of Notre Dame Press, 1983.

Kraybill, Donald. *The Upside-Down Kingdom*. Rev. ed. Scottdale, Pa.: Herald Press, 1990.

Miller, Marlin E., and Barbara Nelson Gingerich, eds. *The Church's Peace Witness*. Grand Rapids, Mich.: Wm. B. Eerdmans, 1994.

Müller-Fahrenholz, Geiko. *The Art of Forgiveness: Theological Reflections on Healing and Reconciliation*. Geneva, Switzerland: WCC Publications, 1997.

Stassen, Glen H. *Just Peacemaking: Transforming Initiatives for Justice and Peace*. Louisville, Ky.: Westminster/John Knox Press, 1992.

Swartley, Willard M., ed. *The Love of Enemy and Nonretaliation in the*

New Testament. Louisville, Ky.: Westminster/John Knox Press, 1992.

Wink, Walter. *Engaging the Powers: Discernment and Resistance in a World of Domination*. Minneapolis, Minn.: Fortress Press, 1992.

———. *Healing A Nation's Wounds: Reconciliation on the Road to Democracy*. Uppsala, Sweden: Life and Peace Institute, 1996.

Volf, Miroslav. *Exclusion and Embrace: A Theological Exploration of Identity, Otherness, and Reconciliation*. Nashville, Tenn.: Abingdon Press, 1996.

Yoder, John Howard. *For the Nations: Essays Public and Political*. Grand Rapids, Mich.: Wm. B. Eerdmanns, 1997.

———. *The Politics of Jesus*. 2d ed. Grand Rapids, Mich.: Wm. B. Eerdmanns; Carlisle, U.K.: The Paternoster Press, 1995.

PEACEMAKING PRACTICE

Lederach, John Paul. *Building Peace: Sustainable Reconciliation in Divided Societies*. Washington, D.C.: United States Institute of Peace Press, 1997.

———. *Preparing for Peace: Conflict Transformation Across Cultures*. Syracuse, N.Y.: Syracuse University Press, 1996.

Sampson, Cynthia, and John Paul Lederach, eds. *From the Ground Up: Mennonite Contributions to International Peacemaking*. Syracuse, N.Y.: Syracuse University Press, 1998.

Yarrow, C. H. Michael. *Quaker Experiences in International Conciliation*. New Haven, Conn. and London, England: Yale University Press, 1978.

Index

A

Accompaniment, 101, 161-162
    See also peace teams
African National Congress (ANC),
        80-82, 120-126
Alinsky, Saul, 44, 45, 46
    Rules for Radicals, 44
Amnesty International, 211. *See also*
        Human rights
Annan, Kofi, 154
Apartheid, 80, 81-84
    rationale for, 85
    struggle against, 82-83, 119-124
    laws:
            Coloured Labour Prefe-
                rence Act, 121, 124
            Group Areas Act, 124
Aristide, President Jean Bertrand,
        163, 169, 171
Asia, 58, 68, 102, 225, 226

B

Balkan Peace Team, 161-163. See also
        Peace teams
Balkans, 161
    Yugoslavia (former), 57, 70,
        105-118, 153-155, 161-164
    Kosova, 98, 191
    Belgrade, 111, 115
    Bosnia, 58, 67-70, 105-117, 168,
        Sarajevo, 70, 107, 112, 116
    Mostar, 109
    Neretva River, 109
    Bihac, 117
    Gorazde, 117
    Pale, 117

Croatia, 70, 106-107, 110-113,
        116-117
    Osijek, 102
Baptist Church, 61, 115, 205
Berdyaev, Nicolai, 88, 89
Berlin Wall, 13, 68
Berlinguer, Enrico, 195
Boehme, Jakob, 48, 49
Boutros-Ghali, Boutros, 154
Brandt, Chancellor Willy, 59, 60
Burundi, 154, 191
Bush, President, 59

C

Caesar, 24, 26, 39, 42
Cambodia, 67, 74, 98, 163, 221
Child Soldiers, 205, 212, 215
Chissano, President Joachim, 196, 201
Christian Peacemaker Teams (CPT),
        102, 161-164, 168-176. *See
        also* Peace teams
Christian church
    Body of Christ, 210, 225
    community, 63-65, 81, 87-89, 207
    early church, 25-27
    new humanity, 207
    peace witness, 154, 155, 159
Cry for Justice Coalition, 163, 169. *See
        also* Peace teams, Haiti
Church of the Brethren, 168, 176, 210,
        220. *See also* Historic peace
        churches
Civil rights movement, 58, 207
Civil society, 63, 96, 197
    citizen's groups, 18, 57, 142
    grassroots peacemaking groups,

60, 64, 98, 99
Clans, racial groups, ethnicity:
  Afrikaner, 80, 85
  Ajuran, 135, 136
  Boran people, 136
  Degodia people, 135, 136
  Griqua people, 122
  Kenyan Somalis, 133, 148
  Khoi-San people, 122
  Nazis, 31, 42, 59, 111
  Nomadic herders/pastoralists,
    133, 148
  Ogaden, 135
  "Blacks", "Whites", "Col-
    oureds", 120-132
  "Contra," 163
Clinton, Bill, 170
Cold War (end of), 9-14, 55, 58, 68, 154,
  219-228
Colombia, 161, 165, 177, 178, 210
Community of St. Egidio, 190-202
Conflict resolution, 119, 163, 177-189,
  190-202
  community-based, 128-148, 156
  just peacemaking initiative, 59,
    62
  in Mozambique, 190-202
  post-conflict situations in,
    177-189
  role of community of faith in,
    96-104
  training, 131, 140, 157, 171, 179.
    See also Peacebuilding
Conflict (causes of):
  ethnic conflict, 57, 67, 103,
    112-114, 128-129, 225
  ethnic cleansing, 83, 108,
    119, 120
  intolerance, 120, 158
  nationalism, 31, 57
  racial conflict, 57, 83, 114, 119,
    128-129
    racism, 31, 120, 121, 158
  religious conflict, 57, 67, 70, 225
    intolerance, 112, 114, 158
  tribalism, 31
    inter-clan conflict, 133-148
Congo, 67, 154, 165
Conscientious objection to military
  service, 205, 210-215

Culture of peace, 9, 19, 95-104
Cycle of violence, 74, 140, 183, 229

D
Demobilization of combatants, 156,
  186-188, 201, 212
Dhlakama, Alfonso, 196
Discipleship, 61-65

E
Early Christian saints, 25-32
East (the), 219, 220
Economic development:
  economic justice, 80, 157
  exploitative, 99
  relationship to peace teams
    work, 164
  relationship to peacemaking,
    147, 155, 188
  relationship to conflict, 128-129,
    135
  right to, 204
  sustainable development, 58, 63
Esquivel, Adolfo Perez, 44, 98
Ethiopia, 133-136
Europe, 44, 48
  Central/Eastern, 18, 58, 102 114,
    220, 221, 225

F
Fellowship of Reconciliation (FOR), 9,
  15, 105-118, 220
Forgiveness:
  as Christian teaching, 28, 30, 203
  as political strategy, 59-60, 66,
    68-78, 227
  spiritual aspect of reconciliation,
    95-96, 188, 229. See also
    Reconciliation
Fox, George, 211
FRAPH, 171
Friends World Committee for Consul-
    tation, 215. See also Quakers
FRELIMO, 191-196, 200

G
Galtung, Johan, 161
Gandhi:
  legacy, 85, 98, 223
  nonviolent actions, 45, 58, 101,
    166-228
  thought, 45, 69, 75-87

Genocide, 103, 106-108, 111-117
Germany, 23, 59, 60, 102, 195
    Oder-Neisse Frountier, 60
    Silesia, Pomerania, East Prussia,
        60. *See also* Berlin Wall
Gersony, Robert, 193
Girard, René, 84
Globalization, 16, 19, 56
Gonçalves, Bishop Jaime (Bishop of
        Beira), 194-197
Gorbachev, President, 58, 59
Goulding, Marrack, 153
Guatemala, 58, 60, 161, 162,177, 190

H
Haiti, 57, 161-171
    Port au Prince, 170, 171
    Jeremie, 169, 171
Harakas, Father Stanley, 27, 28
Historic Peace Churches, 9, 15, 158,
        204-210, 220-228. *See also*
        HPC/FOR
HPC/FOR, 221-229
    HPC/FOR Committee, 11, 14, 16
Human rights, 203-216, 220
    individualism and, 86
    in just peacemaking theory,
        56-58, 66
    monitors of, 169
    movements, 58
    law, 17, 205
        Civil and political rights,
            204
        International Covenant of,
            205
        Economic, social, and
            cultural rights, 204
    in South African Constitution,
        129
    relationship to armed conflict,
        155, 214
    Universal Declaration of, 205
    violations of, 161, 165, 170
        In Mozambique, 191
        In South Africa, 83, 123
        Reporting on, 210-213
    World Conference on, 205
Humanitarian Intervention:
    aid, 101, 156, 195, 201
    military, 57, 155, 165. *See also*

    Peacekeeping
Huntington, Samuel P, 69

I
Image of God (divine image), 206-207,
    211, 224-228
India, 58, 68, 70, 77, 166
Interfaith Cooperation, 80, 109,
    112-113
International Law, 203-205. *See also*
    Human rights law
Interpositioning, 101, 162, 166. *See also*
    Peace teams
Intifadah, 58, 172-174
Islamic Thought, 69, 75-76, 78
Israel/Palestine, 59, 164, 221
    Hebron, 163, 168, 169, 172-176
    Palestine, 37, 38, 58, 66
    Jerusalem, 42, 45, 134
        Fortress Antonio, 42
    Il Ibrahimi Mosque/Cave of
        Machpelah, 172
    Kiryat Arba, 172, 174
Italy:
    Communist Party of, 195
    government of, 196-200
    Rome, 193-201
    Trastevere, 194

J
Janzen, Mark, 13
Jews/Jewish, 29, 38-42, 96, 107-116,
    172, 176
Just War Tradition, 27, 53, 55, 83
Just Peacemaking Theory, 15, 53-67

K
Kaunda, Kenneth, 69, 71, 72
Kennedy, President, 58
Kenya, 98, 102, 133-148, 195-196
    Rift Valley Province, 145, 147
    Wajir District, 133-148
    Mandera, 140, 145
    Garissa, 140, 145
    Nairobi, 140, 157
    Moyale, 145
Khalif, Hamad, 139
Kindom of God, 223-230.
        See also Reign of God
King, Jr., Martin Luther, 40, 59, 71, 223,
    228

Kingdom of God, 62, 65, 228

L
Latin America, 18, 58, 221, 226
League of Nations, 56, 211
Liberation Theology, 80, 81, 86
Love of Enemies, 27-28, 53-55, 83
Luthuli, Albert, 80, 82

M
Machel, President Samora, 192
Machel, Graça, 216
Mandela, President Nelson, 80
Mediators, 139, 197, 202
    third-party, 129, 198
    insider-partial, 165, 166
    use of experts, 200
Mennonite Central Committee, 58,
    102, 144-145
Mennonites, 61, 110, 113, 154, 168, 176,
    210, 220. *See also* Historic
    peace churches
Mexico, 102, 168
    Chiapas, 161
Mohammed, The Prophet, 75, 106
Mondlane, Eduardo, 191
Mozambique, 190, 202, 216
    Parliament of, 200. *See also* FRE-
    LIMO, RENAMO
Mugabe, President Robert, 71, 193
Muslims, 68, 96, 102, 107-116, 143, 172,
    176, 220, 226. *See also* Islamic
    thought, Qu'ran

N
Namibia, 153, 154
Negotiations:
    crisis, short-term, 179
    cease-fire, 163, 200, 221
    in Mozambique, 195-197
    official talks, 185, 186
    UN brokered, 153. *See also* Peace-
    making, Peacebuilding
Nicaragua, 161-163, 188
Non-governmental organizations
    (NGO):
    growth of, 16,18, 99-100
    international (INGO), 60, 216
    faith-based, 100-101, 190-191
    role in Wajir, 136, 145
nonviolence, 40-46, 207, 227

civil disobedience, 176
Jesus' teaching of, 32-47
non-retaliation, 46
nonviolent direct action, 40-43,
    58, 62, 69-78, 164, 169
public witness, 171
religion and, 100
resistance, 34
short-term delegations, 171
strategies of, 228
    Emergency response net-
        works, 163
    Infant formula boycott,
        45-46
    Ahimsa, satya, 77
    Boycotts, 128
    Demonstration, 170
    Zones of peace, 54-57, 103,
        104, 162, 175
in South Africa, 83
unarmed resistance, 31, 50
Northern Ireland, 58, 59, 70, 177
    West Belfast, 177

O
Orthodox Church (Eastern), 26-27, 68,
    87, 109-112
Orthodox Peace Fellowship, 32

P
Peace Brigades International, 102,
    161-166, 176. *See also* Peace
    teams
Peace teams, 102, 161-176
Peace presence, 162, 170-173, 176. *See
    also* Peace teams
Peacebuilding, 223
    community-level, 121, 127
    post-conflict phase, 154, 156,
        177-189
    relationship to activism, 164,165
    relationship to democracy, 119
    spiritual dimensions of, 188
    training for, 100.
Peacekeeping:
    armed, 153-156, 160-162, 223
    civilian, *See* peace teams
Peacemaking:
    in Jesus' teaching, 32-47, 61-62,
        69, 70-71
        Beatitudes, 32, 62

transforming initiatives, 56,
62, 64
role of personal relationships in,
202
role of religious organizations in,
166
role of traditional elders in, 139,
141, 147, 165
role of women in, 138, 165-166
strategies for,
de-escalation, 59
interpositioning, 162
mediation, 156, 163, 179,
191, 197
off-the-record meetings, 214
peace festivals, 143
preventive diplomacy, 156.
See also Nonviolence,
Peacebuilding
Pelikan, Jaroslav, 89
Penn, William, 101
Persian Gulf War, 75, 107, 162
Philippines, 58, 162
Poland, 58-60
Warsaw, 60
Portugal, 191
Colonialism, 191-192
Lisbon, 192
Post-War Recovery, 155, 156
associative interventions, 162
buffer zones, 162
building peace infrastructure,
185
disaster management, 179
dissociative interventions, 162
landmines (clearance of), 156
multi-party elections, 201, 204
Election monitors, 171
relief work, 156, 160
restorative justice, 208, 209
violence prevention, 153, 156. See
also Peacebuilding, Reconciliation
Prayer for enemies, 28-29, 51, 95, 106

Q
Quaker Peace and Service, 144-145
Quaker United Nations Office, 160,
210-216
Quakers (Society of Friends), 49-50,

102, 115, 168, 176, 220. See
also Historic peace churches
Qu'ran, 75, 76, 140

R
Reconciliation:
church work in, 157, 163
in Cambodia, 74
in South Africa, 83-84
post-conflict, 59, 177-189
role of faiths in, 96-97, 227
Refugees:
accompaniment of, 162
as a human rights issue, 215
Bosnian, 108, 112-113
camps, 163
churches' work with, 56, 154
in Kenya, 135-136
Mozambican, 197
repatriation, 156
internally displaced people, 197,
215
Reign of God, 44, 46, 61-65, 80,
223-224. See also Kingdom of
God
RENAMO, 192-200
Roman Catholic Church, 87, 106-112,
176, 190-196, 204-205
Roman Empire, 23-25, 35-40, 46
policy of, 37-38
Rwanda, 14, 57, 68, 154, 165, 179

S
Selly Oaks College, 146
Shanti Sena, 101, 116. See also Peace
teams
Sharp, Gene, 72
Skobtsova, Mother Maria, 31-33
Somalia, 133-136, 154
military intervention, 12, 57, 153
South Africa, 14, 79-91, 119-132, 154,
226
freedom campaign, 58
government of:
National Peace Accord, 129
Reconstruction and De-
velopent Programme,
121, 126-127
Role in Mozambique, 196,
198
Truth and Reconciliation

Commission, 83
Western Cape, 120-132
   Grabouw, 124-127
   Mossel Bay, 126-127
South (the), 219, 220
Soviet Union/Russian Federation, 14,
   18, 30, 58, 192, 212-214
   collapse, 225
   Gulag Archipelago, 30
   Soviet Bloc, 192-198
   Chechnya, 168, 213
Spirituality, 64, 96
   inner light, 51,52
   mysticism, 48-51
   experience of presence of God,
      49-52
   of struggle, 81
St. Giles/St. Egidio, 194

T
Tambo, Oliver, 80
Theology of Reconstruction, 70-90
Track-one Diplomacy, 18,156,160,190,
   199
Track-two Diplomacy, 18,156,160. *See
   also* Peacemaking, strategies
   for; Peacebuilding
Trauma:
   war-related, 70-74, 108, 132, 177
   healing of, 103, 157, 188, 208

U
United States of America (USA),
   105-118
   black theology in, 80
   civil rights movement in, 58, 207
   democracy in, 86
   government of, 59, 114, 193-196,
      200
   Los Angeles, 157, 164, 168
   New York, 75, 153, 172, 201
   peace movements in, 44, 48, 210
   Pennsylvania, 50, 51
   Washington, D.C., 164, 168-169,
      175-176
   in World War II, 31
United Nations (UN),
   Commission on Human Rights,
      215
   Committee on the Rights of the
      Child, 215-216
Department of Political Affairs,
   153
General Assembly, 216
part of just peacemaking theory,
   56-57, 65
relationship with NGOs, 16-17,
   99, 158-159, 166, 211-216
Secretariat / Secretary General,
   154, 155
Security Council, 17, 154, 155
observers, 165-166
ONUMOZ, 200-210
UNESCO, 97, 100
UNHCR, 156
UNICEF, 46, 136, 144
World Health Organization, 46.
   See also Peacekeeping,
   Human rights monitors

V
Victims:
   church support of, 157
   healing for, 208, 229
   in thought of Girard, 83-84
   relationship with victimizers,
      71-78, 229
   solidarity with, 163
Villa-Vicencio, Charles, 80, 81
Wajir Peace Group, 133-148

W
Weapons, 56, 98, 101
   atomic/nuclear, 54, 58-59, 67, 104
   reductions, 62
   systems, 135, 145
   trade, 58, 66, 154
West (the), 70, 75, 86, 96, 165, 209, 226
   society, culture, 207, 219-222
   civilization, 219
   culture, 222
Witness for Peace, 102, 161-163. *See
   also* Peace teams
Woolman, John, 49, 50, 51
World Council of Churches, 9, 11, 220,
   205
   Programme to Overcome Vio-
      lence, 9, 11-12
World War II, 31, 54, 78, 210

Y
Yoder, John Howard, 59

THE CONTRIBUTORS

Dr. Andrea Bartoli is Director of the SIPA International Conflict Resolution Program at Colombia University, New York, USA, and chair of the university's Seminar on Religions and Conflict Resolution. Previously he was Professor of Social Anthropology in the School of Public Health at the University of Rome, Italy. He has been actively involved in conflict resolution and preventive diplomacy since the early 1980s as vice-president of the Community of St. Egidio, especially in Mozambique, Algeria, Guatemala, Kosovo, Albania,and Burundi. He was co-editor of *Somalia, Rwanda and Beyond: The Role of the International Media in Wars and Humanitarian Crises* (Crosslines, 1995).

Dr. Elise Boulding is Professor Emerita of Sociology and former Chair, Department of Sociology, Dartmouth College, Massachusetts. She has been Secretary General of the International Peace Research Association, chair of the Women's International League for Peace and Freedom, and board member, American Friends Service Committee. Her publications include *The Underside of History: A View of Women Through Time* (Sage Publications), and *Building a Global Civic Culture* (Syracuse University Press).

Rachel Brett is Associate Representative in the Quaker United Nations Office, Geneva, Switzerland. She holds a degree in International Human Rights Law from the University of Essex, U.K., and previously taught law at the University of Essex. She was originator and principal researcher of the Essex Human Rights Centre's project on the Organization on Security and Cooperation in Europe. Her most recent publication is *Children: The Invisible Soldiers*, with co-author Margaret McCallum (Stockholm, Radda Barnen, 1996).

Jim Forest is Secretary for the Orthodox Peace Fellowship. Previously he was General Secretary for the International Fellowship of Reconciliation, based in Netherlands. He is author of *Praying with Icons* (Orbis, 1997), *Love is the Measure: A biography of Dorothy Day* (Orbis, 1994), *Living with Wisdom: A Biography of Thomas Merton* (Orbis, 1991), and two books on religious life in Russia, *Pilgrim to the Russian Church* (Crossroad, 1988) and *Religion in the New Russia* (Crossroad, 1990).

Dr. Duane K. Friesen is Professor of Bible and Religion at Bethel College, Kansas. He is author of *Christian Peacemaking and International Conflict: A Realist Pacifist Perspective* (Herald Press, 1986) and a contributor to *Protest, Power and Change: An Encyclopedia of Nonviolent Action from ACT-UP to Women's Sufferage* (Garland Publishing, 1997). Dr. Friesen is a member of the Historic Peace Churches/Fellowship of Reconciliation Consultative Committee.

Robert Herr and Judy Zimmerman Herr are Co-Directors of the International Peace Office for Mennonite Central Committee. Their academic studies were in economic development and theology. Previously they were Mennonite Central Committee administrators for Southern Africa. Their most recent work for publication was a contribution to the book *From the Ground Up: Mennonite Experiences in International Conciliation* (Syracuse University Press, 1998). Judy is a member of the Historic Peace Churches/Fellowship of Reconciliation Consultative Committee.

Doug Hostetter is International/Interfaith Secretary for the Fellowship of Reconciliation USA in Nyack, New York, and director for the Bosnian Student Project. He has worked previously as Executive Secretary for the FOR-USA and as Executive Secretary of the American Friends Service Committee New England Regional Office. He has worked at active nonviolence in Vietnam, Nicaragua, El Salvador, Israel/Palestine, Iraq, and Bosnia. He has published widely in periodicals, and his account of the Bosnian Student Project was published as a Pendle Hill Pamphlet in 1997. He is a member of the Historic Peace Churches/Fellowship of Reconciliation Consultative Committee.

Dekha Ibrahim is Deputy Coordinator of the Nomadic Health Care Project in Wajir District, Kenya. She is the secretary of the Wajir Peace and Development Committee and one of the founders of Wajir Women for Peace. She has conducted peace and mediation training in Africa and has been a trainer at the "Responding to Conflict" program of Selly Oaks College, University of Birmingham, U.K., where she also received her formal conflict resolution training. Formerly she worked as a primary school teacher in Wajir, Kenya.

David Jackman is Associate Representative for the Quaker United Nations Office in New York. He specializes in disarmament, preventive diplomacy, peacekeeping, and postconflict peacebuilding. He has worked as a Programme Associate for Project Ploughshares in Waterloo, Canada, and as an organizer of nonviolence and conflict resolution workshops. He has been a member of the Canadian Friends Service Committee. Publications include articles in various peace movement and church periodicals.

Janice Jenner is a graduate student in the Conflict Transformation Program of Eastern Mennonite University, Harrisonburg, Virginia, where she also teaches classes in cross-cultural learning. From 1989 to 1996 she served as Co-Country Representative for the Mennonite Central Committee in Kenya and was involved in peace and justice work in East Africa.

Kathleen Kern is a volunteer with Christian Peacemaker Teams, with significant involvement in Haiti and the West Bank/Palestine. She is a graduate from Colgate-Rochester Divinity School, New York, and has worked as a curriculum writer for Bible Study Guides for the Mennonite Church for the past eight years. She is author of *When it Hurts to Live* (Faith and Life Press, 1994) and *We Are the Pharisees* (Herald Press, 1995).

Dr. John Paul Lederach is Professor in the Conflict Transformation Program of Eastern Mennonite University, Virginia. He has served as Director of International Conciliation Services for Mennonite Central Committee and continues as a consultant for MCC's work in international conciliation. He has done training in conflict resolution and worked at mediating conflicts in Nicaragua, Somalia, the Phillippines, Northern Ireland, and elsewhere. Among his recent publications are *Preparing for Peace: Conflict Transformation Across Cultures* (Syracuse University Press, 1995) and *Building Peace: Sustainable Reconciliation in Divided Societies* (U.S. Institute of Peace, 1997).

Dr. Lauree Hersch Meyer is Doctor of Ministry Program Director and Associate Professor of Theology at Colgate Rochester Divinity School, New York. She was Professor of Biblical Theology and Interpretation at Bethany Theological Seminary. She has been a participant in ecumenical conversations internationally and through membership in the Faith and Order Commission of the National Council of Churches of the USA. Recent publications include contributions to *The Dilemma of Anabaptist Piety* (Penobscot Press, 1997) and *Should God Get Tenure? Essays on Religion and Higher Education* (Eerdmanns, 1997). Dr. Meyer is a member of the Historic Peace Churches/Fellowship of Reconciliation Consultative Committee.

Dr. Andries Odendaal is Senior Researcher and Trainer in the Saamspan Project of the Centre for Conflict Resolution, Cape Town, South Africa. He was Senior Lecturer in the Faculty of Theology, University of the North, and Regional Coordinator for the Western Cape Peace Committee. Previous publications include a chapter in *New Agendas for Peace Research*, edited by Elise Boulding (Lynne Reinner, 1992), as well as an Occasional Paper published in 1996 by *Track Two* with Chris Spies, titled "Local Peace Committees in the Rural Areas of the Western Cape."

Dr. Gerald Pillay is Professor of Theology and Head of the Department of Theology and Religious Studies at the University of Otago, Dunedin, New Zealand. Previously he was Professor of Church History at the University of South Africa. Dr. Pillay is author of *Religion at the Limits*, *Albert Luthuli* (vol. 1, Voices of Liberation), and a contributor to *A History of Christianity in South Africa* as well as to other volumes.

Dr. Chaiwat Satha-Anand (Haji Qader Muheideen), founder and director of Peace Information Center, teaches political science at Thammasat University, Bankok, Thailand, where he introduced the first university course in Thailand on nonviolence over a decade ago. He is a member of the International Peace Research Association and former convener of their Nonviolence Commission. His most recent publications include *Peace Theory/Cultural Means* (Bangkok: Komol Keemthong Foundation, 1996); *Islam e Nonviolenza* (Torino: Edizioni Gruppo Abele, 1997); and as co-editor, *The Frontiers of Nonviolence* (IPRA Nonviolence Commission; Honolulu: Center for Global Nonviolence; Bangkok: Peace Information Center, 1998).

Lisa Schirch is Assistant Professor in the Conflict Transformation Program of Eastern Mennonite University, Virginia. She is a Ph.D. candidate in Conflict Analysis and Transformation at George Mason University and author of *Keeping the Peace: Exploring Civilian Alternatives in Conflict Prevention* (Life and Peace Institute, Sweden, 1995).

Martin Shupack is Legislative Associate for International Affairs in the Mennonite Central Committee's Washington, D.C. Office. He holds a J.D. degree from Harvard Law School in international law and has worked as a pastor and community organizer in the United States and under the Mennonite Central Committee in Mexico. His publications include articles in the *Harvard Human Rights Journal*, the *Conrad Grebel Review*, and in church publications.

Dr. Dorothee Soelle studied classical philology, philosophy, theology, and German literature and has taught at various German educational institutions from 1954 to 1975. She was Harry Emerson Fosdick Visiting

Professor at Union Theological Seminary in New York from 1978 to 1987. She now works as a freelance writer of theology and poetry in Hamburg, Germany, and as an activist for peace, justice, and creation. She has published numerous books, including most recently *Theology for Sceptics* (Fortress Press, 1995) and *Creative Disobedience* (Pilgrim Press, 1995).

Rev. Chris Spies is Senior Trainer and Researcher in Conflict Resolution for Project Saamspan of the Centre for Conflict Resolution, Cape Town, South Africa. He has served previously as a pastor in the Uniting Reformed Church of South Africa and as Coordinator of the Western Cape Regional Peace Committee. Together with Dr. Andries Odendaal, he has authored an Occasional Paper published by *Track Two* in 1996, "Local Peace Committees in the rural areas of the Western Cape."

Dr. Glen H. Stassen is the Lewis Smedes Professor of Christian Ethics at Fuller Theological Seminary, California, USA. He has served as Co-Chair of the Strategy Committee of the Nuclear Weapons Freeze Campaign and is a board member of the Baptist Peace Fellowship of North America. Dr. Stassen's most recent publications include *Just Peacemaking: Transforming Initiatives for Justice and Peace* (Westminster/John Knox Press, 1992). He is editor of *Just Peacemaking: Ten Practices to Abolish War* (forthcoming from Pilgrim Press,1998) and co-author with John Howard Yoder and Diane Yeager of *Authentic Transformation: A New View of Christ and Culture* (Abingdon Press, 1996).

Dr. Walter Wink is Professor of Biblical Interpretation at Auburn Theological Seminary in New York City. He has also worked as a parish minister and taught at Union Theological Seminary, New York. In 1989-90 he was a Peace Fellow at the United States Institute of Peace. Dr. Wink is author of numerous books and articles, among which is his trilogy, *Naming the Powers*, *Unmasking the Powers*, and *Engaging the Powers* (Fortress Press). He has done teaching in biblical nonviolence in South Africa, Northern Ireland, the former East Germany, South Korea, New Zealand, Mexico, and North America.

About Herald Press, Pandora Press, and Pandora Press U.S.

Responding to challenges and opportunities of a changing publishing environment amid recognition of shared visions, three presses have developed innovative relationships. Herald Press can efficiently produce, distribute, and market books which sell in the thousands. Pandora Press and Pandora Press U.S. are pioneering ways economically to publish shorter runs.

By coordinating their programs, the presses can match their respective strengths with what best suits a given book, share in Herald's ability to provide marketing support, and experience rewarding synergies as the Pandoras enable Herald to support publication of an even wider variety of books that fit the Herald Press mission.

Herald Press

The story begins with **Herald Press**, Scottdale, Pennsylvania. Largest of the presses and long the denominational publisher of the Mennonite Church, Herald publishes books from an Anabaptist-Mennonite perspective that address honestly and creatively such issues as peace and social concerns, a biblical understanding of Christian faith, the mission of the church, and the importance of marriage and family. Herald Press aims to offer church and world the best in thinking and spiritual leadership.

Pandora Press, Kitchener, Ontario, was founded in 1995 to make available, at reasonable cost to publisher and public, short runs of books dealing with Anabaptist, Mennonite, and Believers Church topics, both historical and theological. Pandora Kitchener provided models and inspiration for Pandora U.S.

Pandora Press U.S., Telford, Pennsylvania, was then founded in 1997 by a former Herald Press editor after Herald, though still committed to scholarly books, moved toward publishing fewer. Seeking the light of the gospel in a Pandora's box of question, complexities, opportunities, Pandora U.S. publishes thought-provoking theological and scholarly as well as popular books of interest to Anabaptist, Mennonite, Christian, and general readers.

Though independent, the two Pandoras support each other's programs by consulting on books each press publishes, contracting for each other's services, and coordinating distribution, promotion, and marketing operations to develop distinct but related public images for their similarly-named ventures.